Ophthalmology Board and FRCS Part 2 Exams

Saif Aldeen Alryalat
Editor

Ophthalmology Board and FRCS Part 2 Exams

Eye Yield Clinical

Springer

Editor
Saif Aldeen Alryalat
Department of Ophthalmology
The University of Jordan
Amman, Jordan

ISBN 978-981-96-1516-2 ISBN 978-981-96-1517-9 (eBook)
https://doi.org/10.1007/978-981-96-1517-9

This Springer imprint is published by the registered company Springer Nature Singapore Pte Ltd.
The registered company address is: 152 Beach Road, #21-01/04 Gateway East, Singapore 189721, Singapore

Preface

"Eye Yield Clinical" represents a comprehensive resource meticulously designed to equip ophthalmologists and trainees with the essential knowledge required to excel in clinical exams. This book bridges the gap between traditional ophthalmology textbooks and precise demands of contemporary ophthalmology examinations. Drafted from the latest literature and an extensive pool of ophthalmology questions, "Eye Yield Clinical" has been expertly curated to provide high-yield information critical for exam success. By incorporating insights from updated sources and leveraging the expertise of leading professionals in the field, this textbook offers a streamlined approach to mastering ophthalmology. In the era of expanding question banks and diverse learning platforms, "Eye Yield Clinical" stands out by presenting answers and explanations that align seamlessly with a student's study regimen. This integration not only enhances retention but also ensures that readers are well prepared for the nuances of clinical exams. The book emphasizes frequently missed yet commonly asked exam topics, presenting them through comparative tables, summaries, and clear explanations to highlight the most crucial information. Our authors have diligently addressed longstanding controversies and ambiguities present in other resources, providing clarity and consensus based on the most recent literature. While the primary audience includes ophthalmology residents, students, and fellows preparing for exams, practicing ophthalmologists will also find value in the up-to-date information and evidence-based summaries on nearly all ophthalmology topics. We hope that "Eye Yield Clinical" serves as a valuable companion in your educational journey, helping you achieve excellence in your clinical exams and beyond.

Amman, Jordan　　　　Saif Aldeen Alryalat

Contents

Fundamentals and Pre-exam Eye Yield

1

Alaa Tarazi and Saif Aldeen Alryalat

Abstract

Chapter 1 provides a structured, high-yield review of essential topics in ophthalmology, designed to optimize exam preparation. It covers a wide range of ocular disciplines, including general ophthalmology, retina, glaucoma, cornea, lens, neuro-ophthalmology, pediatrics, and refractive lasers. This chapter offers concise yet comprehensive coverage of key concepts, with a focus on frequently tested material and commonly misunderstood areas. Emphasis is placed on differentiating similar conditions and pathologies, such as visual field defects, corneal disorders, and types of cataracts, ensuring clarity and precision in areas prone to confusion. Additionally, the chapter addresses ocular anatomy, physiology, and management of eye disorders, rectifying common pitfalls. Readers will find detailed explanations on ocular microbiology and pharmacology, equipping them with the tools needed to excel in ophthalmology exams.

Keywords

Retina · Glaucoma · Cornea · Cataract · Pediatric

1.1 Overview

This chapter offers a comprehensive and concise review of essential ocular fundamentals, intended to serve as an indispensable tool for exam preparation. It is particularly designed to focus on high-yield information that is frequently tested, as well as areas often misunderstood or overlooked.

The information covered in this chapter encompasses key concepts across the breadth of ophthalmology, including ocular anatomy and physiology, eye movements, optic nerve disorders, strabismus and amblyopia, eyelid and corneal disorders, retina and vitreous disorders, glaucoma and ocular hypertension, cataract and lens disorders, and ocular microbiology.

Special emphasis is given to distinguishing between similar concepts and pathologies that may be easily confused, such as the causes of different types of nystagmus, visual field defects associated with specific optic nerve disorders, management approaches to different types of strabismus, differentiating features of various corneal disorders, and distinguishing characteristics of retinal disorders and glaucoma.

A. Tarazi (✉)
School of Medicine, The University of Jordan, Amman, Jordan

S. A. Alryalat
Department of Ophthalmology, The University of Jordan, Amman, Jordan

The University of Colorado Anschutz Medical Campus, Aurora, CO, USA

S. A. Alryalat (ed.), *Ophthalmology Board and FRCS Part 2 Exams*,
https://doi.org/10.1007/978-981-96-1517-9_1

Furthermore, this chapter aims to clarify misconceptions and rectify common pitfalls associated with certain topics, such as the roles of medications in ocular diseases, distinguishing features of different types of cataracts and their management, and unique characteristics of various ocular microbes.

1.2 Pre-exam High Yield

1.2.1 General Ophthalmology

The frequency of different eye diseases varies by gender, and Table 1.1 provides a comparison between males and females in terms of which eye diseases are more common. Table 1.2 also compares diseases that are more frequent in either eye; however, this association is fragile. Table 1.3 provides a comparison between different ethnicities and eye diseases.

There are different classes of agents and medications in ophthalmology that are associated with different side effects, as shown in Table 1.4. In Table 1.5, hypersensitivity reaction of different eye conditions is shown (Vaajanen and Vapaatalo 2017).

The retina and optic nerve are supplied by retinal and choroidal arteries and veins. Table 1.6 details different eye-related vascular occlusive diseases and their pathophysiology.

Remember that anterior segment neovascularization is more common in ischemic events, with highest risk in ischemic CRVO (50% in 3 months) and lower in BRVO (2%).

Apart from commonly used procedures in ophthalmology, there are certain procedures that have specific indications, and most are oculoplastic ones, as shown in Table 1.7.

In DCR, the lacrimal bone and part of the maxillary bone are usually removed

Multisystem diseases with ocular involvement might have different findings on cerebrospinal fluid (CSF) analysis, as shown in Table 1.8.

Inheritance patterns of different eye conditions are shown in Table 1.9.

Lasers in ophthalmology can be used for different procedures in glaucoma, retina, and plastics among others. Table 1.10 shows the common lasers in ophthalmology and their wavelength. The most common Nd:YAG emission wavelength is 1064 nm. Starting with that wavelength,

Table 1.1 Conditions that have a higher prevalence in different genders. As a note, this table is a general overview and does not imply that these conditions only occur in the specified gender. Many of these conditions can occur in either gender, although they may have higher incidence rates in one gender over another. Additionally, some of these conditions are rare and should not be considered common conditions for the specified gender

Male	Female
Vascular occlusion	Age-related macular degeneration
Macular telangiectasia type 1 and Coats disease	Retinal arterial macroaneurysms
Retina detachment	Susac syndrome
Central serous retinopathy	Incontinentia pigmenti
Congenital glaucoma	Aicardi syndrome
Peripheral ulcerative keratitis	Posterior vitreous detachment (due to estrogen effect)
Polyarteritis nodosa	Cataract
	Systemic lupus erythematosus
	Duane syndrome
	Exotropia
	Fuchs endothelial dystrophy
	Thyroid eye disease
	Macular hole
	Giant cell arteritis (leading to anterior ischemic optic neuropathy)
	Thygeson's superficial punctate keratitis

Table 1.2 Conditions that have higher prevalence in either eye. As a note, this table is a general overview and does not imply that these conditions only occur in the specified eye. These conditions can occur in either eye, although they may have higher incidence rates in one eye over another. Additionally, some of these conditions are rare and should not be considered as common conditions for the specified eye

Right	Left
Idiopathic juxtafoveal telangiectasis	Duane syndrome
Brown syndrome	

Table 1.3 Conditions that have a higher prevalence in different ethnicities. Please note that this table is a general overview and does not imply that these conditions only occur in the specified racial or ethnic groups. Many of these conditions can occur in any racial or ethnic group, although they may have higher incidence rates in one group over another. Additionally, some of these conditions are rare and should not be considered common conditions for the specified racial or ethnic group

African American	Whites or Caucasians	Asians
Primary open-angle glaucoma	Age-related macular degeneration	Angle closure glaucoma
Hypertensive retinopathy	Disc drusen	Polypoidal choroidal vasculopathy
Sickle cell disease and its retinopathy	Multiple sclerosis	
Systemic lupus erythematosus	Uveal melanoma	
Mooren ulcer (more severe)	Central serous retinopathy	
Ocular sarcoidosis		

[a] African Americans have lower risk of CSR and nuclear cataract (Desai et al. 2003, Storey et al. 2013)

Table 1.4 Systemic effect of different autonomic eye drops

System/drug	Cholinergics (e.g., pilocarpine)	Anticholinergics (e.g., atropine)	Beta-blockers (e.g., timolol)
Heart rate	Decrease	Increase	Decrease
Gastrointestinal	Diarrhea	Constipation	No significant effect
Respiratory	Bronchoconstriction	Bronchodilation	Possible bronchospasm (more common with nonselective beta-blockers)
Urinary	Increased urination	Urinary retention	No significant effect
Musculoskeletal	Enhanced muscle contraction (skeletal)	Decreased muscle contraction (smooth)	No significant effect
Eye	Miosis, accommodation for near vision	Mydriasis, cycloplegia	No significant effect
Salivary glands	Increased salivation	Dry mouth	No significant effect
Sweat glands	Increased sweating	Decreased sweating	No significant effect

Table 1.5 Hypersensitivity reaction of different eye conditions

Type 1 (IgE mediated)	Type 2 (cytotoxic antibodies mediated)	Type 3 (immune complex mediated)	Type 4 (T-cell mediated)
Allergic conjunctivitis	Ocular pemphigoid	Phacoanaphylaxis/ phacoantigenic; marginal keratitis	Sympathetic ophthalmia, granulomatous reactions (e.g., sarcoid or TB), contact dermatitis, phlyctenulosis, white dot syndromes

outputs at 532, 355, and 266 nm can be generated by frequency doubling, frequency tripling, and frequency quadrupling, respectively. For example, selective laser trabeculoplasty (SLT, 532 nm) uses 1046 emission with frequency doubling leading to 532 nm output.

Table 1.11 provides an overview of organisms that may cause different ophthalmic conditions.

Visual field defects that correspond to different disease processes are shown in Table 1.12.

Different sutures are usually preferred for different ophthalmic procedures, as shown in Table 1.13.

Optical coherence tomography (OCT) uses infrared light to assess the reflectivity of different ocular structures, most commonly used for retinal imaging. Layers appear as either hyper- or hyporeflective. Nuclear layers generally appear hyporeflective, while plexiform layers appear hyperreflective.

Table 1.6 Eye-related vascular occlusive diseases and their pathophysiology

Vascular event	Pathophysiology	Neovascularization risk
Branch retinal vein occlusion (BRVO)	Thrombus at arteriovenous crossing	2%
Central retinal vein occlusion (CRVO)	Thrombus proximal to lamina cribrosa	50% for ischemic
Central retinal artery occlusion (CRAO) and branch retinal artery occlusion (BRAO) in old age	Embolus from carotid or vasculitis (e.g., giant cell arteritis)	20% for CRAO and negligible for BRAO
Central retinal artery occlusion (CRAO) & branch retinal artery occlusion (BRAO) in young	Drug abuse, valve abnormalities	20% for CRAO and negligible for BRAO
Anterior ischemic optic neuropathy (NAION)	Non-arteritic: idiopathic small vessel disease (not embolic) Arteritic (i.e., vasculitis)	None
Posterior ischemic optic neuropathy (NAION)		

Table 1.7 Different surgical procedures and their primary aim

Surgery	Aim
The tarsoconjunctival flap advancement (Hughes procedure)	Lower lid >50% full-thickness defect
Lower lid suborbicularis oculi fat (SOOF) elevation	Supports lower eyelid elevation in cases of chronic facial nerve palsy
Quickert-Rathbun sutures (everting suture)	Temporary entropion repair
Hotz procedure	Epiblepharon and entropion in children
Y-plasty or Y-V plasty	Correction of epicanthal folds
Z-plasty	Cicatricial ectropion
Wies procedure	Entropion repair
Gold weight implantation	Lagophthalmos
Eyelid retractor repair	Entropion repair
Fasanella procedure	Horner ptosis
Levator advancement	Levator dehiscence

Table 1.8 Different eye conditions and their peculiar associations

Disease	Definition	CSF association
Multiple sclerosis	Central nervous system demyelinating disease	Oligoclonal bands
Guillain Barré (and its variant Miller Fisher)	Peripheral nervous system demyelinating disease	High-protein low cells (aka albumin-cytologic dissociation)
Neuromyelitis optica (NMO)	Antibody-mediated disease against aquaporin-4	High white blood cells (aka pleocytosis)
Vogt–Koyanagi–Harada (VKH) syndrome	Granulomatous inflammation that involves melanin-pigmented cells	Lymphocytic pleocytosis

In terms of normal physiological loss, on average, the corneal endothelium loses about 0.6% per year (Bourne et al. 1997). Similarly, the retinal nerve fiber layer (RNFL) tends to decrease in thickness by about 0.50 μm or 0.3% each year, especially after the age of 50 years (Wang et al. 2013).

Shaken baby syndrome, a form of abusive head trauma, can have significant ocular implications. The most common eye finding is retinal hemorrhages, and the presence of multilayer multi-aged hemorrhages is highly suggestive for shaken baby syndrome and child abuse (Levin 2010).

Table 1.9 Different eye conditions and their most common mode of inheritance

Disease/syndrome	Inheritance
Phakomatosis (except Sturge-Weber and Wyburn-Mason syndrome)	Autosomal dominant (AD)
Axenfeld-Rieger syndrome and other anterior segment dysgenesis (e.g., PAX6 mutation)	AD
Aniridia (related to PAX6 on chromosome 11)	AD
Marfan	AD
Waardenburg syndrome (WS)	AD
Hereditary hyaloid retinopathies (Stickler, Wagner, Jensen)	AD
Tritanopia	AD
Congenital cranial dysinnervation disorders (Duane, Brown, Mobius, congenital fibrosis of the extraocular muscles)	Mostly sporadic, but AD is the inheritance
Blepharophimosis-ptosis-epicanthus inversus syndrome	May occur as a sporadic or AD disorder
CHED	AD or autosomal recessive (AR)
Wilson disease	AR
Leber congenital amaurosis	AR
Cataract	AD
Congenital glaucoma	AR
Most corneal metabolic disorders (except Hunter syndrome and Fabry disease)	AR
Retinitis pigmentosa (RP)	AR (most common)
Rod monochromatism and Refsum's disease	AR
ICE syndrome	Sporadic
Fabry disease, Hunter, Norrie's disease, choroideremia, Lowe, Alport, Hence-Noonan	X-linked recessive
Aicardi syndrome, incontinentia pigmenti	X-linked dominant (limited to females as males die in utero)
LHON and chronic progressive external ophthalmoplegia (CPEO)	Mitochondrial diseases

The prognosis for retinoblastoma, a type of eye cancer that typically develops in early childhood, is better than often perceived. Less than 5% of treated retinoblastoma patients die of the disease within 2–4 years of onset of symptoms. Moreover, in managing retinoblastoma, cryotherapy has proven to be as effective as photocoagulation for small tumors that are difficult to manage with photocoagulation.

Table 1.10 Commonly used laser types in ophthalmology and their wavelengths

Laser type	Wavelength
Nd:YAG	Infrared, 1064 nm
Femtosecond (FS)	Infrared, 1053 nm
Photodynamic therapy (PDT)	Infrared, 690 nm
Cycloablation	Red to infrared light
Krypton red	647 nm
Micropulse (ML)	532–810 nm
Argon blue-green	488–512 nm
Cross-linking	365 UV light
Photoablation	193 UV light

The treatment approach for melanoma, a type of skin cancer that can also develop in the eye, differs from many other cancers. Chemotherapy, which is often a primary treatment modality for various cancers, is not typically used for melanoma.

Immune checkpoint inhibitors (ICIs) are monoclonal antibodies that target negative regulatory steps in T-cell activation; the most commonly used are against the cytotoxic T lymphocyte-associated antigen 4 (CTLA-4) (ipilimumab, tremelimumab), the programmed death-1 receptor (PD-1) (pembrolizumab, nivolumab, and cemiplimab), and its ligand PD-L1 (atezolizumab, avelumab, and durvalumab). Basically, any -itis (e.g., optic neuritis, uveitis, keratitis) that occurs in a patient on ICI can be related to the ICI (Manson et al. 2019).

Delayed visual maturation syndrome is a specific developmental disorder that applies only to children up to 1 year of age. This condition can delay a child's visual development, but many children with this syndrome eventually gain normal vision. It is noteworthy to consider that the dilator pupillae muscle is immature in infancy. This may result in miotic pupils compared to adults.

Understanding transplacental transmission of infections is critical. Infections like toxoplasma and rubella are most severe if transmission occurs

Table 1.11 Different eye conditions and the organism causing or relating to these conditions

Condition	Organism	Additional information
Acute retinal necrosis	Varicella zoster virus (VZV) in adults, herpes simplex virus 2 (HSV-2) in children	–
Endophthalmitis	Bacillus cereus	Rapid and severe course if untreated, sensitive to intravitreal vancomycin or clindamycin
Endophthalmitis	Gram-positive coagulase-negative (i.e., Staph epidermidis) micrococci	Most common cause of endophthalmitis
Post-cataract surgery endophthalmitis	Staph epidermidis	Most common cause
Dog bites	Polymicrobial; anaerobes, aerobes (both gram-positive and gram-negative), specific species such as *Pasteurella canis*	–
Infection with gram-negative intracellular diplococci (GNID)	Mostly reflect *Neisseria gonorrhoeae*	–
Keratitis after laser ablation	Gram-positive bacteria *Staphylococcus* and *Streptococcus* spp.	–
Chronic, recurrent inflammation following cataract extraction	*Propionibacterium acnes*	Not responsive to gentamicin, has a predilection for capsular bag
Endogenous endophthalmitis	*Klebsiella*	–
Infection	*Bartonella henselae*	Gram-negative bacillus
Orbital cellulitis following bacterial conjunctivitis	*Haemophilus influenzae*	Most frequently associated agent
Infection with intracytoplasmic inclusion bodies	Chlamydia	–
Morax-Axenfeld conjunctivitis	Gram-negative diplobacillary	–
Herpes simplex infection	Herpes simplex	Intranuclear inclusion bodies
Chlamydia infection	Chlamydia	Intracytoplasmic inclusions
Corneal biopsy findings	*Acanthamoeba*	Double-walled cyst form or the trophozoite
Corneal biopsy findings	*Mycobacterium* spp.	Acid-fast pleomorphic rods (rarely cause keratitis)
Fungal infections (on corneal biopsy)	Various fungi	Branching hyphae
Infections (on corneal biopsy)	*Nocardia* spp., *Actinomyces* spp.	Branching filaments

in the first 3 months of pregnancy. However, congenital CMV infection is the most common congenital ocular infection, although it is mostly subclinical, unlike HSV. The infection is acquired during maternal viremia during pregnancy, rather than from the birth canal as in the case for HSV. The most common ocular manifestation of congenital CMV is retinochoroiditis.

Signs of retinopathy (hemorrhages, whitening, exudates, cotton wool spots) in both eyes can be called "Purtscher-like syndrome," which is predominantly in the posterior pole. Vision loss is variable, from one eye to both eyes from minimal to hand motion (Miguel et al. 2013). The pathophysiology proposed includes complement activation and clotting factors due to traumatic or

Table 1.12 Different eye conditions and the typical visual field defects associated with it

Condition	Typical visual field defects
Leber hereditary optic neuropathy (LHON)	Central or cecocentral visual field defects
Primary open-angle glaucoma	Slowly progressive arcuate and peripheral visual field loss
Chronic papilledema	Arcuate defects
Non-arteritic anterior ischemic optic neuropathy (non-AION)	Altitudinal defect, mostly inferior
Chasmal lesion	Bitemporal hemianopia
Retro-chiasmal lesions	Homonymous field defects
Lesions affecting the Meyer loop	Superior incongruous homonymous defects contralateral to the lesion, also known as "pie in the sky" defects

Table 1.13 Ophthalmic procedures and the preferred suture material and size

Procedure	Preferred suture material
Dacryocystorhinostomy (DCR)	5-0 Chromic Gut
Scleral buckle	5-0 Dacron (Ethibond)
Cornea (penetrating keratoplasty, PKP)	10-0 Nylon
Conjunctiva	Vicryl
Pig tube stent for canalicular laceration	6-0 Nylon
Iris suturing and cataract	10-0 Prolene
Squint	Coated Vicryl

inflammatory etiologies. The approach is as follows:

- Make sure that it is not true Purtscher syndrome, by ruling out trauma!
- Exclude hypertensive emergency as the cause of the Purtscher-like retinopathy.
- Systemic diseases, including vascular, autoimmune, and hematologic, then need to be assessed.

Retinal vasculitis is defined generally as the presence of perivascular sheathing on fundus examination and/or vascular leakage or occlusion on FA (Kang and Lee 2014; Ebrahimiadib et al. 2021). Fundoscopic findings include perivascular hemorrhage, perivascular infiltrate, vessel sheathing, vessel caliber abnormalities, nonperfused retina, and retinal neovascularization, but can be subtle or absent when RV is subclinical. Fluorescein angiography findings: Retinal vasculitis manifests as vascular leakage, occlusion of vessels, or vessel wall staining on the angiogram. It can be graded based on central vs. peripheral leakage from vessels and non-perfusion of the retina. It is important to differentiate findings suggestive of disease activity (vasculitis) vs. sequelae of previous vasculitis. It is generally accepted that vascular leakage, either segmental or widespread, is an indicator of inflammation and disease activity. However, although an important indicator of severity, the presence of occlusion or non-perfusion is not a reliable indicator of active disease because it persists after inflammation has resolved (Ref). Leakage from neovascularization also represents sequelae, when it is not at the site of the retinal vessel.

Distichiasis, which is a condition characterized by the growth of extra eyelashes, can be hereditary. Hereditary distichiasis is linked to a mutation in the FOXC2 gene, and lymphedema is a known association. If a lash is pulled out, it typically regrows in about 8 weeks, which is longer than the 2–4 weeks some might expect.

1.2.2 Retina

Spontaneous and familial dialysis typically occurs inferotemporal. In the case of traumatic dialysis, it may also occur superonasal, representing a contra-coup injury to the ora. Notably, lesions predisposing to retinal detachment (RD) are generally found in the superior retina, while benign lesions are located in the inferior retina; examples include retinoschisis, paving stone, and cystoid degeneration. Certain retinal conditions were more frequently found in certain quadrants compared to others, as shown in Table 1.14.

Considerations around the vitreous and silicone oil are important. For instance, patients who

Table 1.14 Retinal quadrants most commonly affected by different conditions

Quadrant	Affected most commonly by
Supero-temporal	BRVO, retinal breaks
Infero-temporal	Dialysis idiopathic
Supero-nasal	Dialysis after trauma
Temporal fundus	MacTel, RAMA, Commotio

have silicone oil in the vitreous experience refractive shifts when measuring axial length. An immersion ultrasound can give an inaccurately high axial length measurement through the dense silicone, resulting in a myopic shift. Conversely, a regression formula application reveals a hyperopic shift in these patients. Furthermore, surface tension, the measure of a liquid's ability to hold together, is higher in gases used for vitrectomy than in silicone. It is also higher in dispersive viscoelastic used in cataract surgery compared to cohesive viscoelastic. Essentially, coatability is equivalent to surface tension.

Retinal pigment epithelium (RPE) defects have a distinct appearance. They exhibit hypo-autofluorescence on fundus autofluorescence (FAF) and hyper-fluorescence on fluorescein angiography (FA). It is also crucial to remember that both Leber congenital amaurosis and enhanced S-cone syndromes are associated with hyperopia. Even though the ABCA4 gene mutation is present in Stargardt's disease, it is not diagnostic, as it is found in 10% of the general population.

The half-life of ranibizumab in the vitreous is approximately 7 days, whereas bevacizumab's half-life is around 3 days. In the context of Best disease, it is a misconception that it is associated with cataracts. Additionally, glaucoma drainage devices (tubes) do not cause corneal neovascularization.

Signs of chronic RD include retinal thinning, a demarcation line, subretinal precipitates, and macrophage activity. Keep in mind that a fixed retinal fold is a sign of proliferative vitreoretinopathy (PVR), rather than chronic RD. In treating pars planitis, steroids, pars plana vitrectomy (PPV), and even cryotherapy are potential therapeutic approaches. Cycloplegia is not typically used.

Other important conditions to consider include multiple evanescent white dot syndrome (MEWDS), which typically presents with an enlarged blind spot on visual field testing, and retinal detachment (RD), which may occur in patients with Jensen's syndrome but not in those with Wagner's syndrome. Cystic retinal tufts carry a high risk of RD; however, the risk of RD in lattice degeneration is only 1%.

Pseudo-cystoid macular edema (pseudo-CME) presents a fundoscopic appearance suggestive of CME but without fluorescein angiography filling and can be caused by nicotinic acid, Goldmann-Favre syndrome, some cases of retinitis pigmentosa (RP), and X-linked retinoschisis. Solar retinopathy does not typically cause CME. Patients with autosomal dominant retinitis pigmentosa (AD-RP) typically retain better vision later in life compared to those with autosomal recessive RP (AR-RP). In the case of cone dystrophy, a full peripheral field is required for diagnosis, in addition to a normal scotopic, abnormal photopic, or flicker ERG. EOG is typically normal as it is a test of RPE function. It is also noteworthy that it is very rare for cone dystrophy to lead to choroidal neovascularization (CNV). Only nephropathic cystinosis presents with retinal deposits, but these are visually and clinically insignificant.

Female carriers of choroideremia are often asymptomatic despite showing patchy depigmentation. Retinopathy of prematurity (ROP) is also noteworthy as about 60% of infants born between 28 and 31 weeks of gestational age develop ROP. Finally, in sickle cell disease, retinal neovascularization occurs, but choroidal neovascularization is rare.

1.2.3 Glaucoma

In the early stages of glaucoma, optic disc hemorrhages (aka splinter hemorrhages) are usually found in the inferotemporal or supero-temporal optic disc regions. This is more associated with glaucoma progression and with normal tension glaucoma.

Considering treatment, it is important to know that almost 10% of patients do not initially respond to timolol, a common medication used in the treatment of glaucoma. Additionally, 5–10% of patients may also experience adverse effects. The most effective additive effect is achieved with a combination of timolol and acetazolamide.

In terms of drug concentrations, mitomycin C (MMC) is typically used in concentrations of 0.02% or 0.2 mg/mL, while 5-fluorouracil (5-FU) is used at 5 mg/mL. Notably, bimatoprost, a prostaglandin analog used in glaucoma treatment, is the only fully synthetic one.

Regarding surgical procedures, argon laser trabeculoplasty (ALT) is not found to be useful for goniosynechialysis. In addition, when performing a gonioscopy, Koppe lines can be seen in cases of angle recession, serving as a potential indicator of the condition.

Primary congenital glaucoma (PCG) is mostly sporadic with 10–40% showing familial with mostly AR inheritance (Leysen et al. 2022). Patients can be screened for mutations in the following genes:

- In PCG with AR inheritance, look for CYP1B1, the most common.
- PCG gene LTBP2 (latent transforming growth factor beta-binding protein 2) within the GLC3C locus. Other mutations of this gene are associated with Weill-Marchesani syndrome and microspherophakia.
- PCG with AD inheritance, ANGPT1 (angiopoietin-1), or TEK (tunica interna endothelial cell kinase, the receptor for ANGPT1, also known as TIE2) is inherited in an autosomal dominant pattern, results in loss of protein function that affects the development of Schlemm canal, and can lead to PCG.
- Congenital glaucoma without anterior segment dysgenesis with AD inheritance can be tested for mutations in MYOC (GLC1A), the gene coding for myocilin, formerly called TIGR. A confirmed MYOC gene should prompt screening for other family members.
- In congenital glaucoma with anterior segment dysgenesis (e.g., aniridia, Axenfeld-Rieger syndrome, Peters anomaly, nail-patella syndrome), the proband should be tested for mutations in FOXC1 (forkhead box C1), PITX2 (paired-like homeodomain transcription factor 2), PAX6 (paired box 6), and LMX1B (LIM homeobox transcription factor 1 beta). Over 80% of patients with aniridia have mutations in PAX6.

Table 1.15 shows different glaucoma-related conditions and the genes associated with them.

Cycloablation can be used with either cryo (aka cyclocryotherapy) or laser (aka cyclophotocoagulation (CPC)) (Table 1.16). The rate of complications is lower with cyclodestructive laser procedures than with cyclocryotherapy.

Minimally invasive glaucoma surgeries (MIGSs) can be divided according to their site of action or placement (Table 1.17): Schlemm's canal, suprachoroidal, and subconjunctival (Otárola and Pooley 2021; Lusthaus 2024). Almost all devices are inserted ab interno, except the PresserFlo.

Table 1.15 Different glaucoma-related conditions and the genes associated with them

Gene	Disease	Note
TIGR/MYOC	Juvenile and adult POAG glaucoma	On GCL1A gene, AD inheritance
Normal tension glaucoma	OPTN	
CYP1B1	Isolated congenital glaucoma	Cytochrome p450 gene (AR inheritance)
Pseudoexfoliation	LOXL1	
Ectopia lentis with glaucoma	LTBP2	Megalocornea with zonular weakness, forward displacement of the lens. Glaucoma here is secondary, with lens removal essential for treatment

Table 1.16 Comparison in different cycloablation, cyclocryotherapy vs. cyclophotocoagulation

Feature	Cyclophotocoagulation (CPC)	Cyclocryotherapy
Mechanism	Laser energy coagulates ciliary body to reduce aqueous humor production	Freezing (cryo) damages ciliary processes to reduce aqueous humor production
Types of energy source	Diode lasers, Nd:YAG lasers, etc.	Cryoprobe
Procedure approach	Transscleral, endoscopic, etc.	Transscleral, external
Clinical considerations	Can be more controlled and precise with various laser types	The freezing process needs to be carefully controlled to achieve desired effects

Table 1.17 Summary of minimally invasive glaucoma surgery (MIGS) trials

Schlemm's canal	Suprachoroidal	Subconjunctival
Trabectome, excimer laser trabeculotomy (ELT), iStent, iStent inject, Hydrus, KDB (Kahook dual blade), GATT	CyPass and iStent Supra	XEN-45 and PresserFlo Microshunt
Inserted through an ab interno method with the assistance of a gonioscopic lens	Allows aqueous to traverse the sclera directly via the intercellular spaces between ciliary muscle fibers and loose connective tissue of the suprachoroidal space	Blep-forming devices
	CyPass was withdrawn due to corneal endothelial damage	Unlike Xen stent, PresserFlo Microshunt is implanted through and ab externo approach requiring conjunctival dissection. Despite this fact, is has been classified by the FDA as a MIGS device

1.2.4 Cornea and Ocular Surface

Corneal nerves may be apparently thickened and more visible in the following (Yin et al. 2023):

- Ocular diseases: Fuchs' endothelial dystrophy, acanthamoeba keratitis, keratoconus, congenital glaucoma, herpes simplex, herpes zoster, posterior polymorphous dystrophy, and corneal transplantation failure
- Systemic disorders: Leprosy (Hansen's disease), primary amyloidosis, pheochromocytoma, Refsum's disease, Marfan syndrome, congenital ichthyosis, ectodermal dysplasia, and neurofibromatosis

About injuries of the Descemet membrane, curvilinear or horizontal tears often point toward primary congenital glaucoma (known as Haab striae). On the other hand, linear tears that are mostly vertical or oblique are often associated with forceps injury sustained during delivery.

Two specific conditions, blepharitis and chlamydia, have known associations with subepithelial infiltrates. Blepharitis often leads to the development of inferior subepithelial infiltrates, while chlamydia is known to cause superior subepithelial infiltrates (SPEs). Lastly, contrary to common misbelief, Thygeson's disease, also known as Thygeson's superficial punctate keratitis, does not show a male predominance.

1.2.5 Cataract and Lens Power

While the most common cause of cataract is age related, different etiologies have been associated with its development and different associations have been described, as shown in Table 1.18.

The use of amiodarone, a medication commonly used to treat heart rhythm problems, can lead to the development of a posterior subcapsular cataract (PSCC). On the other hand, pediatric amyloidosis, a condition characterized by the

Table 1.18 Different conditions and the type of cataract associated with them

Disease	Associated cataract	Notes
Atopic dermatitis	Anterior subcapsular (shield-like) cataract	Usually bilateral, and develops in 10–25% of severe cases by the fourth decade
Acute hyperglycemic attack (classic diabetic cataract)	Snowflake cortical cataract	May resolve or progress to persistent cortical cataract
Blunt trauma	Stellate or rosette-shaped cataract at the posterior capsule axially	Posterior lens capsule might be disrupted
Penetrating trauma (with capsule disruption)	Cortical changes that may remain focal if small or may progress rapidly to total cortical opacification	
Myotonic dystrophy	Christmas tree cataract	90% of patients will develop Christmas tree nuclear cataract by the third decade. Polychromatic iridescent crystals (red and green in color) in the lens cortex, non-visually significant. Hyperopia in 90%
Galactosemia	Oil droplet	Appears within the first few weeks of life, reversed with milk elimination from diet
Neurofibromatosis type 2	Posterior subcapsular cataract	60% of patients
Hereditary fundus dystrophies	Posterior subcapsular cataract	
Chalcosis	Sunflower subcortical cataract	Copper deposition beneath the capsule, non-visually significant
Steroids	Posterior subcapsular cataract	
High myopia	Posterior subcapsular cataract	
Hypocalcemia	Anterior and posterior subcortical cataract	Bilateral, hypocalcemic (tetanic) cataracts are punctate iridescent opacities in the anterior and posterior cortex
Phenothiazines and amiodarone	Stellate anterior subcapsular cataract	Non-visually significant stellate-like deposition on anterior lens capsule
Pilocarpine	Vacuoles at posterior capsule	
Statin and tamoxifen	Cataract	Higher risk with prolonged use
Rubella congenital infection	Nuclear	Bilateral nuclear. Retained nuclei within cells. Induces excessive inflammation if part of the cataract is left. Occurs when mother is infected during the first trimester

Note that hypoglycemia and hypercalcemia are not among the causes of cataract!

abnormal deposition of a protein called amyloid in tissues and organs, does not typically cause cataract. Patients with PSCC often present with worse symptoms for near vision compared to distance vision.

1.2.6 Neuro-Ophthalmology

Ischemic optic neuropathy is most commonly anterior (aka AION), due to small-vessel disease affecting posterior ciliary artery branches to the optic nerve. However, in elderly patients, it is important to rule out arteritis (inflammation of the vessel) etiologies, with giant cell arteritis being the most common. Ischemic events rarely affect the posterior optic nerve.

Retinal ischemic can occur from:

- Retinal artery occlusion, which is an equivalent of stroke and requires stroke evaluation, regardless if it is central or branch.

- Retinal vein occlusion, which is most commonly associated with hypertension and other vascular risk factors. Unlike other vein occlusion in the body, retinal vein occlusion outcome is worse with the use of anticoagulation and antiplatelet (Hayreh et al. 2011).

Chronic relapsing inflammatory optic neuropathy (CRION) is characterized by the rapid onset of pain, followed by subacute vision loss. This condition is more prevalent in females and African Americans, and it often correlates with the presence of MOG-IgG, especially in bilateral disease. In addition, pediatric conditions, including acute disseminated encephalomyelitis (ADEM) and post-viral optic neuritis (mostly post-COVID virus), are now shown to be associated with MOG-Ab (Santoro and Chitnis 2019; Gilardi et al. 2023).

Involuntary facial muscle contraction may include:

- Lid myokymia: Contraction of a single facial muscle, including the lid muscle in the upper or lower, with no further workup warranted.
- Blepharospasm: Contractions of upper and lower lid muscles. Idiopathic and benign if bilateral but require further imaging if unilateral.
- Hemifacial spasm: Contraction of eyelid and facial muscles. Further imaging warranted; it can be due to an intramedullary disease of the pons involving the cranial nerve VII nucleus or fascicle, as seen in children with gliomas.

Electroretinography (ERG) is typically normal in several conditions, including vitelliform dystrophy (pattern dystrophy), dominant drusen, X-linked ocular albinism, and pattern dystrophy. It is abnormal in different conditions:

- About ischemic events, decreased b-wave amplitude is usually associated with such conditions and extinguished ERG in ophthalmic artery occlusion. Meanwhile, increased implicit times can be found in various hereditary conditions. In hereditary conditions such as choroideremia, carriers are usually asymptomatic and have normal ERGs, unlike carriers of juvenile X-linked RP. In choroideremia, central acuity is spared until later in life relative to X-linked RP.
- Outer retinal degeneration conditions, including multiple evanescent white dot syndrome, acute idiopathic blind-spot enlargement syndrome, and acute zonal occult outer retinopathy (AZOOR), result in decreased waveforms on multifocal ERG (mfERG).
- Generalized inflammatory diseases, such as posterior uveitis, may be associated with delay but preservation of amplitude. In fact, a marked 30 Hz flicker delay with high amplitude almost always indicates an inflammatory etiology.

In the context of macular dysfunction, pattern ERG is affected by diseases confined to the macula. A patient with generalized retinal dysfunction sparing the macula will have an abnormal full-field ERG but a normal-pattern ERG. Diseases of ganglion cells, like glaucoma, affect pattern ERG. Multifocal ERG is the best for the assessment of macular dysfunction.

Negative ERG is mostly found in genetic diseases such as congenital stationary night blindness and X-linked retinoschisis and in acquired diseases such as melanoma-associated retinopathy (MAR). A negative ERG with affected a-wave can reflect a central retinal vein occlusion (CRVO). Other causes of negative electroretinogram include siderosis, carcinoma-associated retinopathy, malignant melanoma, and Duchenne muscular dystrophy.

In Best disease, the EOG is almost always abnormal, even in "unaffected," asymptomatic individuals who have the causative genetic variant but have normal-appearing fundi. The light rise of the EOG is typically severely reduced or absent. On the other hand, EOG, which is an RPE function test, is normal in cone dystrophy.

Nystagmus by definition has at least one slow phase. Jerk nystagmus has a slow phase and a fast phase. Pendular nystagmus has only slow phases (Eggers 2019). Table 1.19 shows the patterns of nystagmus and nystagmus-like movements and their localization.

Table 1.19 Different nystagmus and nystagmus-like eye movements, their description, and localization

Nystagmus	Description	Localization
Downbeat	Bilateral conjugate with saccades down	Cervicomedullary junction, mostly Chiari malformation. Idiopathic downbeat nystagmus is GAD antibody related
Upbeat	Bilateral conjugate with saccades up	Brainstem or vermis of cerebellum
Convergence retraction		Dorsal midbrain
Seesaw	One eye rises and intorts, while the other falls and extorts. This is followed by reversal of the vertical and torsional components in the opposite eye	Third ventricular parasellar region (including chiasm issue) (Ref)
Rebound	Horizontal jerk to one side, then slow, then jerk back to same side	Cerebellum
Periodic alternating	Horizontal jerk to one side, then slow, then jerk to the other side within almost 1 min	Cerebellum. Respond to baclofen
Bruns-Cushing		Cerebellopontine angle

Traumatic optic neuropathy is the most common cause of vision loss after blunt trauma with normal eye exam. While mostly nonsurgical, the following etiologies warrant surgical interventions and need to be recognized:

- Optic canal fracture with bony fragment affecting the optic nerve, which requires removal of the bony fragment.
- Foreign body affecting the optic nerve, which requires removal of the foreign body, especially if organic.
- Optic nerve sheath hematoma compressing on the optic nerve, which requires optic nerve sheath fenestration to relieve the pressure.

1.2.7 Pediatrics

Signs that reflect a congenital origin of strabismus include dissociated vertical deviation (DVD), latent nystagmus, and inferior oblique overaction (IOOA). Red flags in strabismus that would suggest an underlying neurological condition include incomitance, ductional deficit, or combined horizontal and vertical.

The optimal angle for primary actions of the ocular muscles is 39° for obliques (secondary at 51°) and 23° for recti (secondary at 67°).

For oblique palsy, the surgical approach depends on the primary complaint. If torsion is the issue, anterior fiber transposition of the affected eye is usually done (Harada-Ito procedure). However, for diplopia (hypo or hyper), surgery can differ. For right oblique paresis, for example, surgery may strengthen ipsilateral depressors or weaken ipsilateral elevators. Opposite procedures can be performed on the other eye. In bilateral superior oblique palsy, the main issue is often cyclotorsion, and bilateral superior oblique tuck is generally the best option.

In Duane syndrome, the typical approach is to recess the recti muscles on the affected side. A lateral Faden procedure can be done for up- or downshift to reduce upshoot in the affected eye on adduction.

For double-elevator palsy, management depends on a forced duction test. If the test is positive, inferior rectus recession is the preferred treatment. If no restriction is present, transposition of the medial and lateral rectus muscles to the superior rectus muscle can be done (Knapp procedure).

Brown syndrome is best treated by superior oblique tenotomy nasal to the superior rectus muscle. This should not be treated by superior rectus recession. It can be managed by simultaneous surgery on the inferior oblique muscle of the

Table 1.20 Duration since birth and the associated ophthalmia neonatorum organism and treatment

Duration	Organism	Treatment	Systemic complications
Within 24 h of birth	Chemical	Observation	
2–4 days	*Neisseria gonorrhoeae*	Systemic ceftriaxone	
5–14 days	Chlamydia	Systemic erythromycin	Pneumonia and otitis media

involved eye and the superior oblique tendon, but not on the superior rectus muscle.

To manage head tilt in nystagmus, the Kestenbaum or Anderson procedure is usually performed, which involves moving the eyes toward the head posture.

It is important to remember that bilateral superior oblique palsy presents with less hyperdeviation and head tilt, but more V-pattern and excyclotorsion, compared to unilateral palsy. Congenital cases generally show fewer symptoms across all categories except fusional vergence when compared to acquired cases.

Phospholine iodide (echothiophate) is a miotic and can cause esotropia. In anisometropic amblyopia, it is recommended to give full cycloplegic correction. Options for managing consecutive esotropia include miotics, reoperation, prisms, and hyperopic correction. Alternate patching should be considered initially post-operation.

Organisms associated with ophthalmia neonatorum are highly associated with the onset of the condition as shown in Table 1.20.

Conflict of Interest None.

References

Bourne WM, Nelson LR, Hodge DO (1997) Central corneal endothelial cell changes over a ten-year period. Invest Ophthalmol Vis Sci 38(3):779–782

Desai U et al. (2003) Central serous chorioretinopathy in African Americans. J Natl Med Assoc 95(7):553–559

Ebrahimiadib N et al (2021) Vascular abnormalities in uveitis. Surv Ophthalmol 66(4):653–667. https://doi.org/10.1016/j.survophthal.2020.12.006

Eggers SDZ (2019) Approach to the examination and classification of nystagmus. J Neurol Phys Ther 43:S20. https://doi.org/10.1097/NPT.0000000000000270

Gilardi M et al (2023) MOG-IgG positive optic neuritis after SARS-CoV-2 infection. Eur J Ophthalmol 33:NP87–NP90. https://doi.org/10.1177/11206721221136319

Hayreh SS, Podhajsky PA, Zimmerman MB (2011) Central and hemicentral retinal vein occlusion: role of anti-platelet aggregation agents and anticoagulants. Ophthalmology 118(8):1603–1611. https://doi.org/10.1016/j.ophtha.2011.04.036

Kang HM, Lee SC (2014) Long-term progression of retinal vasculitis in Behçet patients using a fluorescein angiography scoring system. Graefes Arch Clin Exp Ophthalmol 252(6):1001–1008. https://doi.org/10.1007/s00417-014-2637-z

Levin AV (2010) Retinal hemorrhage in abusive head trauma. Pediatrics 126(5):961–970. https://doi.org/10.1542/peds.2010-1220

Leysen L et al (2022) Genetics in primary congenital glaucoma: implications in disease management and counseling. Eur J Med Genet 65(1):104378. https://doi.org/10.1016/j.ejmg.2021.104378

Lusthaus JA (2024) Imaging of aqueous outflow in health and glaucoma. Justifying the re-direction of aqueous. Eye, pp 1–7. https://doi.org/10.1038/s41433-024-02968-8

Manson G et al (2019) Worsening and newly diagnosed paraneoplastic syndromes following anti-PD-1 or anti-PD-L1 immunotherapies, a descriptive study. J Immunother Cancer 7(1):337. https://doi.org/10.1186/s40425-019-0821-8

Miguel AIM et al (2013) Systematic review of Purtscher's and Purtscher-like retinopathies. Eye 27(1):1–13. https://doi.org/10.1038/eye.2012.222

Otárola F, Pooley F (2021) Minimally invasive glaucoma surgery (MIGS) devices: risks, benefits and suitability. Community Eye Health 34(112):59–60

Santoro JD, Chitnis T (2019) Diagnostic considerations in acute disseminated encephalomyelitis and the Interface with MOG antibody. Neuropediatrics 50(5):273–279. https://doi.org/10.1055/s-0039-1693152

Storey P et al. (2013) Racial differences in lens opacity incidence and progression: the Salisbury Eye Evaluation (SEE) study. Invest Ophthalmol Vis Sci 54(4):3010–3018

Vaajanen A, Vapaatalo H (2017) A single drop in the eye—effects on the whole body? Open Ophthalmol J 11:305–314. https://doi.org/10.2174/1874364101711010305

Wang YX et al (2013) Retinal nerve fiber layer thickness. The Beijing eye study 2011. PLoS One 8(6):e66763. https://doi.org/10.1371/journal.pone.0066763

Yin L et al (2023) Prominent corneal nerves in pure mucosal neuroma syndrome, a clinical phenotype distinct from multiple endocrine neoplasia type 2B. BMC Ophthalmol 23:260. https://doi.org/10.1186/s12886-023-03005-0

2 Clinical Review of Ocular Tumors and Phakomatosis

Mona T. Mohammad and Yacoub A. Yousef

Abstract

Intraocular tumors are categorized based on a variety of factors, including malignant potential, incidence, age of presentation, anatomical location within the eye, tissue origin, relationship to systemic disease, and whether they are primary ocular tumors or secondary deposits from distant cancers. Uveal melanoma (UM) is the most frequent primary intraocular malignancy in adults, with the choroid being the most commonly involved site. In adults, the most prevalent secondary intraocular malignancies are metastatic breast cancer in females and metastatic lung cancer in males. In children, retinoblastoma (RB) is the most common primary intraocular malignancy in children, while secondary intraocular malignancies often result from leukemia, mostly affecting the uveal tract.

Keywords

Tumors · Retinoblastoma · Melanoma · Glioma · Phakomatosis

M. T. Mohammad · Y. A. Yousef (✉)
King Hussein Cancer Center, Amman, Jordan
e-mail: Dm.11804@khcc.jo; yyousef@khcc.jo

2.1 Intraocular Tumors

2.1.1 Overview

Intraocular tumors are categorized based on a variety of factors, including malignant potential, incidence, age of presentation, anatomical location within the eye, tissue origin, relationship to systemic disease, and whether they are primary ocular tumors or secondary deposits from distant cancers. Uveal melanoma (UM) is the most frequent primary intraocular malignancy in adults, with the choroid being the most commonly involved site. In adults, the most prevalent secondary intraocular malignancies are metastatic breast cancer in females and metastatic lung cancer in males. In children, retinoblastoma (RB) is the most common primary intraocular malignancy in children, while secondary intraocular malignancies often result from leukemia, mostly affecting the uveal tract.

2.2 Retinoblastoma

2.2.1 Overview

Retinoblastoma is a malignant tumor of primitive neuroendocrine origin and is the most common primary intraocular malignancy in children. Globally, the incidence of retinoblastoma is 1 in 15,000 to 1 in 20,000 live births (Tamboli et al.

S. A. Alryalat (ed.), *Ophthalmology Board and FRCS Part 2 Exams*,
https://doi.org/10.1007/978-981-96-1517-9_2

1990). Most cases arise before the age of 4 years. About 60% of retinoblastoma cases are unilateral, with bilateral cases typically identified by 12 months of age, whereas unilateral cases are usually diagnosed around 24 months. According to the presence of genetic mutation in RB1 gene (a tumor suppressor gene in chromosome 13), patients are classified into hereditary (in 40% of cases) and non-hereditary (or somatic in 60% of cases) (Cruz-Gálvez et al. 2022).

Hereditary cases are almost always bilateral, while in 15% of unilateral cases, an RB1 gene mutation may be identified. Pinealoblastoma, a tumor of the pineal gland with the same origin as the retina, is sometimes referred to as trilateral retinoblastoma due to the pineal gland being considered a primitive third eye. Advances in understanding the disease and in treatment options resulted in better survival and globe salvage rates.

2.2.2 Retinoblastoma Genetics

Retinoblastoma arises from a photoreceptor cell in the retina and is linked to mutations in the RB1 gene, which normally acts as a tumor suppressor. Individuals inherit two copies of the RB1 gene, one from each parent. The development of retinoblastoma is typically driven by the biallelic inactivation of the RB1 gene on the long arm of chromosome 13 (13q), a key factor in tumor formation known as the two-hit theory. However, in rare cases, retinoblastoma may occur even with non-mutated RB1 genes, due to the activity of the MYCN oncogene. This occurs in fewer than 3% of children with unilateral retinoblastoma and often presents at an earlier age, usually before 6 months.

In hereditary retinoblastoma, a person may inherit an altered RB1 gene from one parent in about 10% of cases, or more commonly, the mutation may arise de novo in an egg or sperm cell or shortly after fertilization. For retinoblastoma to develop, a second mutation in the other copy of the RB1 gene must occur in retinal cells during the individual's lifetime, as explained by Knudson's "two-hit" theory. This second mutation usually happens in early childhood, often leading to retinoblastoma affecting both eyes (Mallipatna et al. 2016).

In contrast, the non-hereditary (sporadic) form of retinoblastoma typically affects only one eye and occurs without a family history of the disease. Individuals with sporadic retinoblastoma are born with two normal copies of the RB1 gene. During early childhood, both copies of the RB1 gene in certain retinal cells acquire mutations. Those with non-hereditary retinoblastoma are not at risk of passing these mutations to their children.

The majority of germinal retinoblastoma mutations are phenotypically manifested as bilateral multifocal tumors; however, about 10–15% of unilateral RB patients have germinal mutation. In unilateral multifocal retinoblastoma, the risk is the same as for bilateral disease since multifocality indicates that multiple retinal cells harbor the mutation. While retinoblastoma has an autosomal dominant inheritance, the molecular action of the gene appears to be recessive. Therefore, it is the loss of constitutional heterozygosity that results in retinoblastoma development. The gene deletion could be simple or functional and in sectional translocation or mosaicism.

2.2.3 Genetic Counseling

The risk of developing retinoblastoma (RB) in future siblings is influenced by the presence or absence of an RB1 gene mutation. If genetic testing reveals no mutation in an affected patient, there is no increased risk for future siblings. However, if an RB1 mutation is identified, the risk of a sibling developing retinoblastoma is approximately 45% due to autosomal dominant inheritance with about 80% penetrance. In cases where genetic testing cannot be performed, the following guidelines apply:

- Children of a parent with bilateral RB: Have a 45–50% chance of being affected.
- Children of a parent with unilateral RB: Have a 5–10% chance of being affected.

- Unaffected parents who have had one child with bilateral RB: Have a 5% chance of having another affected child.
- Unaffected parents who have had one child with unilateral RB: Have around a 1% chance of having another affected child.
- Unaffected parents who have had two or more children with bilateral RB: Have a 45–50% chance of having another affected child.

Table 2.1 shows the risk assessment of offspring according to the presence or absence of family history of retinoblastoma and disease laterality.

2.2.4 Presentation

The most common initial sign of retinoblastoma is leukocoria, occurring in about 60% of cases. This white reflex is due to the tumor extending into the vitreous or causing retinal detachment. The second most frequent presentation is strabismus, seen in approximately 20% of cases (Fig. 2.1). Other, less common signs include a decrease in vision, proptosis, painful glaucoma, heterochromia, hyphema, pseudohypopyon, and nystagmus. In developing countries, where diagnosis is often delayed, patients frequently present with advanced orbital disease, leading to eye proptosis and inflammation.

2.2.5 Clinical Features and Staging Systems

The Reese-Ellsworth (RE) classification system, which predicts the prognosis of retinoblastoma after radiotherapy, was the primary staging system used in the 1960s (Reese and Ellsworth 1963). Later, in the 1990s, a shift towards the use of systemic chemotherapy in conjunction with a variety of focal treatments resulted in the development of the International Classification of Retinoblastoma (ICRB) in which the disease is staged into groups A–E (Table 2.2). This system helps predict which patients with intraocular retinoblastoma are likely to achieve a cure without needing enucleation or external beam radiation treatment (Shields et al. 2006).

The classic fundus exam for a patient with retinoblastoma shows a white retinal mass with either endophytic (towards the vitreous) or exophytic (towards the sclera) growth patterns. There is associated vascularity with overlying telangiectatic vessels and possible feeder vessels. There may be associated subretinal or vitreous seeding of the tumor, with subretinal fluid that may be confined to the tumor or massive causing total exudative retinal detachment (Fig. 2.2).

Diffuse anterior retinoblastoma is a rare variant that involves tumor seeding in the vitreous base and anterior chamber. Patients with this form are typically older than those with classical retinoblastoma, with a mean age of 6.1 years. It is believed that the tumor originates from cone pre-

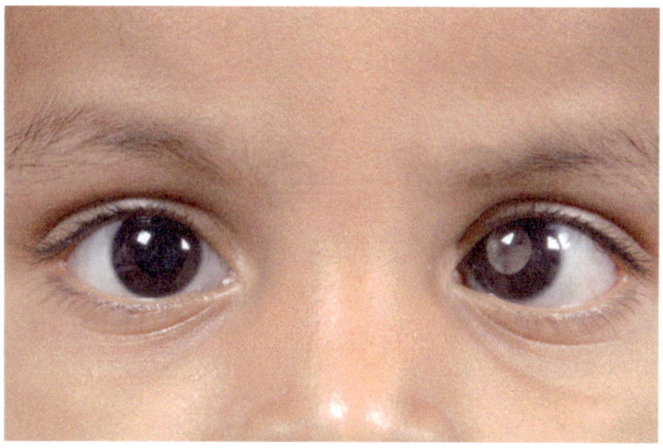

Fig. 2.1 Photo of a child with unilateral left eye retinoblastoma resulting in leukocoria and esotropia

Table 2.1 Risk assessment to develop RB according to family history and disease laterality

	More than one affected person in family	The child has bilateral or unilateral multifocal retinoblastoma	The child has unilateral unifocal retinoblastoma
Siblings of RB child	50%	5%	1%
Offspring of RB child	50%	50%	5–10%

cursor cells. Common presenting symptoms include pseudouveitis, pseudohypopyon, and increased intraocular pressure.

Table 2.2 International classification of retinoblastoma (ICRB)

Group A	Small intraretinal tumors (<3 mm) away from foveola and disc
Group B	Tumors >3 mm, macular or juxtapapillary location, or with subretinal fluid
Group C	Tumor with focal subretinal or vitreous seeding within 3 mm of tumor
Group D	Tumor with diffuse subretinal or vitreous seeding >3 mm from tumor
Group E	Extensive retinoblastoma is characterized by the tumor occupying more than 50% of the globe and may be accompanied by conditions such as irreversible neovascular glaucoma, massive intraocular hemorrhage, tumor extension to the optic nerve or anterior chamber, or presence of phthisis or pre-phthisis

2.2.6 Histology

Histologically, retinoblastoma typically presents as a small blue round cell tumor and may have one of the following patterns:

- **Flexner-Wintersteiner rosettes**: True rosettes that are characteristic of retinoblastoma.
- **Homer-Wright rosettes**: Pseudorosettes that are not specific to retinoblastoma and can be seen in other neuroblastic tumors.
- **Fleurettes**: Curvilinear clusters of necrotic photoreceptors, indicating more differentiation and generally associated with a better prognosis than rosettes.

It is very important to identify high-risk pathological features (HRFs) for any eye with retinoblastoma after enucleation, because the presence of any of those features mandates adjuvant systemic chemotherapy ± radiotherapy to the orbit to

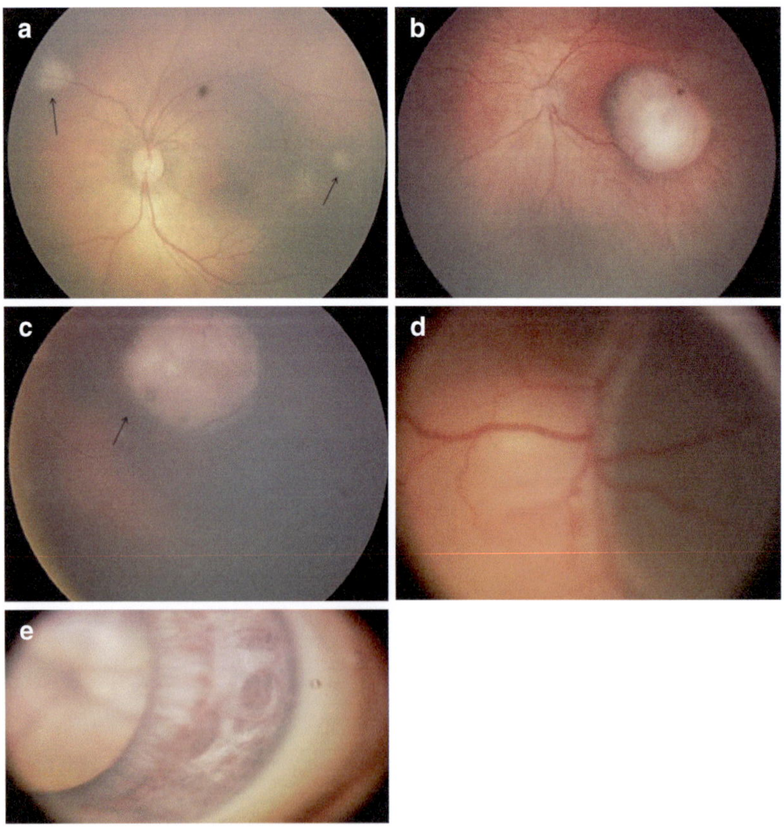

Fig. 2.2 Fundus photos of retinoblastoma: group A two small intraretinal tumors (<3 mm) away from foveola and disc, black arrows (**a**); group B macular tumor >3 mm with subretinal fluid (**b**); group C tumor with focal subretinal seeding within 3 mm of tumor, black arrow (**c**); group D tumor with diffuse subretinal seeding >3 mm from tumor and subtotal retinal detachment (**d**); group E extensive retinoblastoma occupying >50% of the globe with irreversible neovascular glaucoma (**e**)

prevent local recurrence or metastatic disease. These HRFs include tumor invasion of the anterior chamber, iris, or ciliary body; massive choroidal invasion (greater than 3 mm); scleral invasion; involvement of the post-laminar portion of the optic nerve; a combination of focal choroidal invasion (less than 3 mm) and optic nerve invasion; and extraocular tumor extension (Fig. 2.3).

2.2.7 Differential Diagnosis

This includes retinal astrocytic hamartoma, Coats' disease, retinopathy of prematurity, persistent hyperplastic primary vitreous, and medulloepithelioma.

The nature of the red reflux can give some clues to the underlying pathology:

- White color for retinoblastoma
- Orange color for choroidal hemangioma
- Yellow color for Coats' disease
- Blue/gray color for congenital cataract

2.2.8 Treatment

Children with retinoblastoma should be treated by a multidisciplinary team in specialized centers equipped with up-to-date protocols, and modern equipment techniques are available to provide the best management of the disease. Regular follow-up care and monitoring are important to detect any potential recurrence or side effects of treatment.

In general, the primary goals of treatment for retinoblastoma, in descending order of importance, are to save life, globe, and vision of the

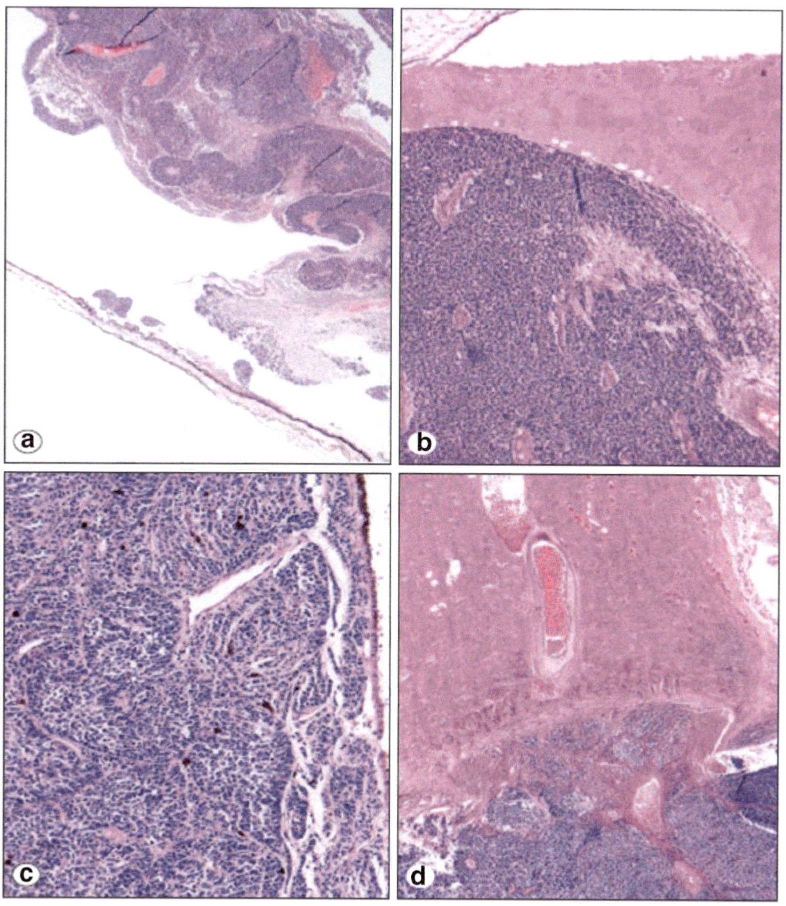

Fig. 2.3 Different pathological features of intraocular retinoblastoma. (**a**) Endophytic tumor growth pattern, with tumor growing towards the vitreous body away from the choroid and sclera (H&E, ×40). (**b**) Exophytic tumor growth pattern associated with (H&E, ×200). (**c**) Massive choroid invasion defined as invasion of the choroid >3 mm in any dimension (H&E, ×400). (**d**) Post-lamina cribrosa optic nerve invasion can be seen in some eyes (H&E, ×200)

patients. There are different treatment options for the disease, and the selection of any treatment modality depends on many factors including disease laterality, stage of the disease, tumor location and any potential for useful vision, and whether the tumor is confined to the globe or extends to the optic nerve, sclera, or other areas such as the orbit, lymph nodes, bones, and central nervous system or has hematogenous metastases.

Treatment options include chemotherapy to shrink the tumor followed by focal consolidation therapy (like laser, cryotherapy, plaque brachytherapy), eye enucleation with orbit implant insertion, or radiotherapy (external beam radiotherapy (EBRT) or brachytherapy using radioactive plaques). Chemotherapy alone cannot cure the disease, but it can regress the tumor to be treatable by other focal therapy (Abramson et al. 2015).

Depending on the stage of the disease, the following treatment guidelines are generally followed:

1. Group A: Focal therapy alone (cryotherapy for small anterior peripheral tumors and (or) laser therapy (argon 532 nm laser and/or 810 nm transpupillary thermotherapy (TTT)) for small posterior tumors).
2. Groups B and C: Systemic chemotherapy (usually 6–8 cycles of carboplatin-vincristine-etoposide (CVE)) for tumor shrinkage followed by focal therapy (cryotherapy for small anterior peripheral tumors and (or) laser therapy (532 and/or 810 nm) for small posterior tumors).
3. Group D: Enucleation if the other eye does not require chemo (i.e., group A or normal); otherwise, treat with systemic chemotherapy followed by focal therapy as above.
4. Group E: Typically requires up-front enucleation without pre-enucleation chemotherapy. This approach is chosen because pre-enucleation chemotherapy can mask signs of extraocular extension, potentially leading to underestimation of the disease's severity and inadequate treatment of systemic metastases. Administering chemotherapy before enucleation in such cases can pose risks, including the possibility of difficult-to-treat systemic metastases.
5. Radiotherapy in the form of external beam radiotherapy (EBRT) is usually reserved as the last option for uncontrolled tumors with potential for vision; it is better to avoid EBRT in patients with germline RB1 mutations because of the increased risk of secondary malignancies, mainly osteosarcomas in the radiation field.
6. Enucleation may be necessary for recurrent tumors when all other treatment modalities, including EBRT, have failed. This approach is used to prevent the spread of the tumor outside the eye or when complications hinder the evaluation and treatment of progressive disease.
7. Pre-chemotherapy cryotherapy, administered 24–72 h before chemotherapy, may be used to enhance drug penetration into the eye, especially in cases of vitreous seeding. However, this approach is not recommended if retinal detachment is present.
8. In the presence of active tumor seeds in the vitreous cavity, intravitreal injection of chemotherapy directly in the vitreous cavity is needed to control vitreous seeding.

2.2.9 Prognosis

Patients with intraocular retinoblastoma generally have an excellent prognosis, with an overall survival rate exceeding 95% in developed countries where modern healthcare facilities are available. The most significant risk factor for a poor prognosis is extraocular extension, through either scleral invasion or optic nerve involvement. Survivors of bilateral retinoblastoma face an increased risk of developing non-ocular malignancies later in life. Genetic predisposition plays a crucial role in this increased risk, and radiation treatment further heightens it. External beam radiotherapy is associated with a higher risk of developing second cancers within the first 30 years of life, with sarcoma being the most common type of secondary malignancy.

2.3 Uveal Melanoma

2.3.1 Overview

Uveal melanoma is the most common primary intraocular malignancy in adults and is known for its high metastatic potential, with about 50% of patients developing metastases. Once metastasis occurs, the cancer can be fatal due to the lack of effective treatments for systemic spread. Typically, metastatic disease is not present at the time of initial detection, making early diagnosis crucial. The global mean age-adjusted incidence is 4.3 per million, with a mean age at presentation of 60 years. Uveal melanoma can affect the iris, ciliary body, or choroid, with the choroid being the most commonly involved site in approximately 90% of cases. The tumors usually present unilaterally and are slightly more prevalent in males (Carvajal et al. 2023).

2.3.2 Clinical Features

Although iris melanomas may be diagnosed earlier because they are more readily visible, posterior (ciliary body, choroidal) uveal melanomas are diagnosed only after patients are evaluated specifically for a visual change or a suspicious lesion detected incidentally during ophthalmoscopy. Iris melanomas are better differentiated and less aggressive compared with posterior uveal melanomas. The types of iris melanoma are circumscribed, diffuse, and tapioca iris melanoma. Circumscribed iris melanomas are characterized by a variably pigmented, well-defined mass in the iris stroma and are more commonly found in the inferior half of the iris. Diffuse iris melanomas are distinguished by progressive iris discoloration, disappearance of iris crypts, and pigment accumulation in the anterior chamber. These conditions are frequently misdiagnosed as pigmentary glaucoma or pigment dispersion syndrome. Tapioca melanoma is a type of iris melanoma with multiple amelanotic nodules on the surface that resemble tapioca pudding. Features suggestive, but not pathognomonic, of iris melanoma include corectopia, ectropion uveae, glaucoma, angle seeding, hyphema, and extraocular extension. It is sometimes difficult to distinguish iris melanoma from nevi, and in such cases, close serial follow-up is required to document the progression of the malignancy.

The presence of sentinel blood vessel, sectorial cataract, and a darkly pigmented mass behind the pupil are suggestive of ciliary body melanoma.

Melanomas in the ciliary body can grow anteriorly into the anterior chamber, displacing the iris root centrally and making the tumor visible on biomicroscopy. In choroidal melanoma, the mass can be either pigmented, mixed, or amelanotic. The shape of the tumor varies across flat, dome, or mushroom configuration and can be associated with overlying orange pigment lipofuscin and/or subretinal fluid (Fig. 2.4).

2.3.3 Ancillary Testing

Uveal melanoma exhibits distinctive features on echography that are highly reliable for accurate diagnosis. According to the Collaborative Ocular Melanoma Study (COMS) report, 88% of tumors showed low to medium reflectivity on ultrasound, often with a mushroom (collar-stud) configuration, or both. The mushroom-shaped "collar-

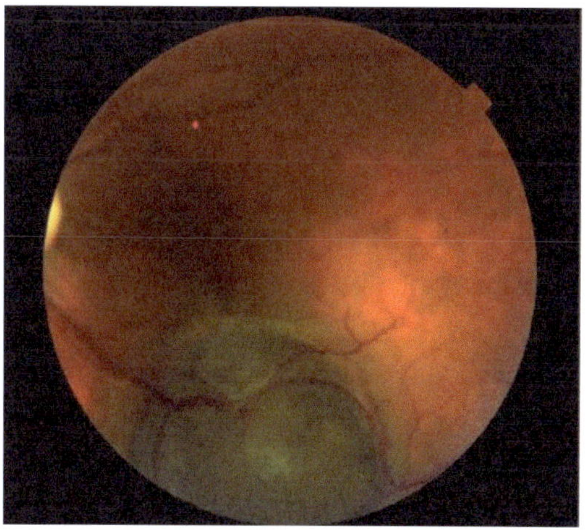

Fig. 2.4 Fundus photo showing dome-shaped melanotic choroidal melanoma with overlying orange pigment lipofuscins and surrounding subretinal fluid

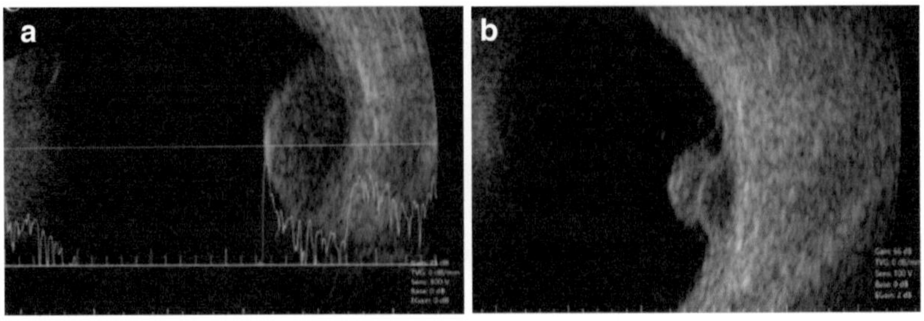

Fig. 2.5 The classic ocular B-scan ultrasound in choroidal melanoma, showing dome-shaped (**a**) or collar-stud (**b**) configuration for a mass with low internal reflectivity and choroidal excavation

stud" configuration is nearly pathognomonic for choroidal melanoma (Fig. 2.5).

Extrascleral extension can be detected using echography if at least 1.5 mm in size. Ultrasound biomicroscopy (UBM) can be employed for anterior uveal lesions. Neuroimaging (MRI, CT) is helpful when a lesion is suspicious for posterior extrascleral extension. Angiographic studies including intravenous fluorescein angiography (IVFA) and indocyanine green angiography (ICGA) can show intrinsic tumor vasculature (double circulation). Abnormal leakage (i.e., hot spots) or blockage (i.e., lipofuscin) may be seen on IVFA. Static perimetry is useful to monitor visual field changes. Certain patients will also undergo optical coherence tomography (OCT) and/or OCT Angio when vision loss occurs secondary to subretinal or intraretinal swelling. Patients with an indeterminate lesion may be a candidate for fine needle aspiration biopsy (FNAB). This decision is made on a case-by-case basis in discussion with the patient.

2.3.4 Systemic Metastatic Disease

Uveal melanoma should be managed with consideration of its systemic nature, as patients need to be evaluated for potential metastatic lesions in addition to local spread. According to the Collaborative Ocular Melanoma Study (COMS) trial, the largest prospective clinical trial for uveal melanoma, only 45% of patients were alive and cancer free 12 years after treatment (Hawkins and Collaborative Ocular Melanoma Study Group 2004). Patients with small or medium-sized tumors rarely have evidence of systemic involvement at initial presentation, while less than 1% of those with large lesions may show systemic disease. The liver is the most common site of metastasis, affecting up to 90% of patients, with other sites including the skin (subcutaneous nodules), lungs, bone, and central nervous system. Routine monitoring typically involves blood tests for hepatic enzymes (AST, ALT, and bilirubin) and imaging studies of the chest and abdomen using ultrasonography or CT. There is no consensus on the optimal frequency and methods for metastatic screening, and current evidence suggests that different screening protocols have not been shown to improve disease-related survival. A recent literature review indicated that routine surveillance for metastasis does not confer a survival benefit. The main benefits of surveillance may be limited to providing reassurance to patients and practitioners and facilitating participation in future clinical trials.

2.3.5 Predictors of Disease-Related Metastasis and Mortality

Monosomy of chromosome 3 and/or amplification of chromosome 8q in choroidal tumors are associated with a significantly higher risk of developing metastases. Conversely, loss of chromosome 1p and gain of chromosome 6p are linked with a better prognosis. Patient age and tumor size are important predictors for time to death from all causes and melanoma-related mortality. Involvement of the ciliary body increases risk, and local recurrence after treatment failure is weakly associated with a higher metastatic rate. Additional high-risk clinical features include extraocular extension, a diffuse growth pattern, a ring configuration, and optic nerve involvement.

Analysis of gene expression has led to the classification of uveal melanomas into two types. Approximately half of ocular melanomas are classified as class 1, which carry a low risk of metastasis. The other half are class 2, characterized by a different gene expression pattern and often showing chromosome 3 monosomy, which indicates a high risk of metastasis. Class 2 tumors are associated with known metastatic risk factors such as ciliary body involvement, a larger basal diameter, older age, presence of exudative retinal detachment, and increased tumor height. The molecular classification of uveal melanoma is considered more predictive of prognosis than clinical, histologic, or cytological factors. However, there are important limitations, including potential inaccuracies due to tumor heterogeneity (i.e., sampling errors), limited availability of molecular genetic tests, and inability to predict progression from class 1 to class 2.

2.3.6 Pathology

Uveal melanoma primarily has two histopathological cell types: spindle cells and epithelioid cells. Spindle cells have elongated nuclei, scant cytoplasm, and a cohesive arrangement. In contrast, epithelioid cells are characterized by round or oval nuclei, abundant cytoplasm, and a discrete, large, and pleomorphic appearance. Many lesions display a mixed cellular population, reflecting a spectrum between these two types (Fig. 2.6). The epithelioid cell type is strongly associated with higher rates of metastasis and mortality, whereas the spindle cell type generally correlates with a better prognosis. Serum immunoassays for biomarkers such as PC-10 monoclonal antibody, osteopontin, S-100 beta, melanoma-inhibitory activity, and human leukocyte antigens can detect malignant uveal melanoma cells in the serum and may indicate the potential for metastasis. However, the direct correlation between these biomarkers and metastatic potential is not always definitive.

Immunohistochemistry (IHC) has improved traditional histologic methods. For example, IHC staining with anti-phospho-histone H3 Ser10 (PHH3) produces higher mitotic counts than traditional hematoxylin-eosin (H&E) staining techniques. Immunopositivity for the proliferation marker Ki-67 can distinguish uveal melanomas that are low versus high risk for metastasis. Most melanomas are diagnosed by H&E alone, but indeterminate specimens can be confirmed using IHC with human melanoma black (HMB)-45, melan-A, tyrosinase, and NK1 C3 stains.

High-risk histologic features for uveal melanoma metastasis and disease-related mortality include the epithelioid cell type, a high mitotic rate, closed periodic acid-Schiff (PAS)-positive loops, mean diameter of the ten largest nucleoli, degree of pigmentation, inflammation, vascular invasion, and tumor necrosis.

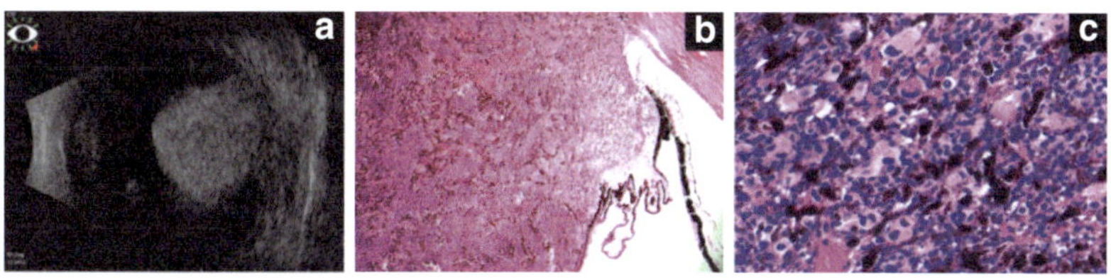

Fig. 2.6 (**a**) B-scan ultrasound shows a mushroom-shaped choroidal lesion associated with overlying retinal detachment and low-to-moderate internal reflectivity suggestive of choroidal melanoma; (**b**) 4× hematoxylin and eosin (H&E) slide (ciliary body malignant melanoma): pigmented predominantly spindle cell tumor arranged in fascicles arising from the ciliary body; (**c**) 40× (ciliary body malignant melanoma): the tumor is of mixed cell type with foci showing large and small epithelioid cells with abundant eosinophilic cytoplasm, prominent nuclei, and inclusions. This tumor exhibits prominent tumor-infiltrating lymphocytes and macrophages. Abundant melanin pigmentation is seen

2.3.7 Staging/Risk Stratification: Tumor-Node-Metastasis (TNM) Classification to Stage Disease

The American Joint Committee on Cancer (AJCC) and the International Union Against Cancer (IUCC) TNM staging systems for uveal melanomas were revised in 2009 (Balch et al. 2009). The clinical (c) and pathologic (p) TNM classifications are distinguished. The former is determined by the clinician prior to treatment while the latter by the pathologist after specimen analysis. Iris melanomas are classified separately from posterior (ciliary body, choroidal) melanomas. Tumor size, ciliary body involvement, and extrascleral extension are used to grade lesions (T). This grade, along with metastasis to regional lymph nodes (N) and distant lymph nodes (M), is used to stage the tumor. The multigene clinical prognostic assay is included in this recent TNM classification.

2.3.8 Treatment

2.3.8.1 Decision to Treat

If the systemic workup is negative, the management options involve serial observation or local therapy (radiation, surgery, or laser) (Table 2.3). Treatment goals are to prevent metastasis, eye salvage, and maintain vision for lesions that are growing or exhibit high-risk features for growth. Overall, surgery and iodine (I-125) brachytherapy were found to result in similar survival rates for patients with medium-sized lesions in the COMS study.

Although most agree that medium and large tumors should be treated promptly, the decision regarding management of smaller indeterminate tumors can be more difficult. Most agree that a small tumor can be observed unless it demonstrates growth or has high-risk features for growth.

High-risk features predictive of subsequent growth in uveal melanoma typically include the presence of orange pigment lipofuscin, visual symptoms, a juxtapapillary location, increased tumor thickness, and presence of subretinal fluid. This approach may change, however, in light of new evidence based on molecular genetic testing. There are currently many clinical trials underway for various systemic therapies to treat metastatic disease, but none have been effective to date. Except for rare cases that may improve after local hepatic resection, there are no effective treatments for melanoma metastasis, and patients succumb to the cancer within 1 year.

2.3.9 Radiation Therapy

In plaque brachytherapy, the plaque is secured over the sclera at the site of the tumor to deliver radiation directly to the tumor with minimal damage to the surrounding tissue (Fig. 2.7). Plaque diameter should be 4 mm wider than the widest basal dimension of the melanoma, in order to provide 2 mm clearance circumferentially (available plaque range 10–22 mm in 2 mm increments). Special notched plaques are used for peripapillary tumors to guarantee tumor control. Tumors with a height of 2–10 mm and basal diameter $<$ 16 mm are eligible for brachytherapy.

Table 2.3 Treatment modalities for uveal melanoma

Laser[a]	Radiation	Surgery
Transpupillary thermotherapy (TTT) diode	Plaque brachytherapy: – (Iodine-125) (I-125) – (Ruthenium-106) (Ru-106) – (Palladium-103) (Pa-103)	Local resection
Photodynamic therapy (PDT)		Enucleation
		Exenteration
	External beam radiation therapy (EBRT)	
	Gamma knife radiosurgery	

[a] Laser is mainly used as adjunctive therapy

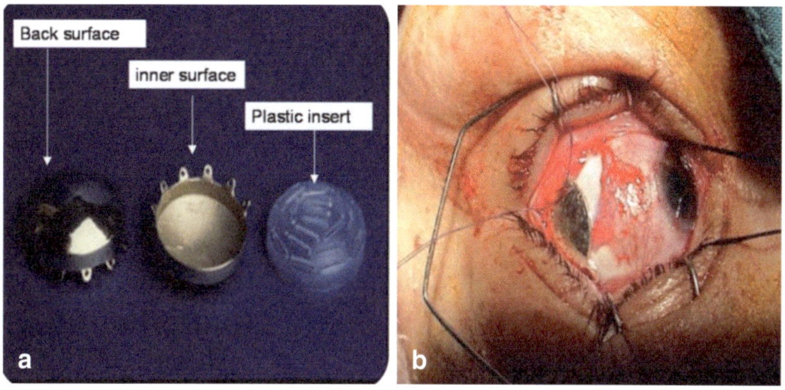

Fig. 2.7 (**a**) The classic round radioactive plaque design. (**b**) Intraoperative photo shows that the plaque is secured over the sclera at the site of the tumor to deliver radiation directly to the tumor with minimal damage to the surrounding tissue

The prescription dose is 85 gray (Gy) to tumor apex (range 75–90 Gy). The dose rate is 50–75 cGy/h, delivered over 4–7 days.

2.3.10 Surgery

Uveal melanoma can be treated by enucleation surgery when the clinical diagnosis is clear. However, when globe-preserving therapy is a viable option, every effort is made to present the risks versus benefits of all options to the patient. Enucleation is usually indicated for large tumors that cannot be controlled with plaque brachytherapy or other forms of radiation. Enucleation is a definitive procedure whereby the entire eyeball is removed with the sclera intact, with disinsertion of the extraocular muscle attachments and the optic nerve. Tumors that have progressed despite prior radiation therapy are often treated by enucleation and rarely by reradiation.

A permanent orbital implant is inserted during surgery, which replaces orbital volume and is covered by the Tenon's fascial and conjunctival layers after the extraocular muscles are attached to it. A temporary plastic conformer is left in place for 6 weeks after which time the ocularist fashions a customized prosthetic shell to rest on the mucous membrane tissue. Some iris or ciliary body melanomas can be excised by local resection. Exenteration is indicated if there is extraocular extension of the melanoma into the orbit.

2.3.11 Chemotherapy

There is no role for systemic chemotherapy in treating the primary intraocular tumor. Systemic therapies including chemotherapeutics, hepatic artery infusion of melphalan, and other agents have not been shown to improve patient survival once metastasis occurs.

2.3.12 Other Therapy

Photodynamic therapy (PDT) and transpupillary thermotherapy (TTT) are noninvasive laser treatments. Both were found to be of limited benefit as primary therapy for choroidal melanoma and are used only as adjunctive therapy for selected cases. Patients with vision loss secondary to macular edema may be treated with intravitreal injection of anti-vascular endothelial growth factor (VEGF) agents (bevacizumab, ranibizumab) and/or steroids.

2.3.13 Differential Diagnosis

Differentiating choroidal melanoma from choroidal nevus is crucial, as choroidal nevus is benign and the most common fundus tumor. Other conditions that must be differentiated from a pigmented choroidal nevus include congenital hypertrophy of the retinal pigment epithelium

(RPE), RPE hyperplasia, combined hamartoma of the retinal epithelium and RPE, and subretinal hemorrhage. An amelanotic choroidal nevus should be distinguished from choroidal metastasis, choroidal granuloma, and choroidal lymphoma. A thorough fundus examination by an experienced clinician, along with imaging techniques such as OCT and fluorescein angiography, is essential for distinguishing choroidal melanoma from these other conditions.

2.3.14 Choroidal Nevus Versus Melanoma

Choroidal nevus originates from melanocytes in the choroidal stroma. It is estimated that 5–10% of the Caucasian population has choroidal nevi, and about 1 in 8845 nevi may progress to uveal melanoma. Typically, a choroidal nevus appears as a flat, homogeneous, slate-gray lesion with a slightly ill-defined border. Over time, it may develop fine drusen on its surface (Fig. 2.8). In some cases, a nevus may be entirely amelanotic. Most nevi are less than 2 mm in thickness. Indicators that a nevus might be evolving into malignant melanoma include a thickness greater than 2 mm, presence of orange pigment on the lesion's surface, and localized secondary retinal detachment.

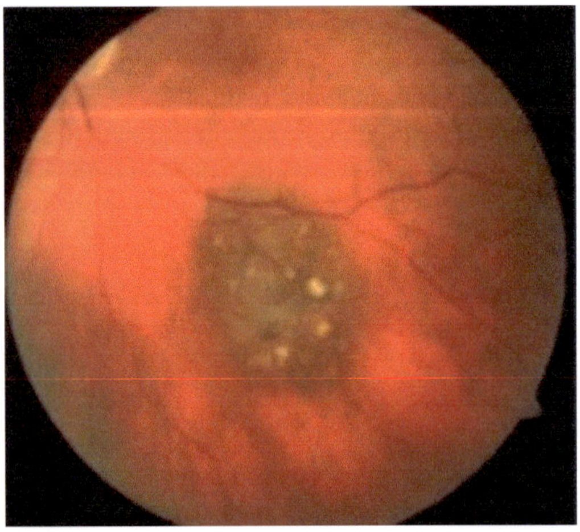

Fig. 2.8 Fundus photo of a typical flat melanotic choroidal nevus with ill-defined borders, and overlying drusen and fibrous metaplasia

Choroidal nevus can exhibit minimal growth, less than 1 mm in base diameter, over many years of follow-up, and this slow growth does not necessarily indicate a transformation into melanoma. A choroidal nevus may also present with a surrounding halo, referred to as a "halo nevus." Patients with a halo nevus generally have a low risk of transformation to choroidal melanoma.

On ultrasonography, a choroidal nevus typically shows high internal reflectivity and acoustic solidity. In contrast, small choroidal melanomas usually have medium to low internal reflectivity and acoustic hollowness. Choroidal nevus generally requires no treatment. Patients with a choroidal nevus should be monitored regularly, and if the lesion shows growth, it should be assessed for potential transformation into early malignant melanoma. Risk factors predictive of this transformation include thickness greater than 2 mm; subretinal fluid; symptoms such as decreased vision, visual field defects, flashes, or floaters; presence of orange pigment; proximity to the optic disc; ultrasonographic hollowness; and absence of a halo or drusen.

A mnemonic to remember the risk factors for ocular melanoma is TFSOM UHHD: "To find small ocular melanoma using helpful hints daily." This stands for Thickness, Fluid, Symptoms, Orange pigment, Margin, Ultrasonographic hollowness, Halo absence, and Drusen absence. Tumors with one risk factor have a 38% chance of growth, while those with two or more factors have a growth rate exceeding 50% within 5 years.

Differentiating choroidal nevus from small choroidal melanoma is crucial. A small choroidal melanoma typically has a tumor thickness of 2–3 mm and shows signs of activity, such as subretinal fluid and/or orange pigment. In contrast, a choroidal nevus is usually less than 2 mm thick and displays signs of chronicity, including drusen, RPE atrophy, RPE hyperplasia, RPE detachment, or fibrous metaplasia. Fluorescein angiography showing hot spots and leakage may indicate growth and potential transformation of a nevus into melanoma (Table 2.4).

Table 2.4 Factors to differentiate choroidal nevus (benign) from choroidal melanoma (malignant)

	Nevus	Melanoma
Size	<2 mm in thickness and <5 mm in diameter	>2 mm in thickness and >5 mm in diameter
Subretinal fluid	No	Yes
Location	Away from disc	Proximity to optic disc <3 mm[a]
Symptomatic (e.g., photopsia)	No	Yes
Drusen and halos	Present	Absent
Lipofuscin orange pigment (mainly on FAF)	Absent	Present
Ultrasound internal reflectivity	High	Low (acoustic hollowness)

[a] 60% of choroidal melanomas are within 3 mm of the optic disc

2.3.15 Choroidal Metastasis

The choroid, due to its rich blood supply, is the most common site of metastasis to the eye, making choroidal metastasis the most prevalent intraocular tumor in adults. The primary cancers that most frequently metastasize to the eye are breast cancer in females (40–47%) and lung cancer in males (21–29%). In many cases, patients with choroidal metastasis have an established diagnosis of systemic cancer at the time the eye lesion is detected. However, in 34% of cases, the choroidal metastasis is identified before the systemic cancer diagnosis. Among patients with unknown primary tumors, the primary sites include lung (7%) and breast (35%), and approximately 50% have no identified primary source. Choroidal metastases are often associated with advanced stages of disseminated disease and generally indicate a poor prognosis.

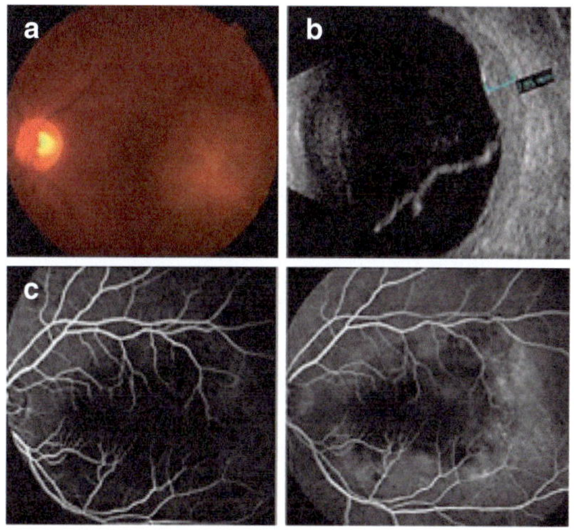

Fig. 2.9 Choroidal metastasis. (**a**) Color fundus photograph of the left eye showing macular amelanotic yellow-white choroidal lesion. (**b**) B-scan ultrasonography showed choroid thickening (2.8 mm) associated with inferior exudative retinal detachment. (**c**) Fluorescein fundus angiograph showed early choroid blockage and late leakage associated with hot spots at tumor margin

The disease can present with various clinical features such as blurry vision, visual field defects, floaters, photopsia, and decreased visual acuity. These symptoms can be unilateral or bilateral, depending on the extent of metastasis. In some cases, patients may not have any ocular symptoms, and the condition may be detected incidentally during routine eye exams. A comprehensive eye examination, including fundus examination, may reveal a yellow-white choroidal mass with surrounding retinal detachment, subretinal fluid, or hemorrhage. The growth is mainly horizontal (infiltrative) as compared to vertical growth of choroidal melanoma (Fig. 2.9). Occasionally, the mass may appear orange, which is typically associated with metastases from renal cell carcinoma, carcinoid tumor, or thyroid cancer. Conversely, a brown-gray appearance is more common with metastatic melanoma. In most cases, the majority of eyes (72%) exhibit a single focus of metastasis.

Imaging studies, including ultrasonography, fluorescein angiography, and optical coherence tomography, are crucial for confirming the diagnosis and evaluating the extent of choroidal lesions. Choroidal metastases typically present with higher reflectivity on A-scan and appear echo-dense on B-scan, in contrast to choroidal melanomas, which usually exhibit medium to low reflectivity on A-scan and are acoustically hollow on B-scan. Additionally, choroidal metastases generally have a significantly lower height-to-base ratio compared to melanomas.

Systemic evaluation, including blood tests, radiological imaging, and biopsy of the primary tumor or metastatic site, may be required to determine the underlying cause of choroidal metastasis. Prompt diagnosis and management can improve visual outcomes and quality of life for patients with this condition.

The treatment for choroidal metastasis is tailored based on the patient's systemic health and the characteristics of the choroidal tumors, including their number, location, and laterality. For patients with poor systemic status or those with resolved or asymptomatic disease, observation may be appropriate. For active, multifocal, and bilateral metastases, systemic therapies such as chemotherapy, immunotherapy, or hormone therapy are considered, as well as whole-eye radiotherapy. For active, solitary metastases, treatment options include plaque radiotherapy, transpupillary radiotherapy, or photodynamic therapy. Enucleation is reserved for cases involving a blind and painful eye. The chosen treatment aims to address both the ocular and systemic aspects of the disease.

2.3.16 Choroidal Hemangioma

Choroidal hemangioma is a benign vascular tumor that arises from the choroid. Choroidal hemangiomas can be classified into two types: circumscribed and diffuse. Circumscribed choroidal hemangiomas are well-defined, dome-shaped tumors that are usually located in the posterior pole of the eye. Typically, choroidal hemangioma is reddish to orange colored. They occur as solitary condition without systemic associations. Diffuse choroidal hemangiomas are flat and diffuse lesions that involve a larger area of the choroid and occur in association with Sturge-Weber syndrome, ipsilateral to nevus flammeus.

Choroidal hemangiomas can be diagnosed through a comprehensive eye exam, including a dilated fundus exam, ocular ultrasound, fluorescein angiography, and optical coherence tomography (OCT).

On ultrasound, hemangiomas appear dome shaped and exhibit high internal reflectivity on A-scan. They also show acoustic solidity on B-scan that is similar to the surrounding choroid, with an echogenic character comparable to that of the normal choroid (Fig. 2.10).

Management of choroidal hemangiomas depends on the size, location, and symptoms of the tumor. Small, asymptomatic tumors may not require any treatment, but larger tumors that cause visual disturbance or threaten the health of the eye may require intervention. Treatment options include laser photocoagulation, photodynamic therapy, plaque radiotherapy for focal lesions, and external beam radiotherapy for diffuse lesions.

Overall, choroidal hemangioma is a relatively rare condition, but it can cause significant visual impairment if left untreated. Early diagnosis and appropriate management can help prevent complications and preserve vision.

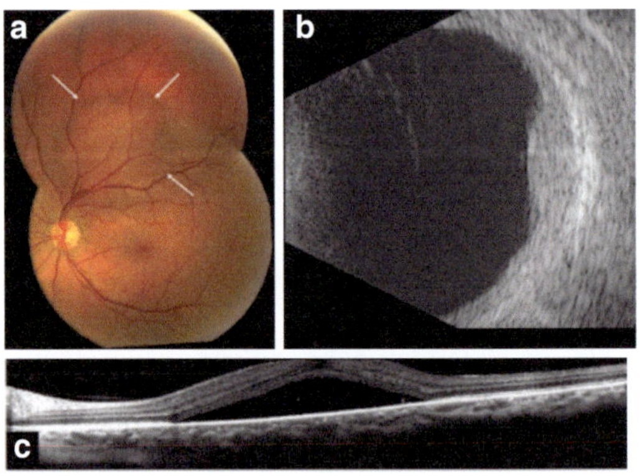

Fig. 2.10 Circumscribed choroidal hemangioma. (**a**) Fundus photo shows well-defined, dome-shaped, reddish to orange-colored tumor. (**b**) Ultrasonography shows a diffuse choroidal mass with medium-to-high internal reflectivity. (**c**) OCT shows the presence of subretinal fluid

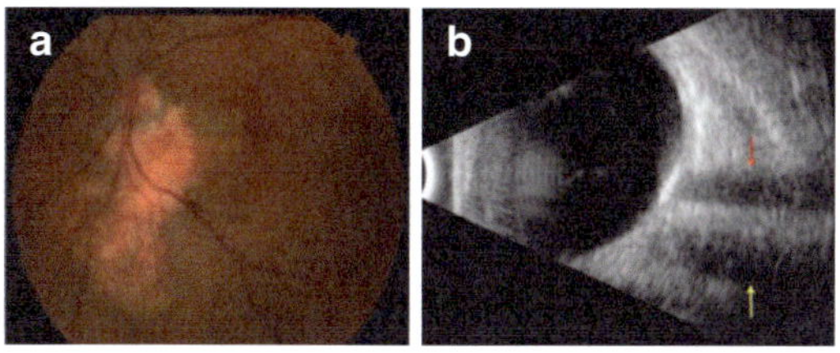

Fig. 2.11 Choroidal osteoma. (**a**) Flat, white-yellow, well-defined, juxta-papillary mass with irregular margins. (**b**) Ocular B-scan shows a placoid lesion with very high internal reflectivity and shadowing (red arrow) giving the characteristic "pseudo-optic nerve"

2.3.17 Choroidal Osteoma

Choroidal osteoma is a benign tumor in which bony tissue replaces the choroid. It usually affects one eye and is more common in young females. The lesions are flat, white-yellow in color with overlying pigments, with well-defined, irregular margins that are commonly located around the optic nerve (juxta-papillary or peripapillary). The diagnosis is mainly clinical. Ocular B-scan shows a placoid lesion with very high internal reflectivity and shadowing giving the characteristic "pseudo-optic nerve" (Fig. 2.11). Other tests, like a brain CT scan, will show the presence of a patch of bone near the optic nerve.

The lesions are usually asymptomatic, but if they grow slowly towards the macula, visual symptoms may develop, primarily as a result of the development of choroidal neovascular membrane (CNV), in which case the patient will require treatment with anti-vascular endothelial growth factor (VEGF) intravitreal injections. Poor vision is also linked to sub-foveal decalcification. Otherwise, choroidal osteoma is asymptomatic and does not require treatment.

2.3.18 Melanocytoma

A melanocytoma (also known as a magnocellular nevus) is a rare benign pigmented tumor and is a derivative of the neural crest. It can appear anywhere along the uveal tract; most commonly, it arises around optic disc. The lesion is typically unilateral dark brown to black, located entirely or partly in the optic disc and may extend to adjacent choroid or retina (Fig. 2.12).

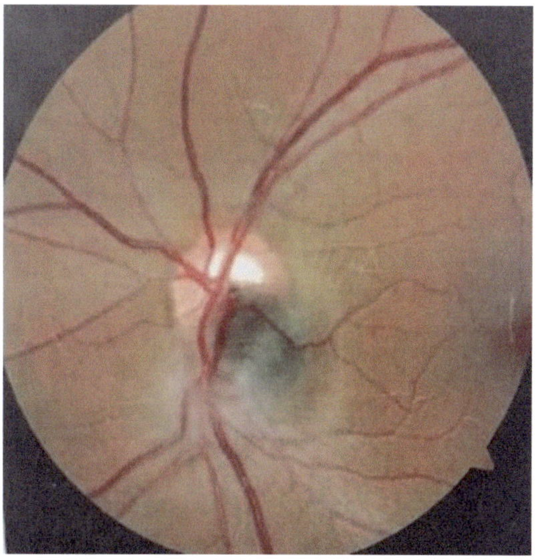

Fig. 2.12 Fundus photo shows that melanocytoma occurs around the optic disc; the tumor is dark brown-black in color, with minimal extension towards the macula

Melanocytomas are typically asymptomatic and are often discovered incidentally during routine eye examinations. However, depending on their size and location, they may cause visual disturbances such as blurry vision or visual field defects. These symptoms usually result from mild exudative retinal changes involving the fovea or neuroretinitis due to tumor necrosis. In rare cases, more severe visual loss can occur due to central retinal vein obstruction or spontaneous tumor necrosis, or even malignant transformation. Given the potential for malignant transformation into melanoma in 1–2% of cases, melanocytomas should be monitored with periodic eye exams.

2.4 Retinal Vascular Tumors

2.4.1 Retinal Hemangioblastoma (Retinal Angioma)

This benign vascular tumor can occur as a solitary lesion sporadically or, more commonly, in association with von Hippel-Lindau (VHL) syndrome, where it tends to be multifocal and bilateral. For patients with retinal hemangioblastoma, genetic testing for a VHL gene mutation is essential, along with pre- and posttest genetic counseling. If the test result is positive, comprehensive clinical screening for additional VHL lesions is necessary. Additionally, screening of family members who may be affected is recommended.

Clinically, retinal hemangioblastomas present as orange-red spherical tumors located in the mid-periphery of the retina, with enlarged and tortuous feeder vessels supplying them. Depending on the tumor size, fluid and lipid leakage can lead to vision impairment through secondary maculopathy or exudative retinal detachment (Fig. 2.13).

Fluorescein angiography is crucial for visualizing the hemangioblastoma's vascular nature and detecting fluid leakage from the tumor.

Complications often arise at later stages of the disease and may include epiretinal membranes, retinal detachment, and vitreous hemorrhage, which can severely impair vision.

Treatment options for small peripheral retinal hemangioblastomas typically involve laser photocoagulation. Larger tumors may be managed with cryotherapy or radiotherapy, including plaque radiotherapy or proton beam irradiation. Photodynamic therapy with verteporfin might also be considered. In advanced cases, additional vitreoretinal surgery may be necessary (Wiley et al. 2019).

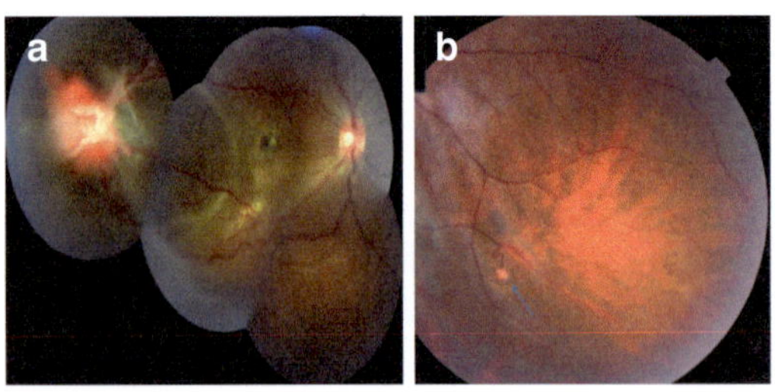

Fig. 2.13 Retinal hemangioblastoma in a patient with VHL. (**a**) Right eye fundus photo shows a large reddish spherical tumor temporal to the macula supplied by enlarged and tortuous feeder vessels. Note the massive subretinal fluid and exudation extending to the fovea that resulted in severe impairment of vision. (**b**) Left eye fundus photo of the same patient shows a small incidental hemangioma (blue arrow)

2.4.2 Retinal Cavernous Hemangioma

Retinal cavernous hemangioma is a benign vascular tumor consisting of clusters of aneurysmatic dilated retinal vessels, often accompanied by varying degrees of retinal gliosis and fibrosis. Unlike retinal hemangioblastomas, cavernous hemangiomas lack a feeding artery and are typically located along the path of a retinal vein. These tumors can be associated with similar vascular anomalies in the central nervous system and with cutaneous vascular malformations. Most retinal cavernous hemangiomas do not cause retinal exudation, are nonprogressive, and usually do not require treatment. Retinal cavernous hemangiomas may bleed into the vitreous in rare instances. Treatment of retinal cavernous hemangiomas is indicated in cases with recurrent vitreous hemorrhage. Laser photocoagulation or cryotherapy may be used.

2.4.3 Retinal Vasoproliferative Tumor

This is a benign retinal tumor that typically presents between the ages of 40 and 60 years, though it can occur at any age. It may be primary or secondary to chronic ocular conditions such as Coats' disease, retinitis pigmentosa, uveitis, or retinal detachment. Clinically, it appears as an orange or pink mass in the peripheral retina, often located inferotemporally, and is associated with retinal vascular changes and exudation. Unlike the retinal angiomas seen in von Hippel-Lindau disease, the "feeder" vessels of these tumors are usually normal or slightly enlarged but not markedly dilated or tortuous. Vasoproliferative tumors can be solitary or multiple, usually found in the pre-equatorial region. The disease may be asymptomatic, but it often progresses slowly, leading to symptoms such as visual loss, metamorphopsia, photopsia, floaters, photophobia, or a red eye due to intraocular inflammation.

Small asymptomatic tumors can be observed; treatment options for symptomatic lesions include PDT laser, cryotherapy, or plaque brachytherapy.

2.5 Racemose Hemangioma (Wyburn–Mason Syndrome)

This is discussed in the next section (Phakomatosis).

2.5.1 Phakomatosis

2.5.1.1 Overview

Phakomatosis refers to a group of rare genetic disorders characterized by the development of hamartomatous or neoplastic lesions in multiple organs, including the eye (Douglas et al. 2019). These disorders are often present at birth or emerge during childhood and can affect various systems in the body. Ocular phakomatosis specifically denotes the involvement of the eye in these conditions. In this overview, we will explore some of the most well-known phakomatosis diseases and their ocular manifestations (Table 2.5):

Neurofibromatosis type 1 (NF1): NF1 is a multisystem disorder caused by mutations in the NF1 gene. Ocular findings in NF1 include Lisch nodules (benign iris hamartomas), optic nerve glioma, choroidal abnormalities, and increased risk of other ocular tumors like optic pathway gliomas. Lisch nodules (iris hamartoma) are a pigmented hamartomatous nodular aggregate of dendritic melanocytes. They are mostly bilateral, have ununiform appearance, are inferiorly distributed, and increase with age, so are present in >90% of patients with NF1 above the age of 20 years (unlike mammillations). Lisch nodules are very rare in NF2. Iris mammillations are unilateral with uniform appearance, and regularly spaced, and mostly at pupillary margin (unlike Lisch nodules). They are mostly sporadic and rarely associated with NF1.

Diagnostic Criteria for NF1

Two or more of the following clinical features signify the presence of NF1 in a patient.

(continued)

- More than 6 cafe au lait macules over 0.5 cm in greatest diameter in prepubertal individuals and over 1.5 cm in greatest diameter in postpubertal individuals
- Two or more neurofibromas of any type or one plexiform neurofibroma
- Freckling in the axillary or inguinal regions
- Optic glioma
- Two or more Lisch nodules (iris hamartomas)
- A distinctive osseous lesion such as sphenoid dysplasia or tibial pseudoarthrosis
- A first-degree relative (parent, sibling or offspring) with NF1 as defined by the above criteria

Absent sphenoid wing is also characteristic for NF1.

Orbital encephalocele arises nasally causing pulsating proptosis, without thrill or bruit. Eyelid neurofibroma can be plexiform (feeling like a bag of worms) or localized (causing S-shaped deformity). They result in mechanical ptosis. They are linked to an increased risk of developing glaucoma in NF1. Plexiform neurofibroma is more specific for NF1.

A new feature that was found to be sensitive and specific is choroidal nodules on near-infrared reflectance (NIR), but not other modalities. The examination of nodules at the optimal cutoff point of 1.5 nodules demonstrated a sensitivity of 83% and a specificity of 96% (Viola et al. 2012). These nodules are believed to consist of proliferating neoplastic Schwann cells arranged in concentric rings around axons.

1. Neurofibromatosis type 2 (NF2): NF2 is characterized by the development of bilateral vestibular schwannomas (also known as acoustic neuromas). Ocular manifestations may include posterior subcapsular cataracts, retinal hamartomas, and epiretinal membranes.

Table 2.5 Specific features for each disease

Disease	Neurofibromatosis 1 (von Recklinghausen disease)	Neurofibromatosis 2	Tuberous sclerosis (Bourneville disease)	Sturge-Weber syndrome (encephalo-facial-cavernous hemangiomatosis)	Von Hippel-Lindau (retino-cerebellar-capillary hemangiomatosis)	Wyburn-Mason syndrome (Bonnet-Dechaume-Blanc syndrome)	Ataxia telangiectasia syndrome (Louis Bar)
Inheritance	AD	AD	AD	Sporadic	AD	Sporadic	AR
Definition	Historically called von Recklinghausen disease	Much less common than NF1	Noncancerous tumors in different organs	Hemangiomatosis disease	Familial neoplastic disease caused by mutation in tumor suppressor gene VHL	Arteriovenous malformation disease	
Systemic manifestation	Tumors (meningioma, glioma, and neurofibroma), cafe-au-lait patches, axillary or inguinal freckles	Bilateral vestibular schwannomas (acoustic neuroma)	Adenoma sebaceum, ash leaf spots, astrocytoma of brain, seizures, tremors, epilepsy, mental retardation, renal cyst, cardiac and lung hamartomas	Nevus flammeus, parietal or occipital leptohemangioma (i.e., at meninges) leading to seizures, hemiparesis, hemianopia	Cerebellar hemangioblastoma, which presents around age 30, is one of the most common manifestations of VHL. Capillary hemangioblastoma (CNS and retina), hypernephroma, pheochromocytoma resulting in hypertension, hepatic, renal, pancreatic cysts. Polycythemia (i.e., high hemoglobin)	Arteriovenous malformation affecting the retina, visual pathways, midbrain, and facial bones	Cerebellar abnormalities. Absent thymus gland and T cells, so recurrent infection
Retinal manifestation	Choroidal nevi, retinal astrocytomas, and optic nerve glioma	Astrocytic hamartoma of RPE and macula, epiretinal membrane	Retinal astrocytoma (occurs in >50% of patients), and retinal achromic patch (punched-out depigmented lesions)	Retinal and choroidal hemangioma (diffuse type is more common)	Retinal capillary hemangioblastoma occurring in 45–85% of patients (50% average), so the best diagnostic modality for VHL is fluorescein angiography	Retinal racemose hemangioma	None

Ocular manifestations	Lisch nodules (i.e., iris hamartoma) and iris mammillations. Tumors along optic nerve tract (up to 25% of patients). Orbital encephalocele and sphenoid dysplasia, prominent corneal nerves, congenital ectropion, lid neurofibroma	Early-onset cataract PSCC (<30%), ocular motor nerve palsy. Optic nerve sheath meningioma, and abnormal ERG	Patchy iris hypopigmentation and iris coloboma	Ipsilateral glaucoma (most common manifestation and cause of visual loss), episcleral hemangioma, and iris heterochromia	–	A large, dilated, and tortuous retinal artery extends from the optic disc into the fundus, directly connecting with a dilated retinal vein before returning to the optic disc	Conjunctival telangiectasias and eye movement abnormalities, occurring later in the disease course

Epiretinal membrane (ERM) in NF2 appears in childhood in almost 80%, with characteristics different from secondary ERMs and with absence of posterior vitreous detachment. It indicates a severe phenotypic form.

2. Tuberous sclerosis complex (TSC): TSC is caused by mutations in the TSC1 or TSC2 genes. Ocular findings in TSC can include retinal hamartomas, also known as astrocytic hamartomas (Fig. 2.14), retinal pigment epithelial changes, and choroidal lesions referred to as choroidal angiomas. The classic triad of symptoms—seizures, mental disability, and cutaneous angiofibromas (adenoma sebaceum)—is present in about 30% of patients and is diagnostic of the condition. Approximately 60% of cases are sporadic, while 40% are inherited in an autosomal dominant manner. Retinal hamartomas are characterized by fibrotic astrocytes with small oval nuclei and long cytoplasmic extensions. They are found in about 50% of TSC patients, with 25% presenting bilaterally. Less commonly, retinal achromatic patches may be observed, which are not well defined but could represent flat astrocytic hamartomas. Intracranial tumors might cause papilledema, multiple cranial nerve palsies, or visual field defects.
3. Sturge-Weber syndrome (SWS): SWS is a disorder characterized by a facial port-wine stain, leptomeningeal vascular malformations, and glaucoma. The ocular manifestations of SWS primarily affect the anterior segment of the eye, including the iris, trabecular meshwork, and ciliary body. Glaucoma is the most common ocular finding in SWS, occurring in 30–70% of patients, typically within the first 2 years of life. It is also the most frequent cause of vision loss in individuals with this syndrome.

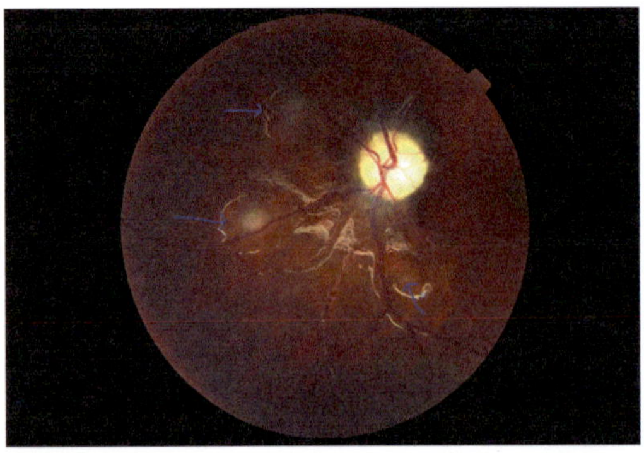

Fig. 2.14 Retinal astrocytic hamartomas: multiple whitish-yellow mass ("mulberry-like lesion") in a patient with tuberous sclerosis. Note the pale optic disc from an old associated brain tumor

4. Von Hippel-Lindau disease (VHL): VHL syndrome is associated with multiple benign and malignant tumors, including ocular manifestations such as retinal capillary hemangioblastomas. These hemangioblastomas can impair vision if they affect the macula or optic nerve. Given the potential aggressiveness of these tumors, annual screening with FFA is recommended for early detection and management. In contrast, von Hippel disease typically involves a solitary retinal capillary hemangioblastoma. VHL syndrome also includes the risk of developing other tumors such as cerebellar hemangioblastomas, pheochromocytomas, and renal cell carcinomas. Regular monitoring and management are crucial for patients with VHL syndrome to address these potential complications.
5. Wyburn-Mason syndrome associated with retinal racemose hemangioma, which is a sporadic condition with ipsilateral AV malformations involving the midbrain, basofrontal region, and posterior fossa. AV malformations may also occur in the maxilla and mandible, so care should be taken while doing dental procedures. Remember that Wyburn-Mason syndrome includes midbrain arteriovenous malformations.
6. Phakomatosis pigmentovascularis (PPV): PPV refers to the coexistence of cutaneous vascular malformations and melanocytic nevi. Ocular involvement in PPV can include eyelid vascular anomalies, choroidal vascular malformations, and conjunctival or episcleral melanocytic nevi.
7. Oculodermal melanocytosis (ODM): ODM, also known as nevus of Ota, is characterized by the presence of bluish-gray pigmentation

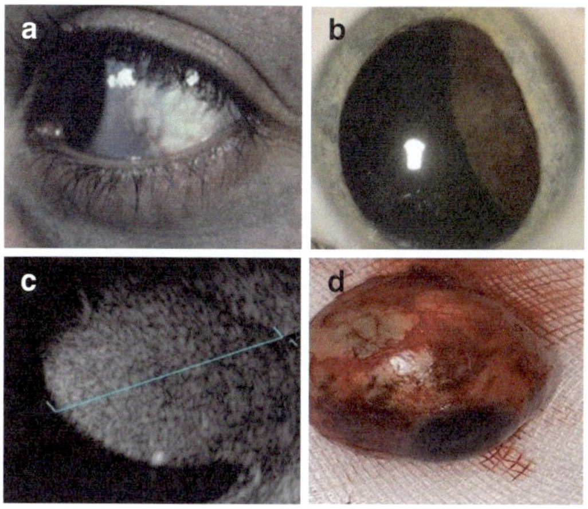

Fig. 2.15 Uveal melanoma in a patient with oculodermal melanocytosis (ODM) (nevus of Ota): (**a**) Melanocytosis over the eyelid and sclera. (**b**) A large melanotic mass in the ciliary body region. (**c**) Ocular B-scan ultrasound shows a large-sized uveal melanoma with moderate internal reflectivity. (**d**) Enucleated eye shows extensive scleral pigmentation

in the ocular and periocular tissues. ODM is associated with an increased risk of glaucoma and melanoma of the uveal tract (Fig. 2.15).

8. Multiple endocrine neoplasia type 2B (MEN2B): MEN2B is a rare inherited cancer syndrome associated with medullary thyroid carcinoma, pheochromocytoma, and multiple mucosal neuromas. Ocular findings in MEN2B can include conjunctival and corneal neuromas, as well as a distinctive appearance of the eyelids and conjunctiva.

It is important to note that the ocular manifestations and severity of phakomatosis diseases can vary widely among individuals. Regular eye examinations and appropriate management by ophthalmologists and other specialists are crucial for early detection and treatment of ocular complications associated with these conditions.

2.5.1.2 Genetics

Except for Sturge-Weber syndrome, which is a sporadic disease, all are inherited. Inheritance is always autosomal dominant (AD), except for ataxia telangiectasia (autosomal recessive AR). Despite the fact that AD is inherited, a portion of each syndrome can be sporadic.

2.6 Optic Nerve Tumors

Optic nerve tumors refer to neoplastic growths that affect the optic nerve or the surrounding structures involved in visual transmission (Miller 2004). These tumors can arise from various cell types and can occur in both children and adults. The most common primary tumor of the optic nerve is the benign glioma. In this overview, we will discuss the types, causes, symptoms, diagnosis, and treatment of optic nerve tumors.

2.6.1 Types of Optic Nerve Tumors

1. **Optic Nerve Glioma**: These tumors originate from glial cells in the optic nerve itself. They are almost always unilateral. They are most commonly associated with neurofibromatosis type 1 (NF1) and typically occur in children. Optic nerve gliomas can be low-grade pilocytic astrocytomas.
2. **Optic Nerve Meningioma**: Meningiomas are tumors that arise from arachnoid cap cells in the meninges (i.e., originate from the optic nerve sheath). Most of these tumors are unilateral, but bilateral cases do occur, more often than glioma. These tumors are typically benign and more common in adults.
3. **Optic Nerve Schwannoma:** Schwannomas arise from Schwann cells, which are responsible for myelinating nerve fibers. Optic nerve schwannomas are rare and can occur at any age. They are often benign tumors.

2.6.2 Causes and Risk Factors

The exact causes of optic nerve tumors are not fully understood, but there are known conditions and genetic factors that increase the risk of developing these tumors. For example, optic nerve gliomas are frequently associated with neurofibromatosis type 1 (NF1). Moreover, genetic mutations and hereditary syndromes can also play a role in the development of optic nerve tumors in certain cases.

2.6.3 Symptoms

The symptoms of optic nerve tumors can vary depending on the location, size, and growth rate of the tumor. Common symptoms include:

1. Gradual or sudden vision loss
2. Decreased visual acuity or blurred vision
3. Visual field defects (such as peripheral vision loss or "tunnel vision")
4. Proptosis
5. Optic disc swelling
6. Headaches
7. Abnormal eye movements or strabismus
8. Nystagmus
9. Other neurological symptoms (depending on tumor involvement)

Chronic compression of the central retinal vein caused by optic nerve tumors can lead to venous stasis retinopathy in some patients. This condition may progress to central retinal vein occlusion (CRVO), development of optociliary shunt vessels, or rubeosis iridis with associated neovascular glaucoma.

2.6.4 Diagnosis

Diagnosing optic nerve tumors involves a comprehensive evaluation by an ophthalmologist or neuro-ophthalmologist, which is also important to distinguish different tumor types (Table 2.6). Diagnostic tests may include:

1. Visual acuity and visual field testing
2. Ophthalmoscopy to examine the optic disc
3. Imaging studies, including magnetic resonance imaging (MRI) and computed tomography (CT) scans, used to visualize the tumor and assess its extent
4. Optic nerve biopsy in certain cases to confirm the diagnosis

The combination of visual loss, optic atrophy, and optociliary shunt vessels is most frequently associated with an optic nerve sheath meningioma. These shunt vessels form to redirect venous blood from the retinal circulation to the choroidal circulation, bypassing the central retinal vein. When present, optociliary shunt vessels are nearly pathognomonic of chronic central retinal vein compression.

Table 2.6 Main distinguishing features between optic nerve glioma and optic nerve meningioma

Features	Optic nerve glioma	Optic nerve meningioma
Tumor origin	Arises from glial cells in the optic nerve	Arises from arachnoid cap cells in the meninges
Prevalence	More commonly associated with neurofibromatosis type 1 (NF1)	Not typically associated with any specific syndrome, but more common in NF2 than NF1
Age of onset	Usually diagnosed in early childhood	Typically diagnosed in adulthood, more in females
Bilateral involvement	Can be unilateral or bilateral	Unilateral, but can rarely be bilateral
Tumor appearance	Generally low-grade pilocytic astrocytomas	Meningiomas, typically benign tumors
Appearance on contrasted images	Kinking of optic nerve	Enhancement, resulting in the "railroad track" or "tram track" sign
Visual impairment	Can cause visual loss, especially if involving the optic chiasm	Can cause visual loss, depending on tumor size and location
Associated symptoms	Neurological symptoms (headaches, seizures)	Uncommon, may cause proptosis
Response to treatment	Some tumors may stabilize or regress	Typically requires surgical resection or radiation therapy
Malignancy potential	Can rarely transform into malignant gliomas	Typically benign tumors with low malignant potential

2.6.5 Treatment

The treatment approach for optic nerve tumors depends on factors such as tumor type, size, location, and individual patient factors. Treatment options may include the following:

1. Observation: In some cases, small, asymptomatic tumors may be monitored closely without immediate intervention.
2. Surgery: Surgical resection may be performed to remove the tumor while preserving visual function.
3. Radiation therapy: Radiation, such as external beam radiation or stereotactic radiosurgery, may be utilized to control tumor growth and preserve vision.
4. Chemotherapy: Systemic or targeted chemotherapy may be considered for aggressive or recurrent tumors.
5. Supportive care: Other treatments and therapies may be employed to manage associated symptoms and complications, such as optic nerve edema or raised intracranial pressure.

Optic nerve tumors require multidisciplinary management involving ophthalmologists, neurosurgeons, neuro-oncologists, and radiation oncologists. The treatment plan is tailored to the individual patient's condition and aims.

Conflict of Interest The authors declare no conflicts of interest.

References

Abramson DH et al (2015) Treatment of retinoblastoma in 2015: agreement and disagreement. JAMA Ophthalmol 133(11):1341–1347. https://doi.org/10.1001/jamaophthalmol.2015.3108

Balch CM et al (2009) Final version of 2009 AJCC melanoma staging and classification. J Clin Oncol 27(36):6199–6206. https://doi.org/10.1200/JCO.2009.23.4799

Carvajal RD et al (2023) Advances in the clinical management of uveal melanoma. Nat Rev Clin Oncol 20(2):99–115. https://doi.org/10.1038/s41571-022-00714-1

Cruz-Gálvez CC et al (2022) Retinoblastoma: review and new insights. Front Oncol 12:963780. https://doi.org/10.3389/fonc.2022.963780

Douglas KAA, Douglas VP, Cestari DM (2019) Neuro-ophthalmic manifestations of the phakomatoses. Curr Opin Ophthalmol 30(6):434–442. https://doi.org/10.1097/ICU.0000000000000609

Hawkins BS, Collaborative Ocular Melanoma Study Group (2004) The Collaborative Ocular Melanoma Study (COMS) randomized trial of pre-enucleation radiation of large choroidal melanoma: IV. Ten-year mortality findings and prognostic factors. COMS report number 24. Am J Ophthalmol 138(6):936–951. https://doi.org/10.1016/j.ajo.2004.07.006

Mallipatna A, Marino M, Singh AD (2016) Genetics of retinoblastoma. Asia Pac J Ophthalmol (Phila) 5(4):260–264. https://doi.org/10.1097/APO.0000000000000219

Miller NR (2004) Primary tumours of the optic nerve and its sheath. Eye 18(11):1026–1037. https://doi.org/10.1038/sj.eye.6701592

Reese AB, Ellsworth RM (1963) The evaluation and current concept of retinoblastoma therapy. Trans Am Acad Ophthalmol Otolaryngol 67:164–172

Shields CL et al (2006) The international classification of retinoblastoma predicts chemoreduction success. Ophthalmology 113(12):2276–2280. https://doi.org/10.1016/j.ophtha.2006.06.018

Tamboli A, Podgor MJ, Horm JW (1990) The incidence of retinoblastoma in the United States: 1974 through 1985. Arch Ophthalmol 108(1):128–132. https://doi.org/10.1001/archopht.1990.01070030134045

Viola F et al (2012) Choroidal abnormalities detected by near-infrared reflectance imaging as a new diagnostic criterion for neurofibromatosis 1. Ophthalmology 119(2):369–375. https://doi.org/10.1016/j.ophtha.2011.07.046

Wiley HE et al (2019) Management of retinal hemangioblastoma in von Hippel-Lindau disease. Retina 39(12):2254–2263. https://doi.org/10.1097/IAE.0000000000002572

3 Clinical Review of Neuro-ophthalmology: Part I

Saif Aldeen Alryalat, Abdee Ryalat, Noor Laylani, and Andrew G. Lee

Abstract

This chapter offers an in-depth clinical review of neuro-ophthalmology, focusing on the interplay between neurological systems and visual disturbances. It begins with an overview of the visual pathway, highlighting how light signals travel from the retina through the optic nerve to the brain's visual cortex. The chapter covers common optic nerve diseases, such as optic neuritis, glaucoma, and ischemic optic neuropathy, detailing their clinical presentation, diagnosis, and treatment. Additional topics include optic disc anomalies, idiopathic intracranial hypertension, pupil disorders, and cranial nerve dysfunction affecting eye movements. This comprehensive guide serves as a crucial resource for ophthalmology trainees and clinicians managing neuro-ophthalmological disorders.

Keywords

Neuro-ophthalmology · Optic nerve diseases · Visual pathway · Optic disc anomalies · Intracranial hypertension

S. A. Alryalat (✉)
Department of Ophthalmology, The University of Jordan, Amman, Jordan

The University of Colorado Anschutz Medical Campus, CO, USA

A. Ryalat
Private Practice, Amman, Jordan

N. Laylani
Department of Ophthalmology, University of Colorado Anschutz Medical Campus, Aurora, CO, USA
e-mail: nalaylani@houstonmethodist.org

A. G. Lee
Department of Ophthalmology, University of Colorado Anschutz Medical Campus, Aurora, CO, USA

Department of Ophthalmology, Neurology, and Neurosurgery, Weill Cornell Medical College, New York, NY, USA

Department of Ophthalmology, Baylor College of Medicine, Houston, TX, USA

Department of Ophthalmology, The University of Iowa Hospitals and Clinics, Iowa City, IA, USA

Department of Ophthalmology, The University of Texas Medical Branch, Galveston, TX, USA

The UT MD Anderson Cancer Center, Houston, TX, USA
e-mail: aglee@houstonmethodist.org

S. A. Alryalat (ed.), *Ophthalmology Board and FRCS Part 2 Exams*,
https://doi.org/10.1007/978-981-96-1517-9_3

3.1 Overview

Neuro-ophthalmology is a specialized field that encompasses the intersection of neurology and ophthalmology, focusing on visual disturbances resulting from the neurological system's dysfunction. It is an area that demands a deep understanding of both ophthalmic disorders and neurological diseases. This chapter aims to provide a comprehensive overview of this complex field and serve as a critical resource for ophthalmology trainees.

The eye and brain's intimate connection forms the basis of neuro-ophthalmology. It starts from the retina, where light signals are converted into neural signals, traveling through the optic nerve and other relay stations before reaching the brain's visual cortex for interpretation. Any disruptions in this pathway can lead to visual disturbances, making the understanding of the visual pathway crucial. This forms the foundation of our discussion in Sect. 3.2, where we explore the intricate journey of light signals from the eyes to the brain.

We then delve into optic nerve diseases in Sect. 3.3. The optic nerve is a critical component of our visual system, responsible for transmitting the neural signals from the retina to the brain. Diseases affecting the optic nerve can have a profound impact on our vision. Here, we discuss the common conditions that affect the optic nerve, including optic neuritis, glaucoma, and non-arteritic ischemic optic neuropathy, along with their clinical presentations, diagnosis, and treatment options.

In Sect. 4.1, we address optic disc anomalies. The optic disc, where the optic nerve leaves the eye, is a critical site to assess in any ophthalmic examination. We cover the most common optic disc anomalies such as optic disc drusen, morning glory disc anomaly, and optic disc coloboma, detailing their features, clinical implications, and management.

Our journey continues with the exploration of idiopathic intracranial hypertension (IIH) in Sect. 4.2. IIH is marked by increased intracranial pressure without any detectable space-occupying lesions or ventricular enlargement. If left untreated, it can result in significant visual impairments. We discuss its pathophysiology, clinical features, and latest management strategies in this section.

Section 4.3 covers pupil-affecting diseases. The pupil's role in controlling the amount of light that reaches the retina is essential in maintaining good vision. Disorders of the pupil can result from a variety of conditions affecting the afferent and efferent pathways, and understanding these conditions is key to the diagnosis and management of these diseases.

The discussion on cranial nerves and eye movements in Sect. 4.4 illustrates the role of the complex neurological control required for coordinated eye movements. Any disruption in these nerves can lead to strabismus or other eye movement disorders.

Finally, we conclude with a miscellaneous Sect. 5.1, where we discuss numerous other conditions and syndromes of neuro-ophthalmological relevance. These include, but are not limited to, cortical visual impairment, visual field defects, and visual hallucinations.

Through this comprehensive exploration of neuro-ophthalmology, the goal is to provide you with the knowledge needed to diagnose and manage neuro-ophthalmological conditions effectively. We hope that this chapter will serve as a stepping stone for further exploration into this fascinating field, encouraging a holistic approach to patient care.

3.2 Visual Pathway

3.2.1 Optic Nerve

The optic nerve originates in the retinal nerve fiber layer and enters the optic disc; travels to the optic chiasm and optic tract; and terminates at the lateral geniculate body (LGB). The optic nerve is divided into four sections over a length of 40 mm including:

1. The intraocular portion (1 mm): Clinically viewed as the optic disc.
2. The intraorbital portion (25 mm): Surrounded by a meningeal sheath and cerebrospinal fluid. The medial and superior recti muscles par-

tially originate from this sheath, which explains the pain experienced with eye movements in patients with optic neuritis.
3. The intracanalicular portion (10 mm): Situated within the optic canal of the lesser wing of the sphenoid bone, making this segment immobile.
4. The intracranial portion (10 mm): Ascending towards the optic chiasma, this section is surrounded only by the pia mater (no dura or arachnoid).

3.2.2 Optic Chiasm

Within the optic chiasm, fibers from the nasal retina decussate and temporal retinal fibers remain uncrossed in the optic tract. The optic chiasm is located inferior to the third ventricle and the lamina terminalis, and superior to the diaphragma sellae, which transmits the pituitary stalk or infundibulum. In approximately 75% of individuals, there can be variations in the positioning of the chiasm, with potential displacements anteriorly or posteriorly. About 53% of the optic nerve fibers decussate, or cross, at the chiasm, where the following occurs:

- Fibers from the nasal retina (representing the temporal visual field) cross at the chiasm, with fibers from the superior retina (representing the inferior visual field) crossing at the upper part and fibers from the inferior retina (representing the superior visual field) crossing at the lower part.
- Fibers from the temporal retina (representing the nasal visual field) pass through the chiasm without crossing.
- Macular fibers predominantly cross at the upper and posterior regions of the chiasm.
- Fibers from the inferior nasal retina loop anteriorly upon crossing, a phenomenon known as the Wilbrand knee. Lesions at this area, where the optic nerve meets the chiasm, can result in a scotoma in the superior temporal field, referred to as a junctional scotoma.
- Compression in the inferior part of the chiasm affects the superior field (by compressing inferior fibers). It will also compress central nasal decussating fibers (temporal retina).

Classical compression on optic chiasm from suprasellar lesion causes bitemporal hemianopsia denser superiorly (Chiu and Nichols 2006). However, if the lesion is compressing optic chiasm anteriorly at the junction of chiasm and the nerve, junctional scotoma occurs, which has two types:

- Junctional scotoma of Traquair: Ipsilateral hemifield defect (which could be nasal or temporal) with ipsilateral RAPD from an ipsilateral lesion compressing the fibers (either nasal or temporal fibers)
- Junctional scotoma: Contralateral superotemporal field defect with ipsilateral optic neuropathy (central scotoma or any other field). Caused by a mass compressing fibers ipsilateral and crossing fibers from the contralateral eye

A mass causing the junctional scotoma of Traquair may progress to cause the junctional scotoma.

Manifestations of chiasmal lesion may include:

- Bitemporal hemianopia along with focal optic atrophy (present in 50% of cases with field defects). As the nasal fibers are affected in the optic nerve bilaterally, the optic atrophy takes on a band-like appearance across the optic nerve head (i.e., band or bow-tie optic atrophy).
- Retinal hemifield slide phenomenon: This nonparetic diplopia arises from the decompensation of a phoria, where significant loss of the temporal visual field in both eyes can interfere with sensory fusion. This disruption causes a phoria to decompensate, leading to near-vision difficulties. The resulting double vision occurs due to the misalignment of the visual fields, known as the "hemifield slide," which results in a failure of fusion.
- Postfixation blindness: Objects located behind the point of fixation are situated in the temporal hemifield of each eye. When these tempo-

ral fields are lost, nothing beyond the point of fixation can be seen. Despite the similar terminology, this condition is not associated with a postfixed chiasm.
- While the majority (80%) of optic chiasms are positioned directly above the sella, there are two anatomic variations that can lead to different visual field loss presentations.

High yield note: Optic chiasmal compression typically causes a bitemporal hemianopia that affects superior fields more than inferior. Chiasmal compression can be associated with postfixation syndrome (blindness beyond point of fixation), hemiretinal slide (a nonparetic diplopia), and band-type optic atrophy. Typical suprasellar lesion compresses the inferior nasal decussating fibers of the chiasm causing bitemporal field defect denser superiorly.

The optic chiasm is most commonly affected by structural lesions, with most common lesions, in descending order, being pituitary adenoma, craniopharyngioma, and meningioma:

Pituitary adenoma: It is a benign tumor of pituitary gland, classified based on size into either microadenoma (<10 mm) or macroadenoma (>10 mm). Optic chiasm is around 10 mm above the normal pituitary gland. Accordingly, microadenoma has low chance compressing the chiasm in majority of cases. For macroadenoma, it slowly compresses the inferior nasal decussating fibers. Accordingly, the most common visual field defect is bitemporal homonymous superior field defect, and only late in the disease, a bitemporal hemianopsia occurs (Lee et al. 2015). Pituitary adenoma can also be classified based on their secreting ability into functioning and nonfunctioning tumor. Lactotrophic adenoma, also known as prolactinoma, is the most common type of functioning pituitary adenoma. It typically affects young to middle-aged adults. In women, excessive prolactin secretion can lead to symptoms such as infertility, amenorrhea (absence of menstruation), and galactorrhea (milk production). In men, it may cause hypogonadism (reduced function of the gonads) and impotence. About a third of primary pituitary tumors do not secrete any hormones (i.e., nonfunctioning) (Ntali and Wass 2018), where the only symptom patient may present with might be visual field defect, increasing the chance of late presentation till significant portion of the field is affected. While pituitary adenoma usually presents gradually, if pituitary apoplexy (i.e., infarction of the tumor) occurred, they may present suddenly with headache, field defect, and hormonal deficiency. It represents an emergency that patients should be aware of. Acute medical management, including hormone administration and surgical decompression, may be necessary.

Craniopharyngioma is a slow-growing tumor arising from vestigial remnants of Rathke's pouch (i.e., pituitary gland embryonic tissue) in the sella. The tumor has a bimodal age incidence including children and older adults. Craniopharyngioma might interfere with pituitary hormones, leading to dwarfism, obesity, and delayed sexual maturity in children, and often presents with visual impairment. As with pituitary adenoma, compression of the optic apparatus can produce optic neuropathy, junctional visual field loss, bitemporal hemianopsia, or optic tract compression (Table 3.1).

Table 3.1 Comparison between pituitary adenoma and craniopharyngioma as causes of optic chiasm compression

	Pituitary adenomas	Craniopharyngiomas
Age	Mainly adults	Bimodal, with peak incidences in children aged 5–14 years and again in older adults aged 65–74 years
Origin	Originate from cells of the anterior lobe of the pituitary gland	Arise from ectoblastic remnants of Rathke's duct
Affected visual field	Optic neuropathy; junctional visual loss; bitemporal field; homonymous hemianopsia	

3.2.3 Optic Tract

The majority of the optic tract, about 90%, forms the lateral root, which terminates at the lateral geniculate body. The remaining 10% of the axons make up the medial root, which ends in the tectum of the mesencephalon, particularly within the superior colliculus and the pretectal nuclei. These fibers are crucial for optic reflexes, such as the pupillary reflex and the vestibulo-ocular reflex. Additionally, some optic tract fibers terminate in the hypothalamus, where they contribute to the regulation of circadian rhythms.

The afferent visual fibers leave the chiasm in the optic tract as crossed and uncrossed fibers:

- Fibers originating from the superior retina (including both the ipsilateral superior temporal retina and the contralateral superior nasal retina) are positioned medially in the optic tract. Fibers from the nasal retina are located towards the anterior portion.
- Fibers from the inferior retina (comprising both the ipsilateral inferior temporal retina and the contralateral inferior nasal retina) are situated laterally in the optic tract. Fibers from the nasal retina are found towards the anterior region.

An optic tract lesion can lead to a contralateral relative afferent pupillary defect (RAPD) due to asymmetric involvement of the nasal fibers. It typically results in a contralateral incongruous homonymous hemianopia, a contralateral RAPD, and a contralateral bow-tie optic atrophy. Bow-tie atrophy is a distinct pattern of optic nerve atrophy featuring atrophy of the nasal fibers of the optic nerve on the side opposite to the optic tract lesion, and atrophy of the upper and lower poles of the optic nerve on the same side as the lesion. Visual acuity and color vision are generally unaffected unless there is bilateral involvement or extension to the chiasm or optic nerve.

High yield note: The homonymous hemianopia secondary to pathology in the retrochiasmal visual pathways (e.g., *optic tract) is characteristically incongruous, while that due to pathology further posterior* (e.g., *the occipital cortex) manifests a higher degree of congruity.*

In optic tract pathology, Wernicke hemianopic pupillary reaction can be appreciated. It is when the pupillary light reflex is normal when the unaffected hemiretina is stimulated; however, it will be absent when the involved hemiretina is stimulated (i.e., light is shone from the hemianopic side) (Takizawa et al. 2017). The clinical utility of the Wernicke pupil is not clearly defined.

3.2.4 Lateral Geniculate Body (LGB)

It is located at the dorsolateral aspect of the thalamus.

- Medial optic tract (from the superior retina and inferior visual field) enters the LGB medially.
- Lateral optic tract (from the inferior retina and superior visual field) enters LGB laterally.
- Macular fibers lie posterolaterally.

The optic tract enters the LGB anteriorly, with the internal capsule situated laterally, the medial geniculate body positioned medially, and the inferior horn of the lateral ventricle located posteriorly. Fibers from the medial optic tract (originating from the superior retina) project medially into the LGB, while fibers from the lateral optic tract (originating from the inferior retina) project laterally into the LGB. Homonymous horizontal sectoranopia, a rare visual field defect, typically results from ischemic damage to the lateral geniculate nucleus (LGN).

3.2.5 Optic Radiations (Geniculo-Calcarine Tract)

The fibers course through the posterior limb of the internal capsule as they leave the LGB to form the optic radiations. These radiations are divided into the following:

- Inferior radiations, originating from the lateral LGB, traverse the temporal lobe (known as

Meyer's loop) to reach the lingual gyrus of the primary visual cortex, situated below the calcarine fissure.
- Superior radiations, originating from the medial LGB, pass through the parietal lobe to reach the cuneus gyrus of the primary visual cortex, located above the calcarine fissure.
- Macular fibers can be found between the two.

The inferior optic radiations form a loop at the tip of the temporal lobe and the calcarine sulcus, known as Meyer's loop. This loop is positioned inferolaterally relative to the anterior tip of the temporal horn of the lateral ventricle.

The optic radiations extend from the LGB to the striate cortex, situated on the medial surface of the occipital lobe, extending both above and below the calcarine fissure. Optic radiation lesions may produce congruous or incongruous partial hemianopias; however, in contrast to the pre-LGB lesion in the optic tract, the homonymous hemianopsia of optic radiation origin will not have associated optic atrophy (band atrophy) or an RAPD.

The optic radiations and visual cortex have a dual blood supply from the middle and posterior cerebral arteries. Three main optic radiations exist.

- **Temporal radiations** consist of inferior fibers of optic radiations that radiate into the tip of the temporal lobe. Their damage will lead to "pie in the sky" superior visual field defect. Their damage may be associated with contralateral hemisensory disturbance and hemiparesis, because of their passage close to the sensory and motor fibers of the internal capsule. Other manifestations of temporal lobe disease include paroxysmal olfactory and gustatory hallucinations (uncinate fits), complex visual hallucinations, and seizures. If the dominant hemisphere is affected, it may also lead to receptive dysphasia.
- **Anterior radiations**: Lesions in the anterior radiations' superior fibers, which pass through the parietal lobe, can cause contralateral homonymous quadrantanopia. Dominant parietal lobe damage may result in acalculia, agraphia, left-right disorientation, and finger agnosia. Nondominant parietal lobe lesions can lead to apraxia, affecting tasks like dressing, and spatial neglect.
- **Main radiations**: In the parietal lobe, the optic radiations are located deep and just outside the trigone and the occipital horn of the lateral ventricle. Lesions in this region typically result in a complete contralateral homonymous hemianopia.

Optokinetic nystagmus (OKN), which is tested using a rotating striped drum, can help determine the cause of an isolated homonymous hemianopia:

- Physiological OKN involves smooth pursuit of a target followed by a saccade in the opposite direction to focus on the next target.
- In cases of parietal lobe lesions, the smooth pursuit pathways towards the affected side are disrupted, causing defective OKN responses. Thus, when the drum rotates towards the lesion side, the OKN response will be asymmetric compared to the normal response when the drum rotates away from the lesion side.
- If the lesion is located in the occipital lobe, the smooth pursuit pathways remain intact, resulting in symmetrical OKN responses.

3.2.6 Primary Visual Cortex

The primary visual cortex, also known as the striate cortex, visual area 1 (V1), or Brodmann area 17, is located on the medial surface of the occipital lobe. It is divided by the calcarine fissure, which runs from the parieto-occipital sulcus to the posterior pole, into the upper cuneus gyrus and the lower lingual gyrus. Since this region is primarily involved in visual processing, Cogan's rule suggests that a patient with an isolated homonymous hemianopia and no other neurological deficits likely has a lesion in the occipital lobe.

Up to 30% of the primary visual cortex is dedicated to the macular region, with the superior macular area represented in the cuneus gyrus and the inferior macular area in the lingual gyrus. The most anterior portion of the striate cortex, adjacent to the parietal lobe, represents the peripheral nasal retina, which corresponds to the temporal crescent of the visual field. This temporal crescent is monocular and can only be seen by the contralateral eye, as it does not have a counterpart in the homonymous visual field of the other eye. Patients therefore can have a homonymous hemianopsia that selectively spares or involves the temporal crescent, and patients may have an isolated monocular temporal crescent from a contralateral occipital lobe lesion.

The *contralateral* cortical representations in the occipital cortex are described below.

- Central field (macular area): Posterior part of occipital lobe lateral to the tip of the calcarine cortex with dual blood supply from the MCA and PCA
- Peripheral field: Anterior part (i.e., tip) of occipital cortex. Supplied by a branch of the PCA
- Monocular temporal crescent

Ischemic lesions of the occipital cortex may produce a macular-sparing congruous homonymous hemianopia due to the representation of the macula in the occipital lobe and dual blood supply. Occlusion of the PCA is responsible for up to 90% of these isolated occipital lobe-related homonymous hemianopic visual field defects. Damage to the tip of the occipital cortex (trauma) can produce a congruous, homonymous hemianopsia, but involvement of the occipital tip produces the macular involvement rather than macular sparing.

Other associated symptoms of visual cortex disease (cortical visual impairment) include:

- Visual unformed or formed hallucinations (Charles Bonnet phenomenon)
- Anton syndrome: denial of cortical blindness
- Riddoch phenomenon: moving visual targets are perceived better than static targets (static-kinetic dissociation)

3.2.7 Summary of Localization of the Visual Pathway and Corresponding Visual Field Defects

1. Optic nerve lesions: Each optic nerve relays visual information from a single eye. Therefore, a lesion located in the anterior part of the optic nerve typically leads to visual field loss in the corresponding (ipsilateral) eye. However, the part of the optic nerve closer to the optic chiasm (distal optic nerve) receives some input from the other eye (contralateral), meaning that a lesion here could lead to visual field loss in both eyes (e.g., junctional scotoma). Optic nerve-related visual field defects can be central (e.g., central or cecocentral scotoma) or peripheral (nerve fiber layer defects). As the nasal and temporal fibers approach the optic chiasm at the junction, monocular hemianopic (nasal or temporal) visual field defects may occur (junctional scotoma of Traquair).
2. Optic chiasm lesions: At the optic chiasm, visual fibers from both eyes (nasal crossing and temporal uncrossed fibers) come together. If a lesion affects the body of the optic chiasm, the most common visual field defect is a bitemporal hemianopia. Typically, a pituitary gland tumor leads to this type of field defect, often being the first clinical sign. Rarely, a binasal hemianopia can occur at the optic chiasm from bilateral compression of the temporal uncrossed fibers (e.g., internal carotid artery dolichoectasia or aneurysms).
3. Post-chiasmal lesions: Lesions of the retrochiasmal pathway produce contralateral homonymous hemianopias, which become more congruent (symmetrical) as the lesion site moves posteriorly. An exception to this rule is an anterior calcarine sulcus lesion, which can result in a contralateral monocular temporal crescent as a visual field defect.
4. Lateral geniculate body (LGB) lesions: Damage to the lateral geniculate nucleus, supplied by the middle cerebral artery, may result in contralateral homonymous hemianopia

paired with significant contralateral sensory loss. Such lesions do not cause a relative afferent pupillary defect (RAPD). Ischemic lesions of the LGB because of the unique blood supply can produce wedge-sparing or wedge-involving homonymous visual field defects that represent the anterior and lateral choroidal artery supply to the LGB, respectively.

5. Visual radiations: Lesions of the inferior optic radiation loops in the temporal lobe (Meyer loop) produce superior homonymous hemianopias ("pie in the sky"), and lesions of the superior optic radiations produce inferior homonymous hemianopias in the parietal lobe ("pie on the floor").
6. Occipital cortex: Lesions of the calcarine cortex can result in congruous homonymous hemianopia with or without macular sparing.

3.2.8 Neurologic Terms and Syndromes for Patients with Cortical Visual Complaints

Agnosia is the inability to recognize objects.

Visual agnosia is being unable to recognize objects visually.

Apraxia is loss of an ability to perform a task despite adequate motor and sensory function.

Ocular motor apraxia is the loss of voluntary movement of the eyes while fixating on a target.

Optic ataxia is a disconnection between visual input and the motor system.

Alexia is the inability to read.

Agraphia is the inability to write.

Acalculia is the inability to calculate.

Prosopagnosia is the inability to recognize familiar faces.

Simultanagnosia is a failure to integrate multiple elements of a scene.

Achromatopsia is the absence of color vision.

Functional visual disorder occurs when visual field defect has no organic cause.

Cerebral achromatopsia is typically caused by lesions of the lingual and fusiform gyri.

Gerstmann syndrome includes homonymous hemianopic field defects with finger agnosia, right-left confusion, and acalculia.

Posterior cortical atrophy can produce an isolated homonymous hemianopsia without a structural lesion on neuroimaging (Alzheimer's disease).

Balint syndrome arises from bilateral lesions in the dorsal parieto-occipital region and is characterized by a triad of symptoms: simultanagnosia, which is the inability to perceive the visual field as a whole; oculomotor apraxia, or difficulty with eye fixation; and optic ataxia, which is the inability to reach for objects using vision. Patients with Balint syndrome may also experience significant neuropsychological impairments. This condition is typically associated with parieto-occipital pathology.

Prosopagnosia, a subtype of agnosia, results from bilateral damage to the inferior occipito-temporal lobes, although it can also occur with damage to the right inferior occipital lobe. This condition is marked by an inability to recognize familiar faces.

Posterior reversible encephalopathy syndrome (PRES), also known as reversible posterior leukoencephalopathy syndrome, is a condition associated with vascular endothelial dysfunction. It commonly arises in patients with malignant hypertension and eclampsia or those on medications such as tacrolimus or ciclosporin. It can also be linked to rare cases of autoimmune diseases. The syndrome may present with cortical visual deficits, but other symptoms such as headaches and seizures are also common.

Anton syndrome: Often due to bilateral occipital lobe infarcts, despite visual impairment, the patient denies visual loss and may confabulate intact vision.

Alexia without agraphia, characterized by an inability to read but an ability to write, is associated with damage to the splenium of the corpus callosum and the left occipital lobe. This condition arises due to a disconnection between the intact right occipital cortex and the angular gyrus in the left parietal lobe, which is crucial for reading. Damage to the left splenium of the corpus callosum impedes the transmission of visual information from the right occipital lobe to the left hemisphere. The primary centers for reading and writing are located in the dominant parietal lobe's angular gyrus. Alexia without agraphia results from the disconnection of the dominant angular gyrus from the bilateral occipital lobe input.

Riddoch phenomenon (aka statokinetic dissociation): can better see moving objects in the blind hemifield; however, static objects may not be detectable.

Palinopsia is seeing a repeat of the same image. The persistence or recurrence of the visual image in time can be hallucinatory (no stimulus present) or illusory (stimulus present). Palinopsia can be seen in occipital or parietal (not temporal) lobe disease.

Cerebral dyschromatopsia, or color agnosia, occurs due to bilateral temporal lobe lesions and is often accompanied by bilateral superior homonymous hemianopia.

A lesion in the right parietal lobe of a right-handed individual typically results in sensory inattention or neglect.

3.2.9 Brainstem Syndromes in Neuro-ophthalmology

Lateral medullary syndrome (Wallenberg syndrome): This syndrome is usually caused by damage to the lateral part of the medulla, most commonly due to a posterior inferior cerebellar artery (PICA) infarct. Symptoms and signs include unilateral Horner's syndrome, nystagmus (rotary) with associated oscillopsia, skew deviation, sensory loss in the ipsilateral face, and sensory loss in the contralateral body (crossed sign).

Benedikt syndrome (paramedian midbrain syndrome): This syndrome arises from damage to the midbrain. It is characterized by ipsilateral oculomotor nerve palsy, contralateral hemiparesis, and contralateral cerebellar ataxia.

Foville syndrome: This syndrome is caused by a lesion in the medial inferior part of the pons. Symptoms include ipsilateral weakness of abduction, facial weakness and analgesia, peripheral deafness, loss of taste in the anterior two-thirds of the tongue, and ipsilateral Horner's syndrome. Other syndromes related to pontine lesions are shown in Table 3.2.

Additional considerations:

- Fourth cranial nerve (CN) palsy with ipsilateral Horner's syndrome suggests cavernous sinus disease.
- Fourth CN palsy with contralateral Horner's syndrome points to a midbrain lesion.

In summary:

- Benedikt syndrome presents with third nerve palsy and contralateral hemiplegia.
- Wallenberg syndrome presents with third nerve palsy, Horner's syndrome, and contralateral hemisensory loss.

Table 3.2 Comparison between different syndromes related to pons lesion

Lesion site	Medial inferior pons	Ventral lower pons	Mid-lower pons	Dorsal lower pons
Syndrome	Foville syndrome	Millard-Gubler syndrome (MGS) (aka ventral pontine syndrome)	Raymond syndrome	–
Manifestation	Ipsilateral abduction weakness, ipsilateral facial weakness and analgesia, ipsilateral peripheral deafness, loss of taste from the anterior two-thirds of the tongue, and ipsilateral Horner's syndrome	Ipsilateral abducens and ipsilateral facial nerve palsy and contralateral hemiplegia	Ipsilateral abducens, contralateral central facial paresis, and contralateral hemiparesis	Isolated abducens nerve palsy

[a] Note that Raymond affects the contralateral face and sometimes spares the facial nerve, while Millard-Gubler affects the ipsilateral facial nerve

- Foville syndrome presents with sixth and seventh nerve palsies and ipsilateral Horner's syndrome.
- Millard-Gubler syndrome presents with sixth and seventh nerve palsies and contralateral hemiplegia.
- Raymond syndrome presents with sixth nerve palsy, seventh nerve palsy, and contralateral hemiplegia.
- Gradenigo syndrome presents with ipsilateral fifth and sixth nerve palsies and suppurative otitis media-related hearing loss.

3.3 Optic Nerve Diseases

3.3.1 Optic Neuritis

Optic neuritis (ON) is a broad term describing inflammation of the optic nerve (Abel et al. 2019). This can be assessed:

- Functionally by assessing optic nerve function, including visual acuity, color vision, visual field, and afferent pupillary function
- Structurally, where the inflammation can be in the intraocular segment, observing optic disc swelling (aka papillitis) on fundus exam, or the inflammation can be in retro-orbital optic nerve, which can be observed on imaging, mostly magnetic resonance imaging (MRI) of the orbit, observing the enhancement of optic nerve

ON can be generally classified into:

- Typical ON, which is multiple sclerosis (MS)-associated ON (50%)
- Atypical ON, which is not associated with multiple sclerosis ON (50%), which can be further classified into:
  - Clinically isolated syndrome (CIS)
  - Antibody mediated, including neuromyelitis optica spectrum disorders (NMOSDs) or myelin oligodendrocyte glycoprotein (MOG) (8%)
  - Other infectious or inflammatory (sarcoid, SLE, GPA, syphilis, TB, zoster)

3.3.2 Typical Optic Neuritis (MS-Associated Optic Neuritis)

A typical optic neuritis usually presents as unilateral, more commonly in females with an average onset around 32 years of age. It is often painful and associated with normal optic disc or mild disc edema. Typically, two-thirds of adult patients have a retro-orbital optic neuritis with normal fundus, while one-third have papillitis. Symptoms may include dyschromatopsia more prominently than acuity loss. Radiographically, there is usually anterior optic nerve enhancement. In contrast, atypical optic neuritis can manifest bilaterally, with a wider age range of onset, often without gender predilection, and may be painless. It can exhibit pronounced disc edema and vitritis, and the vision loss can be progressive over more than 2 weeks, with acuity dropping to 20/200 or worse. Radiographically, there may be extensive enhancement involving more than half of the posterior optic nerve, chiasmal, or optic nerve sheath (Abel et al. 2019). In both cases, a relative afferent pupillary defect (RAPD) is found in up to 90% of instances, either unilaterally or bilaterally but asymmetrically. Pain with eye movement is also frequently reported. Acquired acute color vision deficiency is present in up to 90% of cases. The most common visual field abnormality in optic neuritis is a diffuse reduction in sensitivity across the central 30°, though any nerve fiber layer defect, including altitudinal defects, may also be observed.

ON may be the presenting and only sign of multiple sclerosis (MS) in up to 20% of cases. Most patients with MS eventually suffer ON, but some cases are subclinical and only are demonstrated on imaging or autopsy, where nearly all patients with MS will exhibit evidence of ON demyelination. MRI of the brain and orbit in typical cases of MS-related optic neuritis shows enhancement of the optic nerve and demyelinating white matter lesions in the brain. However, the absence of MS lesions on brain MRI does not rule out MS.

In terms of management of typical optic neuritis, based on optic neuritis treatment trial (ONTT), which only included typical optic neuritis patients, the recommended treatment of idiopathic or MS-related optic neuritis is either no treatment in mild cases (e.g., if visual acuity at presentation is 20/40 or better and visual field loss is mild) or administration of high-dose intravenous methylprednisolone for 3 days to hasten visual recovery. Treatment with an intermediate dose of oral steroids (1 mg/kg/day) should be avoided due to an increased risk of optic neuritis recurrence. Optic neuritis treatment trial showed that all groups had same recovery at 6 weeks, but the IV steroid group had a significantly more rapid recovery. The oral steroid group had more risk of recurrent attack compared to placebo and IV steroids (Newman 2020).

Pediatric optic neuritis differs from the adult variant in several aspects. It occurs equally in males and females, with a higher likelihood of being bilateral, affecting around 70% of cases. Unlike adults, pediatric optic neuritis commonly presents as anterior optic neuritis (60%), with a lower frequency of pain. Approximately two-thirds of cases are attributed to postinfectious or postvaccination causes. Treatment protocols for pediatric optic neuritis largely mirror those for adults, as clinical trials specifically focusing on the pediatric population are lacking. However, despite a potentially worse acute presentation, children tend to have a better long-term visual acuity prognosis compared to adults. Nonetheless, there is still a considerable risk of developing multiple sclerosis (MS), estimated at around 30% overall, albeit lower than in adults. This risk increases if lesions are detected on MRI and with advancing age, highlighting the importance of vigilant monitoring and follow-up in pediatric cases of optic neuritis (Borchert et al. 2017).

3.3.3 Atypical Optic Neuritis

The discovery of antibodies related to MOG and NMOSD led to a new entity of atypical optic neuritis that needs to be considered when a patient presents with the atypical features previously mentioned. NMOSD is an autoimmune, antibody-mediated, inflammatory disease where antibodies form against aquaporin protein 4 (AQP4) in the cell membranes of astrocytes. NMOSD may occur at any age and is characterized by ON that can bilaterally and longitudinally be extensive on contrast-enhanced MRI. The transverse myelitis (demyelination of the spinal cord) is also often longitudinally extensive (three contiguous vertebral segments on spinal MRI) and may occur before, during, or after the ON event. Bilateral long optic nerve segment or optic chiasmal involvement favors NMOSD over MS in cases of ON. Other symptoms of NMOSD include intractable hiccups, nausea, and vomiting, along with insomnia, which can occur from area postrema or hypothalamic involvement of AQP4-rich areas in the brain. In contrast to MS-related ON, IV steroids are recommended for suspected NMOSD, and early and aggressive consideration for plasma exchange (PLEX) should be made in these cases. Immunosuppression rather than immunomodulatory therapy is recommended for NMOSD in consultation with a neurologist (Wingerchuk et al. 2015).

Myelin oligodendrocyte glycoprotein immunoglobulin G-associated disorder (MOGAD) can lead to optic neuritis (ON). MOGAD-related ON tends to be bilateral, recurrent, and often associated with disc edema on clinical examination. MRI findings in MOGAD frequently show perineural rather than parenchymal enhancement, with contrast extending to the optic nerve sheath and surrounding periorbital fat. Treatment typically involves steroids, which are usually effective and may be required for ongoing management, often necessitating a short taper following acute treatment with intravenous steroids (Banwell et al. 2023).

Table 3.3 provides a comparison between optic neuritis in clinically isolated syndrome, MS, NMO, and MOG.

Other etiologies of atypical optic neuritis include the following:

Parainfectious: Parainfectious ON occurs more commonly in children. The clinical presentation of childhood postinfectious ON typically occurs 1–3 weeks after the viral infection. There may be acute and severe visual loss that may be bilateral. Bilateral papillitis is common. Neuroimaging and lumbar puncture may be nec-

Table 3.3 A comparison between optic neuritis in clinically isolated syndrome, MS, NMO, and MOG

	Multiple sclerosis	Neuromyelitis optica	Myelin oligodendrocyte glycoprotein (MOG)
Presentation	Unilateral, mean age of 34 years, Caucasians	Unilateral, female, African American	Bilateral (50%). Up to 85% disc swelling with 50% recurrent. Equal sex
Imaging features	Short segment enhancement mostly in the intra-orbital part	Enhancing lesions over ≥50% of the optic nerve or optic chiasm (long segments). Posterior optic nerve involvement	Extensive perineural enhancement
Biomarkers	Oligoclonal bands in cerebrospinal fluid (CSF) (>80%)	Serum-positive aquaporin 4-IgG CSF pleocytosis	Serum-positive MOG-IgG
Course	90% will regain 90% of vision after attack in 1–3 months	50% will have 20/200 vision or worse. 55% will have a recurrence in 5 years without treatment	10% will have 20/200 vision or worse
Relapse rate	50% (can differ depending on brain MRI)	90%	50%
Spine involvement	Short, ≤1 vertebral segment)	Longitudinally extensive (≥3 vertebral segments)	Longitudinally extensive but short lesions may also be present

essary to exclude papilledema and fulminant intracranial hypertension. IV steroids may be considered, but treatment is often supportive. Exclusion of active infection or alternative etiologies (e.g., NMOSD, MOGAD) is recommended in consultation with a neurologist.

Infectious: Mostly results in optic nerve and retina involvement (aka neuroretinitis); however, isolated infectious optic neuritis has been described with syphilis (Roy et al. 2023) and tuberculosis (Keshavan et al. 2022), in addition to other causes. The optic nerve and retina and immunologically distinct structures are more likely to be involved together in infectious processes and rarely involved together with autoimmune process. Think of it when retina and optic disc are simultaneously involved in one eye (unilateral). While mostly idiopathic (50%), most common effects afterward include bacterial infection (Rickettsia, Lyme, TB, syphilis) and then other pathogen infections (Abdelhakim and Rasool 2018).

Noninfectious, inflammatory ON: Etiologies include sarcoidosis, rheumatologic conditions (e.g., SLE), and other autoimmune disorders that can produce ON.

3.3.4 Ischemic Optic Neuropathy (ION)

ION can be classified into two anatomical types: anterior ION (AION) and posterior ION (PION). AION results from ischemia of the short posterior ciliary arteries, which also supply the cilioretinal artery, leading to acute optic neuropathy with optic disc swelling. In contrast, PION affects the optic nerve behind the optic disc and does not cause disc edema, being referred to as retrobulbar optic neuropathy. The posterior optic nerve receives its blood supply from the surrounding pial capillary plexus, which is fed by pial branches of the ophthalmic artery.

ION can also be divided into arteritic (i.e., vasculitis of the artery) or non-arteritic (NA-AION), as detailed in Table 3.4. The arteritic (A-AION) is almost always associated with giant cell arteritis (GCA) in elderly. Arteritic ION is caused by inflammation and subsequent thrombosis of the short posterior ciliary arteries. GCA can also produce PION in the elderly (Hayreh 2009).

GCA and A-AION or A-PION if left untreated can be blinding, and up to 95% of untreated cases

Table 3.4 Comparison between arteritic and non-arteritic anterior ischemic optic neuropathy

	Arteritic (A-AION)	Non-arteritic (NA-AION)
Prevalence	Less common (5%)	More common (95%)
Most important association	Giant cell arteritis	Hypertension and other vasculopathic risk factors
Severity of vision loss	More likely to be severe (<6/60) but can be variable	Typically less severe (>6/60)
Headache	>70%	10%
Management	Steroids	Modify risk factors

may develop contralateral involvement. Up to 40% of cases suffer permanent vision loss, and earlier diagnosis and treatment make a difference in GCA. The vision loss in GCA is typically more severe (worse than 6/60) than in NA-ION but is variable. Other constitutional symptoms and signs may be present in GCA (e.g., jaw claudication, headache) as well as serum-elevated acute-phase reactants (e.g., erythrocyte sedimentation rate, C-reactive protein, thrombocytosis). Fundus fluorescein angiography (FFA) may show delayed choroidal filling in arteritic ION. NA-ION is mostly associated with HTN and other vasculopathic risk factors.

Patients with GCA may have concomitant polymyalgia rheumatica (PMR), and in the population over the age of 50, the prevalence may be as high as 1 in 200.

3.3.4.1 Anterior Non-arteritic Ischemic Optic Neuropathy

Despite being the most common cause of acute optic neuropathy in patients over the age of 50, it is diagnosed after excluding the arteritic.

The classic presentation of ION is acute, painless unilateral vision loss, which typically develops over a few hours to days, often beginning in the morning. Patients frequently describe the vision loss as blurring or cloudiness, particularly in the inferior field. While most patients experience no pain, headache or periocular discomfort is reported in 8–12% of cases, which can complicate the differentiation from optic neuritis. By definition, optic disc edema is present, usually characterized by segmental hyperemic edema rather than diffuse or pallid edema, which is more common in arteritis conditions.

Etiologies strongly associated with NA-ION include OSA, optic disc drusen, and use of sildenafil. Up to 97% of patients with NA-ION have small optic discs with small or absent optic cups. The exact cause of optic disc edema in AION is not fully understood, but it is generally accepted that the condition results from a compartment syndrome caused by axonal edema in an anatomically crowded optic disc. This typically presents as segmental hyperemic edema rather than diffuse or pallid edema.

Visual acuity is generally good, as detailed in the ischemic optic neuropathy decompression trial (IONDT):

- 30% have normal or only slightly reduced VA.
- 50% of patients had an initial visual acuity of 20/64 or better.
- 66% had 20/200 or better.

Vision can worsen over the 2-week period following initial presentation and typically stabilizes by 2 months.

Loss of color vision is a sensitive sign and correlates with the degree of VA loss. Although round and reactive pupils, RAPD is positive.

The MC field defect is an inferior altitudinal field loss. However, any visual field defect relating to optic nerve damage can occur. Nearly 25% of patients will have central scotoma.

Diagnosis: The diagnosis of NA-ION is primarily clinical. For patients presenting with acute, painless, unilateral vision loss and classic examination findings—such as a hyperemic, swollen optic nerve with peripapillary splinter hemorrhages, and a fellow eye exhibiting a small cup-to-disc ratio—no further testing is necessary.

Risk factors include a small optic disc with a small or absent physiological cup, hypertension (which is very common), diabetes mellitus, hyperlipidemia, collagen vascular diseases, antiphospholipid antibody syndrome, hyperhomocysteinemia, sudden hypotensive events, cataract surgery, and sleep apnea syndrome.

Among the risk factors for non-arteritic AION are migraine, DM, hypertension, but not carotid occlusive disease.

Embolism is not thought to be a common cause of non-arteritic ischemic optic neuropathy. Therefore, carotid artery imaging and echocardiogram are not recommended.

The following risk factors were proved to be significantly associated with NA-ION: male gender, hypertension, hyperlipidemia, diabetes mellitus (DM), coronary heart disease (CHD), sleep apnea, and factor V Leiden heterozygous.

Treatment: The only therapy that can be offered is steroid, despite the nonconclusive evidence, where a recent meta-analysis showed no significant impact of steroids. Decompression or antithrombotics are also ineffective. 40–80 mg of oral prednisone therapy for 2 weeks followed by a tapering regimen is the preferred course. Aspirin does not appear to reduce the risk of involvement of the fellow eye.

The fellow eye has 20–30% risk of being affected.

Main differential diagnoses include arteritic AION and optic neuritis.

Disease course (similar to optic neuritis): Disc swelling gradually resolves, and pallor ensues 3–6 weeks after onset.

Diabetic papillopathy: A unilateral optic neuropathy occurs in diabetic patients, however, not related to severity of DR or control of blood sugar. It is thought to be a form of non-A-AION and has characteristic good vision with absent RAPD, dyschromatopsia, and visual field defects. Dilated optic nerve head vasculature is seen in 50% of cases, and they typically remain on the disc surface and do not extend into the vitreous (unlike NVD). FFA shows leakage around the disc.

***Dyschromatopsia (color vision deficiency) typically correlates with the degree of visual impairment in non-arteritic anterior ischemic optic neuropathy (NA-ION). This differs from optic neuritis, where color vision can be significantly impaired even if visual acuity remains relatively good.

3.3.4.2 Anterior Arteritic Ischemic Optic Neuropathy

Mostly caused by giant cell arteritis (GCA), primarily affecting individuals over 70 years of age and more common in females (about four times more), it is a granulomatous necrotizing arteritis. It predominantly affects large and medium-sized arteries, particularly those branching from the aorta, including the superficial temporal artery (STA), ophthalmic artery, posterior ciliary arteries, and proximal vertebral arteries. The extent and severity of the disease correlate with the amount of elastic tissue in the media and adventitia of the arteries, which is why intracranial carotid arteries are typically spared, as they have minimal elastic tissue.

If GCA is untreated, 30–50% will develop A-AION within a few weeks. However, 20% of A-AIONs develop without preceding GCA.

About 50% of patients with GCA have polymyalgia rheumatica (PMR) at diagnosis, and approximately 20% of PMR patients will develop GCA.

Jaw claudication, characterized by cramp-like pain during chewing due to ischemia of the masseter muscles, is virtually pathognomonic for GCA.

Superficial temporal arteritis is marked by thickened, tender, inflamed, and nodular arteries, though these signs can be subtle.

In arteritic AION, the optic disc typically appears chalky white, pale, and swollen.

Risk factors: smoking, a low body mass index, and early menopause, which may act as independent risk factors. The condition usually affects elderly individuals, with an average age of 70 years, and it is extremely rare in people under the age of 50. Women are affected four times more often than men. The diagnosis of both GCA and polymyalgia rheumatica (PMR) is primarily based on clinical findings.

Diagnosis of GCA: American College of Rheumatology 1990 Classification Criteria for Giant Cell Arteritis:

- Age at disease onset 50 years or older.
- New headache.
- Temporal artery tenderness to palpation or decreased pulsation.
- Erythrocyte sedimentation rate of 50 mm/h or greater (high in 80% of patients).
- Abnormal artery biopsy: biopsy specimen showing vasculitis, with a predominance of mononuclear cell infiltration or granulomatous inflammation, often with multinucleated giant cells (should ideally be performed within 3 days of commencing steroids; if >7 days, histological features may not be present). At least 2.5 cm of artery should be collected. Positive in 85% of patients. Contralateral biopsy might be positive in 5% of patients with negative biopsy on the ipsilateral side.

High ESR does not occur in about 15% of biopsy-proven cases of arteritic AION. It usually remains high even after steroids.

Color Doppler and duplex ultrasonography can reveal a hypoechoic halo around the superficial temporal artery lumen in about 75% of cases. This finding, which results from edema in the artery wall, is often considered pathognomonic for GCA.

Diagnosis of A-AION: Severe visual loss is the rule. However, the upper or lower circulation can be affected leading to an altitudinal visual.

Field defect A-AION affects 30–50% of untreated patients with GCA, of whom one-third develop involvement of the fellow eye (rare to be simultaneous), usually within a week of the first. Posterior ischemic optic neuropathy is much less common. Most cases of A-AION occur within a few weeks of the onset of GCA

Treatment: focuses on preventing blindness in the unaffected eye, as visual loss in the affected eye is unlikely to improve even with prompt treatment. Immediate corticosteroid therapy is crucial because there is a 25% chance that the second eye may also become involved despite early intervention. The risk of contralateral visual loss is high and can occur within days, so corticosteroids should be started immediately. Temporal artery biopsy should follow to confirm the diagnosis and support the need for prolonged corticosteroid treatment in older patients.

GCA is treated with 1 mg/kg oral prednisolone with slow tapering according to ESR/CRP afterward. If A-AION occurs, IV methylprednisolone 500 mg to 1 g/day for 3 days followed by oral prednisolone 1–2 mg/kg/day is usually indicated. Aspirin might also improve the outcome. While treatment will not restore vision in the affected eye, it will reduce the risk of other eye affection. Most patients need treatment for 1–2 years, although some may require indefinite maintenance therapy if they have frequent relapses. Tocilizumab (interleukin-6 inhibitor) can be used to reduce the dependency on steroid and increase the tapering speed (Stone et al. 2017).

High yield note: Amaurosis fugax is a transient monocular vision loss. In ischemic optic neuropathy, the occurrence of amaurosis fugax is a feature or arteritic, rather than non-arteritic.

3.3.4.3 Posterior Ischemic Optic Neuropathy

Very rare, the posterior portion is supplied by the surrounding pial capillary plexus, which in turn is supplied by pial branches of the ophthalmic artery. Initially, the optic disc appears normal, and only optic nerve functions are affected (i.e., impaired function with normal structural appearance) with pallor developing over weeks. It can be classified according to etiology into the following (Hayreh 2004):

- **Non-arteritic** PION shares the same systemic risk factors as non-arteritic NA-ION, but it is not linked to a crowded optic disc. The visual prognosis for non-arteritic PION is similar to that of NA-ION. In some cases, practitioners may prescribe a short course of high-dose systemic steroids if the condition is identified early.
- Postoperative (or perioperative) PION can occur after various surgical procedures, par-

ticularly those involving the heart or spine, with an incidence of about 0.02%. Major risk factors include anemia and intraoperative hypovolemic hypotension. Bilateral involvement is common, and the visual prognosis is generally poor. Early blood transfusion and management of facial or orbital swelling may offer some benefit.

- **Arteritic** PION is associated with GCA and carries a poor visual prognosis.

High yield note: The most common causes of visual loss following bypass surgery are occipital infarction, ischemic optic neuropathy, and pituitary apoplexy, with the former being much more common. It can be differentiated by the presence of pain in apoplexy and pupillary sluggish reaction in ION with disc swelling in AION. Absence of these suggests occipital infarct.

3.3.4.4 Miscellaneous Notes

Non-arteritic ischemic optic neuropathy (NA-ION): Optic nerve decompression surgery (ONDS) demonstrated ineffectiveness in patients suffering from NA-ION when compared to regular monitoring. The observation group noted an improvement of three or more lines of vision in 42.7% of cases, signifying a high potential for spontaneous recovery. The incidence of NA-ION occurrence in the contralateral eye was about 14.7% over a median period of 5.1 years, uninfluenced by factors like age, sex, aspirin usage, or smoking habits.

Central retinal artery occlusion (CRAO): Local intra-arterial fibrinolysis (LIF), compared to conservative standard treatment (CST), did not enhance visual outcomes 1 month posttreatment in patients diagnosed with acute CRAO (≤20 h). LIF had a higher complication rate, however.

Idiopathic intracranial hypertension (IIH): Acetazolamide in combination with weight loss has shown greater improvement in pulsatile midline displacement (PMD) among patients experiencing mild vision loss compared to placebo. Acetazolamide leads to enhancements in visual fields, CSF opening pressure, papilledema, and quality of life, though it does not outperform placebo in managing headaches. The drug is considered safe and well tolerated for IIH patients, even at doses up to 4 g/day.

For giant cell arteritis patients, tocilizumab, an anti-interleukin-6 receptor monoclonal antibody, has proven effective as an additional treatment with prednisolone to decrease the cumulative steroid dosage required.

Central retinal artery occlusion leads to the complete deprivation of blood supply to the entire inner retina unless a cilioretinal artery is present, which occurs in about 15–30% of eyes. Acute branch retinal artery occlusion (BRAO) typically affects the temporal vessels, with visual acuity at presentation varying widely. The combined application of ocular massage and intravenous acetazolamide (500 mg) can significantly lower intraocular pressure (IOP) in a brief period and is a widely employed treatment for acute CRAO and BRAO cases.

A successful paracentesis can also be performed in RAO cases following intravitreal injections. It has been observed that visual recovery from a retinal artery occlusion (RAO) can occur even 3 days post-onset; hence, massage is recommended within this time frame. More than 75% of CRAO patients suffer from generalized atheromatous disease, often linked to hypertension, diabetes mellitus, or both.

The NASCET trial evaluated the efficacy of carotid endarterectomy compared to medical management in patients with symptomatic carotid artery stenosis. Individuals experiencing amaurosis fugax, carotid transient ischemic attacks (TIAs), or mild strokes were randomly assigned to receive either medical management (including daily aspirin) or carotid endarterectomy followed by medical management. Surgery significantly reduced the risk of subsequent stroke in patients with 70–99% carotid stenosis, given that the associated morbidity and mortality rates for angiography and surgery were acceptable (<4%).

Periventricular leukomalacia (PVL) is a condition frequently seen in individuals with a history of prematurity, impacting neuro-ophthalmology. It results in the loss of white matter pathways that transmit visual information from the lateral geniculate bodies to the visual cortex. Radiologically, PVL typically presents with visual field defects and optic disc cupping. Importantly, these defects do not progress over time. Additionally, PVL can lead to horizontal cupping of the optic disc with minimal or absent nasal displacement of vessels. It may also cause thinning of the superior optic nerve associated with inferior visual field defects.

Nonorganic visual loss, or factitious vision loss, can be diagnosed using a variety of tests. These include optokinetic nystagmus, rocking mirror test, and base-up prism test for poor visual acuity (<6/60), and fogging refraction, stereo acuity, and red-green glasses for good visual acuity (>6/60). Stereoacuity testing, in particular, can identify potential malingering as it requires two well-functioning eyes. In cases of suspected nonorganic visual field loss, Goldmann perimetry and confrontation visual field testing can be employed, although modern automated perimetry can often be simulated by patients.

3.3.5 Hereditary Optic Atrophy

It is characterized by bilateral optic atrophy at a young age.

3.3.5.1 Leber Hereditary Optic Neuropathy

Bilateral sequential optic neuropathy presents with unilateral central scotoma with disc swelling or hyperemia in 10–30 years of age. Color vision deficiency with RAPD may be observed. Most common mutations are mitochondrial DNA mutations, including G11778A (up to 90% of patients), with T14484C being less common with better prognosis (good spontaneous visual recovery after attack), and G3460A mutation having worst prognosis. All maternally inherited mitochondrial diseases are with variable expressivity. In LHON, younger age and specific mutations such as 14484/ND6 are associated with better prognostic outcomes. During a dilated fundus examination, optic nerves may appear normal or exhibit hyperemic, "pseudo-edematous" characteristics with peripapillary telangiectasias (Fig. 3.1).

Most patients suffer from permanent bilateral visual loss with a final VA of 6/60 or less. An important finding in LHON is the preservation of pupillary light reflex, despite the severity of disc swelling or the severely depressed visual acuity acutely, which might be due to selective preservation of the pupillary light reflex pathway. Typical visual field loss including central or cecocentral visual field defects is typical. It is associated with loss of hearing and peripheral neuropathy. LHON plus refers to rare variants with additional manifestations such as neuromuscular dysfunction.

Classically, MRI findings in Leber hereditary optic neuropathy have been described as resembling multiple sclerosis, which could present with enhancement of nerves (could be extensive up to chiasm) (Dotti et al. 2008). Neurological manifestations which could include weaknesses is termed "Leber plus" (Kassa et al. 2018).

Treatment for LHON with idebenone, a potent antioxidant approved in the EU, typically begins

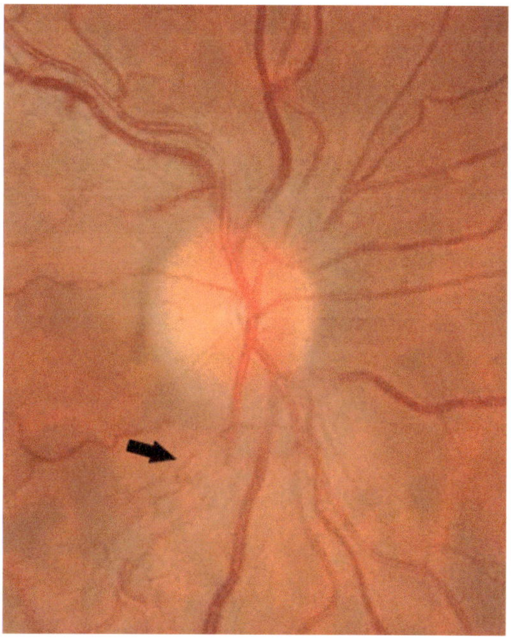

Fig. 3.1 Colored fundus photograph of the right optic disc showing hyperemia with peripapillary telangiectasia (arrow)

promptly at 900 mg/day, divided into three doses, for patients with disease onset within 1 year. Evidence is insufficient to recommend idebenone for chronic patients between 1 and 5 years post-onset of the second eye, and no evidence supports its use beyond 5 years post-onset. In subacute or dynamic cases, treatment at 900 mg/day should continue for at least a year to assess therapeutic response or until improvement plateaus (Zhao et al. 2020). Interestingly, cyanocobalamin (not hydroxocobalamin) forms of vitamin B12 have been reported to worsen outcomes, which contrasts with its potential benefits in other conditions.

3.3.5.2 Dominant Optic Atrophy (Kjer-Type Optic Atrophy, Optic Atrophy Type 1)

It is a common inherited optic neuropathy primarily caused by mutations in the OPA1 gene. It typically manifests as bilateral and insidious visual loss, accompanied by generalized dyschromatopsia, predominantly affecting blue-yellow color perception (tritanopia). Unlike maternally inherited Leber hereditary optic neuropathy (LHON), which primarily affects young males, DOA affects both sexes equally and presents in older individuals. The pathophysiology of DOA involves progressive degeneration of retinal ganglion cells (RGCs) and retinal nerve fiber layer (RNFL), particularly affecting the papillomacular bundle. Mutations in the OPA1 gene lead to mitochondrial dysfunction, which selectively damages RGCs. This mitochondrial impairment is also associated with multisystemic features in about 20% of cases, termed "DOA plus." These may include sensorineural hearing loss, peripheral neuropathy, myopathy, and other neurological manifestations. Diagnosis of DOA is supported by clinical findings such as temporal pallor of the optic discs and reduced RNFL thickness observed on optical coherence tomography (OCT). Genetic testing plays a crucial role, identifying OPA1 mutations in a significant majority (70–90%) of affected individuals (Wong et al. 2023).

Treatment approaches for dominant optic atrophy (DOA) focus on three main areas: pharmacological neuroprotection, gene therapy, and cell-based regenerative therapies involving stem cells. Compared to Leber hereditary optic neuropathy (LHON), treatments for DOA are generally less advanced. Idebenone, originally approved by the European Medicines Agency for treating LHON after acute visual loss, is sometimes used off-label for DOA and is available over the counter (Klopstock et al. 2011). DOA plus refers to cases where optic neuropathy is accompanied by sensorineural hearing loss. Comparative details between **autosomal dominant optic atrophy and LHON** can be found in Table 3.5, outlining their distinctions and similarities.

Behr syndrome AR is diffuse optic atrophy. It is associated with spastic gait, ataxia, and mental handicap. Best visual prognosis is observed among these syndromes.

Wolfram syndrome is also referred to as DIDMOAD (diabetes insipidus, diabetes mellitus, optic atrophy, and deafness). Diabetes mellitus is typically the first manifestation, followed by visual problems and severe visual impairment. Cupping might also be a feature.

3.3.6 Toxic Optic Neuropathy: Nutritional Deficiency

It appears as maculopapular bundle drop, where temporal part of the optic nerve and RNFL are

Table 3.5 Comparison between autosomal dominant optic atrophy and Leber hereditary optic neuropathy

	Autosomal dominant optic atrophy	Leber hereditary optic neuropathy
Inheritance	AD	Mitochondrial (mostly men)
Onset	Insidious bilateral	Acute unilateral sequential
Visual acuity at presentation	20/50 to 20/70	<20/200
Plus syndrome	Hearing loss	MS-like neurological features

affected. Usually, deficiency for months to years leads to the optic neuropathy.

The most common cause is B12 and folate deficiency, where we can check how long they are affected by:

- B12 deficiency, which will have high methylmalonic acid and homocysteine levels as markers of functional deficits of the B12 deficiency
- Folate deficiency, which will have normal methylmalonic acid with high homocysteine as markers of functional deficits of the folate deficiency

Malnutrition resulting from poor dietary habits, improperly managed vegetarian diets, and chronic alcohol abuse are risk factors for optic neuropathies. Another at-risk group includes obese individuals after bariatric surgery. Nutritional optic neuropathy typically presents with painless, gradual bilateral and symmetrical loss of visual acuity, often accompanied by impaired color vision.

Toxic optic neuropathy caused by nutritional deficiency is a progressive condition that typically affects both eyes symmetrically. Patients often experience central blurring and color vision abnormalities (dyschromatopsia) as early signs, while peripheral vision is generally preserved.

Despite these symptoms, the optic disc often appears normal, albeit with mild focal pallor and occasional splinter hemorrhages. While visual acuity may be moderately affected (with a visual acuity greater than 6/60), the loss in color perception is usually disproportionately severe.

This condition can be largely attributed to malnutrition, an overly strict vegan diet, or excessive tobacco and alcohol consumption. In particular, deficiencies in B-complex vitamins—specifically cyanocobalamin (B12), thiamine (B1), and folate—are the main culprits. It is believed that these deficiencies cause mitochondrial damage, leading to the observed symptoms.

Optical coherence tomography (OCT) typically reveals peripapillary thickening and loss of the nerve fiber layer (NFL), despite the macula appearing normal. Although vision recovery can be slow and typically requires dietary improvements and vitamin supplementation, color vision restoration usually takes longer. Because nutritional optic neuropathy typically affects both eyes symmetrically, an RAPD is not typically observed.

Toxic optic neuropathy can also be induced by certain drugs such as antituberculosis medications (isoniazid, ethambutol, and rifampin), methanol, amiodarone, and chloramphenicol. Note, however, that chloroquine drugs primarily affect the macula, unlike the previously mentioned drugs, which affect the disc.

Given its low cost, it is reasonable to conduct vitamin lab testing for patients experiencing bilateral vision problems linked to the optic nerve, even in cases where a hereditary origin is suspected.

A bilateral centrocecal scotoma, a specific type of visual field loss, is commonly seen in nutritional optic neuropathy, particularly in patients with vitamin B12 deficiency or those who abuse alcohol. Blood tests may reveal megaloblastic anemia, indicative of vitamin B12 deficiency, while abnormal liver function tests may be evident in individuals with excessive alcohol consumption.

Ethambutol-induced optic neuropathy, associated with antituberculosis treatment, can develop unusually quickly—even within 1 month of initiating therapy. Central vision loss is the most common visual field defect. Unfortunately, these changes are typically irreversible.

3.3.7 Radiation Optic Neuropathy

It is mostly with dose to optic nerve pathway above 50 Grays, but should also be suspected in lower doses and in cases of total radiation dose of 50 grays (Archer et al. 2019). It has a characteristic enhancement on MRI (Ref). It can also present with papillitis mostly 6–18 months after radiation. Higher risk in chemoradiation, thus, should be suspected with lower doses when concomitant chemotherapy is given. Reports indicated that in some cases, normal imaging may precede RON. It is managed by the following:

- IVMP 1gm for 3–5 days followed by slow tapering of steroid (60–80 mg with 10 mg taper Q2 weeks).
- If optic disc swelling, consider intravitreal injection of anti-VEGF Q6 weeks till improvement.

Fractionated therapy: Over a 10-year period, rates of freedom from optic neuropathy are approximately 96% and 78% when the total optic nerve dose is ≤63 Gy and the fraction dose is ≤1.8 Gy (Bhandare et al. 2005).

Inflammatory optic neuropathy may present with similar imaging abnormalities, but the clinical context, absence of visual recovery, and progressive worsening of vision would suggest radiation-induced optic neuropathy (RON).

Acknowledgements We would like to thank Retina Rocks® for providing the images in this chapter.

Conflict of Interest None.

References

Abdelhakim A, Rasool N (2018) Neuroretinitis: a review. Curr Opin Ophthalmol 29(6):514–519. https://doi.org/10.1097/ICU.0000000000000527

Abel A, McClelland C, Lee MS (2019) Critical review: typical and atypical optic neuritis. Surv Ophthalmol 64(6):770–779. https://doi.org/10.1016/j.survophthal.2019.06.001

Archer EL, Liao EA, Trobe JD (2019) Radiation-induced optic neuropathy: clinical and imaging profile of twelve patients. J Neuroophthalmol 39(2):170. https://doi.org/10.1097/WNO.0000000000000670

Banwell B et al (2023) Diagnosis of myelin oligodendrocyte glycoprotein antibody-associated disease: international MOGAD panel proposed criteria. Lancet Neurol 22(3):268–282. https://doi.org/10.1016/S1474-4422(22)00431-8

Bhandare N et al (2005) Does altered fractionation influence the risk of radiation-induced optic neuropathy? Int J Radiat Oncol Biol Phys 62(4):1070–1077. https://doi.org/10.1016/j.ijrobp.2004.12.009

Borchert M et al (2017) Pediatric optic neuritis: what is new. J Neuroophthalmol 37(Suppl 1):S14–S22. https://doi.org/10.1097/WNO.0000000000000551

Chiu EK, Nichols JW (2006) Sellar lesions and visual loss: key concepts in neuro-ophthalmology. Expert Rev Anticancer Ther [Preprint]. https://www.tandfonline.com/doi/full/10.1586/14737140.6.9s.S23. Accessed 16 Mar 2024

Dotti MT et al (2008) Magnetic resonance imaging findings in Leber's hereditary optic neuropathy. Eur Neurol 32(1):17–19. https://doi.org/10.1159/000116781

Hayreh SS (2004) Posterior ischaemic optic neuropathy: clinical features, pathogenesis, and management. Eye (Lond) 18(11):1188–1206. https://doi.org/10.1038/sj.eye.6701562

Hayreh SS (2009) Ischemic optic neuropathy. Prog Retin Eye Res 28(1):34–62. https://doi.org/10.1016/j.preteyeres.2008.11.002

Kassa R et al (2018) Teaching NeuroImages: Leber hereditary optic neuropathy masquerading as neuromyelitis optica. Neurology 90(1):e94–e95. https://doi.org/10.1212/WNL.0000000000004760

Keshavan A et al (2022) Bilateral optic neuritis as a first presentation of lymph node tuberculosis. Pract Neurol 22(1):51–54. https://doi.org/10.1136/practneurol-2021-003086

Klopstock T et al (2011) A randomized placebo-controlled trial of idebenone in Leber's hereditary optic neuropathy. Brain 134(Pt 9):2677–2686. https://doi.org/10.1093/brain/awr170

Lee IH et al (2015) Visual defects in patients with pituitary adenomas: the myth of bitemporal hemianopsia. Am J Roentgenol 205(5):W512–W518. https://doi.org/10.2214/AJR.15.14527

Newman NJ (2020) The optic neuritis treatment trial. Ophthalmology 127(4):S172–S173. https://doi.org/10.1016/j.ophtha.2019.09.046

Ntali G, Wass JA (2018) Epidemiology, clinical presentation and diagnosis of non-functioning pituitary adenomas. Pituitary 21(2):111–118. https://doi.org/10.1007/s11102-018-0869-3

Roy T, Gupta AD, Islam AR (2023) Optic neuritis presented as the only manifestation of neurosyphilis. Oman J Ophthalmol 16(1):161–164. https://doi.org/10.4103/ojo.ojo_66_22

Stone JH et al (2017) Trial of tocilizumab in Giant-cell arteritis. N Engl J Med 377(4):317–328. https://doi.org/10.1056/NEJMoa1613849

Takizawa G et al (2017) Relative afferent pupillary defects in homonymous visual field defects caused by stroke of the occipital lobe using pupillometer. Neuroophthalmology 42(3):139–145. https://doi.org/10.1080/01658107.2017.1367012

Wingerchuk DM et al (2015) International consensus diagnostic criteria for neuromyelitis optica spectrum disorders. Neurology 85(2):177–189. https://doi.org/10.1212/WNL.0000000000001729

Wong DCS et al (2023) OPA1 dominant optic atrophy: pathogenesis and therapeutic targets. J Neuroophthalmol 43(4):464. https://doi.org/10.1097/WNO.0000000000001830

Zhao X et al (2020) Therapeutic effects of Idebenone on Leber hereditary optic neuropathy. Curr Eye Res 45(10):1315–1323. https://doi.org/10.1080/02713683.2020.1736307

Clinical Review of Neuro-ophthalmology: Part II

4

Saif Aldeen Alryalat, Abdee Ryalat,
Noor Laylani, and Andrew G. Lee

Abstract

This chapter continues the clinical review of neuro-ophthalmology, focusing on critical conditions related to the optic disc, papilledema, pupil disorders, and cranial nerve dysfunction. It begins with a discussion on optic disc anomalies, such as optic disc drusen, morning glory anomaly, and coloboma, detailing their clinical features, implications, and management. The section on papilledema emphasizes its pathophysiology and diagnostic importance in identifying raised intracranial pressure. Pupil-related disorders are explored, including those affecting afferent and efferent pathways, and their role in visual function. The final section covers cranial nerves and eye movements, examining conditions like strabismus and ocular motor dysfunction caused by cranial nerve palsies.

Keywords

Optic disc anomalies · Papilledema · Pupil disorders · Cranial nerves · Eye movement disorders

4.1 Optic Disc Anomalies

This can be broadly classified into congenital and acquired. A group of congenital optic disc anomalies are frequently grouped together, called "cavitary optic disc anomalies." These excavated

S. A. Alryalat (✉)
Department of Ophthalmology, The University of Jordan, Amman, Jordan

The University of Colorado Anschutz Medical Campus, CO, USA

A. Ryalat
Private Practice, Amman, Jordan

N. Laylani
Department of Ophthalmology, University of Colorado Anschutz Medical Campus, Aurora, CO, USA
e-mail: nalaylani@houstonmethodist.org

A. G. Lee
Department of Ophthalmology, University of Colorado Anschutz Medical Campus, Aurora, CO, USA

Department of Ophthalmology, Neurology, and Neurosurgery, Weill Cornell Medical College, New York, NY, USA

Department of Ophthalmology, Baylor College of Medicine, Houston, TX, USA

Department of Ophthalmology, The University of Iowa Hospitals and Clinics, Iowa City, IA, USA

Department of Ophthalmology, The University of Texas Medical Branch, Galveston, TX, USA

The UT MD Anderson Cancer Center, Houston, TX, USA
e-mail: aglee@houstonmethodist.org

S. A. Alryalat (ed.), *Ophthalmology Board and FRCS Part 2 Exams*,
https://doi.org/10.1007/978-981-96-1517-9_4

(bowl-shaped) optic disc anomalies include megalopapilla, peripapillary staphyloma, optic disc coloboma, optic pit, and morning glory disc anomaly (Dutton 2004).

4.1.1 Optic Disc Coloboma

It appears as white excavations, located mostly along the inferior or infero-nasal aspect of the nerve and involving the adjacent retina/choroid (Fig. 4.1). The embryonic fissure of the developing eye is located infero-nasally and extends from the optic nerve to the margin of the pupil. A coloboma is a defect due to the fissure's incomplete closure. It is mostly sporadic but can be autosomal dominant with PAX6 gene mutation. It can be associated with serous retinal detachment affecting visual acuity, but can also be associated with visual field defect. Systemic associations include linear sebaceous nevus syndrome, Goldenhar's syndrome, CHARGE syndrome, and Walker-Warburg syndrome (Lingam et al. 2021). Compared to morning glory syndrome, optic disc coloboma lacks the central fibrous tuft on the optic disc.

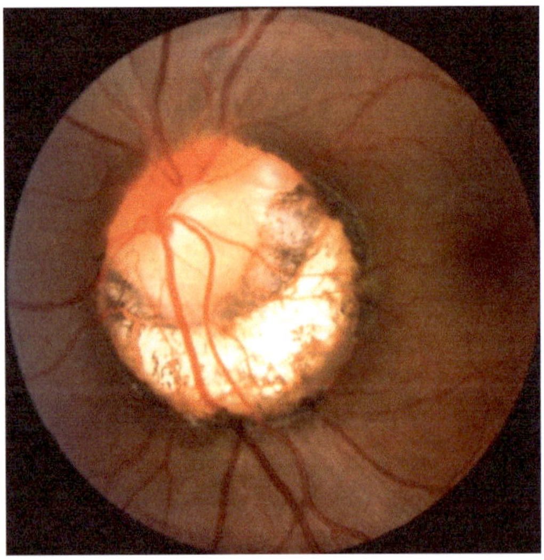

Fig. 4.1 Fundus image showing papillary and peripapillary coloboma. (Courtesy Retina Rocks®)

4.1.2 Optic Disc Pits

These are congenital defects within the optic disc, most commonly temporal (i.e., macular side), but their location poorly correlates with visual field defect. Optic disc appears large and bilateral in 10–15%. It may manifest as a visual field defect with normal central vision. However, almost half eyes may develop serous macular detachment (around the age of 30 years), which spontaneously resolves in 25% (Jain and Johnson 2014). It is characterized by subretinal fluid that extends from the disc elsewhere, unlike other causes that affect posterior or peripheral retina away from the disc. For persistent cases, laser temporal to disc may treat 25%. Definitive management includes vitrectomy with amniotic membrane to close the pit. Histologically, optic pits are composed of herniations of dysplastic retina into a collagen-lined pocket that extends posteriorly, often reaching the subarachnoid space, through a defect in the lamina cribrosa. A comparison between optic disc pits and colobomas is provided in Table 4.1.

4.1.3 Morning Glory Anomaly

It is characterized by a large disc with a central white tuft of glial tissue, a funnel-shaped appearance of the optic nerve and surrounding posterior pole with peripapillary pigmentary changes, and

Table 4.1 Comparison between optic disc pit coloboma

	Optic disc pits	Optic disc coloboma
Pathophysiology	Herniations of dysplastic retina through a defect in lamina cribrosa	Incomplete closure of embryonic fissure
Site	Temporal	Infero-nasal
Serous macular detachment incidence	Higher (50–70%)	Lower

an increased number of straight blood vessels emerging from the periphery of the disc (Fig. 4.2). It is typically unilateral and more common in females. Visual acuity in the affected eye is variable. Serous retinal detachments can occur in 30% of cases. Most cases are isolated; however, it is important to exclude associated structural or vascular anomalies such as encephalocele and moyamoya (a progressive condition characterized by narrowing of the carotid arteries, which may lead to stroke). Such patients should be counseled to have MRI and MRA of the brain. Other systemic associations include PHACE syndrome (posterior fossa malformation, large facial hemangioma, arterial anomalies, cardiac anomalies, and eye anomalies) and neurofibromatosis type 2. *PAX6* gene mutation (AD inheritance) can be responsible.

4.1.4 Peripapillary Staphyloma

Fundus excavation surrounds a relatively normal-appearing optic disc. It is generally unilateral and is accompanied by poor vision, although a bilateral case with normal visual acuity has been reported. Unlike other excavated optic disc anomalies, peripapillary staphyloma is rarely associated with other congenital defects or systemic diseases (Kim et al. 2005; Sanjari et al. 2006). In optic disc coloboma, the optic disc contains the excavation, often accompanied by iris or retina coloboma and frequently associated with systemic disease. In morning glory disc anomaly, the excavation is usually shallower than in peripapillary staphyloma, and there is a centrally located peripapillary glial tuft.

4.1.5 Optic Nerve Hypoplasia

A small optic disc that has a double-ring sign consists of a white ring of visible sclera surrounding a pigmented band thought to consist of migrated pigment epithelium (Fig. 4.3). This condition can vary from mild to severe and is mostly unilateral, although bilateral cases are usually syndromic. A foveola-disc center distance of three or more times the disc diameter strongly suggests hypoplasia. It is mostly associated with maternal age and maternal toxic exposures.

Optic nerve hypoplasia is associated with pituitary abnormalities and septo-optic dysplasia, necessitating urgent endocrine consultation and brain imaging. Risk factors include maternal diabetes, or maternal alcoholism or maternal phenytoin use. The first step upon diagnosing optic disc hypoplasia is endocrine evaluation, along with brain imaging looking for absence of the septum pellucidum with agenesis of the corpus callosum and with pituitary gland abnormalities.

One of the clinical signs occasionally found in this condition is a paradoxical pupil (first constrict to darkness before dilating).

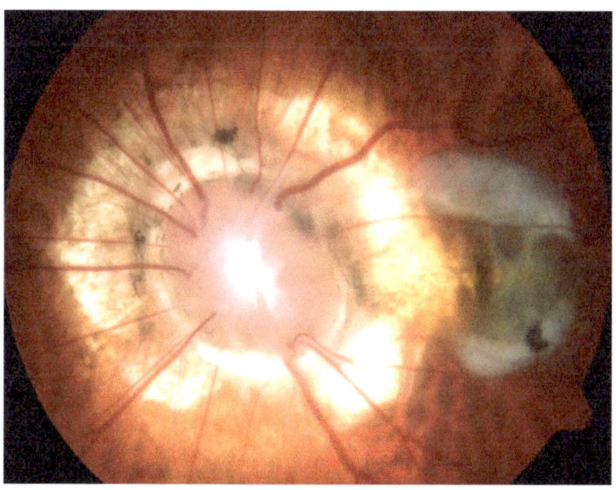

Fig. 4.2 Fundus image showing morning glory disc anomaly. (Courtesy Retina Rocks®)

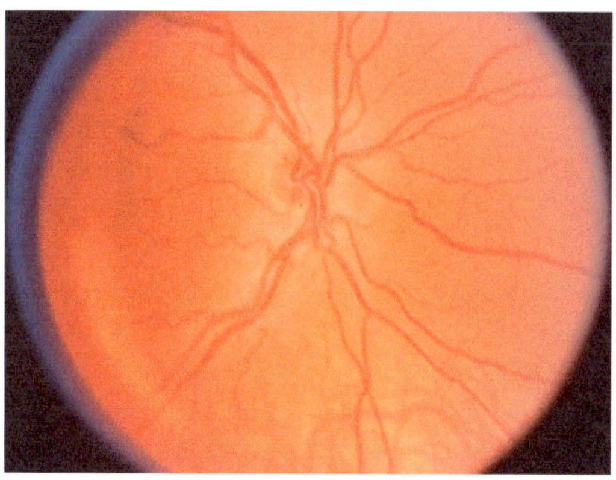

Fig. 4.3 Fundus image showing optic disc hypoplasia. (Courtesy Retina Rocks®)

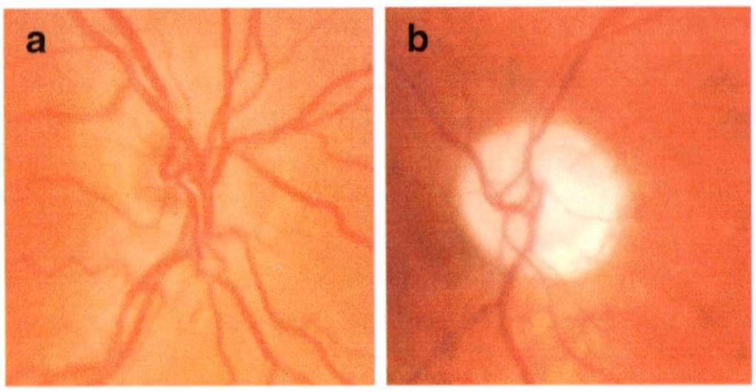

Fig. 4.4 Congenial optic disc hypoplasia (**a**) and acquired optic disc atrophy (**b**). (Courtesy Retina Rocks®)

De Morsier syndrome is a condition characterized by bilateral optic disc hypoplasia, absent septum pellucidum, corpus callosum dysgenesis, and hypopituitarism.

One potential clinical dilemma is differentiating between optic atrophy and congenital optic nerve hypoplasia. Although optic atrophy can be congenital or hereditary, optic nerve hypoplasia is a congenital condition resulting from abnormal development of axons and optic nerve during gestation. The optic disc is smaller in optic nerve hypoplasia (Fig. 4.4). A smaller sized optic nerve however cannot occur on an acquired basis.

4.1.6 Titled Disc

Tilted discs can be classified into two categories based on their etiology: congenital tilted disc syndrome, an anomaly of the eye characterized by inferior or infero-nasal tilting of the optic disc, and myopic tilted disc, an acquired change linked to the progression of myopia (You et al. 2008). Tilted discs are typically assessed subjectively, but can be defined objectively when the ratio of the longest to the shortest diameter of the disc (ovality index) exceeds 1.3. This condition may complicate glaucoma assessment, making measurements of the ganglion cell complex more useful than retinal nerve fiber layer thickness on optical coherence tomography (OCT).

A congenital form called congenital tilted disk syndrome (aka Fuchs coloboma) affects 2% of populations. A bilateral congenital anomaly is associated with a thinning of the retinal pigment epithelium, posterior staphyloma, bitemporal superior visual field defects (20% of cases), and situs inversus of the retinal vessels. Although this may be confused with chiasmal lesions, the visual field defects in TDS can cross the vertical meridian and situs inversus of the retinal vessels:

4.1.7 Disc Drusen

It is an acquired anomaly present in up to 2% of the population, mostly bilateral (75%), asymmetric, and mostly sporadic. It has equal prevalence between male and female and occurs almost exclusively in white ethnicities/Caucasians (>90%). It commonly occurs in the nasal disc and might lead to optic disc elevation, giving the impression of disc swelling, hence called pseudopapilledema. It is associated with visual field loss in 75% of patients, often progressive, where infero-nasal defects are the most common type of visual field loss, though a substantial impact on sight is rare. It is also associated with CNV, vitreous hemorrhage, and anterior ischemic optic neuropathy (AION). No treatment can improve VF defects. They can be found incidentally, but might also be associated with retinitis pigmentosa, angioid streaks, Usher syndrome, Noonan syndrome, or Alagille syndrome (present in 90% of patients). It needs to be differentiated from macular drusen (Table 4.2).

4.1.8 Megalopapilla

It is usually a bilateral AD trait, associated with an enlarged blind spot, but not associated with other anomalies. Despite thinning in NFL, ganglion cell layer is usually normal. Diameter is mostly 2.1 mm or more, or the disc area is greater than 2.5 mm^2.

4.1.9 Myelinated Nerve Fiber Layer

It is present in 1% of population, occurring mostly unilateral (up to 10% bilateral), with almost no systemic associations (Fig. 4.5). Ocular

Table 4.2 Comparison between macular and optic disc drusen

	Macular drusen	Optic disc drusen
Composition	Lipid	Protein and calcium
Occurrence	Elderly with aging	Children with inheritance
Race	Equal	Almost exclusively in whites
Associated diseases	Age-related macular degeneration	Retinitis pigmentosa, angioid streaks, Usher, Noonan, and Alagille syndromes
Vision affection	Central vision	Peripheral vision (mostly infero-nasal)

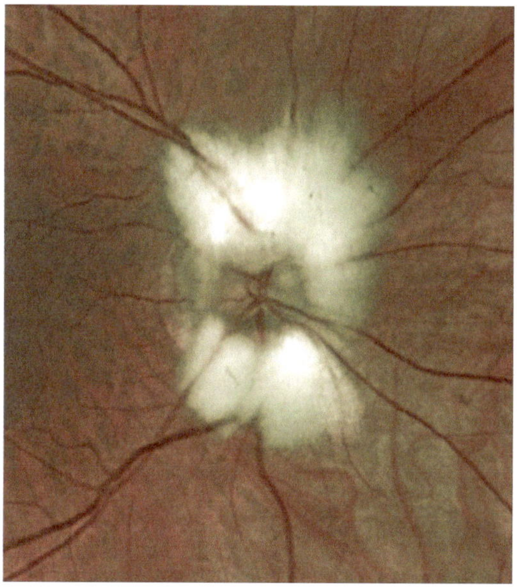

Fig. 4.5 Fundus image showing myelinated nerve fiber layer. (Courtesy Retina Rocks®)

associations include refractive error and amblyopia.

Bergmeister papilla: It represents a remnant of the embryological structure hyaloid artery. The condition is usually asymptomatic and does not interfere with vision; hence, it is often discovered incidentally during routine eye examinations. Its appearance can vary from a small tuft of tissue to a large stalk originating from the optic disc.

4.1.10 Optociliary Shunts

These are usually unilateral anastomoses between the retinal venous and choroidal venous circulations. They occur in about 30% of patients with optic nerve sheath meningiomas (MCC), and can be observed physiologically. They may also be found in conditions such as central and hemicentral retinal vein occlusion, optic nerve sheath meningioma, and chronic glaucoma (i.e., long-standing PXF).

Optociliary shunt vessels are vessels that shunt retinal venous outflow to the choroidal circulation.

4.1.11 Optic Nerve Head Melanocytomas

These are dark brown lesions located on the optic nerve head. While these lesions are usually benign, they can occasionally undergo malignant transformation. They may cause RAPDs and visual field defects and should be monitored to document any growth.

"Pseudo-Foster Kennedy syndrome" is a consequence of anterior ischemic optic neuropathy, in which active disease in one eye is associated with contralateral atrophy in the other eye secondary to a previous episode. It should be distinguished from true Foster Kennedy syndrome, which is uncommon and is classically caused by a frontal space-occupying lesion, characterized by ipsilateral compressive optic atrophy (i.e., pale disc) and contralateral papilledema secondary to raised intracranial pressure.

POEMS (polyneuropathy, organomegaly, endocrinopathy, monoclonal gammopathy, and skin changes) syndrome results from an overproduction of proinflammatory cytokines and vascular endothelial growth factor (VEGF), and elevated VEGF is highly specific for POEMS syndrome. The mandatory criteria for its diagnosis include polyneuropathy and monoclonal plasma-proliferative disorder.

4.2 Papilledema

It is defined as bilateral optic disc swelling caused by increased intracranial pressure (Fig. 4.6). This condition is most commonly associated with idiopathic intracranial hypertension (IIH) (aka pseudotumor cerebri). IIH is diagnosis of exclusion, characterized by elevated intracranial pressure with normal cerebrospinal fluid (CSF) composition and no other identifiable cause of intracranial hypertension on neuroimaging or other evaluations. IIH primarily affects females of childbearing age who are overweight.

There are several accepted criteria to diagnose IIH (Burkett and Ailani 2018), including the modified Dandy criteria:

1. Presence of signs and symptoms of increased intracranial pressure
2. Absence of localizing findings on neurologic examination except those known to occur from increased intracranial pressure (i.e., VI nerve palsy)
3. Absence of deformity, displacement, or obstruction of the ventricular system and otherwise normal neurodiagnostic studies, except for evidence of increased cerebrospinal fluid pressure (>200 mm H_2O); normal neuroimaging except for empty sella turcica, CSF filled optic nerve sheath (enhancement of optic nerve head is allowed, but only the head), and transverse sinus stenosis or collapse (but not thrombosis)

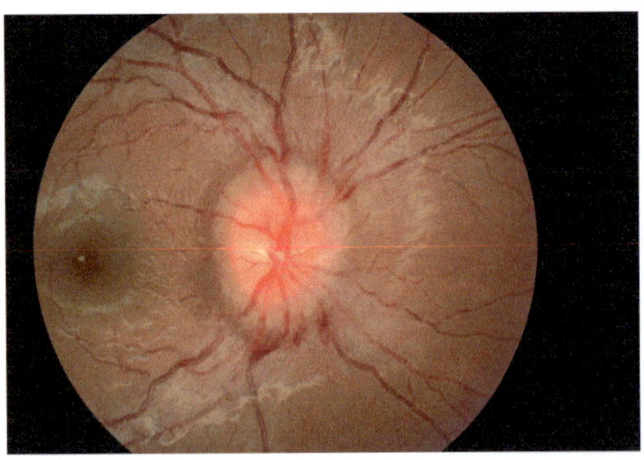

Fig. 4.6 Fundus image showing advanced optic disc edema with inferior hemorrhages. (Courtesy Retina Rocks®)

4. Awake and alert patient
5. No other cause of increased intracranial pressure present

Typically, patients present as bilateral optic disc edema and intact vision. While papilledema is nearly always bilateral, it may be asymmetrical. Acute papilledema is associated with transient vision loss, unilateral or bilateral. A common finding is an enlarged blind spot on the visual field. Visual field loss is the most important indication for the need of treatment.

The pathophysiology of optic disc edema involves the cessation of axonal transport, leading to swelling of the axons. This results in an increase in disc volume due to the enlargement of axons, rather than an accumulation of extracellular fluid, as seen in edema of other tissues. Spontaneous venous pulsation is absent in about 20% of normal individuals and can be difficult to detect even when present, but, if present, may exclude disc swelling.

Features include the following:

- Visual acuity is usually preserved initially, with episodes of transient vision loss mimicking TIA.
- Initial stage (stage 1) includes obscuration of vessels at margin, with nasal part involved initially (away from macula).
- More advanced stage (stage 2) includes complete margin obscuration, filled cup, and appearance of choroidal folds (Paton's lines).
- Obscuration of small and major vessels and hemorrhages signifies advanced stages (stage 3 and above).

Signs can be broadly classified as follows:

- Mechanical clinical signs of optic disc edema are blurring of the optic disc margin, obliteration of the optic cup, anterior extension of the nerve head into the vitreous, and retinal or choroidal folds.
- Vascular clinical signs of optic disc edema are per papillary venous congestion and hemorrhages, nerve fiber layer infarcts (but not NFL edema), and hyperemia of the optic nerve head.

Intracranial noises may occur due to turbulent flow within the cerebral venous sinuses, which can result from elevated intracranial pressure or a fistula. Paton's lines are strain lines that appear around the optic disc in cases of optic disc swelling. The most specific pattern for optic disc swelling is radial lines (there are other three patterns).

Chronic papilledema can lead to a persistent blockage of axoplasmic flow, resulting in visible refractile-appearing areas on the surface of the optic disc. These areas are termed pseudodrusen because, unlike true optic disc drusen, they do not involve calcium deposition.

In patients with IIH and mild visual loss, the combination of acetazolamide and a low-sodium weight-reduction diet compared to diet alone resulted in modest improvement in visual field function (Wall et al. 2014).

Ninety percent of idiopathic intracranial hypertension (IIH) occurs in obese childbearing-age women. Management can be medically by acetazolamide as the first line, with furosemide, topiramate as alternative (all are sulfa drugs), or surgically by optic sheath fenestration, shunting procedures, or venous sinus stenting. Any measure should be accompanied by risk factor alleviation, most importantly weight reduction.

Sulfa allergy myth: The allergy is actually to the hapten (the antigen), and the antigen is "arylamine". This is present in antimicrobials, but not acetazolamide, dorzolamide, and furosemide. The rule is if the previous allergic is life-threatening, do not give any sulfa. If only dermal, counsel the patient that non-antimicrobial sulfa has low risk of allergic, and give a trial dose of Diamox. This is especially important in IIH patients, where Diamox is way more effective compared to others (Shah et al. 2018).

When IIH is accompanied by loss of vision, optic nerve sheath fenestration (ONSF) can alleviate papilledema in the operated eye and, in a significant percentage of patients, in the contralateral eye. However, it may not consistently reduce intracranial pressure, headaches, or diplopia. Unlike lumboperitoneal shunts, which lower intracranial pressure and can cause low-pressure headaches, ONSF does not have this issue. Therefore, ONSF is preferred for patients with visual symptoms, while shunting is reserved for those experiencing headaches.

Please note that tetracycline may increase intracranial pressure.

4.3 Pupil-Affecting Diseases

4.3.1 Overview

Afferent pupillary pathway:

- Begins with the optic nerve and travels to the optic chiasm. From there, the pupillary fibers exit in the first third of the optic tract, bypassing the lateral geniculate ganglion. They then travel via the dorsal root to the pretectum (i.e., do not pass by lateral geniculate), a midbrain area located near the superior colliculus (aka superior brachium). After synapsing in the pretectal region, the fibers travel to both Edinger-Westphal nucleus, which is situated at the level of superior colliculus within the oculomotor nucleus.

Lesion at the superior colliculus will result in the loss of the pupillary reflex without causing a visual field defect. The difference between the afferent light reflex and afferent accommodation reflux is that afferent fibers reach the pretectum via the dorsal root for the light reflux and via the ventral root for the accommodation reflex. There is no clinical condition in which the light reflex is present but the near response is absent.

Efferent pupillary fiber:

- Parasympathetic: Efferent fibers from the Edinger-Westphal nucleus travel to the oculomotor nerve. These nerve fibers pass through the dorsal tegmental midbrain at its superior part, entering the cavernous sinus. They exit with the inferior division of oculomotor nerve, synapse at the ciliary ganglion, and reach the iris constrictor muscle via the short ciliary nerve.
- Sympathetic: Sympathetic fibers originate from the superior cervical ganglia and pass

through the sympathetic plexus above the apex of the lung. They travel to the internal carotid artery within the cavernous sinus and then to the oculomotor nerve. These fibers branch with the long ciliary nerves and ultimately reach the dilator muscle of the iris.

Lesions at any part of the afferent pathway: Disruption of the pathway from the retina to the Edinger-Westphal nucleus will affect both direct and consensual pupillary responses when light is shone on the eye ipsilateral to the lesion (absent if the disruption is complete). However, shining light in the normal eye will produce normal direct and consensual responses. This can be assessed using the relative afferent pupillary defect (RAPD), where a partial afferent defect can be detected. Despite the defect, the pupils will typically remain of relatively equal size. Lesions at any part of the efferent pathway:

Parasympathetic: Disruption in the pathway from Edinger-Westphal nucleus to the iris constrictor muscle will result in pupil dilation (mydriasis) on the side of the lesion (leading to more noticeable anisocoria more in bright light). This will be accompanied by a weak direct response and a normal indirect response in the affected eye, as well as a weak indirect response in the contralateral eye. Since the parasympathetic system controls the pupillary reaction to light, damage to the sympathetic will not impact this reaction, meaning direct and consensual reflexes will remain intact despite the anisocoria. Sympathetic: Disruption in the pathway from superior cervical to the dilator muscle will result in pupil constriction (meiosis), ipsilateral to the lesion (i.e., leading to more noticeable anisocoria in dim light). However, reactions to light (both direct and consensual) will still be preserved, as these responses are mediated by the parasympathetic system.

4.3.1.1 Specific Entities

Anisocoria is associated with defects in the efferent pathway defects rather than afferent pathway, while visual acuity is typically affected in afferent damage but not in efferent damage. Slit-lamp biomicroscopy is particularly useful for identifying iris abnormalities that may suggest causes of anisocoria such as tonic pupil or trauma (e.g., sphincter tear).

Polycoria: Refers to the presence of more than one opening in the iris. True polycoria involves multiple openings that react to light, whereas false polycoria includes extra openings that do not respond to light.

Corectopia: Describes the displacement of the pupil from its normal central position.

Paradoxical pupil: Is when a pupil initially dilates before constricting in bright light or constricts before dilating in dim light. Inherited retinal dystrophies are the most common cause of paradoxical pupils, with stationary night blindness being the most frequent underlying condition. Other causes can include achromatopsia and dominant optic atrophy.

4.3.2 Light-Near Dissociation

The light reflux is typically stronger than the accommodative reflux. Therefore, if the near response is greater than the light response, it indicates a pathologic pupil condition known as "light-near dissociation." This occurs due to a weakness in the light reflux while the near reflux remains intact. Light-near dissociation can be observed in:

- Argyll Robertson pupils
- Aberrant regeneration of the third nerve or ciliary ganglion (e.g., Adie's pupil)
- Dorsal midbrain syndrome (Parinaud syndrome)
- Pineal lesions
- Optic nerve lesion leading to deafferentation

The first step in evaluating light-near dissociation involves using an optokinetic drum. This device help assess pursuit and saccades by rotating downward to produce upward saccades. In patients with dorsal midbrain syndrome, upward saccades often cause convergence-retraction movements of the globes. Additionally, light-near dissociation has been observed in a few case reports involving patients with myotonic dystrophy.

Neutral density filters (NDFs) are useful for quantifying relative afferent pupillary defects. These filters come in 0.3 logarithmic unit steps and help in detecting and measuring the extent of RAPD. The severity size of RAPD can be quantified by the density of the filter needed to balance the pupillary responses between the eyes, with values typically ranging from 0.3 to 1.8 log units. It is put in front of the good eye. NDF can also be used to differentiate between strabismic and organic amblyopia:

- NDF will reduce visual acuity when held in front of eyes with organic causes of vision loss (e.g., AMD, ischemic events).
- NDF will improve visual acuity when held in front of eyes with strabismic amblyopia when using low log unit NDF (e.g., 0.4 log unit NDF).

However, this difference diminishes for high log unit filters (e.g., 3.0 log unit filters), and all eyes have their visual acuity diminish at these levels.

Neutral density filter placed in front of an eye of a healthy adult can mimic certain aspects of amblyopic function (e.g., contrast sensitivity loss, binocular summation, and interocular imbalance).

Absent pupil response to direct and consensual light response occurs when the iris of the affected eye is paralyzed, and this occurs in blunt trauma, third nerve palsy, atropine, and siderosis bulbi.

4.3.3 Horner Syndrome

This condition is caused by an interruption of the sympathetic chain in the head and neck, which may result from central (brainstem), preganglionic, or postganglionic lesions. It presents with ptosis (dropping of the upper and lower eyelids), miosis (constricted pupil that remains reactive to light), and anhidrosis (lack of sweating), with and without conjunctival injection (Table 4.3).

In Horner syndrome, the pupils' size difference in dark conditions is significant if it is greater than 1 mm. This discrepancy vanishes in light. Additionally, dilation delay or lag is pronounced in Horner syndrome. The condition may also affect the lower eyelid due to a potential paralysis of the inferior tarsal muscle, which is sympathetically innervated. As a result, the affected lower eyelid may appear higher than on the normal side, a phenomenon termed "reverse ptosis."

In distinguishing Horner syndrome from congenital ptosis, it is important to note that while the latter affects only the upper eyelid, Horner syndrome affects both the upper and lower eyelids.

It is noteworthy that Horner syndrome can persist following a cluster headache, particularly after multiple episodes. Pharmacological testing

Table 4.3 Comparing Horner syndrome occurring at the first-, second-, or third-order neuron

	Anatomy	Lesions
First order	Hypothalamus to cervical spinal cord C8–T2 (aka ciliospinal center of Budge)	Lateral medullary syndrome, multiple sclerosis, glioma, syringomyelia, or syringobulbia
Second order	Travels through cervical sympathetic chain through the brachial plexus, over the pulmonary apex, and synapses in the superior cervical ganglion	Subclavian artery aneurysm, mediastinal tumors, Pancoast tumor, thyroid malignancies, or surgical procedures in the region
Third order	Enters the cranium within the adventitia of the internal carotid artery into the cavernous sinus to the effector muscles (Müller and dilator papillae)	Lesions of the superior cervical ganglion (trauma, radical neck dissection, or jugular vein ectasia), internal carotid artery dissection or lesions, cavernous sinus pathologies, lesions of the sellar and parasellar regions (invasive pituitary tumors)

in these cases often reveals a postganglionic lesion, indicating that cluster headaches could be a cause of postganglionic Horner syndrome. Generally, any lesion along the sympathetic pathway will result in Horner syndrome on the side of the lesion.

In a clinical examination, a common sign of Horner syndrome is a delay in pupil dilation after exposure to and removal of light. While normal sympathetic function would result in dilation within 2–3 s, in Horner syndrome, this process can take 20–30 s. The condition can also lead to anhidrosis or a lack of sweating. Disruption of the central or preganglionic neurons can lead to anhidrosis on the same side of the face. In contrast, postganglionic lesions at or beyond the superior cervical ganglion may restrict anhidrosis to the forehead. More serious conditions, like Pancoast lung tumors, are usually associated with preganglionic lesions. **Pharmacological testing** can be useful both for diagnosing Horner syndrome and for localizing the lesion:

- **Cocaine**: This drug prevents the reuptake of noradrenaline at the adrenergic synapse. It will not dilate a Horner's pupil but will cause dilation in a normal eye. Therefore, anisocoria of >1 mm after cocaine administration is diagnostic of Horner syndrome, with the smaller pupil being the affected one.
- **Hydroxyamphetamine**: This drug releases norepinephrine from nerve synapses. It will cause dilation of a preganglionic or central Horner's pupil if the postganglionic pathway is intact. However, it will have no effect on a postganglionic Horner's pupil. The test is more sensitive for central lesion than for preganglionic lesions.
- **Phenylephrine, adrenaline, apraclonidine**: These agents act directly on the dilator muscle. They will cause brisk significant dilation in the Horner's pupil associated with postganglionic lesions compared to the unaffected side, due to denervation hypersensitivity (reversal of anisocoria).

Denervation hypersensitivity: This theory explains the exaggerated response of tissue following the disruption of its nerve supply. Instead of neurotransmitters being concentrated at the end plate of the effector organ, they become distributed across the entire membrane, making it hypersensitive to stimuli that act directly on it. In patients with normal pupils, pilocarpine 1% will elicit a response. Therefore, a weaker preparation (0.10%) is recommended to demonstrate denervation supersensitivity.

Screening and Diagnosis of Horner Syndrome: An acute presentation of a headache, mild drooping of the eyelid (ptosis) on one side, and temporary vision loss (amaurosis fugax) should raise suspicion of a carotid artery dissection. In such cases, MRI and MRA of the neck would be the diagnostic methods of choice. A newly onset Horner syndrome in children warrants a screen for neuroblastoma, often through catecholamine testing or MRI. In a patient with anisocoria, the consistent pharmacologic response to pilocarpine use is a small pupil that does not react to light or near stimuli. This distinguishes it from other conditions like Adie's syndrome and Horner syndrome itself. There is no pharmacological test that can differentiate between a central and a preganglionic Horner's pupil. However, accompanying signs can localize the lesion:

- Painful Horner's syndrome is a classical symptom of carotid artery dissection and should be treated as an emergency. It indicates a postganglionic lesion.
- Horner's in combination with a sixth nerve paresis suggests involvement of the cavernous sinus, and a mass in or near the sinus must be ruled out. Brainstem syndromes, such as lateral medullary syndrome, can also be a cause.
- Damage along the rest of the postganglionic neuron: this can affect the nasociliary or long ciliary nerves.

Congenital Horner Syndrome: Normal iris pigmentation fails to develop, leading to heterochromia, with the lighter color indicating the abnormal side. This can also be seen in longstanding Horner syndrome in adults. In adults, central Horner syndrome is often related to stroke, preganglionic Horner syndrome is frequently associated with neoplasm, and postganglionic Horner syndrome may have a vascular cause such as carotid dissection. Additionally, headache syndromes, including migraine, cluster headaches, and trigeminal cephalalgias, might lead to anisocoria. Congenital Horner's syndrome is associated with incomplete ptosis and hemifacial flush when the patient is crying or nursing. In a child with curly hair, limp hair can be observed on the Horner syndrome-affected side.

Anatomical Considerations in Horner Syndrome: In understanding Horner syndrome, certain anatomical details are pertinent. The superior cervical ganglion, a key part of the sympathetic nervous system, is located near the mandible's angle and where the common carotid artery bifurcates. Another critical component, the third-order neuron, is situated near the trigeminal ganglion and the sixth cranial nerve, and it connects with the first division of the trigeminal nerve to enter the eye's orbit. The sympathetic system's effector nerves function in two distinct ways: via the long ciliary nerves, they innervate the iris's dilator muscles and the smooth muscle, known as Müller's muscle, in both the upper and lower eyelids. Additionally, they stimulate vasomotor activity and sweat glands through the external carotid artery.

Pharmacological Management in Horner Syndrome: Apraclonidine, a weak alpha-1 and potent alpha-2 adrenergic agonist, can cause the affected pupil to dilate and possibly elevate the eyelid without affecting the normal pupil when applied topically in Horner syndrome.

4.3.4 Adie's Tonic Pupil

Adie's tonic pupil refers to a condition where the ciliary ganglion, a part of the efferent parasympathetic pathway, becomes damaged. This results in abnormal regeneration of parasympathetic fibers in the short posterior ciliary nerves. Consequently, the pupil exhibits a sluggish light reflex along with a tonic response, meaning it remains constricted for several seconds after the removal of a visual target. Moreover, the affected pupil appears dilated and responds excessively to atropine.

While Adie's tonic pupil generally affects one eye, approximately 8% of cases are bilateral at initial presentation. This condition tends to progress to involve both eyes at an annual rate of 4%. Females are more frequently affected than males, with a 70–30% ratio. Remarkably, about 90% of patients with this condition also demonstrate decreased tendon reflexes.

Unique Features of Adie's Tonic Pupil: A distinguishing characteristic of Adie's tonic pupil is that more fibers innervate the ciliary body than the pupillary sphincter. This difference in innervation underlies the pupillary light-near dissociation observed in these patients. The condition often presents as sectoral palsy, or localized paralysis, of the iris sphincter. Over time, the Adie's tonic pupil typically enlarges to become the larger of the two pupils. For about 2 years, it exhibits hypersensitivity to cholinergic substances. A hallmark diagnostic test involves instilling a low concentration of pilocarpine (0.1–0.125%) into both eyes. The abnormal pupil constricts due to denervation hypersensitivity, while the normal pupil remains unaffected.

Differential Diagnosis for Adie's Tonic Pupil: To distinguish a pharmacological blockade from a third nerve palsy or Adie's tonic pupil, a dose of 0.1% pilocarpine is administered. Unlike in Adie's pupil, the pupil remains dilated in the presence of a pharmacologic blockade and does not overcome this blockade.

A dilated, unresponsive pupil without ptosis or motility dysfunction suggests Adie's pupil. This condition is further characterized by light-near dissociation (poor reaction to light but a robust and prolonged pupillary response to near vision), sectoral palsy of the iris sphincter, and increased sensitivity of the short ciliary nerves to parasympathomimetics such as pilocarpine. It is important to note that there might be a delayed or even absent pupillary reaction to both light and near vision, alongside segmental contraction of the iris sphincter.

Various factors can cause tonic pupil, including diabetes, shingles infection, alcoholism, and Miller-Fisher syndrome, among others. However, isolated optic nerve disease, such as Leber's hereditary optic neuropathy (LHON), does not cause this condition.

4.3.5 Argyll Robertson Pupils

Argyll Robertson pupils (ARPs) are associated with a lesion in the tabes dorsalis, a region that houses the afferent light reflex pathway. The pretectal nucleus may also be implicated. In this condition, the pupils display an absent light response but retain their ability to constrict when focusing on near objects, a phenomenon known as preserved accommodation reflex.

ARPs are typically small and do not respond to atropine. While they are most often bilateral, affecting both eyes (in about 90% of cases), they usually present asymmetrically. Unlike in Adie's tonic pupil, Argyll Robertson pupils do not exhibit a tonic response upon dilation after the removal of a near-visual target.

Associated Conditions and Causes: The ARP is most commonly associated with neurosyphilis but can also be seen in conditions such as diabetes, multiple sclerosis, sarcoidosis, and alcoholism. It typically occurs due to midbrain lesions, which can cause asymmetric pupils. Both acquired and congenital syphilis can lead to the development of ARP.

It is essential to note that asymmetric pupil contraction is a feature of both Adie's tonic pupil and Argyll Robertson pupils.

Diagnosis and Distinguishing Features: In the presence of a pharmacologically dilated eye, the pupil does not constrict either in response to bright light or on accommodation. Additionally, the pupil does not respond to any concentration of pilocarpine. One notable characteristic of ARP is that no other neurological features typically accompany the changes in pupillary response.

4.3.6 Parinaud Syndrome (Aka Dorsal Midbrain Syndrome)

Parinaud syndrome, also known as dorsal midbrain syndrome, manifests bilaterally and is due to a lesion that interferes with the supranuclear inhibition of the oculomotor nerves, leading to aberrant activation. This syndrome is recognized by a triad of symptoms (seen in 65% of cases):

- Upgaze palsy: The vertical gaze centers (riMLF and INC) reside between midbrain dorsally and thalamus. For upgaze, fibers cross through posterior commissure, so damaging one side of dorsal midbrain will affect upgaze bilaterally, unlike downgaze (ipsilateral fibers support ipsilateral downgaze).
- Light-near dissociation: Pretectal fibers between pretectum and Edinger-Westphal nucleus represent the end of the afferent pathway, and the tract for light is different than near (goes ventrally). Damaging these fibers will affect pupillary afferent light reflux (shape is normal as this is afferent fibers).
- Lid retraction: Loss of disinhibition to the levator nucleus within third CN nucleus, leading to bilateral lid retraction, which could be mild.
- Convergence-retraction syndrome when looking upward: Loss of disinhibition to the nuclei of medial, superior, and inferior recti muscles leads to their simultaneous activation, causing globe retraction and nystagmus.

While it localizes to the dorsal midbrain, the etiology can vary. It is mostly vascular in elderly but can be tumor or autoimmune in young and middle age.

4.3.7 Key Symptoms and Signs

In more detail, symptoms of this syndrome include the following:

1. Bilateral lid retraction with superior gaze palsy: This refers to difficulty moving the eyes upward and may become more apparent when the person tries to look up.
2. Convergence deficit: Difficulty in focusing both eyes toward a near object.
3. Globe retraction and nystagmus-like movement: The eyes may draw backward on adduction or upgaze, accompanied by uncontrolled, rhythmic eye movements. This symptom arises due to the simultaneous activation of the superior and inferior rectus muscles.
4. Light-near dissociation: This involves a loss of the light reflex in the pupils but a preserved near-pupillary reflex.

In addition to the key triad, an affected individual may present with dilated or mid-dilated pupils, a remote near point (loss of convergence), exotropia, and even papilledema if a tumor or increased intracranial pressure causes the condition.

Etiology and Associated Signs: The primary cause of Parinaud syndrome varies with age. In children under 10 years, pineal gland tumors are the most common cause, while demyelination is more frequent in middle-aged individuals, and vascular or compressive lesions are common in adults.

Collier's sign, or midbrain-induced neurogenic lid retraction, is a feature of Parinaud syndrome. Furthermore, upward saccades, a type of fast eye movement, in patients with Parinaud syndrome can often induce convergence-retraction of the globes, particularly when stimulated by a downward-rotated optokinetic drum.

Treatment and Prognosis: Treatment for Parinaud syndrome is primarily directed toward addressing the underlying cause. Prognosis varies, but it tends to be worse in cases caused by tumors.

4.3.8 Marcus Gunn Pupil

This term refers to a relative afferent pupillary defect (RAPD) resulting from partial optic nerve injury. The injury can occur anywhere from the retina (as in large retinal detachment) to the optic disc (as in glaucoma), excluding all the way to the brain. Since only the afferent pathway is affected, no anisocoria occurs. Visual acuity is typically impaired. Cataracts do not cause RAPD; however, in the case of very severe cataract, it can enhance the light response in the affected eye, producing RAPD in the contralateral eye.

4.4 Cranial Nerves and Eye Movements

4.4.1 Overview

4.4.1.1 Cranial Nerve III (Oculomotor)

It controls most of the eye muscles, pupil constriction, lens accomodation, and eyelid elevation. CN III starts at the midbrain and then goes ventrally (anteriorly) to the subarachnoid space (close to posterior communicating artery (PCA), where an aneurysm can damage it), then cavernous sinus in the wall, and then the superior orbital fissure (SOF) to the eye (no vertical course, as the eye is almost at the level of midbrain). It then typically divides into superior and inferior divisions after passing through the annulus of Zinn in the orbit, with both divisions passing through the superior orbital fissure within the annulus.

Cranial nerve III injury can occur in different anatomic locations at its course, with different presentations:

- Nuclear and fascicular lesion at the ipsilateral midbrain injury: Present with ipsilateral CN III signs along with accompanying signs depending on other structures involved. Such injury may damage other structures at the midbrain level, where it can involve superior cerebellar peduncle leading to ipsilateral cerebellar signs (Nothnagel syndrome), may also involve red nucleus causing contralateral hemitremor (Benedikt syndrome), or may involve cerebral peduncle causing contralateral hemiparesis (Weber syndrome).
- Cranial nerve in the subarachnoid space: Causes include uncal herniation (i.e., patient is comatose manifest with dilated pupil,

known as Hutchinson sign) and posterior communicating artery (PCA) aneurysm.
- Cavernous sinus and orbital apex: May affect multiple cranial nerves.
- Isolated ischemic infarct: Affects the nerve along its course leading to mostly isolated cranial nerve damage.

Classically, extrinsic damage through an aneurysm or tumor would lead to pupil involving CN III palsy, as parasympathetic pupil fibers are anatomically at the outer region of the nerve, while intrinsic damage by an ischemic infarct would lead to pupil-sparing CN III palsy.

Aberrant Regeneration and Aneurysm Location: Abnormal firing of CN III leading to synkinetic muscle activation, mostly due to miswiring of regenerated fibers. It typically occurs with extrinsic damage in traumatic or compressive lesions due to the breach of endoneurial nerve sheaths and almost nerve in intrinsic microvascular causes.

Cyclic Spasms: Cyclic oculomotor palsy is a rare, nonprogressive disorder characterized by rhythmic spasms and paralysis in the muscles controlled by the third cranial nerve. This congenital condition has a typical pattern lasting about 45 s, with a cycle of third nerve actions superimposed on an apparent third nerve palsy.

4.4.1.2 Cranial Nerve IV (Trochlear)

It primarily controls the superior oblique muscle. It originates in the midbrain, exits dorsally (posteriorly), and then takes a long, round course, which makes it susceptible to palsy from blunt head injuries. It then enters the cavernous sinus wall and proceeds through the superior orbital fissure to the orbit. In adults, trauma is the leading cause of fourth nerve injury, while congenital palsy is the most common cause in children. This injury can result in vertical diplopia with restricted motility in downward and inward rotation. The superior oblique muscle's tertiary action is to abduct or move the eye outward, a function that becomes more pronounced in cases of third nerve palsy, causing an exaggerated outward position of the eye.

Parks three-step test is used for vertical deviation to isolate if the cause is trochlear nerve palsy or not. The three-step test is actually five steps:

- Primary gaze: to assess the laterality of hypertropia
- Horizontal gaze: to assess if the hypertropia is worse with left or right gaze, testing vertical muscles on abduction and adduction
- Head tilt: to isolate the muscle with impaired torsional component
- Double Maddox: to measure the torsional component, where excyclotorsion is expected after isolated CN IV palsy, and an excyclotorsion of >10 PD reflects bilateral palsy
- Positional change, where we use the single Maddox comparing setting vs. supine position, where an improvement of >50% points toward central lesion (i.e., possible skew deviation)

The main aim is to make sure that the vertical deviation is caused by fourth CN palsy vs. not. The typical exam for superior oblique palsy is right hypertropia worse on left gaze and right head tilt, excyclotorsion of 2–10 PD, and no change between supine and setting.

Superior oblique myokymia, characterized by intermittent rapid oscillopsia, is primarily a cyclorotatory phenomenon. Episodes can be initiated by moving the eye into the affected superior oblique muscle's action field.

4.4.1.3 Cranial Nerve VI (Abducens)

It primarily supplies the lateral rectus muscle that controls eye's abduction.

CN VI begins in the pons dorsally, goes ventrally within the brainstem as a fascicle (the only ocular CN with long vertical course), and then goes up to the clivus within the subarachnoid space. It has a long S-shaped pathway. The first bend occurs as the nerve exits from the lower pons. It then travels vertically along the clivus and makes 90° anteriorly to enter Dorello's canal where it pierces the dura and turns anteriorly over the edge of the petrous pyramid, passing through Dorello's canal and under Gruber's ligament.

From there, it enters the cavernous sinus and proceeds through the superior orbital fissure to reach the eye. According to its course and the site of damage, there are six syndromes:

- VI1: the brainstem syndrome, where a complete gaze palsy occurs due to horizontal gaze nucleus damage
- VI2: fascicle
- VI3: subarachnoid, the elevated intracranial pressure syndrome
- VI4: the petrous apex syndrome, where it is accompanied by fifth, seventh, and hearing
- VI5: the cavernous sinus syndrome
- VI6: the orbital syndrome

Ischemic mononeuropathy is the primary cause of an isolated sixth nerve palsy, with affected adults typically noticing improvement within 3 months of onset. For elderly patients (above 70 years), an investigation for giant cell arteritis is warranted if a sixth nerve palsy is present. The sixth cranial nerves ascend the clivus at the base of the skull after converging. If both abducens nerves are sequentially affected, a mass lesion in this location should be suspected, warranting a base-of-skull MRI. In an Asian male presenting with bilateral sixth nerve palsies, nasopharyngeal carcinoma is a possible concern since the ophthalmoparesis may be the first sign of tumor extension along the clivus. In such cases, an otolaryngologic consultation is indicated.

From patients who have their palsy resolved, 85% of patients have complete resolution, while 15% have spread of comitance, where contralateral medial rectus receives less innervation causing esotropia that is comitant on all gazes (usually after few months from injury).

4.4.2 Gaze

Gaze control is moving both eyes simultaneously. The brainstem houses the gaze centers, which are responsible for generating signals that control the muscles responsible for moving the eyes. These include:

- Horizontal gaze centers, which are located in the pons within the sixth cranial nerve (abducens) nucleus and the paramedian pontine reticular formation (PPRF)
- Vertical gaze centers, which are located at the thalamo-mesencephalic junction, where the midbrain and thalamus meet

Key structures in this area include the rostral interstitial nucleus of the medial longitudinal fasciculus (riMLF), the interstitial nucleus of Cajal (INC), and the posterior commissure (PC). Eye movements can be affected by various disorders. Vertical gaze palsy, for example, is characterized by a conjugate limitation of the eyes' movements in upgaze and/or downgaze. Horizontal gaze palsy, on the other hand, is typically indicative of damage to the ipsilateral pontine horizontal gaze center (e.g., a lesion in the right pontine horizontal gaze center would lead to a right gaze palsy; the eyes will be deviated to the left and unable to fully move rightward).

Downgaze palsy can be caused by occlusion of a branch of the posterior cerebral artery (Percheron artery), progressive supranuclear palsy, Whipple's disease, or AIDS. Other conditions like thalamic hemorrhage, acute obstructive hydrocephalus, hypoxic encephalopathy, and massive subarachnoid hemorrhage can cause tonic downward gaze deviations. Progressive supranuclear palsy (PSP) is a neurodegenerative tauopathy primarily affecting vertical saccades, particularly downgaze. It can also impair convergence eye movements and eventually result in global gaze palsy. The artery of Percheron, a rare anatomical variant of the posterior cerebral circulation, can cause bilateral thalamic ischemic strokes when occluded, leading to a clinical triad of vertical gaze palsy, memory impairment, and coma.

Upgaze palsy can be seen in conditions such as Parinaud syndrome, double-elevator palsy, myasthenia gravis, and thyroid eye disease. Among patients with ocular motility problems, the inferior and medial recti muscles are most commonly involved, and upgaze is most commonly affected.

4.4.3 Pursuit and Saccade Movements and Associated Refluxes

These are types of eye movements that allow us to track moving objects and rapidly shift our gaze between different points, respectively.

The excitatory burst neurons for generating horizontal saccades are located in the paramedian pontine reticular formation (PPRF), while the sixth cranial nerve nucleus coordinates horizontal smooth pursuit eye movements. Vertical and torsional saccadic movements are generated by the rostral interstitial nucleus of the medial longitudinal fasciculus (riMLF) in the midbrain.

Saccadic eye movements can reach velocities of up to 800 degrees per second and are triggered by the contralateral frontal lobe. On the other hand, pursuit eye movements may reach velocities of up to 70 degrees per second and are initiated by the ipsilateral posterior parietal lobe. Pursuit movements also have a faster latency than saccadic movements.

The optokinetic response is a combination of a pursuit movement in the direction of the drum or tape movement and a refixational saccadic movement in the opposite direction. For instance, if a drum is moving to the patient's right, the pursuit movement to the right is controlled by the right parietal lobe, while the refixational leftward saccade is mediated by the right frontal lobe. This response can be used to estimate visual acuity and test for supranuclear lesions. If a patient with a right adduction deficit can fully adduct the right eye in response to an optokinetic drum, it indicates a supranuclear lesion.

The oculocephalic reflex, also known as the doll's eye reflex, helps to locate lesions, differentiating between those that are supranuclear to the brain or peripheral to nuclear lesions. The doll's head maneuver can overcome gaze palsies from cortical (supranuclear) lesions but not from infranuclear lesions.

Caloric testing of the vestibular system involves irrigating the ear with warm or cold water. Cold water causes fast-beating eye deviation to the opposite side, while warm water causes deviation to the same side.

The vestibulo-ocular reflex (VOR) involves both the semicircular canals and the otoliths of the utricle and saccule to maintain eye movement during head movement. An impaired VOR can cause difficulties reading print due to the eyes not stabilizing during small head tremors and may cause nystagmus.

Vertical and torsional eye movements are coordinated by the rostral interstitial nucleus of Cajal within the MLF, which also helps maintain oculomotor control and head posture. Saccadic movements require simultaneous activation of both frontal eye fields, with horizontal saccades maturing more rapidly than vertical saccades.

4.4.4 Miscellaneous

Bilateral ophthalmoplegia differential diagnoses include (the pneumonic BMW Car):

- B: Bickerstaff's brainstem encephalitis and botulism
- M: Miller Fisher and myasthenia
- W: Wernicke and Whipple
- Car: Carcinomatous meningitis and cavernous sinus

Myasthenia gravis is the most common cause. Consider history and physical, serology, chest imaging, and EMG (myasthenia gravis section below). It is unlikely when the ophthalmoplegia is associated with pupil abnormality, pain, or proptosis.

Acute peripheral nervous system demyelination (aka Guillain-Barré) can affect the eyes (aka Miller Fisher variant), presenting acutely. Assessment should include detailed history and physical exam, serology with ganglioside antibodies, along with nerve conduction studies showing the demyelination pattern. Miller Fisher syndrome: It presents with a clinical triad of ophthalmoplegia, ataxia, and areflexia, which can present in relatively young age. Bilateral mydriasis is frequently present in typical Miller Fisher syndrome cases. Bilateral symmetrical ophthalmoplegia mostly involves the lateral recti (i.e., mimics CN VI palsy). It might be associated with hyporeflexia and ataxia. It shows positivity for IgG anti-GQ1b antibody in 80% of cases. Cerebrospinal fluid analysis can be normal or can indicate high protein with low white blood cell counts (albumin-cytologic dissociation). Magnetic resonance imaging results of the brain are usually normal, but there can be enhancement of the cranial or spinal nerve roots. It can be managed acutely with intravitreal immunoglobulin (Shaath et al. 2023).

Whipple's disease can present without its classic symptoms, but with prominent parkinsonism and slowed and curved trajectories of vertical saccades (8, 9). The selective deficit in vertical saccades in patients with Whipple's disease is attributed to the involvement of the rostral interstitial nucleus of the medial longitudinal fasciculus (riMLF), which is responsible for vertical saccade generation. While vertical saccades are significantly affected, the horizontal saccades generated at paramedian pontine reticular formation are also often impaired (Shaikh and Ghasia 2017).

Botulism toxicity can cause a fixed dilated pupil, ptosis, ophthalmoplegia, and drooling, among other bulbar symptoms. It should be differentiated from atropine toxicity, which may present with a fixed dilated pupil, tachycardia, flushed dry skin, fever, and agitation.

Oculomotor apraxia is an inability to initiate voluntary horizontal saccades. It is of two types:

- **Congenital oculomotor apraxia** is characterized by the use of horizontal head thrusts past the points of interest, and it may occur in children who have dysgenesis of the corpus callosum.
- **Acquired lesion apraxia** results from bilateral lesions of the supranuclear gaze pathways of the frontal and parietal lobes, such as from bilateral strokes, and is associated with conditions like Balint syndrome.

Congenital ocular motor apraxia is idiopathic and is characterized by increased latency and intermittent failure of horizontal saccadic initiation.

Ocular neuromyotonia is characterized by episodic diplopia lasting 30–60 s, typically occurring after sustained activation of a cranial ocular motor nerve. It is usually associated with a history of radiation therapy for a skull base neoplasm.

The one and a half syndrome is a condition where one eye exhibits horizontal gaze palsy (the "one"), while the other eye shows internuclear ophthalmoplegia (INO) (the "half"). This results in one eye being unable to move horizontally at all, while the other can only move outward, retaining abduction. Formally, it is characterized by a conjugate horizontal gaze palsy in one direction and an internuclear ophthalmoplegia in the other. Potential causes include pontine lesions, demyelinating conditions, and ischemic lesions. **Divergence paralysis** can be associated with Fisher's syndrome, Chiari malformation, pontine tumors, and diazepam (divergence center might be the pons).

Skew deviation: Vertical or torsional diplopia that cannot be isolated to a single muscle or nerve, mostly due to posterior fossa lesion (i.e., three-step test does not localize to fourth palsy; examples include right hypertropia worse with right gaze and right head tilt). Lesions are usually in the brainstem and cerebellum (can be from thalamus to midbrain) and usually ischemic, but compressive tumors and demyelination need to be excluded, especially in younger patients (Walter and Trobe 2021). So, the three-step test will not show a specific oblique palsy, which is why the five-step test is developed to diagnose it (fourth step being Maddox rod, and fifth step is supine exam). It is mostly caused by damage to prenuclear vestibular input to ocular motor nuclei, so any lesion from thalamus to medulla may lead to skew deviation, where a posterior fossa (mostly cerebellum) is usually the cause. The resultant vertical ocular deviation is relatively comitant in nature with normal duction tests (each eye exam is normal). It is associated with:

- Binocular torsional deviation, which can be examined by Maddox rods (the fourth step)
- Abnormal vestibulo-ocular reflex (i.e., abnormality in the otolith), which can be triggered

by examining the deviation in supine position (the fifth step)

- Torticollis
- Tilt in the subjective visual vertical

Its differentials, when a single muscle cannot be isolated as a cause of double vision, are myasthenia gravis and thyroid eye disease among others.

The ocular tilt reaction (OTR) is a particular type of skew deviation. It consists of a triad of vertical deviation, head tilt in the direction of the lower eye, and bilateral ocular torsion in the direction of head tilt.

In lesions above the midbrain, hypertropia is seen on the involved side (no decussation yet).

Ocular motility signs of cerebellar disease are categorized as:

- Proprioceptive abnormalities: manifest by flutter, dysmetria, and instability of gaze
- Defects of vision-dependent functions: manifest by abnormalities of pursuit, vestibular suppression, optokinetic response, and nystagmus

Note that opsoclonus is not among the signs.

Spasm of the near reflex (SNR) occurs when the triad of convergence, miosis, and accommodation persists even when the patient is not focusing on a near object. Patients often present with blurred vision, diplopia, and asthenopia. On examination, they may have an alternating convergent strabismus, abduction deficit, and pseudomyopia. Variable acute esotropia is always present, with greater esotropia at distance fixation compared to near fixation, and there are always limitations in abduction.

Ophthalmoplegic migraine is characterized by episodes of ipsilateral headache followed by palsy of one or more ocular cranial nerves, most commonly the third CN. Unlike typical migraine, ophthalmoplegic migraine is primarily a pediatric condition, occurring in children under 10 years old and affecting males more often than females. Pupillomotor fibers are typically involved, often resulting in residual mydriasis.

A dorsal pontine infarct may include ipsilateral gaze palsy from abducens involvement.

A ventral pontine infarct may include abduction deficit.

In oculomasticatory myorhythmia, patients experience oscillopsia (a sensation that the world is shaking) while chewing due to pendular vergence oscillations that occur with contractions of the masticatory muscles.

4.4.5 Nystagmus

The first step is to describe the movements. Use the following classification:

- Bilateral conjugate when both eyes move together or disconjugate (as in seesaw nystagmus).
- In primary position vs. gaze evoked vs. convergence evoked.
- Describe if there is a fast phase (saccade) and slow phase (pursuit).
- The direction based on the saccade. It is named by the fast phase, worsening with gaze to the fast phase direction (i.e., Alexander's law).

Examine the nystagmus pattern at all gazes. When nystagmus occurs only when one eye is covered, it is termed latent nystagmus (aka monocular nystagmus).

Remember that end-gaze nystagmus can be physiological, and it is related to variation in gaze-holding ability.

When it is saccade without slow phase (aka back-to-back saccade), then it is opsoclonus, and it is called flutter when it is only horizontal and opsoclonus when multidirectional. Opsoclonus is most commonly postinfectious in pediatric and paraneoplastic in adults, but the differential includes infectious (encephalitis), toxicity, or tumor. Brain imaging is warranted to exclude structural lesion in the pons mainly, but also LP for infectious and pan CT for neoplasms.

Nystagmus by definition has at least one slow phase. Jerk nystagmus has a slow phase and a fast phase. Pendular nystagmus has only slow phases.

Table 4.4 provides description of different types of nystagmus and their structural localization.

Common nystagmus types:

Infantile nystagmus is characterized by paradoxical horizontal OKN*, dampening by convergence (so might be accompanied by esotropia), being absent during sleep, being increased by distance fixation, and presence of a null point. Oscillopsia, the sensation of the world moving, is not normally a problem. On testing, horizontal optokinetic nystagmus (OKN) responses may or may not be elicited or may show inversion; that is, instead of the recovery saccade (the "jerk" phase of nystagmus) being in the expected opposite direction to the drum or OKN tape rotation, it is in the same direction. The slow phase moves in the direction opposite that of a rotating optokinetic drum. Vertical saccades, however, are generally preserved.

Spasmus nutans is an acquired form of nystagmus that occurs within the first 2 years of life. It presents as a clinical triad of (1) bilateral, small-amplitude, high-frequency nystagmus; (2) head bobbing; and (3) torticollis. The head movements are considered compensatory mechanisms that improve vision by reducing the frequency and asymmetry of the nystagmus. Increased amplitude occurs in abduction. An idiopathic form spontaneously resolves by age 3 years, offering a good prognosis. Secondary causes include glioma of the optic nerve, anterior visual pathway, empty sella syndrome, and porencephalic cyst. The nystagmus is usually in all directions and asymmetrical (disconjugate).

Congenital motor (efferent) nystagmus often has a family history, with mostly X-linked inheritance. Presentation is about 2–3 months after birth and persists throughout life. VA is generally better than with sensory deficit nystagmus, at 6/12–6/36. There is low-amplitude pendular nystagmus that may convert to jerk nystagmus on side gaze.

Latent nystagmus is associated with infantile esotropia and DVD. There is no nystagmus with both eyes open, but horizontal nystagmus becomes apparent when one eye is covered; the fast phase is in the direction of the uncovered eye.

Manifest latent nystagmus is a type of horizontal jerk nystagmus which increases in amplitude when one eye is covered. It occurs in strabismus, amblyopia, or uniocular pathology such as cataract.

Seesaw nystagmus is a type of disjunctive nystagmus characterized by one eye elevating and intorting while the other eye depresses and extorts. The eye movements are typically pendular, slow, and low frequency, as well as similar in amplitude between the eyes. It is most commonly observed in patients with large tumors in the parasellar region, which can compress the optic chiasm and cause bitemporal hemianopia.

Table 4.4 Nystagmus classification according to their characteristic appearance and potential localization

Nystagmus	Description	Localization
Downbeat	Bilateral conjugate with saccades down	Cervicomedullary junction, mostly Chiari malformation. Idiopathic downbeat nystagmus is GAD antibody related
Upbeat	Bilateral conjugate with saccades up	Brainstem or vermis of cerebellum
Convergence retraction		Dorsal midbrain
Seesaw	One eye rises and intorts while the other falls and extorts. This is followed by reversal of the vertical and torsional components in the opposite eye	Third ventricular parasellar region (including chiasm issue) (Ref)
Rebound	Horizontal jerk to one side, then slow, then jerk back to same side	Cerebellum
Periodic alternating	Horizontal jerk to one side, then slow, then jerk to the other side within almost 1 min	Cerebellum. Respond to baclofen
Bruns-Cushing		Cerebellopontine angle

Sensory nystagmus occurs in eyes with poor visual acuity.

Nystagmus may sometimes localize to the site of etiology. Types of nystagmus that localize to a site or an etiology are the following:

- Upbeat nystagmus: This can result from lesions of the anterior vermis and lower brainstem, as well as from drug effects and Wernicke's encephalopathy.
- Downbeat nystagmus: This may be localized to anatomic structures at the craniocervical junction (e.g., Arnold-Chiari malformation), spinocerebellar degeneration or cerebellar atrophy, and may be seen in certain intoxications (alcohol, lithium, anticonvulsants).
- Vestibular nystagmus: This type originates within the vestibular system and includes periodic alternating nystagmus (PAN) and rebound nystagmus (detailed below). It is almost always horizontal, and fixation decreases the nystagmus.
- Seesaw nystagmus: While it can be congenital, it is most commonly found in patients with large parasellar tumors, often craniopharyngiomas. Acquired seesaw nystagmus is frequently accompanied by bitemporal hemianopia.

Nystagmoid movements (i.e., nystagmus-like syndrome, but not considered true nystagmus):

- Convergence–retraction nystagmus is a jerk nystagmus due to the co-contraction of extraocular muscles, often the medial recti. It can be induced by rotating an ***OKN drum downwards***; the upward refixation saccade is associated with medial rectus contraction, bringing both eyes nasally in a convergence movement. So its direction can be thought of as upward (i.e., fast-phase direction). It is classically associated with retraction of the globe into orbit. It is a component of Parinaud dorsal midbrain syndrome; causes include lesions of the pretectal area such as pinealoma and vascular accidents.
- Ocular flutter and opsoclonus: Voluntary flutter, often mistaken for nystagmus, is marked by irregular, brief, and fatigable bursts of rapid-frequency and low-amplitude eye movements without slow phase. Voluntary flutter typically occurs in patients with nonorganic motility disturbances. These conditions involve saccadic oscillations without intersaccadic interval; ocular flutter oscillations are purely horizontal, while in opsoclonus, they are multiplanar. Causes include viral encephalitis and myoclonic encephalopathy in infants ("dancing eyes and dancing feet"), and it can have a transient idiopathic occurrence in healthy neonates or may be drug induced. Both ocular flutter and opsoclonus may be linked to malignancies such as metastatic neuroblastoma in children or small-cell CA of the lung in adults. In adults, the most common cause of opsoclonus is paraneoplastic syndrome associated with small-cell carcinoma of the lung.

Rebound nystagmus occurs with cerebellar lesions. It is a primary position nystagmus, which is provoked by prolonged eccentric gaze holding, and appears after the eyes are returned to primary position.

Periodic alternating nystagmus (PAN) is a conjugate horizontal jerk nystagmus that periodically reverses direction. During the active phase, the amplitude and frequency of nystagmus first progressively increase and then decrease. This is followed by an interlude lasting 4–20 s during which time the eyes are steady and may show low-intensity, often pendular movements. A similar sequence in the opposite direction occurs thereafter, with the whole cycle lasting between 1 and 3 min. PAN can be congenital or result from cerebellar disease, ataxia telangiectasia, and drugs such as phenytoin. It is often seen in posterior fossa disease, particularly cerebellar, and can also localize to the craniocervical junction (e.g., Arnold-Chiari malformation). In young patients, the most likely cause of PAN is demyelinating disease such as multiple sclerosis. Therefore, PAN can be caused by cerebellar lesions, demyelination, ataxia telangiectasia, or Arnold-Chiari malformation, but not by parasellar lesions.

In pendular nystagmus, one eye elevates and intorts while the other depresses and extorts. It can be due to parasellar tumors (often with bitemporal hemianopia), syringobulbia, and brainstem stroke.

Alexander's law describes the increased frequency and amplitude of nystagmus movements accompanying gaze in the direction of the fast phase. So, an upbeat nystagmus is the most prominent upgaze.

Opsoclonus is also referred to as "saccadomania" or dancing eyes. Neuroblastoma patients with opsoclonus have excellent survival.

Horizontal saccades are markedly slow in patients with a previous history of optic neuritis.

The saccadic movement that is often affected in progressive supranuclear palsy (PSP) is downward saccades. This is in distinction to the dorsal midbrain syndrome (Parinaud syndrome), where upward saccades are generally affected.

Monocular nystagmus in a neonate can be chiasmal and hypothalamus glioma, blind eye, MS, and spasmus nutans.

In the management of downbeat nystagmus (which usually presents in Chiari malformation), clonazepam, baclofen, gabapentin, base-out prisms, memantine, and 3,4-diaminopyridine are options.

Voluntary flutter, often mistaken for nystagmus, is characterized by irregular, brief, and fatigable bursts of rapid-frequency and low-amplitude eye movements that lack a slow phase. It is typically observed in patients with nonorganic motility disturbances.

Ocular bobbing is a vertical jerk that is most commonly caused by pontine dysfunction. This means that the oculocephalic reflex will be abnormal.

Acknowledgements We would like to thank Retina Rocks® for providing the images in this chapter.

Conflict of Interest None.

References

Burkett JG, Ailani J (2018) An up to date review of Pseudotumor Cerebri syndrome. Curr Neurol Neurosci Rep 18(6):33. https://doi.org/10.1007/s11910-018-0839-1

Dutton GN (2004) Congenital disorders of the optic nerve: excavations and hypoplasia. Eye (Lond) 18(11):1038–1048. https://doi.org/10.1038/sj.eye.6701545

Jain N, Johnson MW (2014) Pathogenesis and treatment of maculopathy associated with cavitary optic disc anomalies. Am J Ophthalmol 158(3):423–435. https://doi.org/10.1016/j.ajo.2014.06.001

Kim SH et al (2005) Peripapillary staphyloma: clinical features and visual outcome in 19 cases. Arch Ophthalmol 123(10):1371–1376. https://doi.org/10.1001/archopht.123.10.1371

Lingam G et al (2021) Ocular coloboma—a comprehensive review for the clinician. Eye (Lond) 35(8):2086–2109. https://doi.org/10.1038/s41433-021-01501-5

Sanjari MS, Falavarjani KG, Kashkouli MB (2006) Bilateral peripapillary staphyloma, a clinicoradiological report. Br J Ophthalmol 90(10):1326–1327. https://doi.org/10.1136/bjo.2006.096362

Shaath DS, Scheidt AF, Stiff HA (2023) Sudden-onset bilateral mydriasis in a young girl. JAMA Ophthalmol 141(8):792–793. https://doi.org/10.1001/jamaophthalmol.2023.2585

Shah TJ, Moshirfar M, Hoopes PC (2018) "Doctor, I have a sulfa allergy": clarifying the myths of cross-reactivity. Ophthalmol Therapy 7(2):211–215. https://doi.org/10.1007/s40123-018-0136-8

Shaikh AG, Ghasia FF (2017) Novel eye movement disorders in Whipple's disease—staircase horizontal saccades, Gaze-evoked nystagmus, and esotropia. Front Neurol 8:321. https://doi.org/10.3389/fneur.2017.00321

Wall M et al (2014) The idiopathic intracranial hypertension treatment trial. JAMA Neurol 71(6):693–701. https://doi.org/10.1001/jamaneurol.2014.133

Walter E, Trobe JD (2021) The clinical and imaging profile of skew deviation: a study of 157 cases. J Neuroophthalmol 41(1):69. https://doi.org/10.1097/WNO.0000000000000915

You QS, Xu L, Jonas JB (2008) Tilted optic discs: the Beijing eye study. Eye (Lond) 22(5):728–729. https://doi.org/10.1038/eye.2008.87

Clinical Review of Neuro-ophthalmology: Part III

5

Saif Aldeen Alryalat, Abdee Ryalat, Noor Laylani, and Andrew G. Lee

Abstract

The final part of the neuro-ophthalmology clinical review covers a range of miscellaneous conditions that affect the eye and surrounding structures. It explores thyroid eye disease, myasthenia gravis, and internuclear ophthalmoplegia (INO), highlighting their neuro-ophthalmic manifestations. Additionally, the chapter examines eyelid and facial contractions, sagging eye syndrome (SES), and chronic progressive external ophthalmoplegia (CPEO). Carotid-cavernous fistula (CCF) and cavernous sinus pathology are discussed for their impact on ocular function. Visual phenomena, primary headaches related to the eye, and electrophysiology are included to broaden the understanding of complex neuro-ophthalmic disorders. The chapter concludes with an exploration of Marcus Gunn jaw-winking syndrome, providing insights into its rare presentation.

Keywords

Thyroid eye disease · Myasthenia gravis · Internuclear ophthalmoplegia · Carotid-cavernous fistula · Marcus Gunn jaw-winking

5.1 Miscellaneous

5.1.1 Thyroid Eye Disease

An immunological mechanism with two main phases described, a dynamic phase of progressive

S. A. Alryalat (✉)
Department of Ophthalmology, The University of Jordan, Amman, Jordan

The University of Colorado Anschutz Medical Campus, CO, USA

A. Ryalat
Private Practice, Amman, Jordan

N. Laylani
Department of Ophthalmology, University of Colorado Anschutz Medical Campus, Aurora, CO, USA
e-mail: nalaylani@houstonmethodist.org

A. G. Lee
Department of Ophthalmology, University of Colorado Anschutz Medical Campus, Aurora, CO, USA

Department of Ophthalmology, Neurology, and Neurosurgery, Weill Cornell Medical College, New York, NY, USA

Department of Ophthalmology, Baylor College of Medicine, Houston, TX, USA

Department of Ophthalmology, The University of Iowa Hospitals and Clinics, Iowa City, IA, USA

Department of Ophthalmology, The University of Texas Medical Branch, Galveston, TX, USA

The UT MD Anderson Cancer Center, Houston, TX, USA
e-mail: aglee@houstonmethodist.org

S. A. Alryalat (ed.), *Ophthalmology Board and FRCS Part 2 Exams*,
https://doi.org/10.1007/978-981-96-1517-9_5

deterioration representing active inflammation (which plateaus and then improves in around 18 months) and the final static or "burnt-out" phase, represents the residual fibrosing sequelae. Accordingly, disease activity (representing degree of inflammation: CAS scale) and disease severity (representing the degree of damage: EUGOGO classification) should be differentiated. Active inflammation needs treatment with steroid and other anti-inflammatory agents, while inactive disease complications require rehabilitation or surgical corrections (Bartalena et al. 2021).

Patient Assessment

- Eyelid: Lagophthalmos (inability to close the eyelids on normal rather than forced eyelid closure) with Bell's reflux assessment, lid lag (asymmetrical decrease in the normal downward movement of the lids during downgaze)
- Exophthalmometer: Useful for follow-up tracking
- Motility and associated double vision (Bahn-Gorman scale)
- Corneal epitheliopathy
- Optic nerve function: Visual acuity; color vision and discrimination, RAPD, and fundoscopy for disc appearance and choroidal folds
- Clinical activity score

Although a subtotal thyroidectomy may provide primary treatment of dysthyroid state, it will not have an effect on the eye findings (except lid retraction). So, it is not part of the treatment, especially in acute cases.

Lid retraction is the most common sign in Graves' ophthalmopathy.

In the early stages of thyroid eye disease, it may present with intermittent diplopia, generally worse in the morning, secondary to orbital congestion.

Thyroid eye disease is one of the most common causes of choroidal folds, which are often horizontal with respect to the macula.

Thyroid orbitopathy may result in optic neuropathy (estimated to occur in 5% of patients with thyroid eye disease).

5.1.1.1 Clinical Activity Scales

A *clinical activity score* (CAS): by assessing two symptoms:

- Orbital ache: periorbital or retro-orbital pain
- Gaze-evoked pain:

Five Signs

- Conjunctival redness: Any redness is considered graded according to the area affected (trace, <50%, >50%). Dilated vessels over the insertions of these muscles are common and almost pathognomonic.
- Eyelid erythema:
- Eyelid edema: Fullness and skin thickening.
- Chemosis: Differentiated from conjunctivochalasis.
- Swelling of the plica or caruncle: The plica is the fold of conjunctiva lying adjacent to the caruncle.

Score of above 3 (4 and above) is considered for active thyroid (PPV >80%).

The Bahn-Gorman scale categorizes diplopia into four grades. Grade I involves intermittent diplopia that occurs only when the patient is fatigued. Grade II is characterized by inconstant diplopia, appearing only on lateral or upward gaze. Grade III refers to constant diplopia present in straight and level gaze, which can be corrected with prisms. Finally, grade IV is constant diplopia that cannot be corrected with prisms.

5.1.1.2 Severity Scale

Mild TED: Only a minor impact on daily life that has insufficient impact to justify immunomodulation or surgical treatment. They usually have one or more of the following:

- Minor lid retraction (<2 mm)
- Mild soft tissue involvement
- Exophthalmos <3 mm above normal for race and gender
- No or intermittent diplopia and corneal exposure responsive to lubricants

Moderate-to-severe GO patients without sight-threatening GO whose eye disease has sufficient impact on daily life to justify the risks of immunosuppression (if active) or surgical intervention (if inactive). They usually have two or more of the following:

- Lid retraction ≥2 mm
- Moderate or severe soft tissue involvement
- Exophthalmos ≥3 mm above normal for race and gender (18–21 Caucasians, 21–23 African-Americans)
- Inconstant or constant diplopia

Sight-threatening (very severe) GO patients with dysthyroid optic neuropathy and/or corneal breakdown

Eyelid Assessment

- MRD1 is the distance between the center of the pupil and upper lid margin in primary gaze (normally the upper lid covers 1 mm of the iris, leaving 4 mm distance from the margin to reflux (MRD1)).
- MRD2 is the distance between the center of the pupil and lower lid margin in primary gaze (normally the lower lid at the tip of the iris, leaving 5 mm distance from the margin to reflux (MRD2)).
- Levator function measures the movement of upper lid from up to down (normally >10 mm).

5.1.1.3 Diagnosis

The diagnosis can be established in a patient with eyelid retraction in addition to supporting signs or symptoms. High-risk patients for TED are patients with unstable hormones, those who are smokers (dose-response), and those with high TSHR-AB. Note that other antibodies are less sensitive and specific, with high percentage (10–30%) present in normal population.

On non-contrasted CT: Measurement of muscle and fat tissue size and the extent of compression on optic nerve.

On ultrasound: Muscle size measurement.

On contrasted MRI: To assess the enhancement of extraocular muscles, the temporal muscles are considered the reference standard because they are spared from Graves' disease and because of their structural similarity and close anatomical relationship to the EOM.

This patient was presented with progressive optic neuropathy for over 1 year with no obvious lid retraction or proptosis, but with mild abduction deficit. His vision deteriorated over the year from 20/40 to CF in the right eye:

The image shows enlargement of inferior and medial recti mainly (with sparing of tendons), explaining the restricted motility to upgaze and abduction.

5.1.1.4 Treatment

Mild disease should be managed symptomatically; cases with modified risk factors (smoking and hormone control) with active mild disease can be offered selenium.

Moderate-severe: The aim in moderate-severe active disease is to shorten inflammatory phase and decrease its complications. Surgeries should be avoided due to the changes during the inflammatory phase, and stick to patching and prisms. Inactive disease should be offered rehabilitation and surgery if needed. Active moderate-severe disease: An intermediate dose of IV glucocorticoids, that is, a starting dose of 0.5 g IV methylprednisolone once weekly for 6 weeks, followed by 0.25 g once weekly for 6 weeks and a cumulative dose of 4.5 g should be used in most cases of moderate-to-severe and active GO (0.75 followed by 0.5 is only reserved for severe diseases). If IV steroid is not available, the dose is 1 mg/kg body weight, which is gradually tapered down by 5–10 mg/week until withdrawal (4–6 months); however, oral regimen has significantly more side effects due to the sustained steroid dose. Second-line therapies include cyclosporine and azathioprine combined with steroids teprotumumab, rituximab, tocilizumab, or orbital radiotherapy.

Dysthyroid optic neuropathy (DON): The patient needs urgent treatment with IV steroids for 3 consecutive days, and if there is no improvement within 1–2 weeks, surgical decompression is done.

Orbital radiotherapy is regarded as an effective second-line treatment for moderate-to-severe and active GO, especially when combined with glucocorticoids, particularly in the presence of diplopia and/or restriction of extraocular motility. However, the supporting evidence is primarily derived from observational studies, which provide level III evidence.

Thyroid iodine radiotherapy can cause or worsen TED in 15%. Prophylactic treatment with oral steroid for 2–3 months can reduce this risk. It is considered in patients with TED or high-risk patients without TED. The doses are 0.5 mg/kg for high risk and 0.1 mg/kg for lower risk.

Selenium: In an *RCT* that included mild active disease with <18 months since dx, 6-month selenium supplementation should be given to patients with mild and active GO. Improved manifestation and QoL can be observed with sodium selenite (200 μg) (91.2 μg selenium) daily for 6 months, an effect that is maintained.

The risk of TED is highest after radioactive iodine, then after subtotal thyroidectomy, and least after total thyroidectomy.

5.1.1.5 Clinical Trials

Teprotumumab for the Treatment of Active Thyroid Eye Disease: Teprotumumab is given as IV infusion at Q3 weeks. It reduces mainly proptosis (>2 mm), but also CAS (>2) and diplopia per Gorman score (>1 grade). The main effect can be seen at 6 weeks (i.e., after three doses) and includes hearing loss (reversible in the clinical trial), in addition to infusion-related reaction. Usually, eight doses are given per course (Douglas et al. 2020).

Proof-of-Concept and Randomized, Placebo-Controlled Trials of an FcRn Inhibitor, Batoclimab, for Thyroid Eye Disease: Batoclimab is given at Q1 week subcutaneously. Usually six doses are given over 6 weeks. While there was a decrease in proptosis, there was also a dose-dependent increase in LDL, which led to early trial termination (Kahaly et al. 2023).

5.1.2 Myasthenia Gravis

This affects the postsynaptic membrane at the neuromuscular junction, nicotinic receptors (only skeletal muscle); however, other autonomic and smooth muscles include muscarinic receptors (despite both being Ach neurotransmitters) (Gilhus et al. 2019). No pain, pupil involvement, or proptosis is expected in MG; however, 5–15% have concomitant thyroid abnormality. Oculobulbar is most frequently affected due to high concentrations of NMJ.

Females are twice affected early on (20–40 years), with male predominance in older ages (>55 years). Ptosis is the most common ocular manifestation in myasthenia gravis (though lid retraction may occur). Seventy-five percent of all myasthenics will have eye findings at presentation; up to 50% will have ocular myasthenia only; this is mainly due to high end plate-to-muscle ratio in ocular muscles. Chest imaging is essential in workup, although thymoma is only present in 10% of cases. Thymectomy is important even without thymoma evidence. If ocular signs remain isolated for more than 2 years, the disease is likely to remain clinically ocular; however, late conversion to generalize MG is possible. 5% will have an overlap between myasthenia and Graves. The clinical appearance of ptosis with exotropia and the underaction of the medial rectus would be most suspicious for myasthenia gravis.

The lateral rectus muscle is the most frequently involved among the extraocular muscles.

Note that accommodation or pupillary functions are not typically affected in MG. Nystagmus is never a feature for myasthenia gravis.

When Ach-R-Ab is absent, the term becomes seronegative myasthenia gravis. 50–70% of seronegative myasthenia gravis cases have positive anti-MuSK antibodies. MuSK-myasthenia gravis represents 6% of all cases of myasthenia gravis.

Difficulty breathing and swallowing are the feared manifestations that might suggest systemic MG, where a significant number of pure ocular cases convert to generalized MG.

Bimodal age distribution: Asians develop juvenile form, while Caucasians develop senile form.

Signs include the following:

- Enhanced ptosis (or curtain effect): occurs when elevation of one eyelid leads to ptosis or worsening of existing ptosis in the opposite eyelid, as described by Hering's law. The

"Cogan's lid twitch" is a prominent clinical sign where the upper eyelid rapidly shoots upward and appears to "twitch" momentarily after a sustained downward gaze, before returning to its resting position.
- Forced eyelid closure test: involves the patient squeezing their eyes shut for 5–10 s and then opening them. When the patient fixes their gaze on a target in the primary position, a positive test is indicated by an upward overshoot of the eyelid followed by a downward drift. Orbicularis weakness is a characteristic sign of OMG and, in some cases, can lead to incomplete eyelid closure in what is known as the "peek sign."

Ice-pack test (with 2–3 min of ice pack on eyelid, ptosis improves by >1 mm for a few seconds) is 75% sensitive with high specificity. Cogan's lid twitches are a sign of myasthenia gravis (MG), elicited by instructing the patient to maintain downward gaze for 15 s and then gaze upward, finally returning to primary gaze. Cogan's sign is present when the affected lid briefly "twitches" upward on returning to primary gaze.

Myasthenia gravis antibodies (Table 5.1):

- First line: anti-Ach-R-Ab (which has blocking, modulating, and binding types) in 85%
- Second line: anti-MuSK (most dangerous) in 10%
- Third line: anti-striated, anti-titin, anti-LRP4 in 5%

Single-fiber EMG is the best type of EMG, which will show fatigability (>90% sensitive). The other option is conventional ERG with repetitive stimulation (only up to 50% sensitive).

Chest CT is indicated upon diagnosis (except for MuSK-positive patients, as thymoma is rare).

Eighty percent of patients with MG have detectable antibodies against the acetylcholine (ACh) receptor (AChR). However, a small percentage of patients have antibodies against muscle-specific kinase (MuSK) or lipoprotein receptor-related protein 4 (LRP4) instead. Anti-LRP4 antibodies may be less MG specific than those against AChR and MuSK, and this subgroup of MG is less well established than the others.

The Tensilon test, which uses intravenous edrophonium (an acetylcholinesterase inhibitor that can cause bradycardia), has a sensitivity of 85% for ocular myasthenia gravis (MG) and 95% for systemic MG. This test is diagnostically useful for MG as it enhances neuromuscular transmission. The most reliable indicators of a positive response to edrophonium are observable improvements in ptosis or ocular misalignment.

Vertical diplopia is more common than horizontal diplopia in myasthenia gravis (so vertical recti are more likely affected).

5.1.2.1 Management

Four modalities exist:

- Symptomatic treatment with ACh-esterase inhibitors (pyridostigmine/Mestinon): Onset of action within 15 min with peak in 2 h.
- Steroids: Onset of action within 1 month. However, an initial worsening is expected, so a strategy of incremental dosing with alternate days might lead to less symptomatic worsen-

Table 5.1 Antibodies associated with myasthenia gravis syndrome and their sensitivities and characteristics

	Sensitivity	Association with thymoma presence	Other
Acetylcholine receptor (AChR)-*binding* antibodies	90%	More likely	More in systemic disease
MuSK protein antibodies	50% of those negative for AChR antibodies	Less likely	More in systemic disease
Antibodies against skeletal muscle (e.g., anti-titin)	80–90% of those with thymoma, and one-third of those without	More likely	Suggestive of a severe disease

ing. Here is the strategy by a landmark RCT: "an alternate-day dose of oral prednisone starting at 10 mg, which was increased in 10-mg steps every 1–2 weeks till symptoms were controlled (up to 100 mg on alternate days)" (Wolfe et al. 2016).
- IVIG or plasmapheresis: Within a day.
- Thymectomy: Months to years (consider in all thymoma patients, resistant generalized myasthenia, almost no role for isolated ocular).

In all patients, consider exacerbating factors:

- Drugs that may exacerbate control (e.g., beta-blockers) or lead to myasthenia crises (e.g., botulinum)
- Acute events, like infections (so consider immunization)

The rule of thumb is to assume that any medication may exacerbate unless proven otherwise, so close follow-up is required after each medication.

For mild-to-moderate disease, you can start with ACh-esterase inhibitor. For severe or myasthenic crises, go for IVIG/plasmapheresis followed by steroids.

Immunotherapy-related myasthenia symptoms typically start following receiving 1–4 treatment cycles, with a median time of 7 days for the development of respiratory failure from the first symptom onset of MG.

Pyridostigmine is generally less effective in MuSK-positive patients and for the control of diplopia.

Always make sure that the patient is not taking a medication that might exacerbate myasthenia (from beta-blockers to antibiotics); review its table.

Steroids are better for ocular myasthenia than Mestinon.

It is worth noting that the randomized trial of thymectomy in myasthenia gravis did not include patients with isolated ocular myasthenia.

Lambert–Eaton myasthenic syndrome is mediated by antibodies against presynaptic voltage-gated calcium channels; in 60%, this is a paraneoplastic phenomenon associated with a lung tumor, less commonly affecting ocular structures. It shows a negative Tensilon test.

5.1.3 Internuclear Ophthalmoplegia (INO)

Internuclear ophthalmoplegia (INO) is a condition that affects conjugated lateral gaze, leading to impaired adduction in the affected eye. When attempting to look toward the side opposite the affected eye, the affected eye shows minimal or no adduction, while the opposite eye abducts with accompanying nystagmus.

Ipsilateral absence or slowing of ipsilateral adduction and contralateral abduction nystagmus: The lesion affects the ipsilateral MLF at the side of impaired adduction. Field of gaze with the largest ocular misalignment is contralateral to the brainstem lesion within the medial longitudinal fasciculus (MLF).

The lesion causing MLF can be localized by observing if convergence is preserved or not as follows:

- If convergence is intact, the lesion is probably in the pons anteriorly (aka caudal).
- If convergence is absent, the lesion is probably at the thalamo-mesencephalic junction and posteriorly (aka rostral).

A bilateral INO produces bilateral adduction lag, bilateral abducting nystagmus, and vertical gaze nystagmus, which is most noticeable during upgaze, as described by Alexander's law. This condition typically localizes to the pons. The two most common causes of INO are demyelination and stroke.

Convergence remains intact if the lesion is anterior and discrete, but it becomes impaired if the lesion is posterior or extensive. Variations include the following:

- One-and-a-half syndrome is characterized by gaze palsy on the affected side, typically due to abducens nucleus lesion, combined with damage to the MLF. This results in a gaze palsy in the direction of the lesion (e.g., left

gaze palsy in left lesion), limited adduction on the same side due to MLF involvement, and inability of one eye to adduct or abduct, while the contralateral eye can only abduct. This syndrome usually indicates in the pons, commonly caused by demyelination in younger patients and ischemia in older patients. MRI is the preferred diagnostic tool. An example of this syndrome is a lesion affecting both the medial longitudinal fasciculus and the ipsilateral abducens nucleus or the parapontine reticular formation (PPRF). The condition results from a unilateral lesion of the paramedian pontine reticular formation or the abducens nucleus on one side, causing the conjugate gaze palsy toward the side of the lesion, and interruption of internuclear fibers of the ipsilateral medial longitudinal fasciculus after crossing the midline from its site of origin. Wall-eyed bilateral internuclear ophthalmoplegia (WEBINO) is characterized by dissociated abducting nystagmus, impaired convergence, and supranuclear vertical gaze palsy. This condition results from a midbrain lesion that damages the bilateral medial longitudinal fasciculus and pretectum, which are supplied by the anteromedial perforators of the posterior cerebral artery. The convergence deficit associated with WEBINO leads to bilateral exotropia and abducting nystagmus.
- Some patients with myasthenia gravis (MG) will present with a pseudo-INO that closely resembles true INO. The presence of other associated motility disorders, particularly ptosis or fatigability of adduction, should lead to a Tensilon test for further evaluation.

Pseudo-one-and-a-half syndromes can also occur in conditions such as myasthenia gravis, Wernicke's encephalopathy, or Guillain-Barré syndrome.

5.1.4 Eyelid and Facial Contractions

These can be either contraction of muscle or a group of muscles (dystonia), including myokymia (contraction of one lid or one muscle), blepharospasm (bilateral contraction of upper and lower lids), facial spasm (contraction of multiple muscles of the face), and Meige syndrome (eye and face muscles). All these contractions cannot be inhibited by the patient (i.e., not suppressible).

Blepharospasm is a bilateral progressive condition and a form of focal dystonia (involuntary muscle contractions) in eyelid protractor muscles leading to episodic closure of the eyelids. Etiology is related to *basal ganglia dysfunction.* It is more common in females during 40–60 years. Most are primary, but the most common secondary is Meige syndrome. In blepharospasm, symptoms can be relieved upon distraction by talking, touching the temples or the forehead between the eyes, or chews on glasses.

Symptoms often start as mild and infrequent spasms that progress over time to forceful and frequent contractures of the eyelids. In advanced cases, this can lead to functional blindness from inability to temporarily open the eyes, making it a progressive disease. The first-line treatment is to modify and alleviate exacerbation, like bright light (wearing sunglasses) and ocular surface disease (using lubrication). If symptoms persist, periodic injection of botulinum toxin into the eyelid protractor muscles is recommended.

Eyelid protractor muscles: the orbicularis oculi, corrugator supercilii, and procerus muscles.

Severe cases of essential blepharospasm may result in entropion (NOT ectropion). It is managed by botulinum toxin injection. More severe cases may be managed by myectomy, either surgical or chemical (permanent denervation via doxorubicin). Systemic medications can also be used (e.g., benzodiazepine). Lid crutches are not used for blepharospasm.

Meige syndrome is a rare form of dystonia that represents a combination of two forms of dystonia, blepharospasm and oromandibular dystonia (OMD). The patient has frequent forced spasms of the eye, jaw, tongue, and lower facial muscles.

Hemifacial spasm initially begins by brief spasm of the orbicularis oculi, which later spreads along the distribution of the facial nerve. It most commonly occurs because of compression of the facial nerve in the cerebellopontine angle by anomalous aberrant vessels (demonstrated in 90%). Neuroimaging is required here, followed by surgical decompression if vessels are found. Such contractions are present at sleep (unlike blepharospasm, which is also asynchronous).

Note that hemifacial spasm is characteristically unilateral, whereas apraxia of the eyelid opening,essential blepharospasm, and Guillain-Barré syndrome cause bilateral abnormalities.

Facial myokymia is the continuous unilateral twitching/contraction of small bands or strips of facial muscle. The most common cause is MS in adults and pontine glioma in children, representing an intramedullary disease of the pons involving the seventh nerve nucleus or fascicle.

Facial myokymia and hemifacial spasm occurring in patients with multiple sclerosis are linked to an ipsilateral pontine MRI lesion in a small percentage of cases. While facial myokymia typically resolves on its own, hemifacial spasm can persist in some patients and may require treatment. Note that blepharospasm is mostly bilateral, unlike myokymia and hemifacial spasm.

Undulating movements of the eyelid are typical of eyelid myokymia, which is usually a benign and self-limited condition when it occurs alone. If the myokymia extends to other facial muscles, it suggests a broader involvement of the facial nerve, often associated with pontine lesions. When optic disc pallor is also present, consider multiple sclerosis, as it may be linked with both facial myokymia and optic neuropathy. Superior oblique myokymia presents as intermittent visual disturbance that can be described as "shaking and tilted vision." While largely idiopathic, it has been associated with neurovascular compression of the trochlear nerve by an adjacent artery; thus, neuroimaging is required during assessment. While no treatment was agreed upon, the anticonvulsant gabapentin has been used successfully.

Summary of pathophysiology:

Benign essential blepharospasm: dysfunction of the basal ganglia.

Hemifacial spasm: facial root exit zone in the cerebellopontine angle.

Facial myokymia: intramedullary disease of the pons involving the CN VII nucleus or fascicle.

5.1.5 Sagging Eye Syndrome (SES)

Acquired, adult horizontal and/or cyclovertical strabismus can result from age-related orbital connective tissue degeneration. This condition, known as superior eye syndrome (SES), is characterized by significant displacement of all four rectus muscle pulleys away from the orbital center and elongation of the EOMs. Typical clinical findings in SES include generalized sag of the levator aponeurosis, leading to superior sulcus deformity (64%) and aponeurotic blepharoptosis (29%). Most patients with SES show symmetrical limitation of supraduction, although they generally have full horizontal ductions and clinically normal horizontal saccadic eye velocities. Rupture of the SR-LR band is observed in over 90% of cases. Patients with acute or chronic onset of binocular diplopia suggestive of SES, without additional acute neurologic deficits, may not require an urgent neurologic evaluation.

5.1.5.1 Sagging Eye Syndrome Vs. Heavy Eye Syndrome

Sagging eye syndrome occurs in elderly patients who are 70 years or older, and their symptoms include mild-to-moderate distance esotropia with full abduction, and a high lid crease or ptosis (due to mechanical age-related displacement of pulleys inferiorly).

Heavy eye occurs earlier in life than SES in high myopia patients who often show greater esotropia without ptosis.

5.1.6 Chronic Progressive External Ophthalmoplegia (CPEO)

It is a painless, progressive, bilaterally symmetric motility disease that initially affects the upgaze, but progresses to include all muscles and lead to frozen globe. Ptosis can also be observed. It begins in young adulthood and is a mitochondrially inherited disease. This condition is characterized by a progressive course without remission or exacerbation. Due to symmetrical loss of eye movement, diplopia is rare; however, difficulties with reading may occur due to insufficient convergence. Systemic associations can be seen in Kearns-Sayre syndrome (KSS). **Kearns-Sayre syndrome (KSS)** (aka oculo-cranio-somatic disorder) is a severe form of the CPEO that is mitochondrially inherited and involves a combination of the already described CPEO as well as mild pigmentary retinopathy in both eyes, cardiac conduction abnormalities, and cerebellar ataxia, with an onset before the age of 20 years.

For a clinical diagnosis of Kearns-Sayre syndrome (KSS), in addition to ophthalmoplegia and retinopathy, patients should exhibit at least one of the following three additional manifestations: cardiac conduction abnormalities (i.e., heart block), elevated cerebrospinal fluid protein, or cerebellar dysfunction. Unlike myasthenia gravis, KSS presents with progressive course, rather than intermittent symptoms. Edrophonium, which can cause bradycardia, should not be administrated to a patient under consideration for KSS until a cardiac evaluation has been conducted.

For both CPEO and KSS, progressive generations have severe disease due to more abnormal genes inherited.

Orbital apex syndrome is characterized by the presence of optic nerve dysfunction which can include decreased vision, an afferent pupillary defect, and/or dyschromatopsia; this condition is not typically seen in cavernous sinus syndrome because the optic nerve passes through the optic canal, not the cavernous sinus.

In contrast, the hallmark of ophthalmoplegia resulting from a lesion in the cavernous sinus is multiple, ipsilateral ocular motor nerve dysfunction involving any combination of the third, fourth, fifth, and sixth cranial nerves as well as sympathetic fibers. If only one oculomotor nerve is affected, it is usually the sixth nerve, which is the only ocular motor nerve not protected by the dural wall of the cavernous sinus.

Tolosa-Hunt syndrome is characterized by idiopathic, sterile inflammation primarily affecting the cavernous sinus along and the nerves within it (e.g., palsy of third, fourth, or sixth, or a combination of them). On MRI, it appears as enhancing mass. Patients with Tolosa-Hunt syndrome usually experience rapid and dramatic relief of pain with corticosteroid therapy, although improvement in motility may take weeks or even months.

5.1.7 Carotid Cavernous Fistula (CCF)

This should be suspected whenever corkscrew conjunctival vessels are seen or in cases of chronic red eye. It can be associated with other findings, including high IOP, proptosis, and choroidal detachment (Jadhav et al. 2023). There is abnormal communication between arteries and veins within the cavernous sinus. The prominent finding is enlargement of superior ophthalmic vein (SOV), where high pressure in cavernous sinus will cause high pressure in the veins (retrograde into SOV or anterograde into cerebral venous sinuses), leading to high ICP.

The mean diameter of SOV is approximately 2 mm, highly variable from 1 to 2.9 mm, often asymmetric (up to 75% of individuals); however, a diameter of >2.5 mm can be considered a reasonable cutoff for SOV dilation. It is not specific to CCF, and causes can include increased intracranial pressure, orbital diseases (e.g., thyroid eye disease), and vascular etiologies (mainly CCF).

It is classified based on the tear location: direct fistulas (Barrow type A) and dural, or indirect fistulas (Barrow types B, C, and D). By direct, we mean the tear is in the internal carotid artery itself within the cavernous sinus. The indirect can be from meningeal artery branches of ICA (Barrow B), ECA (Barrow C), or both (Barrow D).

It is classified also into high vs. low flow (an angiographic classification). Angiographically, high-flow fistulas are characterized by rapid filling of the cavernous sinus through the fistula with minimal or no filling of the intracranial vasculature. In contrast, low-flow fistulas exhibit slower filling of the cerebral venous system through the fistula, while intracranial arteries remain well filled. Angiography helps identify the drainage pattern of the fistula—whether it drains anteriorly via the superior ophthalmic vein (SOV), posteriorly via the inferior petrosal sinus (IPS), or a combination of both—and can also reveal whether there is reflux into cortical veins.

Based on the reflux or retrograde flow, CCF can be classified into Cognard 1 and 2a when there is no vein reflux or Cognard 2b to 5 when there is a reflux (need surgical intervention).

The MCCs of direct CCF are trauma, iatrogenic, and EDS type 4. Indirect CCFs (dural CCF) usually occur in postmenopausal, hypertensive women arising from dural branches of either ICA or ECA.

Mostly patients present with orbital symptoms secondary to anterior drainage, including arterialization of conjunctival veins (aka corkscrew vessels), high IOP from episcleral vein (according to Goldman equation), and proptosis. But they can also present with nerve palsy and resultant diplopia.

MRI with contrast can show the dilated SOV. CTA has 90% sensitivity, and MRA has 80% sensitivity. Angiogram is the gold standard when there is high suspicion despite normal imaging.

5.1.8 Primary Headaches Related to Eye

According to the *International Headache Society (IHS)*, there are four main types of primary headaches:

(1) Migraine, (2) tension type, (3) trigeminal autonomic cephalalgia, and (4) others. Each of these primary categories has further second- and third-degree diagnoses (e.g., retinal migraine is 1.2.4). The main two types that may present to ophthalmic clinic are:

- **Migraine and its subtypes:** These are often associated with visual phenomena.
- **Trigeminal autonomic cephalalgia:** These are characterized by periorbital pain and autonomic stimulation.

5.1.8.1 Migraine

Migraine with aura or aura without migraine: The visual aura that migraine patients may experience can range from monocular tunnel vision to total vision loss (lasting hours rather than few seconds in amaurosis fugax), geometric or bolt-like colors or scotomas (geometric jagging and scintillating scotoma), and polyopia (multiple images in one eye). The duration of the attack is crucial in differentiating the migraine (5–60 min) from TIA which lasts for seconds, especially in cases of aura without headache. The IHS provides the following specific description of migraine aura: a zigzag figure near the point of fixation that may gradually spread right or left and assuming a laterally convex shape with an angulated scintillating edge, leaving absolute or variable degrees of relative scotoma in its wake. In some cases, scotoma without positive phenomena may occur; this is often perceived as having an acute onset but usually enlarges gradually upon closer inspection.

IHS gave separate description for retinal migraine (1.2.4) vs. migraine aura without headache (1.2.2) (Table 5.2):

- **Retinal migraine** affects one eye and is usually followed by a headache on the same side. This type is considered more serious and requires thorough evaluation to rule out other causes of monocular blindness.
- **Migraine aura without headache** affects both eyes, does not progress to a headache, and presents with more varied visual symptoms. While typically less concerning from a medical standpoint, it can still be distressing for the patient.

5.1.8.2 Trigeminal-Autonomic Cephalalgias (TACs)

TACs are characterized by unilateral headache accompanied by prominent cranial parasympa-

Table 5.2 Comparison between retinal migraine and migraine aura without headache

Criteria	Retinal migraine	Migraine aura without headache
Affected eyes	One eye only	Both eyes
Associated headache	Typically follows visual symptoms; may also occur before or during	No headache (also called "acephalgic" or "silent" migraine)
Duration of visual symptoms	Usually less than an hour	Typically, 20–30 min
Type of visual phenomena	Partial or complete temporary blindness	Flashing lights, zigzag lines, blind spots (scotomas), etc.
Risk	Higher risk; considered more serious as it can signify underlying vascular issues	Generally less concerning medically, but still distressing for the patient
Other aura symptoms	Usually not present	Can include tingling, auditory or olfactory hallucinations, difficulty speaking, etc.
Diagnosis	Requires eye exam and possibly imaging to rule out other causes	Often based on patient history if other causes can be excluded

Persistence of migraine aura for more than 60 min may suggest migrainous infarction (documented on imaging) or persistent aura without infarction

Table 5.3 Comparison between the two main types of trigeminal-autonomic cephalalgias, including cluster headache and paroxysmal hemicrania

Criteria	Paroxysmal hemicrania	Cluster headache
Pain duration	Shorter, usually 2–30 min per attack	Longer, often 15 min–3 h per attack
Frequency of attacks	More frequent, often several times a day, up to 20 or more	Less frequent, typically 1–3 attacks per day during a cluster period
Pain intensity	Severe, but usually less intense than cluster headaches	Often described as extremely severe, sometimes called "suicide headaches"
Response to indomethacin	Typically responds dramatically to indomethacin	Does not respond to indomethacin

thetic features such as lacrimation, rhinorrhea, conjunctival injection, ptosis, and miosis. The two main types that need to be differentiated are cluster headache and paroxysmal hemicrania. They both affect one side with autonomic features, but they differ as shown in Table 5.3.

The third type is short-lasting unilateral neuralgiform headache attacks, which occur as sawtooth frequency of attacks.

Primary headache should not be considered when it starts close to disease or trauma. Also, if the headache intensity and characteristic acutely change, consider a secondary cause.

5.1.9 Visual Phenomena

Hallucinations are visual perception without external stimulus. Need to make sure that no delusional aspect occurs:

- The patient needs to have insight into the hallucination, knowingly it is not real.
- Should not have auditory component (no hearing).
- No other psychiatric diagnosis, not on drugs.
- Need visual acuity and field exam, in order to rule out Charles Bonnet syndrome.

Illusion is when an external stimulus is perceived differently.

Visual hallucinations are broadly classified into two categories (Degueure et al. 2022):

- Simple (elementary or non-formed) hallucinations or complex (formed) hallucinations. Simple hallucinations manifest as lights, colors, lines, and shapes or geometric designs.
- Complex hallucinations differ in that these present as formed images of objects, animals, people, and lifelike scenes.

Charles Bonnet syndrome is an example of complex visual hallucinations. Hallucinations from occipital lobe are simple, while those from parietal or temporal are complex.

Charles Bonnet syndrome is complex and vivid hallucinations that occur with visual impairment with patients having insight into that being unreal (the patient must not be hearing their voices or interacting with these hallucinations). AMD is the most commonly associated pathology, but can occur in up to 60% of visually blind in one or both eyes and 15–20% of glaucoma patients with visual field defects (Menon 2005).

5.1.9.1 Migraine Visual Aura

It can be either positive (formed/unformed images perceived in the field) or negative (missing area in the field, scotoma). It can be monocular or binocular.

While migraine is the most common cause, its typical features are binocular (as it is brain in origin where fibers from both fields exist), minutes up to one hour, zigzag geometric lines (scintillating scotoma), alternating sides and patterns, and gradual spread from the center to periphery or vice versa. The classic description of the fortification spectrum involves a zigzag pattern that appears near the point of fixation, builds up over several minutes, and gradually spreads from the center to the periphery, assuming a convex shape. This phenomenon is explained by cortical spreading depression, a slowly propagating wave of depolarization followed by suppression of cortical activity.

Red flags include locked on one side (suggests lesion), monocular* (retinal migraine vs. lesions), and seconds or hours. Moreover, any change in a preexisting typical aura should prompt investigation.

* A binocular photopsia may be perceived as monocular in the eye ipsilateral to the temporal defect.

Patients who have very stereotyped visual auras that always occur in the same location in the visual field may harbor a cerebral lesion in the contralateral visual cortex. Indicated tests include visual field (may show defects that localize) and brain imaging (may show the lesion).

Migraineurs may experience a variety of episodic or persistent visual disturbances in addition to the classic fortification spectrum, including micropsia where objects appear too small, Alice in Wonderland syndrome with episodes of distorted body image, palinopsia or persistence of visual images, scintillating scotomas which are negative scotoma in the middle of fortification spectra, and "visual snow" which presents as persistent television-like static. Persistent positive visual phenomena such as visual snow are often not responsive to prophylactic treatment with migraine medication.

Visual seizures, when originating in the occipital lobe, often consist of multicolored, circular, and spherical patterns that last on the order of minutes.

5.1.9.2 Occipital Seizure

Ictal elementary visual hallucinations are stereotyped for each patient, usually lasting for seconds. They primarily consist of multiple, brightly colored, small circular spots, circles, or balls. These hallucinations mostly appear in a temporal hemifield, often moving contralaterally or in the center, where they may be flashing. They may multiply, increase in size during the course of the seizure, and progress to other nonvisual occipital seizure symptoms and, more rarely, to extra-occipital manifestations and convulsions. Blindness typically occurs usually from the onset, and postictal headaches, often indistinguishable from migraine, are common (Panayiotopoulos 1999).

5.1.9.3 Visual Snow

Visual snow (VS) is characterized by the bilateral presence of dynamic, flickering dots affecting the entire visual field, often resembling snow or pixelated television static. Visual snow has a unique "syndrome" of visual disturbances. This syndrome is defined by its persistence for longer than 3 months and the presence of at least three additional visual symptoms, which include palinopsia, entoptic phenomena, photophobia, and nyctalopia (night blindness) (Schankin et al. 2014). Up to 60% of individuals with visual snow also experience migraines, and a smaller percentage have tinnitus. Differential diagnoses for visual snow include recreational drug use, bilateral optic neuropathy, or central brain lesions. However, the most common cause is idiopathic. Anticonvulsants, particularly lamotrigine, have been frequently tried and shown the highest efficacy in case reports. Despite these visual disturbances, most patients with visual snow have normal best corrected visual acuity, perimetry, and fundoscopy. Palinopsia: Persistence or repetition of the image after removal of stimulus, which is different from afterimage. Afterimages are brief, physiological visual remnants caused by prolonged exposure to a stimulus, while palinopsia is a pathological repetition of images that persists or recurs even after the stimulus is gone. It is most commonly idiopathic (60%) but can occur with brain lesions or migraine headaches. Usually, it is a neurological disease from migraine or epilepsy, but can be from drugs (trazodone, stimulants). The approach should begin with excluding drugs and then CNS/visual pathway causes. An entopic (i.e., inside the eye) phenomena represent a spectrum of enhanced vision:

- Blue-field entoptic phenomenon: seeing around 20 dots moving when staring on the sky, presumably representing WBCs
- Floaters: seeing vitreous materials
- Spontaneous photopsia
- Self-light of the eye, described by patients as swirls or luminous clouds of orange or violet color moving centrifugally or centripetally

5.1.9.4 Dysphotopsia After Cataract Surgery

If it happens directly after cataract surgery, the differential would be:

- Negative dysphotopsia due to *shadow from the IOL*, manifested by a dark crescent or curved shadow that can appear similar to a scotoma in the peripheral temporal field of vision
- Floaters due to PVD
- Ischemic optic neuropathy

Check RAPD, and examine the retina; if all are negative, then it is mostly IOL related.

Bilateral sequential vertical streaks of light for a few seconds occur due to peripheral retinal tractions. Note that migraine usually causes bilateral simultaneous lights that are of minutes' duration.

A phosphene is the phenomenon of seeing light without light entering the eye. Normally, the retina perceives light when a photon converts 11-cis-retinol to all-trans, which will block Na channel leading to hyperpolarization. Drugs, mainly ivabradine, a cardiac Na blocker, may cause phosphene by blocking these channels in the retina.

5.1.10 Electrophysiology

Electrophysiology plays a crucial role in the evaluation of the visual system. It involves the measurement of electrical potentials in response to visual stimulation, contributing significantly to the diagnosis and assessment of various ocular and systemic diseases. These tests, including the electrooculogram (EOG), electroretinogram (ERG), and visual evoked potential (VEP), provide valuable insights into different components of the visual pathway.

- EOG is particularly useful for evaluating the retinal pigment epithelium (RPE), measuring the trans-RPE potential. Despite the c-wave in ERG also evaluating the RPE potential, it is not clinically employed. A significant advantage of EOG is that it does not require electrodes to touch the eye surface.
- ERG includes pattern ERG, which serves as a measure of ganglion cell function, offering vital information in diseases like glaucoma, which primarily affects these cells. In contrast, an abnormal flash ERG response is more commonly associated with outer retinal disorders, reflecting the test's sensitivity to photoreceptor function. Another recently developed form of ERG is multifocal ERG (mfERG), which generates a topographic ERG map of

central retinal cone-system function, making it beneficial in diagnosing macular dysfunction and assessing central retinal involvement in generalized retinal diseases.
- VEP measures the integrity of the afferent visual pathway and can be used to assess visual acuity, necessitating the correction of refractive errors prior to testing.

The conventions used in electrophysiological readings typically include "P" for positive hyperpolarization of the curve or "N" for a negative depolarization deflection. The number following "P" or "N" denotes the expected time of the peak response since the stimulus onset. The nature of the stimulus used varies among tests. For ERG, the standard stimulus is flash light, with checkerboard used in pattern ERG. Conversely, in VEP, pattern checkerboard is the primary stimulus, while flash VEP is secondary. EOG always uses flashlight stimulus.

Interpreting changes in these tests can aid in diagnosing and monitoring a variety of conditions. For instance, ischemic events are generally linked with decreased b-wave amplitude, while an increase in implicit times can suggest hereditary diseases. Conditions causing outer retinal degeneration, like multiple evanescent white dot syndrome, acute idiopathic blind-spot enlargement syndrome, and acute zonal occult outer retinopathy (AZOOR), lead to decreased waveforms on mfERG. Conversely, inflammatory diseases often present with a delay but preservation of amplitude. Understanding these electrophysiological responses thus allows clinicians to better manage their patients' visual health. Table 5.4 shows a comparison between electrooculogram (EOG), electroretinogram (ERG), and visual evoked potential (VEP).

Characteristic changes of electrophysiological studies can reflect the underlying disease process, where:

- Ischemic events are usually associated with a decreased b-wave amplitude.
- Increased implicit times may be found in various hereditary conditions.
- Extinguished ERG is seen in ophthalmic artery occlusion.
- Carriers of choroideremia are usually asymptomatic and have normal ERGs, unlike carriers of juvenile X-linked RP. Central acuity is spared until later in life in choroideremia relative to X-linked RP.
- EOG results in Best disease are almost always abnormal, even in "unaffected," asymptomatic individuals who have the causative genetic variant but have normal-appearing fundi. The light rise of the EOG is typically severely reduced or absent (Arden ratio (light:dark) of 1.5 or less).
- Causes of outer retinal degeneration, such as multiple evanescent white dot syndrome, acute idiopathic blind-spot enlargement syn-

Table 5.4 Comparison between the main three electrophysiological study types, including electrooculogram (EOG), electroretinogram (ERG), and visual evoked potential (VEP)

	Visual evoked potential (VEP)	Electroretinography (ERG)	Electrooculography (EOG)
Method	Six electrodes placed at occipital cortex	Ocular contact lens electrode and occiput electrodes	Electrodes around the eye and on occiput
Primary stimulus	Checkerboard (pattern)	Flash light	Flash light
Function measured	Optic nerve function and VA	Overall retinal layers (i.e., inner and outer retina)	Localized macular function
Main indices	P100 latency and N75-P100 amplitude	Amplitude and latency of a, b, and c waves	Arden ratio
Types	Pattern (main), flash, and sweep	Flash field (main), pattern, and multifocal	None
Main indications	Optic neuropathy assessment and VA assessment in children and amblyopia	Retinal ischemic events, retinitis pigmentosa, and hydroxychloroquine toxicity	Diagnosis of Best disease (vitelliform macular dystrophy)

drome, and acute zonal occult outer retinopathy (AZOOR), lead to decreased waveforms on mfERG. mfERG has superior diagnostic value compared to other electrophysiological studies.

Generalized inflammatory disease, such as posterior uveitis, may be associated with delayed but preserved amplitude in diagnostic tests. In particular, a significant delay in the 30 Hz flicker delay with a high amplitude almost always indicates an inflammatory etiology.

5.1.11 Cavernous Sinus Pathology

Involvement of the third, fourth, fifth (V1 and V2 divisions), sixth, and sympathetic nerves can indicate a lesion in the cavernous sinus. A mid-dilated pupil that neither reacts to light nor dilates in darkness usually signifies impairment of both parasympathetic and sympathetic innervation of the pupil. This finding, along with other symptoms, can best be explained by a cavernous sinus lesion. Meningioma and internal carotid artery aneurysm are the most common causes, especially when there is a slowly progressive history.

Consider fungal infection (e.g., mucormycosis) in diabetic or immunocompromised patients with cavernous sinus pathology.

Tolosa-Hunt syndrome: It is an idiopathic granulomatous inflammation in the cavernous sinus. It is suspected when a pathology involves facial pain (V1 and/or V2) and any of the cranial nerves III, IV, and VI, as this will localize to cavernous sinus. The next step is to show evidence of inflammation in the cavernous sinus through imaging or biopsy. Excluding secondary causes is essential, and response to steroid should be observed within few days. If the optic nerve function is involved, then this further localizes to orbital apex.

CN VI palsy with Horner syndrome is called Parkinson sign, and it represents cavernous sinus lesion.

5.1.12 Marcus Gunn Jaw-Winking Syndrome

This is present mostly as unilateral ptosis that retracts upon mastication. Most are congenital, but acquired cases exist. Male and female are affected equally.

This condition involves a connection between the motor branches of the muscles of mastication and superior division of oculomotor nerve, which controls the levator palpebrae superioris, even though the muscles themselves are normal. It is an example of synkinesis, where abnormal innervation connects two groups of normally unrelated muscles, causing them to contract together. However, it is not synkinesis resulting from aberrant regeneration. This form of synkinetic ptosis is typically unilateral and not hereditary. It is characterized by intermittent elevation of the ptotic eyelid, coinciding with the contraction of the ipsilateral external pterygoid muscle, which moves the jaw toward the opposite side.

As this condition generally improves with age, it can be monitored with observation while keeping an eye on the affected eye for amblyopia. In severe and persistent cases, surgery may be considered. However, attempting to repair only the ptosis without addressing the jaw winking could result in an exaggeration of the aberrant eyelid movement to a level above the superior corneal limbus. So, surgical options include:

- Levator muscle myectomy above the Whitnall's ligament (solve the reflux, but not the ptosis)
- Bilateral excision of the levator muscle and bilateral frontalis suspension
- Unilateral levator muscle excision and frontalis sling only on the affected side

In severe and persistent cases, surgery may be considered. However, attempting to repair only the ptosis without addressing the jaw winking could result in an exaggeration of the aberrant eyelid movement to a level above the superior corneal limbus.

Sarcoidosis most commonly affects facial nerve due to involvement of parotid gland and subsequent compression.

5.2 Conclusion

In conclusion, neuro-ophthalmology, as detailed in this chapter, is a complex and crucial field in clinical ophthalmology that intertwines both the neurological and ophthalmological aspects of medical science. We started this chapter by providing an overview, setting the foundation for understanding the nuances of this field. In the sections following the overview, we delved deeper into the intricacies of the visual pathway, exploring how visual information is transmitted from our eyes to our brains, which is integral in diagnosing and treating various visual impairments. We also discussed optic nerve diseases and optic disc anomalies, both of which can have profound implications on a patient's vision. Next, we explored idiopathic intracranial hypertension (IIH), a critical condition that, when untreated, can lead to severe visual consequences. We examined its causes, clinical features, diagnostic criteria, and management. We then looked at various diseases affecting the pupil, emphasizing the importance of the pupil in regulating light entry and contributing to the quality of vision. Understanding these diseases is pivotal in the diagnosis and management of various ophthalmic conditions. Our discussion on the role of cranial nerves in eye movements highlighted the complexity of the visual system and the delicate coordination required for proper visual function. Any disruption in these nerves can lead to strabismus or other eye movement disorders. Finally, under miscellaneous section, we discussed numerous other conditions and syndromes of neuro-ophthalmological relevance. Through this comprehensive exploration of neuro-ophthalmology, the objective is to provide ophthalmology trainees with a well-rounded understanding, encouraging a holistic approach when diagnosing and treating patients. The goal is to underscore the importance of correlating clinical findings with a patient's history and symptoms, ensuring effective management and treatment. As we conclude this chapter, we hope that it serves as a vital resource, ensuring a high yield of knowledge for upcoming exams and beyond.

Acknowledgements We would like to thank Retina Rocks® for providing the images in this chapter.

Conflict of Interest None.

References

Bartalena L et al (2021) The 2021 European Group on Graves' orbitopathy (EUGOGO) clinical practice guidelines for the medical management of Graves' orbitopathy. Eur J Endocrinol 185(4):G43–G67. https://doi.org/10.1530/EJE-21-0479

Degueure A et al (2022) An unusual presentation of vivid hallucinations. Cureus 14(5):e25441. https://doi.org/10.7759/cureus.25441

Douglas RS et al (2020) Teprotumumab for the treatment of active thyroid eye disease. N Engl J Med 382(4):341–352. https://doi.org/10.1056/NEJMoa1910434

Gilhus NE et al (2019) Myasthenia gravis. Nat Rev Dis Prim 5(1):1–19. https://doi.org/10.1038/s41572-019-0079-y

Jadhav S, Padmalakshmi K, Bhende M (2023) Red eye and choroidal detachment in an older woman. JAMA Ophthalmol 141(7):687–688. https://doi.org/10.1001/jamaophthalmol.2023.1513

Kahaly GJ et al (2023) Proof-of-concept and randomized, placebo-controlled trials of an FcRn inhibitor, Batoclimab, for thyroid eye disease. J Clin Endocrinol Metabol 108(12):3122–3134. https://doi.org/10.1210/clinem/dgad381

Menon GJ (2005) Complex visual hallucinations in the visually impaired: a structured history-taking approach. Arch Ophthalmol 123(3):349–355. https://doi.org/10.1001/archopht.123.3.349

Panayiotopoulos CP (1999) Elementary visual hallucinations, blindness, and headache in idiopathic occipital epilepsy: differentiation from migraine. J Neurol Neurosurg Psychiatry 66(4):536–540. https://doi.org/10.1136/jnnp.66.4.536

Schankin CJ et al (2014) "Visual snow"—a disorder distinct from persistent migraine aura. Brain 137(5):1419–1428. https://doi.org/10.1093/brain/awu050

Wolfe GI et al (2016) Randomized trial of thymectomy in myasthenia gravis. N Engl J Med 375(6):511–522. https://doi.org/10.1056/NEJMoa1602489

Clinical Review of Pediatric Ophthalmology and Strabismus: Part I

6

Nisreen Abushehab, Jamila G. Hiasat, Saif Aldeen Alryalat, and Almutez Gharaibeh

Abstract

This chapter explores key conditions affecting vision in children, focusing on amblyopia, strabismus, and esotropia. Amblyopia results from poor visual development, often due to misalignment or occlusion. The chapter discusses its causes, early diagnosis, and effective treatment strategies, including patching and vision therapy. Strabismus, characterized by misalignment, is examined for its impact on binocular vision and depth perception, with an analysis of treatment options such as surgical intervention and corrective lenses. Additionally, the chapter addresses other pediatric conditions, including esotropia, outlining its different types and management strategies for each. The role of pediatric ophthalmologists in multidisciplinary care and the latest advancements in diagnostic and therapeutic approaches are also discussed, underscoring the significance of these interventions for optimal visual outcomes in children.

Keywords

Pediatric ophthalmology · Amblyopia · Strabismus · Esotropia · Visual development

6.1 Postnatal Ocular and Visual Development

The growth and development of the human eye follow an algorithm. Although it is beyond the scope of this discussion to cover, it is important to keep in mind the following:

- At birth, the fovea is not fully developed, and visual acuity is roughly 20/200. The retina is almost fully developed at birth, apart from macular region which continues to show variation of thickness over age.
- Myelination of the optic nerve reaches lamina cribrosa, starting at 7 months of intrauterine life. The bony orbit continues to grow after birth until the age of 10 years.

N. Abushehab (✉)
Department of Ophthalmology, Ministry of Health, Amman, Jordan

J. G. Hiasat
Division of Pediatric Ophthalmology and Strabismus, UPMC Children's Hospital of Pittsburgh, Pittsburgh, PA, USA

Department of Ophthalmology, University of Pittsburgh School of Medicine, Pittsburgh, PA, USA
e-mail: Hiasatjg@upmc.edu

S. A. Alryalat
Department of Ophthalmology, The University of Jordan, Amman, Jordan

The University of Colorado Anschutz Medical Campus, CO, USA

A. Gharaibeh
Department of Ophthalmology, The University of Jordan, Amman, Jordan

S. A. Alryalat (ed.), *Ophthalmology Board and FRCS Part 2 Exams*,
https://doi.org/10.1007/978-981-96-1517-9_6

- The axial length of the globe has a mean of roughly 16 mm at birth and continues to increase with age.
- The average horizontal diameter of the cornea is 9.5–10.5 mm in a newborn with steeper keratometric values compared to adults.
- The lens is proportionately large in comparison to the globe. The dilator pupillae muscle is immature at birth, which is responsible for miotic pupils at a very young age.
- Infants can show signs of visual fixation as early as 4 weeks and follow objects of interests by 2 months of age.
- Stereopsis and accommodation begin to develop at the age of 4 months.
- Vertical movements are seen at 6 months.
- Intraocular pressure is lower in infants.

  In a 1-month-old infant, neonatal eye movements are present; visual fixation is evident, and preferential viewing can reveal vision from 20/200 to 20/400; and horizontal movements are normal, but vertical movements are not fully developed until age 6 months.

6.2 Basic Anatomy and Motor Physiology of Extraocular Muscles (EOMs)

Ocular position: When the eye is looking straight ahead with the visual axis parallel to the sagittal axis of the head, the eye is in primary position. Orbits diverge 23′ from the visual axis.

Muscle action is the result of muscle contraction when the eye moves from primary position. Horizontal muscles have one action, while vertical and oblique muscles have three actions: vertical, horizontal, and torsional.

The most robust action is termed primary action, followed by the less obvious secondary and tertiary actions.

Vertical recti and obliques are not aligned with the visual axis, necessitating **a certain degree of rotation to perform their primary functions, including the primary action (Table 6.1 and Fig. 6.1).**

Table 6.1 Extraocular muscle anatomical origin, insertion, length, and actions

	Origin	Anatomic insertion (mm)	Approximate muscle and tendon length (mm)	Primary action	Secondary action	Tertiary action
Medial rectus (MR)	Annulus of Zinn	5.5	40, 4	Adduction (primary position)	–	
Lateral rectus (LR)	Annulus of Zinn	6.9	40, 8	Abduction (primary position)	–	
Superior rectus (SR)	Annulus of Zinn	7.7	40, 6	Elevation (abducted 23′)	Intorsion (67′ adducted)	Adduction
Inferior rectus (IR)	Annulus of Zinn	6.5	40, 7	Depression (abducted 23′)	Extorsion (67′ adducted)	Adduction
Superior-oblique (SO)	Orbital apex above annulus of Zinn (sphenoid bone)	Posterotemporal to equator	32 and 26 (longest tendon)	Intorsion (39′ abducted)	Depression (51′ adducted)	Abduction
Inferior oblique (IO)	Lacrimal fossa (maxillary bone)	Under inferior border of lateral rectus (macular area)	37, 1 (shortest tendon)	Extorsion (39′ abducted)	Elevation (51′ adducted)	Abduction

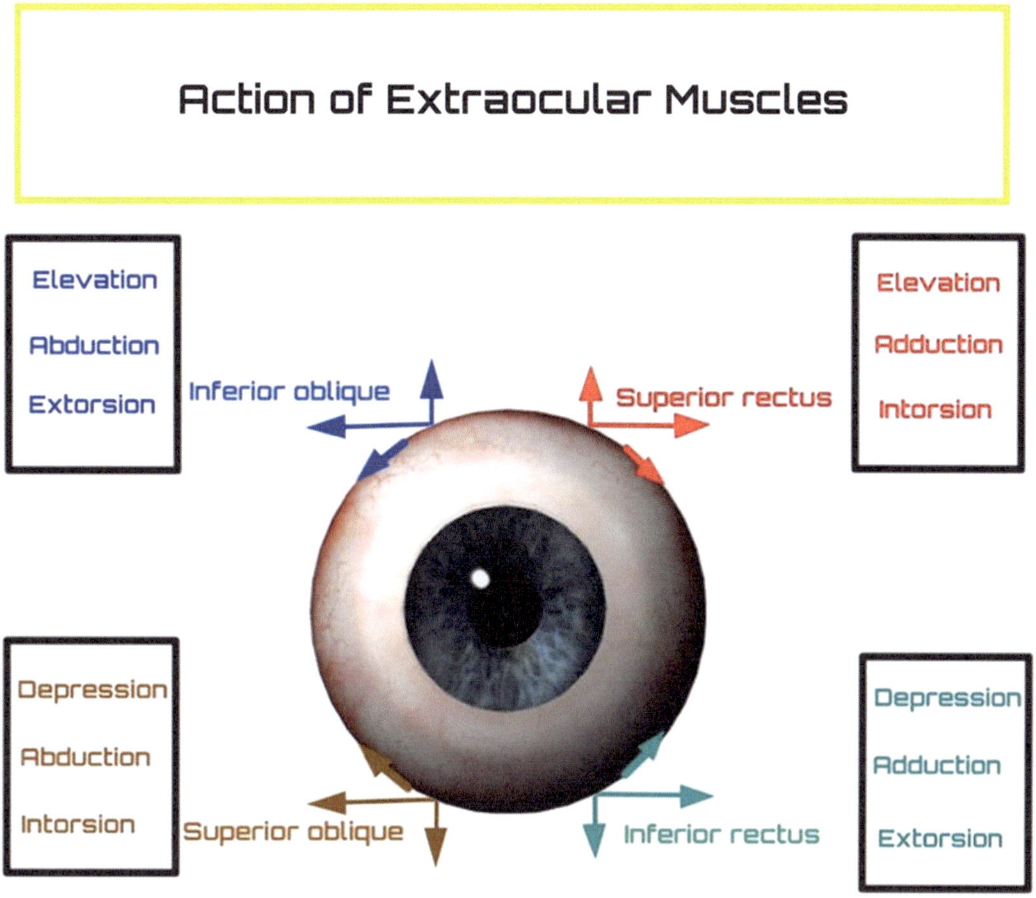

Fig. 6.1 Actions of extraocular vertical muscle

1. Vertical recti insert anterior to the equator, forming a 23° angle with the visual axis.

   Obliques insert posterior to the equator, forming a 51° angle with the visual axis.

6.2.1 Ocular Movements

The rotation of the globe occurs along the axes of Fick. The X-, Y-, and Z-axes meet at the center to produce ocular movement (Fig. 6.2). X and Z traverse through the equator of the globe and form Listing's plane. Y-axis passes through the center of the pupil perpendicular to it.

1. Horizontal X-axis: around which elevation and depression occur.
2. Anteroposterior Y-axis: around which intorsion and extorsion occur.

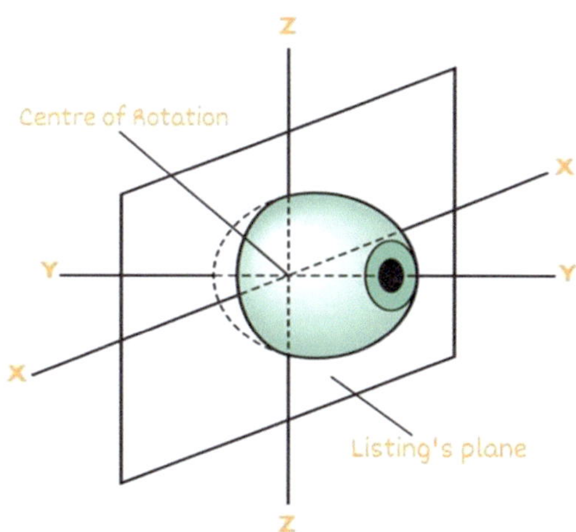

Fig. 6.2 Axes of ocular movements

3. Vertical Z-axis: around which abduction and adduction occur.

The main three ocular movements:

- **Ductions are** monocular movements without regard for the movement of the fellow eye.
- **Versions** are binocular, simultaneous, conjugate movements of both eyes.

Vergences: Binocular, simultaneous, disjunctive movements, meaning the eyes move in opposite directions. Convergence involves simultaneous adduction, or inward turning of the eyes, while divergence refers to the outward movement of the eyes from a convergent position.

Anatomical points with clinical relevance:

1. Recti tendons insert around the limbus, forming a circle called spiral of Tillaux. The spiral of Tillaux marks the approximate location of the ora serrata. The recti muscle insertion is the thinnest location of sclera, which increases the risk of perforating injury during strabismus surgery.
2. The superior and inferior rectus muscles are distinctly bound to the upper and lower eyelid by the fascial extension from its sheath; thus, surgery on them may lead to a change in the eyelid position (e.g., retraction in cases of rectus muscle recession surgery).
3. Inferior oblique is unique: it is the only muscle with an anterior anatomic origin, and approximately 10% may have more than one muscle belly. This explains residual inferior oblique overaction after a successful IO recession.
4. The anterior fibers of the superior oblique primarily control torsion, while the posterior fibers are responsible for its depressor effect. This distinction explains the different surgical approaches to the SO muscle.

(continued)

5. The nerve that supplies the inferior oblique muscle enters the lateral side, crossing the inferior rectus muscle; surgery can damage the nerve. This nerve also carries parasympathetic fibers, so damage to it may result in pupil dilation.
6. Obliques run below recti. It is important to separate SR from SO while doing strabismus surgery.
7. Tenon capsule separates the intraconal fat that present 10mm from limbus, so penetrating posterior tenon capsule during strabismus surgery (10mm or beyond) may lead to fat prolapse, and fat adherence syndrome (FAS) subsequently.

6.2.2 Vascular Supply of EOM

Extraocular muscles are the most vascularized and most innervated muscles in the body (10× than a regular striated muscle). The ratio of nerve fibers to muscle fibers is very high, approaching 1:3.

Branches of the ophthalmic artery:

The lateral muscular branch supplies the lateral rectus, superior rectus, superior oblique, and levator palpebrae superioris muscles, while the medial muscular branch, larger than the lateral, supplies the inferior rectus, medial rectus, and inferior oblique muscles.

The anterior ciliary arteries provide the main blood supply to the rectus muscle, with each muscle receiving at least two anterior ciliary arteries, except for the lateral rectus, which has only one anterior ciliary artery and contributes the least to the anterior segment circulation.

The oblique muscles do not have anterior ciliary arteries and do not contribute to the anterior segment circulation.

Vortex veins are closely associated with the insertion of superior and inferior rectus muscles.

6.2.3 Nerve Supply of EOM

Extraocular muscles are innervated by the third, fourth, and sixth cranial nerves as follows:

1. Lateral rectus is innervated by the abducent nerve (sixth).
2. Superior oblique is innervated by the trochlear nerve (fourth).
3. Medial, superior rectus muscles are innervated by the superior division of the oculomotor nerve, while the inferior rectus and inferior oblique are supplied by the inferior division (third).
4. The superior rectus is the only muscle supplied by the contralateral oculomotor nucleus.

The EOMs can be divided into two distinct layers, an orbital layer (OL) and a global layer (Table 6.2).

Agonist/antagonist and synergist muscles: The muscle that moves the eye in a specific direction is called an agonist, while the muscle that moves the eye in the opposite direction is called the antagonist (e.g., MR and LR). These are within the same eye that work together to move the eye in the same direction, like the SO and IR.

Hering's law of yoke muscles: Normally, the movements of the two eyes are in the same direction. It explains that when both eyes move in the same direction, the muscles responsible for this coordinated movement, known as yoke muscles, receive equal innervation to ensure synchronized action. This law highlights the balance between the muscles in each eye during movement. In contrast, Sherrington's law focuses on the relationship between agonist and antagonist muscles within the same eye, stating that when an agonist muscle contracts, a corresponding inhibitory signal is sent to the antagonist muscle to relax, allowing for smooth and precise eye movements.

6.3 Dysfunction of the Motor Mechanisms

Strabismus is the term for ocular misalignment and can take two basic forms: heterotropia where there is a manifest misalignment, and a heterophoria where there is a latent strabismus with good alignment maintained by motor fusion.

In the presence of strabismus, motor adaptation occurs to maintain binocular single vision; it may result in abnormal head posture, which can be:

- Face turn mainly to compensate a horizontal deviation as a result of horizontal recti palsy or restriction
- Head tilt mainly to indicate an abnormal cyclovertical muscle action
- Chin up or down mainly to compensate a vertical deviation as a result of vertical muscle palsy or restriction

Table 6.2 Differences between orbital layer and a global layer of extraocular muscles

	Orbital layer	Global layer
Site	Outer (facing orbital wall) thinner	Inner (facing globe) thicker
Action	Rotating eye on pulleys	Primary eye position and globe rotation
Fibers	Small-diameter fibers with more mitochondria and abundant vessels (red fibers)	Larger-diameter fibers with less mitochondrial content and fewer vessels
Insertion	Insert at the pulley (penetrate the tenon)	Insert at the sclera (does not penetrate tenon)
Percentage of singly innervated	80% of fibers are singly innervated	90% of fibers are singly innervated
Resistance to fatigue	Resistant to fatigue, but highly affected by botulinum injection	Amenable to fatigue, but less affected by botulinum injection
Fiber color	Darker color (mostly red fibers)	Lighter color

6.4 Approach to Understand Sensory Mechanism

Binocular single vision (BSV) or binocular fusion is to use both eyes together and merge images into one single image. Two fundamental aspects are motor fusion and sensory fusion.

BSV starts to develop as early as 3 weeks of age. Abnormal visual stimulation through blurred image or strabismus early on results in absent or poor BSV.

6.4.1 Worth's Grades of Binocular Vision

1. Simultaneous perception
2. Fusion
3. Stereopsis

6.4.2 Fusion

6.4.2.1 Sensory Fusion

Corresponding retinal points are areas on the retinas of both eyes that are equidistant from the foveal center, meaning they have zero binocular disparity. Normal retinal correspondence (NRC) occurs when images of objects align on these corresponding retinal points, resulting in the perception of a single image (Fig. 6.3). If images fall on non-corresponding retinal points, the brain perceives them as double, leading to diplopia, which then triggers feedback mechanisms to correct any misalignment of the eyes. In addition to NRC, the images must be sufficiently similar in size, brightness, and sharpness to permit sensory fusion. Unequal images (aniseikonia) present a challenge to fuse (e.g., unilateral aphakia with spectacle correction).

6.4.2.2 Motor Fusion (Vergence Movements)

Motor fusion is the vergence movements that allow for images to fall and be maintained on a corresponding retinal point. Retinal disparity outside the Panum's area simulates these fusional eye movements to maintain single binocular image.

6.4.3 Stereoscopic Vision

An empirical horopter is a conceptual line in space around the fixation point where objects project onto corresponding retinal points (4.4), resulting in zero disparity and single binocular image. Points along this horopter will not induce stereopsis because they have the same disparity as the fixation point.

Disparities that deviate from zero are categorized as crossed or uncrossed. *Crossed disparities* occur with objects in front of the horopter (near objects), while *uncrossed disparities* occur with objects behind the horopter (far objects).

Panum's area is a zone around the horopter, where images are still perceived as single despite being projected onto slightly non-corresponding retinal points (Fig. 6.4). This area is narrowest at the fixation point and expands peripherally. Images falling outside Panum's area are perceived as double, a phenomenon known as physiological diplopia.

Stimulation of disparate retinal areas for objects within Panum's fusional area will produce three dimensional stereoscopic visions.

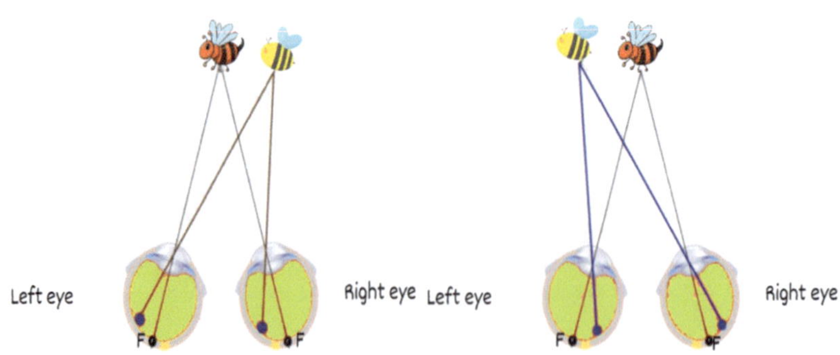

Fig. 6.3 Points on the nasal retina of one eye correspond to points on the temporal retina of the other eye

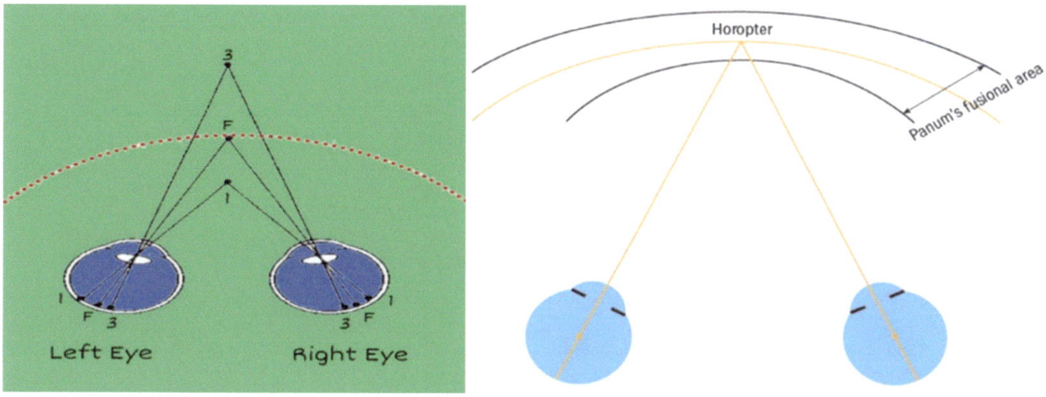

Fig. 6.4 The concept of horopter. (I) Crossed disparity, (F) objects on a horopter will stimulate corresponding retinal points (i.e., zero disparity), (3) uncrossed disparity

While stereopsis requires binocular vision, it occurs with or without bifoveal binocularity (i.e., bifoveal binocular single vision). So, stereopsis can occur with anomalous binocular single vision, when a fovea in one eye corresponds to an extrafoveal point on the other eye.

Stereoacuity is a quantitative measure of stereopsis; it represents the smallest horizontal retinal image disparity that gives rise to depth perception.

Stereopsis is measured in seconds of arc. 1 arc degree = 60 min of arc

1 min = 60 s of arc. Normal stereoacuity = <60 s of arc (the lower the value, the better the stereoacuity).

Test to measure stereopsis includes random dot tests (e.g., TNO, Frisby), which provide a more reliable assessment of BSV (up to 15 arc seconds) than contourbased tests (e.g., Titmus). Note: Stereoacuity tests that start with the letter **T** (**T**NO, **T**itmus), green-red, or polarized glasses are needed, respectively, to complete the corresponding test.

6.4.4 Accommodation and Vergence

Accommodation is a method for changing the eyes' refractive power to produce a clear retinal image (image blur is the main stimulus for accommodation).

Vergence: Disjunctive movement, simultaneous, synchronous, adduction, or abduction of both eyes.

The accommodative convergence/accommodation (AC/A) ratio is the magnitude of AC that happens for each diopter of accommodation (A).

1. Fusional vergence refers to the disconjugate eye movements that adjust for retinal image disparity. Fusional convergence addresses exophoria, while fusional divergence addresses esophoria. Fatigue or illness can diminish **the fusional vergence mechanism,** potentially leading to the development of a tropia from a previously controlled phoria. Normal fusional convergence: about 20–25 Δ at distance and 25–30 Δ at near.
2. Normal fusional divergence: about 6–8 Δ at distance and 8–10 Δ at near.
3. Normal vertical fusion: 2–3 Δ at near and distance.
4. Cyclovergence: about 8°.

6.5 Mechanism of Sensory Adaptation

Strabismus or blurred image can result in disruption of binocularity. The neurodevelopmental changes of the visual system are called sensory adaptations. Sensory adaptations can happen in the mature and immature visual systems.

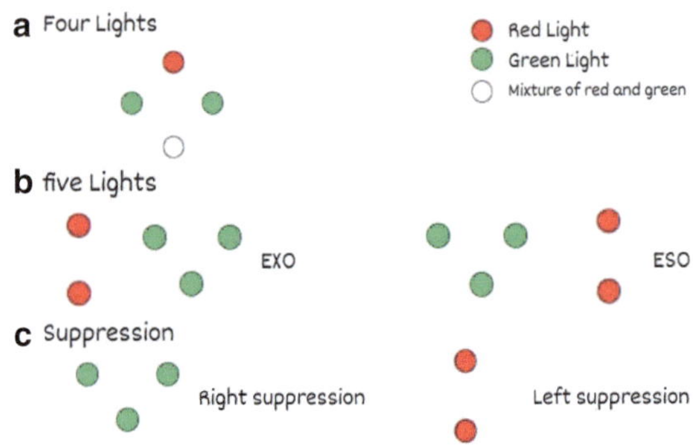

Fig. 6.5 Worth 4-dot test: (**a**) BSV or harmonious ARC with manifest deviation, (**b**) diplopia: uncrossed (esotropia) and crossed (exotropia), (**c**) right or left suppression

6.5.1 Suppression

It is the active central inhibition of one eye's visual input and occurs only during binocular viewing. Unlike amblyopia, which remains even when the better eye is closed, suppression is specifically a binocular phenomenon.

Suppression can be either *central or peripheral*. Central suppression involves the inhibition of the image from the fovea of deviating eye to avoid confusion, while peripheral suppression involves the inhibition of the image from the peripheral retina to avoid diplopia. Suppression can be *monocular or alternating*, and facultative or constant.

6.5.2 Abnormal Retinal Correspondence (ARC)

It is a cortical adaptation that allows for some degree of binocularity despite the presence of a manifest strabismus. One of the factors that determine which compensatory mechanism will occur is the angle of deviation. The lesser the deviation angle, the higher the chance for ARC presence.

Tests to Assess ARC:

1. Worth 4-dot test
2. Bagolini striated glasses
3. Base-out prism test
4. Afterimage test
5. Synoptophore: a difference between the subjective and objective angles (the angle of anomaly) that indicates that the patient has a form of ARC
6. The red filter test

6.5.3 Amblyopia

This is discussed later in the chapter.

6.5.4 Monofixation Syndrome (Microtropia)

Sub-optimal binocular vision is due to development of central suppression scotoma (<3°) with compensatory peripheral fusion, commonly as a result of a small angle strabismus (<8PD) or blurred image due to refractive error, partial cataract, etc. Amblyopia is common; however, the majority of patients have stereopsis up to 60 arc seconds.

Patients with monofixation syndrome will fuse at near with Worth 4-dot test and suppress the non-dominant eye at distance (Fig. 6.5). With Bagolini glasses, the patient will report a gap in the center of the line presented to the deviated eye.

In the base-out 4-prism diopter test, when the prism is placed in front of the non-fixating eye, no ocular motor response is observed. This is because the displaced image falls within the suppression scotoma of the non-fixating eye and is thus not perceived.

Bagolini striated glass test is a subjective clinical test to asses binocularity; a linear streak of light is shown to each eye oriented 90° apart and centered on the fixation light. Seeing the lights cross as an X means that the patient has normal vision and NRC. Through this test, suppression, microtropia, diplopia, and manifest deviations can be noted.

Worth 4-dot test consists of two green lights, one white light, and one red light. The patient wears red-green glasses, with the **r**ed lens over **r**ight eye and green lens over left eye. Flashlight is used at near (33 cm) and distance (6 m) (Fig. 6.5).

Eccentric fixation: which is usually a monocular phenomenon, unlike ARC which occurs during binocular viewing. In eccentric fixation, the eye uses a part of the retina other than the fovea for fixation. This condition is often seen in strabismic amblyopia and is associated with reduced visual acuity.

ARC is tested for and recorded simultaneously in both eyes because it is a binocular phenomenon. Eccentric fixation, a monocular phenomenon discovered by examining just one eye, is not always connected to it. The presence of eccentric fixation can have a major impact on the test outcomes because some ARC tests require independent stimulation of each fovea.

Confusion: Visual confusion occurs when two objects separated in visual space project their images to corresponding retina areas. Clinically significant visual confusion is rare.

Diplopia: Perception of two different images of the same object, and results from simultaneous stimulation of non-corresponding retinal point or disparate retinal point.

Visual acuity tests in children: Depending on the child's age, developmental stage, and cooperation, a visual acuity testing method should be used:

- Tests for preverbal patients: ability to fix and follow; optokinetic nystagmus (OKN); fixation preference; preferential looking tests; visual evoked potentials
- Tests for verbal patients: HOTV test; Snellen optotypes; Allen pictures; LEA Symbols Kay's picture tests; Tumbling E test

6.6 Measurement of Ocular Deviation and Ocular Movements (Motor Examination)

Strabismus is a condition where visual axis deviates from bifoveal fixation. There can be a manifest deviation (heterotropia) or a latent strabismus (heterophoria) as we have discussed before.

The examination of strabismus includes detection, estimation, and measurement of the deviation.

After testing in primary gazes, the measurements should be repeated in all nine gazes. Observation of head posture as well as additional version and duction testing establishes whether deviation is comitant or incomitant.

The angle of strabismus can be broadly tested by

1. Light reflex tests (Fig. 6.6)
   (a) Hirschberg's test

   It is used as an initial screen for strabismus and in uncooperative patients (e.g., babies and blinds). It is least accurate among the tests.
   - Patients' attention is critical, and the patient should be able to fixate on a light with central fixation OU.
   - Patient should be fixating on an accommodative target preferably with both eyes open.
   - They may be slightly decentered nasally in both eyes because of the physiological positive angle kappa.

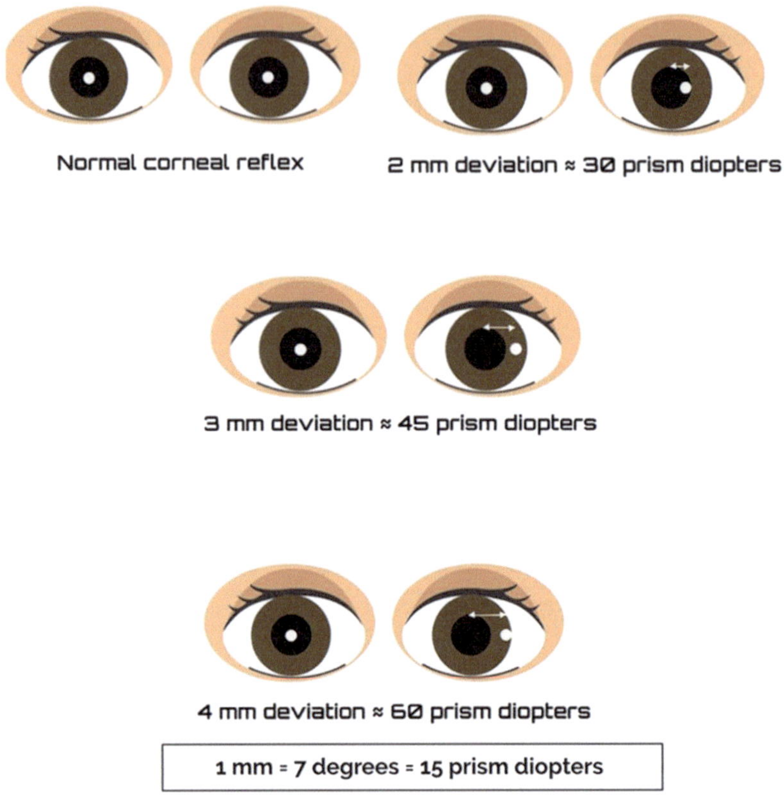

Fig. 6.6 Corneal light reflux test (aka Hirschberg's test): If light is at pupil margin (i.e., 2 mm from center), then it is 30PD; in the middle of iris (i.e., 4 mm), it is 60PD; while if at limbus (i.e., 6 mm), then it is 90PD. **1 mm = 15PD = 7°**

- Asymmetric angle kappa can lead to asymmetric reflex displacement, which can be distinguished from a true tropia using cover-uncover tests. A temporal displacement of the reflex indicates esotropia, while a nasal displacement suggests exotropia. An inferior displacement points to hypertropia, and a superior displacement indicates hypotropia.

> Krimsky test: Centralizing the light reflux using prisms in front of the *fixating eye*. As the patient fixates on an accommodative target, a prism is positioned in front of the fixing eye with the apex pointing in the direction of deviation. Prism power is increased or decreased to make the light reflex symmetrical in both eyes.
>
> Modified Krimsky test: Centralizing the light reflux using prisms in front of the *non-fixating eye*.

(continued)

> Both tests provide a rough estimate of the deviation, and it can be misleading in patients with large angle kappa.

b-bruckner reflex

Bruckner reflex is a screening test used in children. It is performed by using the direct ophthalmoscope and targeting it in both eyes simultaneously as in distant direct ophthalmoscopy.

Brighter red reflex is seen in deviated eye in strabismus, anisometropia, retinal pathology, or media opacities.

2. Cover-Uncover Tests:

> The Bruckner test compares the intensity of the light reflex between both eyes. In the presence of strabismus, brighter reflex is seen in deviated eye, as the light is reflected off the less pigmented peripheral retina.

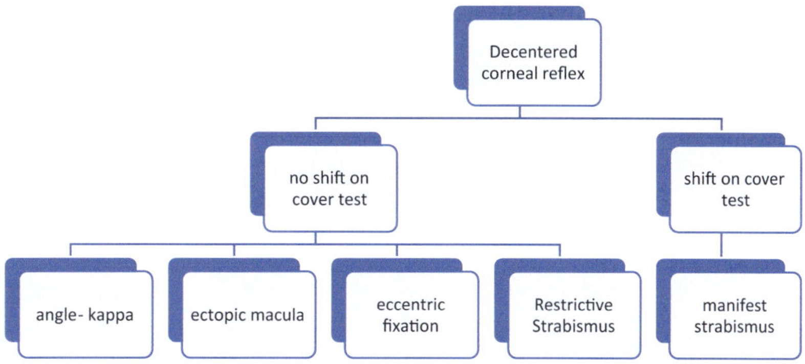

Fig. 6.7 Approach to decentered corneal reflex

(a) *Start with cover test*: Cover test is used to pick up tropias. Distance measurements are done at 6 m and near at 33 cm preferably with an accommodative target held at eye level. In the cover test, the light reflex is shown in both the eyes, and the examiner covers the apparently fixating eye while the patient fixates at an accommodative target; note the refixation shift in the uncovered eye (fellow eye).

After covering one eye, observe for a shift in the uncovered eye.

In case of no shift, cover the opposite eye and observe the uncovered eye (fellow eye) for tropia. If there is no movement/shift of either eye after covering and uncovering each eye, it implies orthotropia with no manifest squint. However, it might not rule out a phoria.

(b) *Uncover test*: Observe for corrective movement (i.e., phoria) in the eye which is *under cover*.

We start with this test if there is no manifest deviation, to detect phoria.

3. Alternate cover test

The alternate cover test disrupts fusion and manifests the phorias, and hence is more dissociating, in addition to tropia. In this test, we hold the occluder over one eye for several seconds and then rapidly move it over the other eye.

Alternate cover test for total deviation (i.e., manifest and latent)

Points to remember (Fig. 6.7):

- The cover test picks up tropias, and the uncover test may pick up phorias.
- Cover-uncover test should not be done too slowly as that may manifest a phoria due to prolonged occlusion causing dissociation.
- Other conditions which can be picked up by cover test are latent nystagmus, pseudoptosis, pseudostrabismus, and eccentric fixation.

4. Prism alternate cover test

Alternate cover testing is then performed over the prism. If there is residual deviation, prism power is increased. The point of neutralization is no movement on alternate cover test. The deviation measured in prism diopters.

For comitant deviations with full ductions, a prism can be placed in front of either eye or even split between the eyes to measure the deviation. However, when dealing with an incomitant deviation due to ocular restriction or muscle paresis, considerate is important to distinguish between the **primary and secondary deviations from accurate measurement**.

Primary deviation refers to the amount of deviation of the restricted or paretic eye, when the non-paretic eye is fixing on an object. Secondary deviation is the deviation of the "good" or non-paretic eye, when the restricted or paretic eye is fixing on an object. In incomitant strabismus, the secondary deviation is always greater than primary deviation due to Herring's law of equal innervation.

5. Simultaneous prism cover test

   A prism of approximate power (from Hirschberg) is placed in front of the deviating eye, and an occluder is placed over the fixing eye simultaneously. If the eye behind the prism does not move, it implies that the deviation is neutralized. Keep increasing prisms in case there is a shift behind the prism till there is no refixation movement.

   Quantification of a tropia only, with no contribution from a phoria, is by simultaneous prism-cover test.

   General principles:

   (a) Prisms are placed with the apex/base oriented to neutralize the deviation such that the apex is toward the direction of deviation. Apex in for esotropia, out for exotropia, down for hypotropia, and up for hypertropia.
   (b) Maintain dissociation by occluding one eye always, even while changing prisms.
   (c) Prisms should not be stacked over one another if they are of the same orientation. Vertical prisms can be stacked horizontally.
   (d) Measurement of deviation is done in nine cardinal positions of gaze.
   (e) When measuring a deviation with prisms, the eye without the prism is considered the fixing eye, while the eye looking through the prism is the non-fixing eye. This holds true regardless of the patient's fixation preference or whether amblyopia is present .Refractive correction should be worn by the patient, and if refractive error is newly corrected, 2–3 weeks should be allowed for the patient to adapt to his/her glasses.
   (f) All prism reflex tests are affected by high refractive power. Plus glasses always measure less than the actual deviation (both in esotropia and exotropia); minus glasses always measure more than the actual deviation (both in esotropia and exotropia). Effect is significant when refractive error is more than five.
   (g) A plus lens is really 2 prisms stacked base to base, and a minus lens is 2 prisms stacked apex to apex.

> 1. Remember 3M mnemonic: minus measures more, in both exotropia and esotropia.
> 2. "Plus" measures "less" in both exotropia and esotropia.

6.7 Amblyopia

Amblyopia, also known as functional amblyopia, is a condition characterized by a unilateral or, less commonly, bilateral reduction in best corrected visual acuity, resulting from abnormal visual development.

The disruption in neurodevelopment occurs due to abnormal visual stimulation, which can be caused by factors such as blurred retinal image, or strabismus, where there is a strong fixation preference for one eye, leading to cortical suppression of the nondominant eye. Children under the age of 8 are particularly susceptible to strong cortical suppression, allowing them to eliminate double vision.

6.7.1 Definition of Amblyopia

Amblyopia is defined as two Snellen lines' difference or more between the two eyes. Amblyopic patients have aggravated crowding phenomenon (because of visual cortex impairment), so their VA is poorer when assessed by full line (i.e., not individual letters).

6.7.2 Classification

Three main types of amblyopia (Table 6.3):

6.7.2.1 Strabismus Amblyopia

Strabismus amblyopia arises from competitive or inhibitory interaction between neurons that receive non-fusible input from the two eyes. Amblyopia is most likely to develop in cases where the strabismus is constant and non-alternating.

Patients with strabismus who exhibit alternate fixation and suppression are less prone to developing amblyopia, but they may still experience

Table 6.3 Comparison between different amblyopia types and their characteristics

Amblyopia type	Etiology	Notes
Strabismus amblyopia	Unilateral constant deviation	Often associated with constant esotropia
Refractive amblyopia	Anisometropia	Myopia >–3.00 D Hyperopia >+1.00 D Astigmatism >1.50
	High isometropia (bilateral cases)	Myopia >–8.00 Hyperopia >+5.00 Astigmatism >2.50 D
Deprivation amblyopia	Along visual axis Along visual pathway	Ptosis, cataract Coloboma, optic nerve pathway

abnormal binocular function. Strabismus amblyopia is characterized by constant cortical suppression, which weakens neuronal connections to the deviated eye. This form of amblyopia affects about 50% of patients with congenital esotropia, a condition involving a constant tropia. However, it is relatively rare in individuals with intermittent strabismus, such as intermittent exotropia, or those with incomitant strabismus, such as Duane's syndrome and Brown's syndrome. These patients often maintain central fusion by adopting a compensatory head posture, which helps prevent amblyopia.

6.7.2.2 Anisometropic Amblyopia

Anisometropic amblyopia occurs when different refractive errors in each eye lead to a defocused retinal image. Recent studies in the United States suggest that it may be more common than strabismus amblyopia. Most patients with anisometropic amblyopia retain good stereopsis and peripheral fusion, often presenting with monofixation syndrome.

Note

1. Better vision in mesopic conditions might be seen in conditions like anisometropic amblyopia.

6.7.3 Isoametropic Amblyopia

Isoametropic amblyopia, also known as bilateral ametropic amblyopia, is characterized by a bilateral decrease in visual acuity due to chronically defocused retinal images caused by similarly large uncorrected refractive errors in both eyes. Significant hyperopia (exceeding 4.00–5.00 D) and myopia (exceeding 5.00–6.00 D) are common risk factors. Additionally, bilateral high astigmatism greater than 2.50 D–3.00 D can result in a loss of resolving ability specific to the chronically blurred meridians, leading to meridional amblyopia.

6.7.4 Visual Deprivation Amblyopia

This is the least common form of amblyopia, but the most severe and challenging form of amblyopia to treat. It arises from an eye abnormality that obstructs the visual axis or interferes with central vision. The most frequent cause of visual deprivation amblyopia is congenital or early acquired cataracts; but other causes include blepharoptosis, periocular lesions obstructing the visual axis, corneal opacities, and vitreous hemorrhage. Severe cases of deprivation amblyopia are often associated with sensory nystagmus, such as in the case of unilateral congenital cataract.

Figure visual deprivation amblyopia

Even in bilateral cases, untreated visual deprivation amblyopia can result in visual acuity of 20/200 or worse. In children under 6 years old, dense cataracts that occupy the central 3 mm or more of the lens can lead to severe amblyopia. However, similar lens opacities acquired after the age of 6 generally cause less visual harm.

Reverse amblyopia, also known as occlusion amblyopia, is a form of visual deprivation amblyopia that can develop in the initially dominant eye if it is excessively patched during treatment.

6.7.5 Treatment Principles

Mnemonic "CAR" amblyopia: correction of refractive errors; amblyopia therapy; removal of the opacities of the media.

The basic strategy for treating amblyopia is to (Chen and Cotter 2016):

1. Provide a clear retinal image, either refractive error correction or clearing media.
2. Correct ocular dominance as early as possible during the period of visual plasticity (birth to 8 years).

Patients with unilateral amblyopia will have strong dominance for the "good eye" and will suppress the amblyopic eye.

There are two ways to switch fixation to the amblyopic eye:

1. Occlude the dominant eye.
2. Blur the vision of the dominant eye (penalization).

1. Occlusion

   Occlusion therapy (patching) is commonly used to treat unilateral amblyopia. The sound eye is covered, obligating the child to use the amblyopic eye.
2. Penalization

   Penalization is a technique used to blur the vision of the stronger, or sound, eye in order to force the amblyopic eye to take over fixation.

   This method is effective only if fixation successfully shifts from the sound eye to the amblyopic eye. Blurring the sound eye can be achieved through different methods:

   (a) Optical penalization: This involves overprescribing plus power in the sound eye, which blurs its vision and encourages the amblyopic eye to fixate.

   (b) Atropine penalization is a stronger form of penalization, particularly useful in cases of dense amblyopia. Atropine is used to induce cycloplegia (paralysis of the ciliary muscle), which blurs vision in the sound eye. This method is most effective when the good eye is hypermetropic by at least +3.00 diopters, as the cycloplegia will blur the vision sufficiently to make the amblyopic eye take over fixation, especially for near tasks. Keep in your mind:

   - Discontinuation occlusion therapy can sometimes lead to a recurrence of amblyopia, especially when the condition is associated with strabismus and suppression of diplopia. To help restore binocularity, it may be beneficial to reduce occlusion to part-time and prescribe full hyperopic correction.
   - Patients with amblyopia often demonstrate better scotopic vision (low light), as shown by improved acuity when tested with a **neutral density filter**. A mild relative afferent pupillary defect (RAPD) is also common in amblyopia. Although a central depression in the visual field has been reported, it is extremely difficult to detect using standard-sized test targets. If a central scotoma is identified on a standard visual field test, it suggests another underlying cause.
   - Iatrogenic amblyopia is rare when patching is limited to less than 5 hours per day.
   - Dense amblyopia can cause a mild RAPD, but the defect is typically subtle.

     (Other common causes include visual tract disease and extensive unilateral retinal disease.)

6.8 Art of Glass Prescription in the Pediatric Age Group

In children, the primary concern is to clear the retinal image to prevent amblyopia.

1. Refractive error occurs when there is a failure to focus the light on the retina.
2. A child by the WHO definition is a person who is between the age of 0 and 16 years.
3. The leading cause of visual impairment in children is uncorrected refractive errors.

Remember

1. Emmetropia

   It is the refractive condition in which parallel rays of light from a distant object are focused directly on the retina when the eye is not accommodating. In an emmetropic eye, the far point is at infinity, and infinity is conjugate with the retina.
2. Ametropia

   It is the absence of emmetropia and can be either refractive or axial.
3. Anisometropia

   It is a condition where there is a significant difference in refractive error between the two eyes. It is typically defined by a difference in spherical equivalent refraction (SER) of 1 diopter or more between the eyes (SER difference ≥1.00 D).
4. Aniseikonia

   It is a binocular condition in which the apparent sizes of the images seen with the two eyes are unequal.

Through the course of infancy and early childhood, the human eye experiences dramatic anatomical and physiological development. Throughout the first year of life, the eyes expand most rapidly.

So, when dealing with the pediatric age range, one should be very skilled in assessing the refractive condition; you should keep in your mind normal values of refractive error with age and process of emmetropization.

Emmetropization is both an active and a passive process. The passive process is that of proportional enlargement of the eye in the child, and the active process means error stimulates the eye to correct it and it requires normal visual experience.

Emmetropization fails when refractive errors are outside normal range for age and the risk of amblyopia and strabismus is increased. Emmetropization continues at a slower rate after the age of 3 until around 6 years of age. Proper care must be given for spectacle prescription during critical period.

What is the principle of cycloplegic refraction?

Determination of total refractive error during temporary paralysis of ciliary muscles from using cycloplegic eye drops which otherwise does not manifest on subjective noncycloplegic refraction.

When we need cycloplegic refraction (Table 6.4):

It is mandatory to relax accommodation before attempting refraction in children. Incomplete cycloplegia often leads to over- or underestimation of refractive errors.

For infants less than 12 months, the dilating drops of choice are 0.5% (or 0.25%) cyclopento-

Table 6.4 Comparison between different cycloplegic agents

Agent	Adult and pediatric doses	Onset of cycloplegia	Duration of cycloplegia
Tropicamide	1%	20 min	8 h (can take up to 24 h)
Phenylephrine	10% and 2.5%	Up to 15 min	6 h
Cyclopentolate	1% and 0.5%	15–60 min	24 h (mydriasis takes 3–7 days)
Atropine	1%, should be avoided in infants	Hours	Days–weeks

late and 2.5% (or 1%) phenylephrine. **Note that atropine drops should be avoided in young infants because of the potential for anticholinergic adverse effects. For infants older than 1 year, cyclopentolate 1% with 2.5% phenylephrine is usually used.**

Tropicamide, cyclopentolate, and atropine agents have similar side effects, including dry mucous membranes, flushing, and tachycardia, with highest frequency for atropine.

Considerations in spectacle prescription for pediatric patients:

You should keep in mind these questions when you prescribe spectacles in children less than the age of 6 years:

1. Is refractive error within the normal range for the child's age? Is this error significant for the visual needs for the child depending on his age?
2. Will this error emmetropize?
3. Is this error amblyogenic?
4. Will this error cause any effect on the strabismus if present?

6.8.1 Guidelines for Spectacle Prescription in Myopia

Myopia carries a relatively low risk of amblyopia, and symmetric myopia prescriptions should only be based on the patient's visual needs depending on age. Low-to-moderate myopia may not require a prescription for infants because infants are not expected to see distance object, if myopia exceeds -4 D; it is likely to result in visual blur and amblyopia and therefore requires a prescription. High myopia is defined as myopia higher than 6 diopters. Tables below detail the management of isometropia myopia (Table 6.5), anisometropic myopia (Table 6.6), isometropia hyperopia (Table 6.7), anisometric hyperopia (Table 6.8), isometropic astigmatism (Table 6.9), and anisometropic astigmatism (Table 6.10).

Table 6.5 Management of isometropic myopia according to age

Infants (0–1) year	<5.00 D, no need to prescribe >5.00 D, needs prescription (reduce by 1–2 D) Undercorrect because emmetropization does occur for myopia
Toddlers (1–3) years	<4.00, no need to prescribe >4.00, needs prescription (reduce by 1–2 D)
Preschool age (3–6) years	<3.00, no need to prescribe >3.00, needs prescription (reduce by 1–2 D) If it improves VA and the child appreciates it. Can give full correction at this age
School age (above 6 years)	– Full prescription must be given to prevent amblyopia – In very high myopia (≥10 D), full correction can be barley tolerated so undercorrection is recommended

Table 6.6 Management of anisometropic myopia according to age

Infant (<1 years)	Give prescription if myopic anisometropia >3D
Toddler (1–3 years)	Give prescription if myopic anisometropia >2.5 D
Preschool children	Give prescription if myopic anisometropia >2D
School age	Give prescription if myopic anisometropia >2 D

Table 6.7 Management of isometropia hyperopia according to age

Infant <1 year	When error is ≥3.50 D partial or 2/3 prescription is advised if patient is orthotropic Full cycloplegic correction is given when error is ≥2 D in patients with esotropia
Toddler (1–3 years)	Correction is given when error is ≥3.5 D partial or 2/3 prescription is advised if patient is orthotropia Full cycloplegic correction is given when error is ≥2 D in patients with esotropia
Preschool (3–6 years)	When an error is ≥2.50 D partial or 2/3 prescription is advised if the patient is ortho Full cyclocorrection given when error is ≥1.50 D in patient with esotropia
School age (above 6 years)	≥1.50 D in the school years (without symptom) is indicated for correction (full or near-full correction may be given at this age as emmetropization has essentially ended)

Table 6.8 Management of anisometropia hyperopia according to age

Infant (0–1 year)	<2.50 D, no prescription needed ≥2.50 D, prescription needed, partial if orthotropia, full if esotropia
Toddlers (1–3 years)	<2.00 D, no prescription needed >2.00D, partial prescription if orthotropia, full prescription if esotropia
Preschool age	<1.50 D, no prescription needed >1.50 D, prescription need, partial prescription if orthotropia, full prescription if esotropia
School age >6 years	1—Cycloplegic refraction is always recommended when hyperopia is present in initial retinoscopy 3—At school age, a child is expected to be nearly emmetropic 4—Isometropic error (≥1.50 D) in the school years (without symptom) is indicated for correction given full or near full 5—A full- or near-full correction may be given at this age as emmetropization has essentially ended 6—Hyperopic anisometropia (≥1.00 D) needs full correction

Table 6.9 Management of isometropic astigmatism according to age

When to consider prescribing	What to prescribe
<2.50 D in infant >2.50 D at 15 months of age upwards	No need to prescribe (Give partial correction up to 3–4 years)
≥2.00 D at 2 years of age upwards	Give partial cylinder up to 3–4 years, after which give full cylinder
≥1.50 D at 4 years upwards	Give full cylinder
≥0.75 D at school age without symptoms	Give full cylinder

Table 6.10 Management of anisometropic astigmatism according to age

Infants (0–1 year)	<2.50 D, no need to prescribe >2.5 D, need prescription, give 2/3
Toddlers (1–3 years)	>2.00 D, no need to prescribe >2.00 D, if amblyopic, give full If no amblyopia, give 2/3
Preschoolers (3–6 years)	<1.50 D, no need to prescribe >1.50 D, if amblyopic, give full If no amblyopia, give 2/3
School age (above 6 years)	<0.75 D, no need to prescribe >0.75 D, need to prescribe full

6.8.2 Anisometropic Myopia (6.6)

It can be harmful to overcorrect for myopia since it can result in accommodative spasm, which can induce severe asthenopia and esotropia.
Intermittent divergent strabismus is the only situation in which over-minused spectacles may be recommended. In order to correct exotropia, accommodative convergence is induced using minus glasses.

6.8.3 Guidelines for Spectacle Prescription in Hypermetropia

General rules:

1. If there is no esodeviation or sign of decreased vision. Correction of low hyperopia is not required. When esophoria or esotropia is present, hypermetropia needs to be fully corrected.
2. Moderate-to-high degrees of hypermetropia require correction to achieve good visual acuity.
3. To prevent refractive amblyopia in the more hypermetropic eye, more than 1 D of hypermetropic anisometropia must be corrected.
4. High hyperopia is defined as >+5.

6.8.4 Guidelines for Spectacle Prescription in Astigmatism

Studies show that 30–50% of infants less than 12 months of age have significant astigmatism, which decline over the first few years of life, becoming stable by approximately 3–5 years of age. Large cylinders in infancy will usually emmetropize. *About 2.00 D astigmatism is normal in infants and 1.50 D astigmatism in toddlers and preschoolers, and correction is not needed unless the astigmatism is associated with high myopia or high hyperopia. School-age children with 1.0–1.5 D of astigmatism may benefit from correction.*

The visual system may not be highly sensitive to uncorrected astigmatism in the first year of life. However, from around 1 year of age, uncorrected astigmatism, especially oblique astigmatism (oblique astigmatism degrades visual acuity more and is more amblyopiagenic), can be associated with meridional amblyopia.

In 3–4 years old, 1.50 D or more of astigmatism is associated with poorer recognition acuity.

Astigmatism anisometropia had to be greater than 1.50 D before amblyopia occurred.

Oblique astigmatism at any age is more amblyogenic than regular astigmatism.

Oblique astigmatism of 1.00 D and greater must be corrected from 1 year onwards.

6.9 Horizontal strabismus

6.9.1 Pseudostrabismus

It is the illusion of strabismus when none exists. Pseudoesotropia is more common than pseudoexotropia.

Pseudoesotropia can occur in:

1. Wide nasal bridge (most common)
2. Prominent epicanthal folds (semilunar fold of skin at the medial canthus)
3. Small interpupillary distance
4. Myopia
5. Negative angle kappa (angle formed by pupillary axis and visual axis at the pupil) where corneal light reflex appears to be on the temporal side of the pupillary center

Pseudoexotropia can occur in:

1. Hypertelorism, which is widely set eyes with wide interpupillary distance (most common).
2. Positive angle kappa, where macula is dragged temporally and corneal reflex appears nasally. It is mostly seen in retinopathy of prematurity as a result of temporal dragging of the macula; it can also be seen in ectopic macula resulting from toxocara retinal scars, high myopia, or congenital retinal folds.

6.9.2 Angle Kappa

Normally, the angle kappa is slightly positive with 5′ (Fig. 6.8), meaning that the macula is temporal, so light reflex on the cornea appears deviated nasally, giving the impression of exotropia.

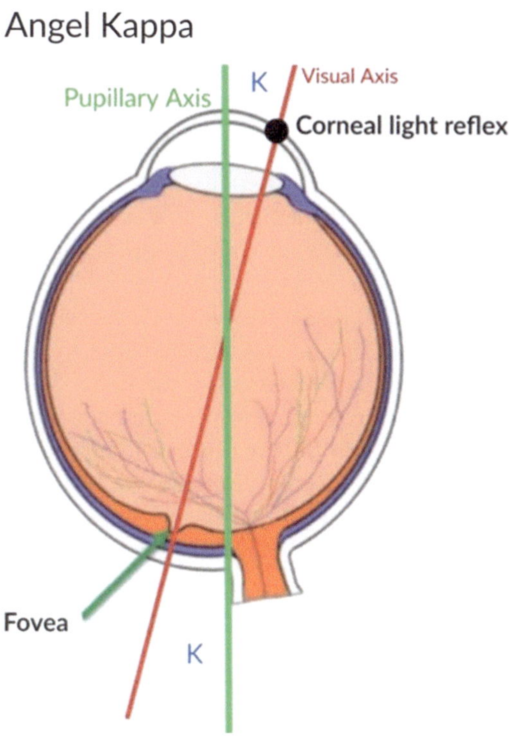

Fig. 6.8 Representation of angle kappa

Large positive angle kappa and negative angle kappa give the impression of exotropia and esotropia, respectively.

The visual axis is an imaginary line that connects object in space, and the center of the fovea is different from the anatomical axis; pupillary axis is an imaginary line perpendicular to the cornea. The angle between the two axes is the angle kappa, which is mostly 5′. It is normal (aka positive) when the macula is temporal to the center of the retina (Fig. 6.9).

6.9.3 Esotropia

Esotropia prevalence is 3.3% in pediatrics. It is classified as follows:

6.9.3.1 Infantile Esotropia (Congenital Esotropia)

It is a large-angle esotropic deviation that presents before the age of 6 months and represents nearly 50% of all cases of esotropia.

Note

There is a term small angle neonatal esotropia, which is esotropia of small, variable angle (15–35 PD), with an onset from birth to 2 months of age. Approximately 30% will resolve spontaneously by 6 months of age.

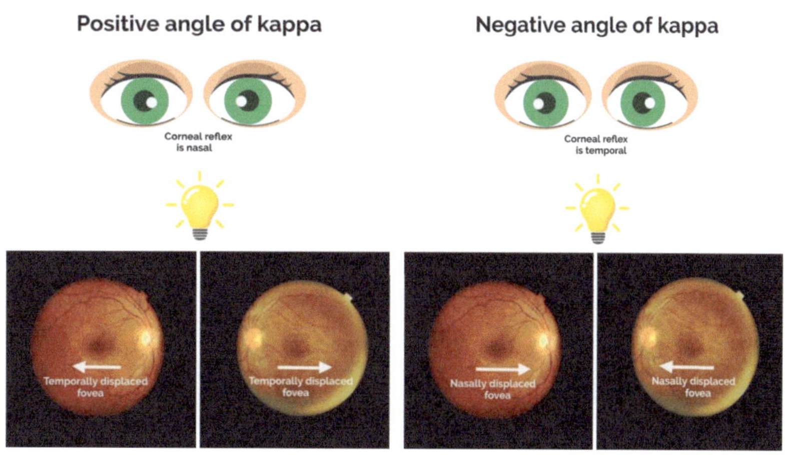

Fig. 6.9 Relation of angle kappa on corneal light reflux and foveal displacement

Clinical Features of Congenital Esotropia

- Large angle constant esotropia (≥40 PD), usually with mild limited abduction that disappears in monocular duction testing.
- Onset from birth to 6 months of age.
- Spontaneous resolution is rare.
- Amblyopia is common (30–50%); most cases have fixation preference with one eye.
- Not associated with high refractive error, up to +2.25 sphere (i.e., not accommodative).
- Note that high AC/A ratio is not typical in infantile form.
- Associated motor phenomena (usually present after 2 years of age):

    1. Inferior oblique overaction (IOOA) (60%).
    2. Dissociated vertical deviation (DVD) (40%) which violates the Hering's law. Present at all gazes, usually asymmetric between the eyes and intermittent.

        * DVD and IOOA (resulting in V pattern mostly) mimic bilateral sixth nerve palsy, usually develop after 1 year, and are present in 80% by the age of 3 years.
    3. Latent nystagmus (40%): This signals poor monocular vision and usually improves binocularly (congenital motor nystagmus).
    4. Asymmetrical optokinetic nystagmus.

        Monocular asymmetrical OKN

        Asymmetry optokinetic nystagmus normally presents in all infants up to age of 6 months and then becomes symmetrical. In patients with congenital esotropia, it remains asymmetrical.

        Asymmetry means abnormal response when drum rotates from nasal to temporal, and normal response when drum rotates from temporal to nasal.
    5. Cross fixation: Alternate fixation of either eyes, and cross fixate for lateral targets (i.e., right eye for left targets and vice versa).

Management

In general, congenital esotropia needs to be surgically corrected to allow binocular vision as soon as possible. The strabismus surgery of choice is bilateral MR recession.

First Line of Treatment Is Amblyopia Management

Amblyopia should be treated before surgery by patching the dominant eye until the patient can maintain good fixation with the nondominant eye, as this treatment can influence the angle of strabismus.

Follow-up is necessary to test for changes in fixation preference, as just 1 or 2 weeks of patching can sometimes reverse fixation preference in young infants.

Timing of Surgery for Congenital Esotropia

Most studies recommend early surgery for congenital esotropia, and to be performed between 6 months and 1 year of age in order to achieve peripheral fusion and measurable stereoacuity.

The Congenital Esotropia Observation Study (CEOS) showed that spontaneous resolution was rare (2–4%), and if there is constant large-angle esotropia (≥40 PD) with the angle stable or increasing on at least two examinations, two or more weeks apart, *early surgery should be considered*.

Intermittent small-angle esotropia (<30 PD may improve with observation with spectacles if needed) may resolve in approximately one-third of cases.

Surgery needs to be balanced between early surgery (at 6 months) that improves binocularity and stereopsis but with higher reoperation rate (some may switch to exo) and between delayed surgery (2–3 years) with fewer surgeries but worse binocularity.

In general, the eye in infantile esotropia should be surgically aligned by the age of 12 months and very latest by the age of 2 years.

Note: Presence of high diopter hyperopia may reflect an accommodative component, and diagnosis is likely to be an infantile accommodative esotropia; see later.

Surgical Procedure

Bilateral medial rectus (MR) muscle recessions (measure from the limbus) using the near deviation as the target angle.

Prognosis of Congenital Esotropia

Motor alignment is achieved in about 80% of surgical cases.

If alignment is within 8 PD of orthotropia and is achieved before the age of 2, approximately 60–80% of patients will achieve some degree of peripheral fusion and gross stereopsis, often referred to as monofixation syndrome. If alignment is achieved after the age of 2, the likelihood of obtaining significant binocular fusion is reduced.

The timing of strabismus surgery for congenital esotropia remains controversial, with recent data suggesting that earlier surgery may lead to better stereopsis outcomes.

Differential Diagnosis (Fig. 6.10)

Differential Diagnosis of Infantile ET with Limited Abduction

1. Duane's syndrome
2. Congenital fibrosis syndrome
3. Congenital sixth nerve palsy (very rare—usually transient, resolving by 4 months of age)
4. Infantile myasthenia gravis

6.9.3.2 Infantile Accommodative Esotropia

Patients with infantile accommodative esotropia are usually highly hypermetropic. They must accommodate a considerate amount to see clearly. Convergence is linked with accommodation; when they overaccommodate, they overconverge, thus developing an esotropia.

> Every child with eye misalignment that does not correct by the age of 4 months should have complete ophthalmic examination.

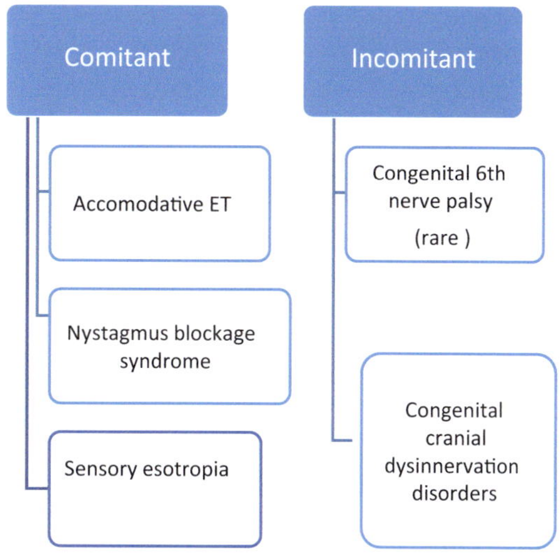

Fig. 6.10 Differential for esotropia with onset before 6 months of age

Clinical Features

- Acquired esotropia, onset at 2 months to 1 year of age
- Hypermetropia >+2.50 sphere (usually +3.00 to +6.00 sphere)
- Variable deviation, often intermittent

Management

Prescribe the full hypermetropic correction.

Evaluate and treat amblyopia after spectacles are prescribed. If a residual esotropia persists (>10 to 15 PD), after prescribing full hypermetropic correction, then we consider partly accommodative esotropia, and surgical correction is indicated.

6.9.3.3 Accommodative Esotropia

- It occurs from 6 months to 7 years of age (mostly between 2 and 3 years of age) with the deviation for near fixation being larger than that for distance.
- Hypermetropia ranging from 2.00 to 7.00 D (rarely more than +7.00 D because of lack of

accommodation at high degrees of hyperopia).
- Most neonates are not yet accommodating (as the accommodative reflux is not present at birth), so the accommodative esotropia is acquired when the infant starts to accommodate to bring vision in focus.
- Accommodative esotropia is usually intermittent at onset, but may become constant.
- Accommodative esotropia occurs when uncorrected hyperopia leads the patient to accommodate excessively to sharpen the retinal image. This increased accommodation results in increased convergence of the eyes. If there is insufficient fusional divergence to counteract this convergence, esotropia develops.
- There is evidence that some highly hyperopic patients are protected from accommodative esotropia despite an appropriate unaided focusing effort due to a low AC/A.

There are three types of accommodative esotropia:

1. Refractive accommodative esotropia
   (a) *Refractive accommodative ET (fully accommodative esotropia)*

      It is due to uncorrected hypermetropia with normal AC/A ratio (AC/A ratio ≤5)

      It is an intermittent esotropia (angle at distance = near) which is related to accommodative effort appearing at near and at stress. With an onset of 1–3 years, having hyperopia of +3D to +6D, the deviation is always variable, and esotropia regresses on all positions with hyperopia correction, and there is a tendency of the deviation to diminish with decreased accommodation with age.

   (b) *Refractive accommodative ET with high AC/A (AC/A ratio >5)*
      - Excessive convergence response for the amount of accommodation required to focus while wearing their full cycloplegic correction.
      - An intermittent esotropia appearing at near and at stress.
      - They usually have hyperopia, but can occur with any refractive error.
      - The esotropia regresses for far with full hyperopia correction and disappears (or becomes <10PD) with plus correction (usually +3.00) for near.
2. Partially accommodative with high AC/A ratio (mixed type)
   - Most common type
   - Residual esotropia after full hyperopic correction, measured more at near

   Microtropia and bilateral inferior oblique overaction are common.

   The condition usually requires surgical correction after correction of ametropia. The surgical correction as soon as possible aims to restore binocular vision with spectacles.
3. Nonrefractive accommodative esotropia (high AC/A) ratio

   It is a condition that is diagnosed when an emmetropically corrected patient—regardless of refractive error, though hypermetropia may be present—exhibits orthotropia at distance fixation but shows more than 10 prism diopters of esotropia at near fixation. This condition can be fully corrected with a +3.00 diopter add lens over each eye. Usually, the esotropia is more pronounced at near fixation to distance fixation. Nonrefractive accommodative esotropia can be treated with bifocal lenses, miotics, or surgical (e.g., bimedial recession).

   Two types:

   (a) Nonrefractive with convergence excess ET
      - ET is caused by an abnormally high accommodative convergence/accommodation (AC/A) ratio.
      - A normal near point of accommodation (accommodation is normal).

   (b) Nonrefractive hypoaccommodative ET
      - ET for near fixation due to increased accommodative effort to overcome a weakness of accommodation (remote near point of accommodation).
      - In both conditions, patient is orthotropic with BSV for distance. The

deviation is greater for near fixation with suppression and is unrelated to the refractive error.

It is treated by prescribing straight top executive bifocal lenses with the near addition or surgically (bilateral medial rectus recession ± Faden).

Treatment of Accommodative Esotropia

Our aim is to discourage the accommodative innervational effort needed for clear vision, whether such effort is essentially normal, excessive, or required because of subnormal accommodative response.

The goal of treatment for esotropia is to reduce the manifest deviation to within 8 PD or less. Achieving this level of alignment allows for the development of at least peripheral fusion and may potentially enhance fusional amplitudes.

1. The first step is to prescribe full hypermetropic correction; the goal is to align with the patient wearing full hypermetropia and obtain binocular fusion (significant refractive error that needs glass is more than +2.00 sphere).
   (a) Corrects the esotropia for both distance and near to within 8 PD—residual angle that allows for peripheral fusion and surgical correction is not indicated.
   (b) Corrects the esotropia for distance, but there is a residual esotropia of more than 10 PD for near—suspected high AC/A ratio accommodative esotropia that is treated with either bifocal glasses or surgery.
   (c) Residual esotropia more than 10 PD for both distance and near—partially accommodative esotropia: surgery is indicated.
2. Anticholinesterase Miotics
   (a) It is an option to reduce the angle without glasses. Pilocarpine causes contraction of the ciliary muscle, thereby keeping the eye in an accommodative state.
   (b) Miotics are an alternative method of facilitating accommodative effort. As such, it can be used to treat accommodative esotropia by reducing the drive for convergence.
   (c) Disadvantage applies to anisometropic hyperopia, because facilitation of accommodation will be directed to the needs of the less hyperopic eye, doing little to remove a source of amblyopia. Furthermore, miotics do not compensate for an astigmatic component of the refractive error.

Important Point in Accommodative Esotropia Treatment

1. When the child can maintain near vision without tropia through the near add (+3 add), the near add can be reduced as to wean from glasses and allow the child to develop divergence amplitude, so keep full cycloplegia prescription for far, and reduce the near add from +3 to +2 and assess if only phoria is present.
2. Bifocals are prescribed for esotropia when the patient can fuse at distance but exhibits esotropia at near while wearing full hyperopic correction.
3. Fully accommodative esotropia requires full cycloplegic refraction, as even a small esotropia can disrupt binocular fusion.
4. Some practitioners attempt to reduce the plus power in an effort to wean patient spectacles, but there is no evidence to support that reducing plus power increases the likelihood of outgrowing the need for glasses. However, data shows that providing full plus correction does not hinder the natural reduction of hypermetropia. Reducing the plus power often results in a small esotropia, which can compromise the development of binocular fusion.
5. Once full-time spectacle wear begins, esotropia may increase when the child is not wearing glasses. This is because the child exerts a strong accommodative effort to achieve an image as clear as the one experienced with refractive correction.
6. Before diagnosing a patient with partially accommodative esotropia, you need to make sure that they fully wear their glasses and the cycloplegia refraction was done with full cycloplegia, so repeat cycloplegic refraction at the next visit.

7. The prismatic diopter difference between near and far that is **considered significant is 10PD** (termed clinically significant difference); if the difference is less, then this is considered equal near and far.

For the long-term management of both refractive and high AC/A ratio accommodative esotropia, it is important to note that hyperopia usually increases until age 5–7 years before it begins to decrease.

6.9.3.4 Acute-Onset Comitant Non-accommodative ET

This should be carefully differentiated from paralytic strabismus paying careful attention to motility limitation and near-distance deviation difference. There is no other associated ocular abnormality. Neuroimaging should be considered. Surgical correction is indicated (bilateral medical rectus recession).

6.9.3.5 Cyclic Esotropia

Intermittent esotropia can present in a cyclic pattern, usually occurring every other day in a 48-h cycle, although variable intervals and 24-h cycles have also been documented. On strabismus days, fusion and binocular vision are usually absent or defective, while there is improvement on the orthotropic days. Surgical treatment is generally effective, with the amount of surgery based on the maximum angle of deviation present when the eyes are esotropic. Cyclic esotropia can be either congenital or acquired and does not respond to hyperopic correction.

6.9.3.6 Sensory Esotropia

Sensory ET develops as a result of one eye's poor vision. If the underlying reason of poor vision is treatable, treatment includes amblyopia therapy as well as surgical correction.

6.9.3.7 Divergence Insufficiency

It can manifest in two forms: primary isolated divergence insufficiency and secondary divergence insufficiency. The primary form, also known as age-related distance esotropia, is a benign and slowly progressing condition that typically affects patients over 50 years old. In contrast, the secondary form is rare and associated with neurologic abnormalities such as pontine tumors, increased intracranial pressure, or severe head trauma and is likely due to mild sixth nerve paresis. Both forms of divergence insufficiency present with a greater deviation at distance than at near and are generally comitant, making them difficult to distinguish from sixth nerve palsy.

6.9.3.8 Sixth Nerve Palsy

It can occur acutely due to infection, trauma, tumor, or ischemic events. It is often associated with a compensatory head turn toward the side of the affected lateral rectus muscle. It often resolves within weeks, during which patching may prevent amblyopia if face turn is not present. In childhood, almost 70% of abducens palsies can be accounted for by trauma, primary intracranial tumors (especially pontine gliomas and cerebellar astrocytomas), and congenital or postinfectious etiologies. It is important to perform duction eye movements rather than version. Deficit is noticed better when the unaffected eye is occluded. Moreover, the esotropia is worse for distance than near.

Muscle sequelae of right sixth nerve palsy are:

1. Overaction of the left medial rectus (yoke muscle overaction)
2. Contracture of the right medial rectus
3. Secondary inhibitional palsy of the left lateral rectus

Management of Right Sixth Nerve Palsy

Injecting botulinum toxin into the right medial rectus can help reduce its contracture. If the angle of deviation is small, a base-out Fresnel prism placed over the paralyzed eye can assist in fusing the double images. For patients without inhibition of the left lateral rectus, surgical option includes:

(a) Recession of the left medial rectus combined with resection of the right lateral rectus (affected muscle)
(b) Faden operation on the left medial rectus

In cases with fully developed muscle sequelae, the recommended surgery is recession of the right medial rectus combined with resection of the right lateral rectus.

6.9.3.9 Spasm of the Near Reflux

It is a substitution of a convergence movement for a gaze movement during horizontal versions, often leading to intermittent esotropia. Patients may exhibit combinations of excessive convergence, increased accommodation, and miosis. This condition can present as acute esotropia alternating with orthotropia. Cycloplegia is useful in managing this condition. The presence of new myopia (pseudomyopia) supports the diagnosis, although it can be different to confirm if the spasm is intermittent. However, the presence of miosis on attempted lateral gaze is an important diagnostic clue.

6.9.3.10 Residual Esotropia

Residual angle esotropia >15 PD after surgery for esotropia

6.9.3.11 Consecutive Esotropia

It occurs mostly after exotropia surgical procedure; always consider occlusion if visual acuity is also affected and the angle is >10PD.

Strabismus fixus convergence or "heavy eye" syndrome (HES)

It is a cause of acquired esotropia typically occurring in the context of high myopia. Patients with this condition often present with diplopia due to progressive esotropia and hypotropia, accompanied by limited abduction and elevation. While esotropia and hypotropia are most common, cases involving exotropia and hypertropia have also been reported. It is due to lateral rectus muscle infero-displacement and superior rectus nasal displacement. It shows no association between the amount of hypotropia and of anisometropia (Hennein and Robbins 2021).

Conflict of Interest None.

References

Chen AM, Cotter SA (2016) The amblyopia treatment studies: implications for clinical practice. Adv Ophthalmol Optom 1(1):287–305. https://doi.org/10.1016/j.yaoo.2016.03.007

Hennein L, Robbins SL (2021) Heavy eye syndrome: myopia-induced strabismus. Surv Ophthalmol 66(1):138–144. https://doi.org/10.1016/j.survophthal.2020.06.001

7 Clinical Review of Pediatric Ophthalmology and Strabismus: Part II

Nisreen Abushehab, Jamila G. Hiasat, Saif Aldeen Alryalat, and Almutez Gharaibeh

Abstract

This chapter continues to delve into pediatric ophthalmology, beginning with an exploration of exotropia, including its causes, diagnosis, and management. It also discusses divergent strabismus (DVD) and its implications for binocular vision. The chapter then addresses incomitant ocular motor apraxia (IOOA), emphasizing its impact on ocular alignment and movement. Rare syndromes such as congenital fibrosis of the extraocular muscles (CFEOMs), monocular elevation deficiency (MED), and Möbius syndrome are examined, highlighting their clinical features and associated ocular anomalies. Finally, the chapter discusses nystagmus, detailing its various types, underlying causes, and management strategies. By providing a comprehensive overview of these conditions, the chapter aims to enhance understanding and improve outcomes in pediatric ophthalmic care.

Keywords

Exotropia · Nystagmus · Binocular vision · Pediatric vision disorders · Rare conditions

7.1 Exotropia

Exophoria X, intermittent exotropia X (T), and constant exotropia XT are often seen as a continuum within the same spectrum, characterized by progressively weakening fusional control, influenced by factors such as alertness, general health, anxiety, and their level of cooperation during examination. Exotropia often becomes apparent as the amplitude of accommodation and tonic convergence begin to decline, though it can occur in infancy. As exophoria begins to decompensate, the patient may experience symptoms as diplopia, asthenopia, or photophobia, which arise due to absence of near clues that help control the deviation. If the deviation persists, suppression develops, leading to the loss of these symptoms. It has worse prognosis and is less common in children than esotropia. It occurs spontaneously in blind eye or amblyopic eyes (aka sensory exotropia).

N. Abushehab (✉)
Department of Ophthalmology, Ministry of Health, Amman, Jordan

J. G. Hiasat
Division of Pediatric Ophthalmology and Strabismus, UPMC Children's Hospital of Pittsburgh, Pittsburgh, PA, USA

Department of Ophthalmology, University of Pittsburgh School of Medicine, Pittsburgh, PA, USA
e-mail: Hiasatjg@upmc.edu

S. A. Alryalat
Department of Ophthalmology, The University of Jordan, Amman, Jordan

The University of Colorado Anschutz Medical Campus, CO, USA

A. Gharaibeh
Department of Ophthalmology, The University of Jordan, Amman, Jordan

S. A. Alryalat (ed.), *Ophthalmology Board and FRCS Part 2 Exams*,
https://doi.org/10.1007/978-981-96-1517-9_7

Table 7.1 Difference between infantile exotropia and infantile esotropia

	Esotropia	Exotropia
Prevalence in pediatric	More common (>50%)	Less common
	Infantile esotropia	Infantile exotropia
Prevalence in adults	Same	Same
Gender	Equal	Female predominance
Neurological associations	Rare	More common
Course	Mostly constant	Mostly intermittent
Amblyopia and diplopia	More common (>50%)	Rare
If starting after 6 months	Congenital esotropia	Infantile/constant exotropia
Role of genetics	Present	Absent
Role of miotics	Improve	Worsen

7.1.1 Congenital Exotropia (Infantile)

In contrast to infantile esotropia, minimal to no refractive error and neurological and ocular abnormalities present in 50% of cases (Table 7.1).

7.1.1.1 Clinical Features

1. It is a rare condition.
2. Onset by 6 months of age, usually present at birth at first few weeks.
3. Mainly constant exotropia.
4. Large angle >40 PD.
5. Poor fusion associated with amblyopia more than intermittent exotropia.

7.1.1.2 Etiology

Unknown

7.1.1.3 Treatment

- Correct amblyopia if present.
- Surgery for XT after 6 months of age; bilateral lateral rectus recession can be done to correct misalignment.

Note:
Infantile exotropia characteristics similar to infantile esotropia, including limited binocular potential (poor fusion potential), oblique dysfunction with associated alphabet pattern, latent nystagmus, and DVD.

7.1.2 Intermittent Exotropia

Most common form of XT (75% of all exotropia)

Onset: typically, in first few years of life (2–3 years)

Most common symptoms:

1. Blur vision.
2. Asthenopia.
3. No diplopia (mostly the image from the deviated eye is suppressed and the patient does not report diplopia).
4. Monocular eye closure in bright sunlight as protective mechanism (the diplopia develops upon looking at bright sun, leading to closing of one eye to compensate, a phenomenon called diplophotophobia).
5. Mild amblyopia occasionally occurs in intermittent exotropia, but severe amblyopia is uncommon.

   Excellent stereopsis is expected with well-controlled intermittent exotropia, and this stereopsis is better than what is observed in monofixation syndrome.

Exophoria usually breaks to exotropia with inattention and with stimulation, more on far than near. The deviation often becomes manifest with fatigue, visual inattention, or illness when fusional compensatory mechanisms are compromised.

The difference between exophoric and intermittent exotropia is that the tropic spontaneously breaks, while the phoria breaks only with stimulation.

Exodeviation control may be categorized as follows (progression of exotropia):

1. Good control: Stage of latent deviation (phoria)

   Exotropia is only apparent after cover testing, and the patient quickly resumes fusion without blinking or refixating.
2. *Fair control: Stage of intermittent exotropia (distance deviation > near deviation)*

   Exotropia becomes evident after fusion is disrupted by cover testing, and the patient resumes fusion only after blinking or refixating.
3. *Poor control: Stage of constant exodeviation (inadequate fusional convergence leads to constant exotropia)*

   Exotropia manifests spontaneously and may remain manifest for an extended time.

   Remember that miotics are useful in accommodative esodeviation (causes myopic shift, so corrects hyperopia but worsens myopia), but are likely to make an intermittent exotropia worse.

   The most common cause for constant exotropia is the decompensation of intermittent exotropia. In intermittent exotropia, high AC/A ratios develop as a fusional mechanism to manage near work.

7.1.2.1 Classification of Exotropia

1. Basic exodeviation
2. Convergence insufficiency pattern
3. Divergence excess pattern
4. Simulated divergence excess pattern

Basic Intermittent Exotropia

Deviation at distance is within 10 prism diopters of the near deviation.

Patients with this condition typically exhibit normal tonic fusional convergence, accommodative convergence (normal AC/A ratio), and proximal convergence.

It is associated with both divergence excess and convergence insufficiency.

It is also known as mixed-type exodeviation.

Convergence Insufficiency

Near deviation is 10 prism diopters greater than the distance deviation (15% of exotropia). It occurs in older children, where they have intermittent exotropia for near more than far. It is accompanied by a decrease in near point of convergence and convergence amplitude. They often report asthenopic symptoms near work. It can be partially managed by orthoptic exercises and managed ultimately with medial rectus resection.

Divergence Excess Pattern

This is a subtype of intermittent exotropia in which distance deviation is 10 prism diopters greater than the near deviation.

Before making a diagnosis of divergence excess, a patch test should be done, and if the far exotropia is still higher than near, then it is considered a *true divergence excess*; otherwise, it is termed *simulated divergence excess*, and it is managed similar to the intermittent basic exotropia.

True Divergence Excess

Sixty percent of patients with true divergence excess had a high AC/A ratio (prone to postoperative overcorrection at near if the distance measure is used as a surgical target angle), and 40% had a normal AC/A ratio.

Bifocal glasses (+3 add for near) can be used for a high AC/A ratio and should be discussed preoperatively with patients who have true divergence excess. It is managed mainly by lateral rectus recession, as it is too tight in those patients.

True divergence excess (60% of all divergence excess!)→ Far > near > 10 PD → high AC/A ratio → bifocal should be tried → overcorrection expected in 75% of cases (worse prognosis) leading to consecutive esotropia.
High AC/A ratio usually responds to refractive error correction and minus overcorrection, but they may convert to esotropia with surgery correction.

So, all patients with suspected divergence excess should undergo refraction, 30-min occlusion test. If true divergence excess is suspected, the next step is to trial a bifocal with a +3.00 D add lens to assess if the patient has a high AC/A ratio. If the near deviation increases significantly, approaching the distance deviation with the +3.00 D add, it indicates a high AC/A. This is crucial because patients with a high AC/A ratio are at risk of overcorrection (with a chance of 75% overcorrection) if surgery is performed based on the full distance deviation . Parents should be informed about the poor prognosis associated with this condition and the potential need for bifocal to manage the high AC/A ratio postoperatively.

Prognosis should be done before surgery and of the possible need for bifocals to decrease the high AC/A ratio postoperatively.

Simulated or Pseudo-Divergence Excess

In cases where there is a larger exotropia at distance than near, the near deviation increases to within 10 prism diopters of the distance deviation after 30–60 min of monocular occlusion (i.e., during a patch test).

As these patients have increased tonic fusional convergence at near, the prolonged monocular occlusion reduces tonic fusional convergence, revealing the full latent deviation.

Some recommended half-an-hour patching for the diagnosis of a pseudo-divergence excess type of exodeviation. Patch test is used to uncover the total angle of deviation and determine the target angle for surgery. It suspends the tonic fusional convergence and hence differentiates true divergence from pseudo-divergence excess. Patching for 30 min is now considered appropriate. Other types of exotropia are the following:

7.1.3 Sensory Exotropia

Sensory esotropia or exotropia may occur secondary to sensory deficit and poor vision.

Causes: any cause that leads to poor vision such as marked anisometropia as unilateral high myopia, retinoblastoma (22% present with strabismus), unilateral cataract, etc.

7.1.4 Consecutive Exotropia

It occurs in some children after surgery for esotropia.

Treatment:
Correct refractive error if present
Occlusion
Surgical correction

All forms of exotropia should be monitored, and some require treatment. Young children with intermittent exotropia and good fusional control should be followed without surgery, sometimes with patching treatment trials. Deviations that are present most or all of the time often require treatment. Amblyopia is uncommon in patients with intermittent exotropia, but, if present, should be treated.
Surgical intervention is considered if the deviation is constant, intermittent with poor control and/or a large angle that preclude binocular fusion.

1. Nonsurgical
   Remember (Four Os)

> Patients with good and stable control for intermittent exotropia are observed with no surgical interventions.

   (a) Optical correction
      Spectacles with full minus and astigmatism correction, hypermetropia, and partial correction to achieve best corrected VA with least plus
   (b) Over-minus correction if the cycloplegic refraction is low hypermetropia to encourage accommodation and convergence and improve control
   (c) Occlusion: part-time patching of the preferred eye or alternating
   (d) Orthoptic exercise (convergence insufficiency)
      1. Pencil push-up
      2. Base-out prism
2. Surgical
   Surgery is reserved for patients who have manifest exotropia >50% of daytime, with the success rate of ~50% (i.e., achieving remnant tropia <10 PD).

   For exotropia, surgical approaches vary based on the deviation type and other factors. Some surgeons prefer bilateral surgery when the distance deviation exceeds the near deviation. In contrast, unilateral surgery is preferred when the near deviation is greater than the distance deviation. If the poor vision is present in one eye, unilateral surgery on that eye is typically chosen. Bilateral surgery is often recommended for patients with an A or V pattern.

7.1.4.1 Augmented Surgical Correction for Intermittent Exotropia

Prediction of the surgical success rate for X(T) can be challenging, with many patients experiencing a recurrence of exotropia (more than half after 5 years). In managing exodeviation surgically, there is consensus that an initial overcorrection is a key factor for success. This approach induces diplopia, which stimulates fusional vergence and helps patients move beyond their previously established temporal suppression scotoma.

Differential diagnoses of incomitant exotropia:

1. Congenital third nerve palsy
2. Duane syndrome (patients with type 2 can present with exotropia, usually accompanied by deficient adduction and a head turn away from the affected side)
3. Congenital fibrosis syndrome
4. Craniofacial abnormalities
5. Ocular myasthenia gravis (may be comitant)

7.2 Vertical Strabismus

Keep the following in your mind:

An oblique muscle overaction can be:

Primary: True overaction can be accompanied by A or V patterns.

Secondary: Due to weakness in its antagonist oblique muscle (palsy), patterns do not usually exist.

7.2.1 Superior Oblique Palsy

Superior oblique muscle palsy (fourth or trochlear nerve palsy) is the most common isolated cyclovertical muscle palsy encountered by ophthalmologists. The most common cause is closed-head trauma. It is accompanied with variable manifestation, which includes one or all of the following:

1. Hypertropia of the affected eye in primary position
2. Hypertropia increased on adduction
3. Esotropia mainly on downgaze (upon reading), leading to V-pattern esotropia

4. Excyclotorsion in primary and more on downgaze

They might have diplopia, which is usually worse upon gaze to the contralateral side (right gaze in left oblique palsy). So, as a compensatory mechanism, they usually have a head tilt to the contralateral side (the normal side); the symptoms worsen if the head tilts to the ipsilateral side (right head tilt in right oblique palsy). The compensatory head tilt makes the affected eye in a position where it extorts when looking in the opposite gaze direction, and depression occurs in abduction (secondary to ipsilateral rectus muscle action). It can be congenital or acquired (Table 7.2).

***Paradoxical head tilt (i.e., to the ipsilateral side of muscle palsy) occurs in cases of severe palsy, so by head tilt to the same side, the image from this ipsilateral eye will be out of the field and ignored.

7.2.1.1 Congenital Superior Oblique Paresis

- Congenital superior oblique palsy often arises from a defect in the fourth nerve nucleus or in the motor portion of the fourth cranial nerve. The exact cause of this condition is unknown. In some cases, the superior oblique paresis is associated with a lax tendon and, in rare cases, an absent superior oblique tendon. Although congenital superior oblique palsy is present at birth, its clinical signs often first appear in late childhood or adulthood due to high vertical fusion amplitude. Fusional control weakens over time, leading to a manifest deviation later in life. Personal photographs may reveal a long-standing head tilt opposite to the side of the hypertropia.
- Patients often adopt a compensatory head tilt away from the side of the palsy to reduce the deviation and maintain binocular fusion. This can lead to facial asymmetry from chronic head tilt.
- The condition is commonly associated with ipsilateral inferior oblique overaction and relatively less superior oblique underaction. Congenital cases have higher vertical fusional amplitude and fuse large hypertropias up to 35 PD compared to acquired cases.
- Congenital unilateral cases generally have less excyclotorsion compared to acquired cases.

7.2.1.2 Acquired Superior Oblique Palsy

- Acquired superior oblique palsy most commonly results from closed-head trauma. Since the trochlear nerves exit the midbrain close together, trauma usually affects both nerves, but the paresis may be asymmetric.
- In acquired superior oblique paresis, versions are generally normal; there is minimal inferior oblique overaction, but patients experience significant extorsional diplopia.
- Classically, there is little to no hypertropia in the primary position. For example, in bilateral acute superior oblique palsy, a right hypertropia is observed on head tilt to the right and in left gaze, while left hypertropia is seen on head tilt to the left and in right gaze. This can create a V pattern (arrow) type with an esotropia in downgaze and more extorsion in downgaze.
- Patients often report torsional, vertical, and horizontal diplopia that worsens in downgaze.

Table 7.2 Comparison between congenital and acquired superior oblique palsy

	Congenital	Acquired
Fusional amplitude	Higher (>6)	Lower (4–6)
Excyclotorsion	Lower	Higher
V pattern	Less	More
Binocular single vision	Better	Worse

7.2.1.3 Unilateral vs. Bilateral Superior Oblique Palsy

Bilateral superior oblique palsies are often associated with severe head trauma and can be difficult to diagnose, especially when symptoms are highly asymmetric. Key indicators of bilateral involvement include a greater esodeviation observed in downgaze, a hyperdeviation that shifts between right and left when the head is tilted or when gazing sideways, and significant excyclotorsion. In contrast to unilateral palsies, bilateral cases usually present with minimal or no hyperdeviation in the primary gaze and large degrees of excyclotorsion. Compared with a unilateral palsy, bilateral superior oblique palsies usually have little if any hyperdeviation in primary gaze. In contrast to unilateral superior oblique palsies, bilateral cases often do not have a head tilt (Table 7.3).

> Normally, the fovea is located 0.3 disc diameters below the horizontal line passing through the center of the disc. In excyclotorsion,
>
> Subjective excyclotorsion can be measured by bilateral Maddox rod or the synoptophore.

7.2.1.4 Surgical Management of Superior Oblique Palsy

- Surgery for congenital superior oblique palsy is recommended for significant head tilt, hypertropia causing asthenopia, and symptomatic diplopia. While the timing of surgery is debated, observation is advised if the head tilt is mild and binocular fusion is preserved.
- In acquired cases: conservative observation is recommended for at least 6 months with surgery considered if the symptoms do not resolve spontaneously.
  (a) For acquired unilateral case palsy, prism can manage small, fairly comitant deviations with minor torsion. Surgical intervention is reserved for significant deviations that may be incomitant or exhibit substantial torsion.
  (b) For bilateral cases, strengthening procedures such as anterior and temporal transposition of the superior oblique tendon are typically used to enhance the muscle's cyclotorsional function. If esotropia and vertical hypertropia are also present, bilateral superior oblique tuck procedure should be considered.

So to summarize, fourth nerve palsy can be treated by three surgical approaches:

1. Strengthening of the superior oblique such as tucking:
   Bilateral severe SOP "arrow" pattern (>15 PD of esotropia in downgaze) esotropia in downgaze is the main concern, along with hypertropia and excyclotorsion. Symptomatic diplopia is usually present.
2. Harada-Ito procedure
   In traumatic bilateral superior oblique paresis with extorsion, excyclotorsion is the main concern. Esotropia >8–10 PD in downgaze and no significant hypertropia in the primary position are usually present.

Table 7.3 Comparison between unilateral and bilateral superior oblique palsy

	Unilateral SOP	Bilateral SOP (mostly acquired)
Hyperdeviation (hypertropia)	More (large hypertropia)	Less
V-pattern esotropia (not exo)	<10 pd	More than 10 pd
Excyclotorsion (extorsion)	Less	More (>10°)
Head tilt, chin depression	Compensatory tilt to other side Minimal chin depression	Absent head tilt Chin depression present
Alternate hypertropia or diplopia	Absent	Present
Head tilt test (three-step test)	Positive (head tilt to the affected shoulder)	Positive (head tilt to the more severe side)

Table 7.4 Comparison between inferior oblique palsy and Brown's syndrome

Features	Inferior oblique muscle palsy	Brown's syndrome (i.e., superior oblique pulley system abnormality)
Forced duction test	Negative	Positive
Strabismus pattern	A pattern	None or V pattern
Superior oblique muscle overaction torsion	Usually, significant intorsion	None or minimal
Head tilt test*	Positive	Negative

Harada-Ito procedure is an advancement (strengthening) of the anterior fibers of the superior oblique muscle. This procedure will correct torsion and possibly some of the esodeviation in downgaze. However, it will not significantly affect the vertical deviation on side gaze.

Bilateral medial rectus recessions (small) with infraplacement one-half tendon width may be done after SO surgery to correct residual ET.

3. Weakening of ipsilateral inferior oblique (myectomy or recession)

   If vertical deviation is the concern: inferior oblique weakening procedure is indicated.
4. Weakening of the contralateral inferior rectus (recession)

If the hypertropia in the primary position exceeds 15–20 PD, an isolated inferior oblique recession alone will be insufficient to correct the hypertropia. In such cases, contralateral inferior rectus recession should also be performed.

*** Remember that a fourth nerve nucleus of one side supplies the opposite muscle, as the fourth CN crosses to the other side upon emergence from the nucleus.

For example, signs of right superior oblique palsy might be from the right fourth nerve or left fourth nucleus lesions.

7.2.2 Inferior Oblique Palsy

- It is rare and can be confused with Brown's syndrome or primary superior oblique overaction.

Clinical Features

- Limited elevation in adduction
- Marked superior oblique overaction
- Negative forced duction
- A-pattern esotropia
- Positive head tilt test

Inferior oblique palsy can be either congenital or acquired. Congenital inferior oblique paresis is often unilateral and associated with significant hypophoria in the primary position that can be fused (Table 7.4). Acquired inferior oblique paresis, on the other hand, leads to cyclovertical diplopia and necessitates a neurological evaluation.

- Mydriasis and accommodative paresis indicate damage to the parasympathetic supply to the globe, which travels with the nerve to the inferior oblique (partial third nerve palsy).
- Patient with left inferior oblique palsy will manifest as a right hypertropia worse in right gaze and right head tilt.

7.2.2.1 Three-Step Test (Parks-Bielschowsky Three-Step Test)

A patient with right hypertropia can have either palsy of ipsilateral depressors (i.e., inferior rectus or superior oblique) or palsy of contralateral elevators (i.e., superior rectus or inferior oblique).

The diagnosis of right superior oblique muscle palsy can be established by the three-step test (also called *Parks-Bielschowsky three-step test*) (Manchandia and Demer 2014):

The test is indicated in the diagnosis of isolated cyclovertical muscle palsies in patients with hyperdeviations.

In cases of long-standing deviations, spread of comitance occurs, and the results of the three-step test are less reliable making the localization of the affected muscle more difficult.

The Test Is Contraindicated in:
1. Patients with restrictive strabismus
2. Previous strabismus surgery, especially of the cyclovertical extraocular muscles because the test can easily be misinterpreted
3. History of C-spine instability or deformity

The Three-Step Test:

Step 1: Determine which eye is higher on primary: there is an equilibrium between muscle that elevates the eye (SR, IO) and the muscles that depress the eye (IR, SO)

Step 2: Determine in which gaze the hyperopia is worse: On abduction, the SR is the main elevator, and IR is the main depressor. On adduction, the IO is the main elevator, SO is the main depressor, and the eyes are vertically aligned by the equilibrium between those muscles.

Step 3: Determine at which head tilt hypertropia worsens: there is an equilibrium between muscles that intort the eye (SR, SO) and muscles that extort the eye (IR, IO). On RT head tilt, the RT eye intorts and the LT eye extorts; on left head tilt, the LT eye intorts, and the RT eye extorts.

Remember that the superior vertical muscles (SR, SO) are intortors, and the inferior vertical muscles (IR, IO) are extortors.

An example is shown in Fig. 7.1.

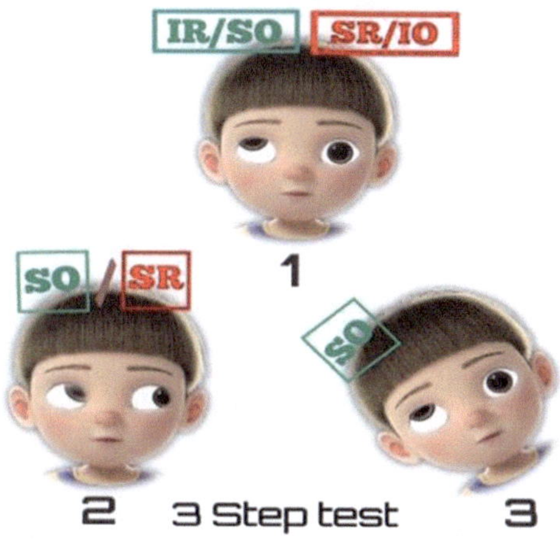

Fig. 7.1 Example of a three-step test, where (1) hypertropia of the RT eye in 1ry position: either depressor is palsy (IR, SO) or elevator of the other eye is palsy (SR, IO). (2) In left gaze, the RT eye is still hypertropic, so superior muscle palsy (SO same eye or SR on the other eye). (3) Hypertropia increases on head tilt to the same side, so right superior oblique palsy

Three-step test to make it easy:
1. Which eye is hypertropic
2. If hypertropia increases when looking nasally >> superior muscle palsy (SO same eye, SR other eye)

(continued)

If hypertropia increases when looking temporally >> inferior muscle palsy (IR same eye, IO other eye)

3. If hypertropia increases with head tilt to the same side >> oblique muscle palsy (SO same eye, IO other eye)

If hypertropia increases with head tilt to the other side >> vertical muscle palsy (IR same eye, SR other eye)

7.2.3 Brown's Syndrome (Superior Oblique Tendon Sheath Syndrome)

Brown's syndrome causes vertical deviations, with characteristic restriction of elevation in adduction due to abnormalities of the tendon-trochlea complex. It is unilateral or bilateral (10% of cases), congenital or acquired (most are congenital), and intermittent or constant (spontaneous resolution may occur). Some may be a form of congenital cranial denervation disorder (CCDD).

There is a tendency to affect the right eye.

Clinical Features

Remember "brown eyes addiction"

Br: Brown's

e: defect in elevation

Add: in adduction

1. Deficient elevation in adduction (passive)
2. Minimal or less deficient elevation in abduction
3. Positive forced ductions
4. Minimal or no superior oblique overaction
5. Y-pattern mostly in bilateral cases (marked divergence in upgaze)

Other Features:

1. Downshoot in adduction
2. Widening of palpebral fissure on adduction
3. Ortho or hypo in primary position
4. Head posture (chin up)
5. Audible click

7.2.3.1 Classification (Pathophysiology)

Congenital Brown's syndrome is more common than acquired Brown's syndrome and may be considered part of congenital cranial dysinnervation disorders. Congenital Brown's syndrome is a constant, stable condition that may, though rarely, resolve spontaneously.

- *Helveston theory*:
- The tendon of superior oblique does not function like a cord through a pulley, but rather acts like a telescope, with its component part of the tendon sliding over each other. During the contraction and relaxation of the superior oblique muscle, the central tendon fiber of the tendon moves more extensively than the peripheral fibers.
- *Wright hypothesis*
- Stiff muscle tendon complex (which could be a type of CFEOM)
  (a) Short superior oblique tendon
  (b) Stiff (inelastic) superior oblique tendon

Acquired Brown's syndrome (Table 7.5): Orbit and sinus imaging is recommended in acute-onset cases.

Differential Diagnosis of Brown's Syndrome:

1. Inferior oblique palsy
2. Double-elevator palsy (DEP)
3. Fracture orbital floor with entrapped muscle
4. Congenital fibrosis extraocular muscle (CFEOM)
5. Graves' disease

Management:

Observation is the most common conservative management option, as spontaneous resolution is likely in intermittent and acquired cases but less likely in long-standing congenital cases.

An MRI scan should be performed on patients with acquired Brown's syndrome to rule out orbital pathology. Since many of these cases will resolve on their own, conservative treatment without surgery is the preferred option. Treatment is available for inflammatory Brown's syndrome with either a local cortico-

Table 7.5 Cause of acquired Brown's syndrome

Cause of acquired Brown's syndrome	Examples
Peritrochlear scarring and adhesions	Chronic sinusitis, trauma, blepharoplasty and fat removal, and lichen sclerosus
Tendon-trochlear inflammation and edema	Idiopathic inflammatory (pain and click), trochleitis with superior oblique myositis, acute sinusitis, systemic inflammation as adult rheumatoid arthritis, juvenile rheumatoid arthritis, systemic lupus erythematosus often causing intermittent Brown's syndrome which resolves spontaneously
Superior nasal orbital mass	Glaucoma implant and neoplasm
Tight or inelastic superior oblique muscle	Thyroid disease (inelastic muscle), peribulbar anesthesia (inelastic tendon), Hurler-Scheie syndrome (inelastic tendon), and superior oblique tuck (short tendon)

steroid injection or oral anti-inflammatory drugs.

7.2.3.2 Surgery

Surgery Indications:

1. Hypotropia in primary, severe limitation of elevation in adduction
2. Anomalous head posture: severe chin up, face turn

1. SO tenotomy or tenectomy
   - Results in a consecutive SO palsy in more than 50% of cases (45–80%).
   - Results are unpredictable in all patients because of inferior oblique overaction that is frequently followed.
   - Note:
   - In an SO tenotomy performed nasal to the SR, the cut ends of the tendon may scar into the sclera, potentially creating a new insertion at the nasal border of the SR. This issue can be minimized by carefully preserving the intermuscular septum along the nasal border of the SR and to approach through a superotemporal fornix incision.
2. Split SO tendon elongation
3. Lengthening the SO tendon, it can be achieved by using a loosely tied nonabsorbable suture between the cut ends of the superior oblique tendon or a silicone expander which is inserted between the cut ends.

SO tendon elongation procedure has reduced the incidence of consecutive superior oblique palsy to <10%.

7.2.4 Dissociated Vertical Deviation (DVD)

It is an ocular motor disorder characterized by a slow, upward drift with excyclotorsion of non-fixating eye when the other eye is fixating a target. Typically, DVD contradicts *Hering's law of motor correspondence*, as there is no hypodeviation of the fellow eye on cover testing.

7.2.4.1 Etiology

DVD occurs in any condition that interrupts binocular single vision and usually appears at the age of 2 years and rarely before the age of 1 year.

Patients with DVD generally have poor binocular single vision. It mostly occurs on top of horizontal strabismus, with esotropia being the most common, also seen in exotropia and even in orthotropia.

It is usually bilateral but asymmetrical (unilateral cases are commonly associated with deep amblyopia).

DVD may be:

1. Manifest (spontaneously visible)
2. Latent (only seen when the eye is covered, i.e., dissociated)

Anomalous head posture is reported in 30% of patients with DVD, and it is a motor adaptation to maintain binocular single vision; the deviation of the eye increases with contralateral head tilt.

Vertical deviation of DVD is usually variable and difficult to measure. Bielschowsky's phenomenon (aka graded density filter bar): as the density of the filter bar increases (less light enters the eye), the eye drifts up, and as the density of the filter bar is decreased, the eye comes down. It is used to differentiate DVD from IOOA.

7.2.4.2 Treatment

1. Observation for patients with latent and mild DVD.
2. Surgery is indicated when there is a large manifest DVD and anomalous head posture. The surgical treatment can be planned based on the grade of the DVD and the presence or absence of inferior oblique (IO) overaction:
   1. Manifest DVD with no IO overaction—superior rectus recession ± inferior rectus resection

2. Manifest DVD with IO overaction—recession with anteriorization of IO

Differential Diagnoses of DVD:

1. Inferior oblique overaction

   The important differentiating points between IOOA and DVD include the following:

   1. Hyperdeviation is maximum in adduction in IOOA, and never on abduction, while it is almost of similar degrees in all positions of gaze in DVD.
   2. Recovery movement occurs when eye is uncovered, and a slow downward drift is noticed in DVD.
   3. V pattern is associated with IOOA, while it is absent in DVD.
   4. Superior oblique underaction is usually associated with IOOA, but in DVD, superior oblique may overact.
   5. An extorted fundus can be seen in IOOA, while it is absent in patients with DVD.
   6. Bielschowsky's phenomenon is present in DVD, while it is absent in IOOA.
   7. DVD is often associated with latent nystagmus.
2. Skew deviation

   The important differentiating points between skew deviation and DVD include the following:

   1. In skew deviation, there is intortion of the higher eye and extortion of the lower eye, while in DVD, the higher eye extorts.
   2. Skew deviation is associated with brainstem or cerebellar lesions, but DVD is associated with any condition that interrupts BSV.
   3. Vertical diplopia is associated with skew deviation, while DVD is not associated with diplopia.
   4. Seesaw nystagmus is associated with skew deviation, while DVD is associated with latent nystagmus.

7.2.5 Inferior Oblique Muscle Overaction (IOOA)

It manifests as over-elevation of the eye in adduction and is often associated with horizontal deviations. It is reported in 70% of patients with esotropia and 30% of patients with exotropia and can lead to a V-pattern strabismus.

There are two types of IOOA:

1. Primary type is frequently bilateral, and its etiology is unclear.
2. Secondary type is unilateral; it is due to ipsilateral superior oblique (SO) palsy or contralateral superior rectus palsy.

The head tilt test can help distinguish between primary inferior oblique overaction and inferior oblique overaction secondary to superior oblique palsy. A positive head tilt test suggests superior oblique palsy, while a negative head tilt test indicates primary inferior oblique overaction.

Management:

Note that the primary position deviation is not affected by surgery on oblique muscles.

The available weakening procedures for the inferior oblique include myotomy, recession, myectomy, and anterior transposition. Anterior transposition is preferred in cases with DVD or 4+ IOOA.

Causes of over-elevation and over-depression on adduction (Table 7.6)

Figure grade of inferior oblique overaction

Table 7.6 Causes of over-elevation and over-depression on adduction

Causes of over-elevation on adduction	Causes of over-depression on adduction
IOOA, associate with fundus extorsion, V pattern	SOOA, associate with fundus intorsion, A pattern
DVD	Brown's syndrome
Duane	Duane
Large angle XT in the other eye	Large angle XT in the other eye
Lateral rectus muscle pulley heterotropia	Lateral rectus muscle pulley heterotropia

7.2.6 Superior Oblique Myokymia

Definition:

"Unilateral rotary nystagmus": It is a paroxysmal, monocular (very rarely bilateral), high-frequency (10–12 s), low-amplitude rotary nystagmus due to bursts of contraction of the superior oblique muscle (intermittent spontaneous firing of one superior oblique muscle) that result in oscillopsia and diplopia.

Sign and Symptom:

- Intermittent bursts of brief torsional and/or vertical diplopia and blurred vision last for a few seconds to minutes due to abnormal involuntary movement of superior oblique muscle; the attacks could occur at any time and multiple times a day and could resolve for years and then return.
- Best observed by a direct ophthalmoscope or on slit lamp to detect the intermittent incyclotorsion and could be heard by stethoscope.

Etiology:

1. Mostly benign condition, idiopathic of unknown etiology. There is some evidence that it is a response to the regeneration of damaged trochlear nerve axons; some cases of superior oblique myokymia occur after recovery from SO palsy, but it is not aberrant regeneration.
2. Rarely associated with midbrain lesion, lesions of the cerebellopontine angle, or head trauma.
3. May be secondary to neurovascular compression of trochlear nerve by an adjacent artery; SOM may, in some cases, fall under the umbrella of "neurovascular compression syndromes," similar to the pathogenesis of hemifacial spasm and trigeminal neuralgia.
4. Rarely associated with family history of multiple sclerosis.

Neuroimaging is not recommended if there are no additional neurologic complaints or abnormalities. However, patients who do not respond to medical treatment should undergo contrast-enhanced MRI studies for further investigation.

Treatment:

Numerous systemic medications including carbamazepine, baclofen, benzodiazepines, and beta-blockers have been tried. Topical beta-blockers also had a short-term success in some patients.

Surgery might be necessary if medical treatment is ineffective in controlling symptoms or not tolerated. Any connection between the affected SO and the globe must be cut out for the procedure to be successful such as in SO tenotomy, SO tenectomy, and Harada-Ito procedure.

> Superior oblique myokymia is a tremor of superior oblique muscle. Patient experiences repeated brief episodes of uniocular shimmering or shaking of images (jumping), which lasts from seconds to minutes.

7.2.7 Skew Deviation

It is an acquired vertical misalignment of the eyes associated with vertical diplopia, typically <5 prism diopters, and may include torsional components. It is usually a comitant *hypertropia* of a supranuclear origin, *resulting from a disturbance or imbalance in vestibular input to the ocular motor nuclei*. Skew deviation can sometimes be incomitant, mimicking a partial third or fourth nerve palsy (Table 7.7).

It is often the initial sign of diseases affecting the brainstem, cerebellum, or peripheral vestibular system and its afferent projections.

Etiology:

- Cerebellar disease
- Lesion in midbrain (e.g., dorsal midbrain syndrome)
- Vascular lesion of pons and medulla oblongata (Wallenberg's syndrome)
- Diseases of the vestibular nuclei in the medulla (e.g., lateral medullary syndrome)
- Disease of medial longitudinal fasciculus (e.g., internuclear ophthalmoplegia)

Table 7.7 Comparison between ocular tilt response and superior oblique palsy

	Ocular tilt response	Superior oblique palsy
Hypertropia	Comitant and does not change with head tilt	Incomitant worse on gaze to opposite side, worse on ipsilateral head tilt
Head tilt	Pathological head tilt	Compensatory head tilt to allow BSV
Torsion	Bilateral torsion, conjugate toward lower eye No or minimal torsional diplopia	Unilateral excyclotorsion of hypertropic eye Torsional diplopia
	Associated with other neurological signs (gaze-evoked nystagmus, gaze palsy, ataxia)	Usually no associated neurological signs except if caused by brain trauma

Triad of Ocular Tilt Response:
Head tilt
Vertical (skew) deviation
Ocular torsion

So keep in your mind that skew deviation is a vertical deviation mimicking superior oblique palsy.
In skew deviation, the hypertropic eye intorts and hyperopic eye extorts. In superior oblique palsy, the hyperopic extorts.

7.2.8 Monocular Elevation Deficiency (MED)

It is a rare sporadic condition in which there is a limitation of elevation of the affected eye. Most cases are congenital. It can be due to either:

1. Tight or contracted inferior rectus (+ve forced duction)
2. Weakness of elevator muscle SR or IO (−ve forced duction)

Characterized by
1. Pseudoptosis in 75% of cases and can be associated with true ptosis in 25% of cases.
2. Chin-up head posture to maintain fusion.
3. 25–30% are ortho in primary position.
4. The Bell's phenomenon is generally absent in cases involving inferior rectus restriction and superior rectus palsy. However, it is usually present in cases of MED resulting from supranuclear defects.
5. Marcus Gunn jaw winking is present in 25% of patients.

Management Depends on Forced Duction Test:
1. In patients with a positive forced duction test, inferior rectus recession is the first choice of management.
2. If there is no restriction, transposition of the medial and lateral rectus muscles to the superior rectus muscle can be performed (Knapp procedure).

7.3 Congenital Cranial Dysinnervation Disorders (CCDDs)

Congenital cranial dysinnervation diseases are developmental abnormalities of one or more cranial nerves (CNs) along with nuclear hypoplasia, nerve misdirection, and/or absent nerves. CCDDs are nonprogressive conditions present since birth. It may be isolated or familial where genetic abnormalities have been identified. Secondary structural alterations of the extraocular muscles, such as stiffness or contracture, are frequently the result of abnormal innervation.

CCDDs Include
1. Duane syndrome
2. Congenital fibrosis of the extraocular muscles
3. Möbius syndrome
4. Congenital CN VII palsy

7.3.1 Duane Retraction Syndrome

Duane syndrome is a congenital oculomotor disorder with a prevalence of about 1/1000 in general population:

- Most common type of CCDD.
- Female predominance (in 60% of the cases).
- 70% of cases are isolated, and 30–40% of cases are associated with other congenital anomalies. Hypoplasia of sixth nerve nucleus can be present.
- Amblyopia is not common (10–14%) as it is usually compensated by head posture.
- Eye movements in Duane syndrome violate Sherrington's law.

1. Isolated Duane syndrome:
   - Mostly sporadic in 90% of the cases (commonly unilateral), but 5–10% are inherited as AD (commonly bilateral).
2. Syndromic
   (a) Okihiro syndrome (Duane-radial ray syndrome)
   (b) Goldenhar syndrome
   (c) Wildervanck syndrome
   (d) Möbius syndrome
   (e) Holt-Oram syndrome

7.4 Classification (Huber's)

This classification takes electromyographic (EMG) evidence of differing etiologies:

1. Duane syndrome type 1 (DRS I) 60%, mimicking sixth nerve palsy
2. DRS type 2 Limited adduction
3. DRS type 3 Limited abduction and adduction

Clinical Features:
1. Ipsilateral face turn
2. Ortho or may be esotropia in primary position (Table 7.8)

   Limited abduction

   Lid fissure narrowing in adduction, widening in abduction

   On EMG, it shows absence of electrical activity in the ipsilateral lateral rectus muscle on abduction, with paradoxical activity on adduction.

Duane syndrome type 2 (DRS II), the least common, 15%

Clinical Features:
1. Limited adduction
2. Normal or mildly limited abduction
3. In primary position, straight or slight exotropia
4. Poor adduction as lateral rectus contract against medial rectus

Duane syndrome type 3 (type III), 25 % of cases

Characterized by:
1. Limited adduction and abduction
2. Mostly orthotropic in primary position

Clinical Features of DRS:
- Poor convergence.
- Sudden upshoot or downshift of the globe (mimicking SOOA or IOOA). This is known

Table 7.8 Comparison between Duane type 1, sixth nerve palsy, and congenital esotropia

	Duane 1	Sixth nerve palsy	Congenital esotropia
Diplopia	Absent (head tilt may compensate)	Present	Absent
Eso angle	Smaller (<30PD)	Larger (>30PD)	Larger (>30PD)
Forced duction	+ve	−ve	−ve
Comitant	No	No	Yes
Globe retraction/palpebral fissure changes	+ve	−ve	−ve
Limited abduction	+ve	+ve	–
Limited adduction	+ve (slightly limited)	−ve	−ve

as leash or bridle phenomenon and may be due to slippage of globe which allows the MR to act as elevator, caused by a tautness or leash effect from the lateral rectus muscle.
- Widening of palpebral fissure with abduction (oculomotor stimulation).
- Compensatory head posture to maintain BSV: a face turn to the side of the affected side in DRS type I.
- Ocular associations of DRS: cataract, heterochromia, microphthalmia, crocodile tears, and Marcus Gunn jaw winking.
- Systemic associations: seizures, bone abnormalities (syndactyly, polydactyly), agenesis of genitourinary system, sensory neural deafness, and cafe au lait spots.

Management of DRS:
- Amblyopia management if present (mostly anisometropic amblyopia)
- Observation
- Indication for surgery:
  - Strabismus that interferes with BSV in forced primary position
  - Significant abnormal head posture
  - Severe palpebral fissure narrowing, upshoot or downshoot on adduction

Surgical Management for Unilateral Duane:

Type 1: medial rectus recession on the affected side; surgery on lateral rectus could exacerbate globe retraction.

Type 2: lateral rectus recession on the affected side.

Type 3: bilateral recession of both recti for severe globe retraction that might be present.

In general, muscle resection in Duane syndrome is generally avoided as it might exacerbate globe retraction.

A lateral rectus Y split is effective in reducing upshoot or downshoot in cases of DRS.

> Medial rectus contracture is uncommon in Duane syndrome in congenital sixth nerve palsy; it is common and results in esotropia in primary position.

7.4.1 Congenital Fibrosis of the Extraocular Muscles

Congenital fibrosis of the extraocular muscles (CFEOMs) is a rare, nonprogressive, group of cranial nerve and associated nuclei developmental disorders that cause dysinnervation and consequent aberrant EOM anatomy, with limitation and restriction caused by the replacement of hypoplastic muscles by fibrous tissue.

CFEOM I: AD inheritance, most common. This type predominantly involves CN III, and it is typically characterized by bilateral ptosis, severe restriction to upgaze, exotropia, and a chin-up head posture.

CFEOM II: AR inheritance with bilateral CN III and IV dysgenesis, and it is typically characterized by exotropia with limited adduction.

CFEOM III: AD inheritance with variable penetration. It can be unilateral or asymmetrical. CFEOM III is often associated with other neurological abnormalities, and it is typically characterized by bilateral ptosis and involvement of extraocular muscle innervated by CN III.

7.4.2 Möbius Syndrome

Möbius syndrome is a rare neurological condition, which is sporadic, nonprogressive, and characterized by both CN VI and CN VII dysgenesis, which affects both muscles that control facial expression and eye movements, and other cranial nerves are sometimes affected.

Clinical Features:
1. Horizontal gaze palsy is present in 50% of cases, resulting from involvement of both the paramedian pontine reticular formation (PPRF) and the sixth cranial nerve (CN VI) palsy. This condition is characterized by the absence of abduction of either eye beyond the midline, with no deviation in the primary position. Bilateral sixth nerve palsy with convergent strabismus occurs. Cross fixation is present which leads to contraction of medial rectus and positive force duction test.

2. Bilateral Facial Palsy.
3. Vertical gaze movements are normal, and Bell's phenomenon is intact.
4. Other cranial nerves may be affected. The hypoglossal 12th nerve may be involved so that the tongue is shrunken and relatively immobile. The trigeminal 5th nerve may be affected as well as 8th, 9th, and 10th cranial nerves.
5. Other features: Limb abnormality and chest abnormality with absence of pectoralis muscle are common. Micrognathia, microstomia, cleft palate, syndactyly, and mild intellectual disabilities may be associated with Möbius syndrome.

Patients with Möbius syndrome exhibit one of three patterns of ocular motility involvement, which are likely related to the severity and timing of the in utero insult:

- Orthotropia in the primary position with marked deficits in both abduction and adduction, seen in 40% of cases.
- Esotropia with cross fixation and sparing of convergence, occurring in 50% of cases.
- Large exotropia with absence of convergence, present in 10% of cases.

7.5 Nystagmus

Nystagmus is a rhythmic biphasic oscillation of the eyes (Papageorgiou et al. 2014). It is a regular, repetitive to-and-fro movement of the eyes (horizontal, vertical, or torsional) with two phases:

1. Slow drift from the target of interest
2. Corrective saccade back to the target

Nystagmus must be evaluated for the underlying reason because it is a sign rather than a diagnosis. Remember the description of nystagmus (Table 7.9).

Doctors are never felt worried.

D: Direction (horizontal or vertical), dissociate (or conjugate)

A: Amplitude

N: Null point

F: Frequency

W: Waveform (pendular or jerk)

Table 7.9 Nystagmus description

Amplitude	Amplitude is the excursion of the nystagmus and described as Fine: <5° Moderate: 5–15° Large >15°
Intensity	Amplitude × Frequency
Null zone	Head position at where nystagmus is minimized
Frequency	Frequency is the number of to-and-fro movements in 1 s, described as cycles/s or Hertz (Hz) Slow: 1–2 Hz Medium: 3–4 Hz Fast: 5 Hz or more
Conjugate/dissociated	Conjugate: when its direction, frequency (number of oscillations per unit of time), and amplitude (magnitude of the eye movement) are similar in both eyes Dissociated: when it differs in any one of the parameters between both eyes
Jerk/pendular	Jerk nystagmus: which is characterized by a slow movement in one direction followed by rapid corrective movement in the opposite direction. The nystagmus is named based on the direction of the fast phase. For example, in right jerk nystagmus, the slow phase moves left, followed by a fast "jerk" movement to the right. Pendular nystagmus: involves the eyes oscillating back and forth with equal speed in both directions, without a distinct slow or fast phase

Nystagmus characteristics may change with gaze direction. Pendular nystagmus can become jerk nystagmus on the side gaze. Jerk nystagmus can have a *null point* or *null zone* (gaze position in which the intensity [frequency × amplitude] is diminished and the vision improves), or it can decrease in intensity with gaze in the direction opposite that of the fast-phase component (analogous to Alexander's law for vestibular nystagmus)

Nystagmus comes in a wide variety of forms, each of which describes a particular variation of the cause.

Classification of Nystagmus:

1. Age of onset: early-onset (congenital, latent, spasmus nutans) and late-onset acquired nystagmus
2. Nature of movement and underlying cause: pendular, jerk
3. Plane of movements: horizontal, vertical, torsional
4. Effect of fixation block: latent (appears only upon covering one eye), manifest, latent manifest
5. Causes: either physiological or pathological

7.5.1 Early-Onset Nystagmus (infantile or congenital)

- Infantile or congenital nystagmus (infantile nystagmus syndrome (INS))
- It is a relatively rare condition present since birth to the age of 6 months (mostly develops 2–3 months of age). Congenital nystagmus has many underlying causes and usually becomes apparent during the first few months of life.
  1. Congenital motor nystagmus:
     (a) Binocular horizontal nystagmus (mixed pendular and jerk; when INS has a jerk waveform, it shows an exponential increase in velocity during the slow phase).
     (b) Conjugate movements of both eyes with the presence of null point, resulting in abnormal head position.
     (c) Benign and visual acuity is usually normal.
     (d) Convergence dampens nystagmus. INS can be confused with nystagmus blockage syndrome in which esotropia and nystagmus happen to coexist.
     (e) Abduction and fixation exacerbate the nystagmus (increase its amplitude). It can be associated with latent nystagmus.
     (f) Inverse paradoxical response to OKN stimulus in 2/3 of patients (fast phase of jerk is in the direction of moving OKN drum).
     (g) Exponential increase of slow-phase eye movement.
     (h) While mostly somatic, X-linked mutations in FRMD7 gene are described.
     (i) May be seen in isolation or associated with strabismus and afferent visual defects.
     (j) Oscillopsia is not present.
  2. Congenital sensory nystagmus:
     – Secondary to an early-onset, bilateral abnormality of the pregeniculate afferent visual pathway, resulting in poor visual acuity.

Can be:

- Wandering or roving nystagmus (i.e., absence of fixation) with visual acuity <20/200
- – Pendular nystagmus is noted in patients with better visual acuity
- – Jerk nystagmus if better than 20/100

Ocular albinism is associated with macular hypoplasia with poor visual acuity, nystagmus, and strabismus. Sometimes, it is associated with high refractive errors.

7.5.1.1 Treatment of Congenital Nystagmus

Medical treatment can be in the forms of base-out prisms to induce convergence as it might dampen the nystagmus and could improve visual acuity. Use of prisms to shift the viewing position to the null point is also an option.

Surgical treatment of nystagmus by performing extraocular muscle surgery to place the null zone in primary position (Kestenbaum procedure) or recessing all four rectus muscles to decrease tension (large recession procedure).

- Spasmus nutans

  Spasmus nutans syndrome: rare condition that manifests during the first 2 years of life and usually improves spontaneously in the third or fourth year of life.

  It presents as a triad of:

  1. Small-amplitude, high-frequency (“shimmering”), binocular asymmetric (increased

amplitude in abduction), disconjugate nystagmus. It may be horizontal, vertical, torsional, or rotatory. Spasmus nutans often presents with a very asymmetric nystagmus, and it may be monocular.
2. Head nodding.
3. Torticollis (head tilt or turn):

May be associated with amblyopia. Spasmus nutans may appear to be entirely monocular and raise the suspicion of chiasmal or hypothalamic lesions such as anterior visual pathway glioma, central lesions as empty sella syndrome, and porencephalic cyst. Neuroimaging is recommended.

- Infantile monocular nystagmus:

Transient, high-frequency, and low-amplitude monocular nystagmus.

Infantile monocular (latent) nystagmus mostly occurs in blind eyes (usually due to visual loss and often secondary to optic neuropathy, posterior fossa tumors, optic nerve, chiasmal and/or hypothalamic gliomas). It usually presents as a vertical pendular nystagmus. Neuroimaging is warranted.

Note:

Heimann-Bielschowsky phenomenon is a type of monocular vertical nystagmus, characterized by slow, coarse, pendular, with variable amplitude. It typically occurs in an eye that has suffered profound visual loss and may develop years following monocular visual impairment.

In cases of bilateral visual loss, bilateral nystagmus is noted, with nystagmus more prominent in the eye with poorer vision.

- Latent nystagmus (fusion maldevelopment nystagmus syndrome) (FMNS)

1. Latent nystagmus is generally benign. Latent nystagmus can be a cause of blurred vision when testing vision monocularly.
2. Nystagmus which appears or markedly enhances when one eye is occluded.
3. Conjugate, horizontal jerk nystagmus is a marker of fusion maldevelopment, typically resulting from infantile-onset strabismus or less commonly decreased vision in one eye, such as in amblyopia.
4. Latent nystagmus is often found in patients with congenital esotropia, regardless of whether the esotropia is corrected. It may also be observed after surgery for infantile esotropia, likely due to the early disruption of binocular function.
5. Latent nystagmus is characteristically dampened in adduction and worsened in abduction.
6. The fast phase is toward the fixating eye, so the direction of the nystagmus in both eyes changes with the viewing eye.
7. Exponential decrease of velocity of slow phase on electronystagmography (ENG).
8. Usually bilateral especially when associated with congenital esotropia.
9. Manifest latent nystagmus is latent nystagmus that can be seen without occlusion.

7.5.2 Acquired Nystagmus

May be physiological or pathological (Fig. 7.2). Oscillopsia is usually present.

May be localizing nystagmus which includes the following:

1. Seesaw nystagmus: parasellar and midbrain lesions.
2. Vertical downbeat nystagmus: cervicomedullary junction
3. Vertical upbeat nystagmus: pons and midbrain lesions
4. Convergence retraction: dorsal midbrain lesions
5. Spasmus nutans: chiasmal glioma

7.5.2.1 Physiological Nystagmus

Vestibular Nystagmus

1. Caloric nystagmus

Demonstrated by caloric test:

When cold water is introduced into one ear, the fast component of horizontal nystagmus beats away from the stimulated ear. Conversely, warm water causes the fast component to beat toward the ear. If cold water is applied to both ears, the fast component of the

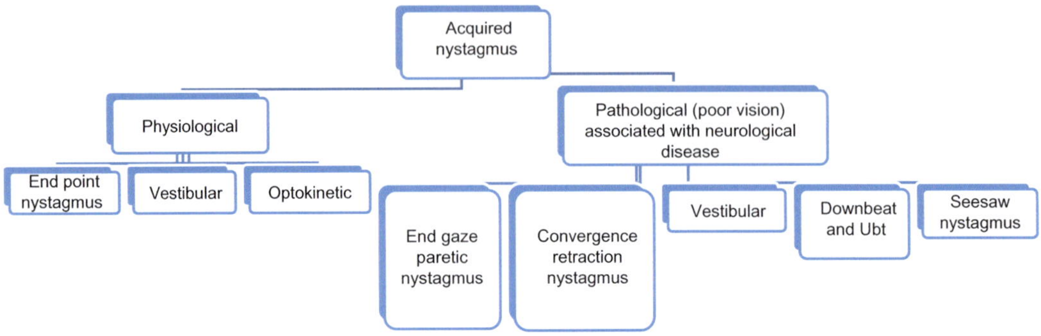

Fig. 7.2 Differential for acquired nystagmus in pediatrics

Table 7.10 Optokinetic nystagmus responses and their relevant differential

Abnormal OKN	Organic blindness, INO, dorsal midbrain lesion, lesion in central saccadic frontal lobe
Asymmetrical OKN (poor response when drum rotate from nasal to temporal)	Unilateral parieto-occipital lesion, unilateral peripheral vestibular lesion, latent nystagmus which is associated with congenital esotropia
Reverse or inverse OKN (paradoxical response) (the direction of fast recovery phase is similar to the direction of drum rotation)	Congenital motor nystagmus

nystagmus beats upwards, while warm water in both ears causes the fast component to beat downwards.

2. Rotatory nystagmus, also known as vestibule-ocular response or Doll's eye maneuver, occurs due to:

   Stimulation of the vestibular labyrinth or nerve during head rotation. When the head is rotated, a slow phase of eye movement occurs in the direction opposite to the head movement, followed by fast phases in the same direction as head movement. This mechanism helps stabilize retinal images as the head moves.

Optokinetic Nystagmus

Jerk nystagmus is induced by moving a full visual field stimulus.

- Slow phase (pursuit): eye follows the target.
- Fast phase (saccade): eye refixates on the next target.
- Uses (Table 7.10):
- Functional visual loss evaluation

  Visual acuity/potential evaluation in children

  Determine the cause if isolated homonymous hemianopia

Gaze-Evoked Nystagmus

Jerk waveform eye movement that occurs in extreme gaze (angle of gaze >45°).

Pathological (if persistent and asymmetrical) as in:

- Lesions in brain stem, cerebellum, and less commonly cerebral lesions. Anticonvulsants are described as a cause.

Note: Unlike end-gaze nystagmus, which is conjugate, transient with low amplitude of under 4°. Gaze-evoked nystagmus is sustained, has a larger amplitude, and may be asymmetric. End-gaze nystagmus tends to be more prominent with age and is usually benign. In contrast, gaze-evoked nystagmus is often associated with downbeat nystagmus and is generally considered pathological.

7.5.2.2 Pathological Nystagmus

Convergence Retraction Nystagmus (Parinaud Syndrome)

Irregular jerky nystagmus in which both eyes converge and retract on attempted upward gaze.

7.5.2.3 Downward optokinetic drum is used to elicit convergence retraction nystagmus.
Causes: dorsal midbrain lesions, pinealoma.

Seesaw Nystagmus

- Defined as pendular nystagmus with elevation and intorsion of one eye simultaneous with depression and extorsion of other eye; this is followed by reversal of cycle, so that the eyes move like a seesaw.
- Disconjugate nystagmus that has both vertical and torsional components.

Causes:

- Parasellar lesions, most often craniopharyngioma, pituitary tumors, lesions in chiasma, third ventricle, and/or diencephalon.
- Bitemporal hemianopia can be present. Patients usually have a disabling oscillopsia that responds poorly to treatment.

Periodic Alternate Nystagmus (PAN)

Also known as central vestibular instability nystagmus, this type of nystagmus is characterized by conjugate, horizontal jerk movements. It can be either congenital or acquired. The fast phase of nystagmus beats in one direction for about 1–2 min, followed by a neutral phase lasting for 10–20 s. The nystagmus then reverses direction, with the fast phase beating in the opposite direction due to a shifting null point, for another 1–2 min. This cycle of alternating directions continues to repeat.

Some children adopt an alternating head turn due to change in the null point position.

- Causes: vestibular and posterior fossa lesions, Arnold-Chiari malformation, craniocervical junction, cerebellar disease, ataxia telangiectasia, drug (e.g., phenytoin, ethanol).

Vertical Upbeat Nystagmus

Jerk nystagmus with fast-phase beating upwards in primary position.

Often worsens in upgaze.

Causes: structural lesion in brainstem as lesions of medulla (as medulloblastoma), pontomedullary junction (lower brainstem), anterior cerebellar vermis, lesion in fourth ventricle, and cerebellar degeneration. Less common causes include demyelinating diseases and encephalitis.

- May be treated with base-up prisms to force the eyes to look downward and therefore dampens nystagmus.

Vertical Downbeat Nystagmus

Jerk nystagmus with fast-phase beating downward in primary position.

Often worsens in downgaze.

Oscillopsia is usually prominent.

Causes: lesions at craniocervical junction (foramen magnum), Arnold-Chiari malformations, syringobulbia, drugs (e.g., lithium, alcohol, anticonvulsant, anxiolytic), Wernicke's encephalopathy, hydrocephalus.

May be treated with base-down prisms to force the eyes upward and therefore dampens nystagmus.

Note:

- Ocular conditions that result in congenital nystagmus include ocular albinism, Leber's congenital amaurosis, congenital stationary night blindness, and optic nerve hypoplasia.

Nystagmus is often associated with disruption of early binocular visual development (congenital esotropia, congenital unilateral cataracts).

7.5.3 Nystagmus-Like Disorders (aka Nystagmoid Movements)

These are not considered pure forms of nystagmus as the slow phase is absent. These represent disorders of saccades and include:

- Ocular bobbing

  Rapid, conjugate down movements followed by slow drift back to midline. May be associated with horizontal gaze palsy. Light near reflex is intact.

  Causes: Pontine lesions, toxic-metabolic conditions (metabolic encephalopathy) or cerebellar lesions.
- Ocular flutter

  Rapid horizontal involuntary binocular conjugate saccades without intersaccadic intervals.

  Causes: viral and para-infectious autoimmune encephalitis, paraneoplastic disorder associated with neuroblastoma.
- Opsoclonus

  Rapid multiplanar involuntary binocular conjugate saccades that occur without intersaccadic interval. Associated with eye blinking, facial twitching, myoclonus, and ataxia. Often presents with very high frequency and large amplitude, with no clear direction for fast phase.

  Causes: acute post-infectious cerebellar ataxia, viral encephalitis, and paraneoplastic manifestations of neuroblastoma and drug (e.g., lithium, cocaine).

Opsoclonus and Flutter:

- Bursts of Binocular conjugate saccades in the horizontal plane (ocular flutter)
- Bursts of Binocular conjugate saccades in all planes, horizontal and vertical (opsoclonus).
- These eye movements are distinctive in being visible under closed lids and during sleep. Acute onset is usually associated with a para-infectious cause, while subacute onset is associated with a paraneoplastic cause.
- Neuroblastoma with ocular flutter or opsoclonus has a better prognosis than neuroblastoma without ocular flutter or opsoclonus.

7.5.4 Treatment of Nystagmus:

Treat underlying cause.

To relieve the symptoms, the null point should be moved toward the fixation, either through prisms (where the apex is directed against the head posture) or through strabismus surgery, known as Kestenbaum or Anderson procedures.

Nystagmus surgery involves recession and resection of the horizontal extraocular muscles to adjust the eye positions in relation to head turn. For instance, in case of nystagmus with a left head turn, the Kestenbaum or Anderson procedures would include recessing the left medial rectus and the right lateral rectus muscles. Conversely, the r and procedure would involve resection of the left lateral rectus and the right medial rectus muscles.

7.6 Alphabet Patterns

7.6.1 Types of Pattern Strabismus

1. A and V Pattern:

   An A or V pattern is found in 15–25% of horizontal strabismus cases and may occur due to relative contributions of the superior rectus and inferior oblique to elevation or of the inferior rectus and superior oblique to depression and are abnormal.

   V-pattern strabismus exists when the magnitude of deviation is less convergent or more divergent in upgaze, mostly due to IOOA.

   An A-pattern strabismus exists when the magnitude of deviation is more convergent or less divergent in upgaze, mostly due to SOOA.

We can find V pattern (most common pattern of strabismus) in:

1. Infantile esotropia
2. Bilateral superior oblique palsies
3. Craniofacial malformations

We can find A pattern (second most common type of pattern strabismus) in:

1. Exotropia
2. Patient with spina bifida
2. Less common variations of pattern strabismus include the following:
   (a) Y pattern: Both eyes diverge in upgaze with normal ocular alignment in primary position and downgaze. It is mostly associated with inferior oblique overaction, and it can also occur in pseudo-inferior oblique overaction due to anomalous innervation of the lateral rectus muscles in upgaze (no fundus torsion and no superior oblique underaction).
   (b) X pattern: Both eyes diverge in primary position, and it increases in both upgaze and downgaze. It is seen in patients with large-angle exotropia, mostly due to contracture of the lateral rectus muscles.
   (c) Lambda patterns: Both eyes diverge in downgaze with similar horizontal deviation in primary position and upgaze; it is mostly associated with overdepression in adduction in cases of SOOA.

X and Y patterns result from pseudo-overaction of the inferior oblique muscles, and weakening them would not collapse the pattern.

A-pattern exotropia would be less XT on upgaze and more XT on downgaze (in SOOA).
V-pattern exotropia would be more XT on upgaze and less XT on downgaze (in IOOA).
Y pattern would be ortho in primary and downgaze but XT on upgaze.
X pattern would be ortho in primary and upgaze but XT in downgaze.

7.6.2 Etiology of Pattern Strabismus (Table 7.11)

Horizontal, vertical, and oblique muscle dysfunctions; craniofacial malformations; and orbital pulley system abnormalities among other less common causes have been implicated.

An inferior displacement of lateral rectus pulley can resemble an inferior oblique overaction and V pattern. A superior displacement can resemble a superior oblique overaction and A pattern.

7.6.3 Examination of Pattern Strabismus

1. Abnormal head posture: can manifest as chin elevation in cases of V-exotropia or A-esotropia, while chin depression may be observed in A-exotropia and V-esotropia.
2. Overelevation or overdepression in adduction: the examiner should look specifically for apparent oblique muscle overaction.
3. Deviation measurement is conducted in primary position, 25 degrees upgaze, and 35 degrees downgaze. An A-pattern deviation is considered clinically significant if the difference between upgaze and downgaze exceeds 10 prism diopters. For V-pattern deviations, a difference >15 prism diopters is deemed clinically significant.
4. Orbital imaging may be considered in patients with craniofacial or orbital muscle pulley abnormalities.

7.6.4 Management of Pattern Strabismus

1. Weakening of oblique muscle if overreaction is present.
2. Vertical transposition of horizontal muscle, where medial rectus muscles are moved toward the "apex" of the pattern (i.e., upward in A pattern and downward in V pattern), while the lateral rectus muscles are moved toward the open end. Remember MALE.
3. Pattern strabismus associated with craniofacial anomalies is complex and often difficult to manage.
4. Horizontal transposition of vertical rectus muscles (temporal displacement to decrease pattern esotropia) is rarely done.
5. Y pattern: inferior oblique muscle-weakening procedure or superior transposition of the lateral rectus muscles can improve this pattern.

Table 7.11 Comparison between A-pattern and V-pattern strabismus

	A pattern	V pattern
Oblique muscle dysfunction	Superior oblique overaction	Inferior oblique overaction
Vertical muscle dysfunction	Inferior rectus underaction and overaction of its yoke muscle, superior oblique	Underaction of superior rectus and overaction of its yoke muscle, inferior oblique
Horizontal muscle dysfunction	Medial rectus underaction in downgaze and lateral rectus underaction in upgaze	Overaction of medial rectus in downgaze and lateral rectus in upgaze
Anatomical factors	Hydrocephalus with frontal bossing, can simulate superior oblique overaction Up-slanting palpebral fissures	Extorsion of rectus muscle pulleys with primary orbital anomalies such as Crouzon and Apert syndromes Down-slanting palpebral fissure
Orbital muscle pulley dysfunction	LR insertions are higher than MR insertions	MR insertions are higher than LR insertions

6. X pattern: recession of the lateral rectus muscles alone usually improves the pattern.
7. λ pattern: superior oblique weakening if there is overdepression in adduction suggestive of SOOA. Vertical transposition of horizontal rectus muscles may be effective in cases of no oblique dysfunction.

> So keep in your mind: An alphabet pattern with significant oblique overaction should be corrected by oblique weakening. In the absence of oblique overaction, transposition of the recti should be undertaken using the mnemonic (MALES): Medial rectus is toward the apex, and lateral rectus is toward the empty space.

7.7 Abnormal Head Posture (AHP)

Paresis or paralysis of an extraocular muscle may result in diplopia if acquired. In early-onset strabismus, diplopia usually is not a complaint due to image suppression. In acquired strabismus, a patient often attempts to maintain binocular fusion by adopting abnormal head posture. If a horizontal deviation is present, a face turn will be present. With a vertical deviation, chin depression or chin elevation is noted, and if a cyclovertical deviation occurs, a head tilt is present and usually away from the affected side (Table 7.12).

7.7.1 Torticollis

This can be muscular (e.g., congenital muscular torticollis) or ocular. Muscular torticollis is mostly due to a birth injury to sternocleidomastoid muscle.

Torticollis that persists during sleep or remains evident even when one eye is closed is a key indicator for identifying non-ocular causes of torticollis. The presence of facial asymmetry denotes chronicity of torticollis

Ocular torticollis differential diagnosis:

In cases of superior oblique palsy, Brown's syndrome, DVD, nystagmus, specific head postures to compensate for their condition and improve vision.

Example: With right superior oblique palsy, the patient may turn their head to the left, position it downward, and tilt it toward the left shoulder to minimize diplopia and maintain binocular fusion.

7.7.2 Facial Asymmetry

It can include muscular and ocular etiologies: torticollis (most common cause if left untreated for a long time), trauma, and facial palsy.

Conflict of Interest None.

Table 7.12 Abnormal head posture and their differential

Chin elevation	Chin depression	Face turn	Head tilt
– A-pattern esotropia – V-pattern exotropia – Ptosis – Inferior rectus entrapment – Thyroid eye disease – Bilateral Brown's syndrome – Intranuclear ophthalmoplegia – Upbeat nystagmus	– V-pattern esotropia – A-pattern exotropia – Bilateral superior oblique palsy – Downbeat nystagmus	Associated with horizontal deviation: – Sixth nerve palsy: toward the affected side – Duane syndrome – Congenital nystagmus (null point) – Oblique muscle palsy: toward the unaffected side – Brown's syndrome: toward unaffected side	Associated with cyclovertical deviation: – Superior oblique palsy: head tilt and face turn to unaffected side – Inferior oblique palsy: head tilt and face turn to affected side – Brown's syndrome: head tilt toward the affected side – DVD: head tilt toward the affected side

References

Manchandia AM, Demer JL (2014) Sensitivity of the three-step test in diagnosis of superior oblique palsy. J Am Assoc Pediatr Ophthalmol Strabismus 18(6):567–571

Papageorgiou E, McLean RJ, Gottlob I (2014) Nystagmus in childhood. Pediatr Neonatol 55(5):341–351

8 Clinical Review of Pediatric Ophthalmology and Strabismus: Part III

Nisreen Abushehab, Jamila G. Hiasat, Saif Aldeen Alryalat, and Almutez Gharaibeh

Abstract

This chapter continues the exploration of pediatric ophthalmology, focusing on critical interventions and conditions that affect vision in children. It begins with thoroughly examining strabismus surgery, covering preoperative assessment, surgical techniques, and potential postoperative complications. The discussion then shifts to retinopathy of prematurity (ROP), detailing its pathophysiology, risk factors, screening protocols, and current treatment options to prevent vision loss. Additionally, the chapter explores congenital infections such as rubella, herpes simplex virus, and toxoplasmosis, highlighting their impact on ocular health. Through this comprehensive overview, the chapter seeks to enhance clinical understanding and improve management outcomes for strabismus and related pediatric ocular conditions.

Keywords

Strabismus surgery · ROP · Congenital infections · Conjunctivitis · Screening

8.1 Approach to Strabismus Surgery

In the management of strabismus patient, keep in your mind (Cestari and Hunter 2012):

1. Amblyopia management (patching, etc.)
2. Refractive error correction
3. Surgical correction of strabismus

Ocular misalignment is corrected by strabismus surgery through four distinct mechanisms:

- Slackening a muscle—recession
- Tightening a muscle—resection, plication
- Reducing moment arm—Faden procedure
- Changing vector force by transposition

N. Abushehab (✉)
Department of Ophthalmology, Ministry of Health, Amman, Jordan

J. G. Hiasat
Division of Pediatric Ophthalmology and Strabismus, UPMC Children's Hospital of Pittsburgh, Pittsburgh, PA, USA

Department of Ophthalmology, University of Pittsburgh School of Medicine, Pittsburgh, PA, USA
e-mail: Hiasatjg@upmc.edu

S. A. Alryalat
Department of Ophthalmology, The University of Jordan, Amman, Jordan

The University of Colorado Anschutz Medical Campus, CO, USA

A. Gharaibeh
Department of Ophthalmology, The University of Jordan, Amman, Jordan

S. A. Alryalat (ed.), *Ophthalmology Board and FRCS Part 2 Exams*,
https://doi.org/10.1007/978-981-96-1517-9_8

8.1.1 Weakening Surgeries for Recti Muscle

- Recession for recti muscle: it moves the muscle insertion closer to the origin creating a muscle slack, which makes the muscle less tight and reduces the arc of contact.
- The muscle slack reduces muscle strength according to Starling's length–tension curve.
- Recession has its greatest effect in the field of action of the muscle.
- Posterior fixation suture (Faden): also known as retroequatorial myopexy.
- Faden weakens the rotational force of a rectus muscle when the eye rotates towards the Faden muscle, without affecting the primary position of the eye. This means that it only affects the muscle when in action.
- This procedure does not affect the primary position of the eye.
- The muscle belly is sutured to globe posterior to its insertion farther than the limit of its arc of contact (12–14 mm posterior to the rectus muscle insertion).
- Irreversible because of fibrosis.
- It reduces the moment arm only when the eye rotates towards the muscle that is sutured.
- Best suited for MR muscle as it has the shortest arc of contact, it is less effective for the lateral rectus (LR) muscle due to its long arc of contact (this technique is used exclusively for recti muscle).

  Indications for a Faden:

  (a) Paralytic strabismus: In case of an LR palsy, Faden of the contralateral MR is done to produce progressive weakening in adduction to match existing weakening in abduction in the affected eye. It is used when the patient is orthotropic in primary position but has diplopia on gaze towards paretic muscle (in patients with right lateral rectus palsy, Faden is done on the left medial rectus).
  (b) Duane's retraction: contralateral MR.
  (c) Nystagmus blockage syndrome: MR.
  (d) Convergence excess esotropia (near esotropia with high AC/A): both MR.

- Marginal myotomy:
- Several cuts are made alternatively at the two borders of the muscle to weaken a muscle.

8.1.2 Weakening Surgeries for Oblique Muscle

- Tenotomy.

  This is useful for weakening superior oblique muscle; temporal conjunctival incision is made and reflected nasally. This helps to keep the nasal intermuscular septum intact and reduce tendon scarring. The main indication for tenotomy is Brown syndrome.
- Superior oblique tendon expander of Wright.

  A segment of silicone 240 retinal band is inserted between the cut ends of SO tendon. Most can be managed with 5–6 mm length of band. It is also used in Brown syndrome.
- Myotomy: a weakening procedure for inferior oblique muscle where muscle is cut in the middle. It can be ineffective as ends of the muscle can reattach.
- Myectomy

  It is an effective surgery and a strong weakening procedure. It is useful for weakening inferior oblique muscle, in which the portion of muscle around 6–8 mm is cut and removed. This reduces the chance of reattachment of the muscle to the globe.
- Inferior oblique recession

  This produces slackening of inferior oblique. The IO is inserted at a point 2 mm lateral and 3 mm posterior to the lateral end of IR insertion.

  Indications for inferior oblique weakening procedure:

  (a) V-pattern esotropia
  (b) Secondary inferior oblique overaction as in ipsilateral superior oblique palsy
  (c) Contralateral superior rectus palsy
- Graded recession with anterior transposition for oblique muscle:

  It is recommended for IO overaction. The basis is that the more anterior (in relation to inferior rectus insertion) the IO insertion, the greater the weakening effect.

- Extirpation-denervation

  The nerve to the IO is located on the posterior border of the muscle and can be hooked and cauterized. This results in muscle laxity. The procedure can also be combined with myectomy. Anteriorization of IO-J deformity

  In "J" deformity, the inferior oblique is disinserted and reattached at inferior rectus insertion. This is neither a weakening nor a strengthening surgery, but it changes the action of inferior oblique from elevator in adduction to anti-elevator at primary position. This occurs because the neurofibrovascular bundle of the inferior oblique inserts into the posterior fibers and can act as a tether, holding the eye down.

  It is mainly a surgery for DVD and some cases of significant IOOA 4+. The main complication of this procedure is the postoperative severe limitation of elevation called "the anti-elevation syndrome."

8.1.3 Strengthening Surgeries for Recti Muscle

- Resection:

  It is the most common procedure for muscle strengthening and involves excision of the tendinous part of recti muscle.

  For MR—maximum limit is 6 mm. For LR—maximum limit is 8 mm.

  Note:

  Superior and inferior rectus resection will narrow the palpebral fissure due to their close relationship to superior–levator complex and lower eyelid retractors.

- Advancement:

  It is not a primary operation, and it is done on previously recess muscle. Advancement of a muscle means disinserting a previously recessed muscle and reattaching closer to its original insertion.

- Plication

  Fold piece of the muscle around itself, and suture to sclera, in contrast to resection shortening of the muscle that occurs without cutting or disinserting the muscle. In plications, the anterior ciliary artery circulation is theoretically preserved.

  Possible advantages of rectus muscle plication include a lower risk of "lost" muscles and anterior segment ischemia.

8.1.4 Strengthening Surgeries for Oblique Muscle

- Harada-Ito procedure

  It involves selective strengthening of anterior (one-quarter to one-third of SO fiber) through anterior and lateral displacement of anterior SO fiber, which is then reattached at 8 mm posterior to superior border of lateral rectus; this will induce intorsion (enhance incyclotorsion action) without too much change in depression and abduction.
- Indication: torsional diplopia, as seen in a partially recovered SO palsy with a significant degree of extorsion. Patients with bilateral traumatic superior oblique paresis often experience partial recovery, resulting in extorsion and esotropia in downgaze, but without significant oblique dysfunction or a hypertropia in the primary position.
- Tucking:
- It shortens the muscle by folding the muscle and suturing the folded muscle to muscle. It is mainly used for bilateral superior oblique muscle palsy to improve depression on adduction (may induce transient pseudo-Brown syndrome-like manifestation due to limited elevation on adduction).

8.1.5 Adjustable Suture Technique for Strabismus Surgery

It is a method in which muscles may be repositioned after initial surgery (Nihalani and Hunter 2011). It is usually used to increase the likelihood of success with a single operation in patients with unpredictable outcomes, such as those undergoing reoperations. However, this technique alone does not guarantee long-term satisfactory alignment. During the procedure, surgery is completed with externalized sutures and slip knots, allowing for the muscle position to be adjusted during the early postoperative days or within just a few hours. While this technique can be successfully used in children, it often requires additional general anesthesia. Relative contraindications include patient anxiety and a history of prior vagal episodes. Transposition surgery in strabismus is based on changing the location of the muscle insertion, so the muscle pulls the eye in a different direction. Transposition surgeries can be used to treat:

(a) A rectus muscle paresis
(b) A lost muscle
(c) Pattern deviation

8.1.6 Transposition Surgery in Strabismus

8.1.6.1 Hummelsheim Procedure

It is used for sixth nerve palsy and involves half-tendon transfer technique. In this procedure, a muscle hook is utilized to separate the superior and inferior rectus muscles from their insertion sites by approximately 14 mm. The temporal halves of these muscles are then disinserted and moved towards the lateral rectus muscle. Finally, these transposed halves are sutured to the sclera adjacent to the insertion of the lateral rectus. This technique aims to correct the misalignment resulting from sixth nerve palsy by adjusting the muscle forces on the eye.

8.1.6.2 Knapp Procedure

This involves a full-tendon transfer and was initially described for the management of double-elevator palsy. However, it can also be applied in cases of sixth nerve palsy. One potential complication of this procedure is anterior segment ischemia. Complication of transposition surgery:

1. Anterior segment ischemia occurs more in full-tendon width transposition (Knapp) than split tendon (Jensen and Hummelsheim).
2. Induces unwanted deviations (torsional or vertical or horizontal) especially if there is asymmetric muscle transposition done

8.1.6.3 Jensen's procedure

It can be used to treat sixth nerve palsy. In this procedure, the muscle bellies of the superior rectus, inferior rectus, and lateral rectus muscles are partially split to half their tendon width, extending 12–14 mm from their insertion, with the aid of a muscle hook. Unlike other procedures, the muscles are not disinserted. The split tendons are then transferred and secured to the adjacent muscles (superior with lateral rectus and inferior with lateral rectus) using nonabsorbable suture.

Advantage of this procedure is that it preserves the anterior ciliary arteries, thereby reducing the risk of anterior segment ischemia.

8.1.7 Botulinum Toxin Chemo-Denervation

Clinical trials using botulinum toxin for the treatment of strabismus have shown this agent to be most effective in the following conditions:

1. Small- to moderate-angle esotropia and exotropia (<40Δ).
2. Postoperative residual strabismus (2–8 weeks following surgery or later).
3. Acute paralytic strabismus (especially sixth nerve palsy). Botox is given to ipsilateral medial rectus to eliminate diplopia temporarily.
4. Active (but not chronic fibrosed phase) thyroid eye disease (Graves' disease) or inflamed or pre-phthisical eyes, when surgery might be inappropriate.
5. As a supplement to medial rectus muscle recession for large-angle infantile esotropia or lateral rectus muscle recession for large-angle exotropia. Botulinum toxin injection is generally not effective in patients with large deviations, restrictive or mechanical strabismus (such as that caused by trauma, chronic thyroid eye disease), or secondary strabismus where a muscle has been overly

recessed. It is also ineffective in treating A- and V-pattern strabismus, DVDs, and chronic paralytic strabismus. The effects of injection usually last around 6 months. In children, long-term ocular realignment may occur due to contracture of the direct antagonist combined along with motor and sensory adaptations that help restore some degree of binocularity.

The most common complication of botulinum injections is ptosis, followed by secondary vertical strabismus.

8.1.8 Complications of Strabismus Surgery

Intraoperative Complication

1. Surgery on the wrong muscle which may occur because of globe rotation.
   - The inferior oblique and lateral recti are most frequently confused.
2. Hemorrhage may occur due to inadvertent injury to vortex vein, especially during inferior oblique surgery.
3. Disruption of the muscle sheath and damage to the muscle during dissection are frequent causes of bleeding.

   Topical vasoconstrictors, bipolar cautery, and careful dissection help to decrease risks of bleeding.
4. The oculocardiac reflex.

   Sinus bradycardia can occur due to traction on the EOMs during surgery, especially when hooking the medial rectus muscle. In its most severe form, this reflex can lead to asystole. Surgeon must be aware of the potential to induce the oculocardiac reflex when manipulating a muscle and should be prepared to release tension immediately if the heart rate drops excessively. Administrating intravenous atropine and other agents can protect against this reflex.
5. Scleral perforation

   It is one of the most dangerous complications of strabismus surgery, during muscle reattachment. This can occur when the needle passes too deeply through the sclera. Risk factors include thin sclera, high myopia, inexperienced surgeons, and re-surgeries. The needle may penetrate into the suprachoroidal space or pass through the choroid and retina. In most cases, this results in a small chorioretinal scar without significantly affecting vision. If vitreous escapes through the perforation site, the patient will need vitreoretinal evaluation. Surgeons may apply immediate local cryotherapy or laser therapy.
6. Lost or slipped muscle

   Slipped muscle: The tendon retracts posteriorly inside the muscular sheath. The sheath is still empty and fixed to the sclera at the insertion site.

   Lost muscle: The lack of any connection between the muscle tendon and its sheath with the sclera. The clinical manifestations of a lost muscle are more severe and appear earlier than those of a slipped muscle. Magnetic resonance imaging (MRI) is preferred for locating the muscle and determining whether it remained attached to the globe. The medial rectus is most commonly affected and is difficult to retrieve because it lacks fascial connections to the oblique muscles, which could otherwise prevent it from retracting posteriorly. This complication may occur during muscle disinsertion if the suture is not placed properly.

Postoperative Complication

1. Overcorrection (consecutive strabismus), undercorrection (residual strabismus) mostly due to improper surgical dosage calculations or preoperative assessment
2. Excessive conjunctival scarring, which may limit duction
3. Changes in refractive error

   Most commonly induced astigmatism when strabismus surgery is performed on recti muscles of the same eye.
4. Postoperative infections

   Rarely occurs as preseptal cellulitis, orbital cellulitis, or endophthalmitis.
5. Ocular surface complications

   Corneal dellen: secondary to disruption of tear film regularity.

   Inclusion cyst: arises from inadvertent burying of conjunctiva while approximating the edge.

Prolapsed tenon's capsule: Prolapsed or exposed tenon's tissue which may be secondary to inappropriate apposition of the conjunctival margins.

6. Diplopia:

   It occurs in older children and especially in adults. Surgery can move the image of the fixation object in the deviating eye out of a suppression scotoma. Abnormal retinal correspondence may cause transient paradoxical diplopia in the presence of orthotropia. Patient may overcome the diplopia by fusion or the diplopia may persist.
7. Change in palpebral aperture:

   This can occur following strabismus surgery on the horizontal and vertical rectus muscles. Recession of a horizontal rectus muscle typically results in widening of the palpebral aperture (PA), while recession tends to decrease its height. Similarly, after surgery on the vertical rectus muscles, recession can cause widening of the palpebral aperture, whereas resection may lead to narrowing.
8. Anterior segment ischemia:

   It is a rare but serious complication, with the risk increasing when three or more recti muscles are operated in the same eye simultaneously. Early signs include cells and flare in the anterior chamber, corneal epithelial edema, and folds in Descemet's membrane. More severe cases may present with an irregular pupil and iris atrophy.
9. Retinal detachment

   Intraoperative scleral perforation during muscle reattachment may cause postoperative retinal detachment. The risk of retinal detachment depends on the depth of the needle penetration.

8.2 Retinopathy of Prematurity (ROP)

Normally, retinal vascularization begins at around the 16th week of gestation, starting at the optic nerve head and extending towards the periphery. This process is usually completed in the nasal retina by about 36 weeks of gestation and in the temporal retina by around 40 weeks.

ROP incidence according to weight:

1000–1250 g —> 50%
750–1000 g —> 80%
<750 g —> 90%

ROP incidence according to gestational age:

28–31 weeks —> 60%
<28 weeks —> 80%

8.2.1 Criteria for Exam

Current evidence suggests screening infants with the following (Dogra et al. 2017):

1. Gestational age of 30 weeks or less
2. Infants with a birth weight of ≤1500 g
3. Selected infants with a birth weight between 1500 and 2000 g or gestational age of >30 weeks with an unstable clinical course

Initial screening should be performed at 31 weeks' postmenstrual age in infants with gestational ages of 26, 6/7 weeks or less at birth, and at 4 weeks' chronological age in infants with gestational age of 27 weeks or more at birth.

Zones

Zone I: small circle of the retina around the disc. The radius is twice the distance from optic nerve to fovea.

Zone II: the ring-shaped section of the retina surrounding zone I, which extends to the ora serrata on the nasal side.

Zone III: is a crescent-shaped area of temporal retina.

Stages

Stage 1: ROP is a demarcation line that separates normal retina from avascular retina.

Stage 2: is a ridge which has height and width that separates normal retina from avascular retina.

Stage 3: is the growth of fragile new abnormal blood vessels.

Stage 4: includes mild tractional RD, with 4a (the RD does not involve the fovea) and 4b (the RD involves the fovea).

Stage 5: is end-stage tractional total RD (while stage 4 does not involve the whole retina).

Plus disease is when retinal arterioles and venules are dilated and tortuous.

Combining zones and stages, ROP can be divided into threshold and pre-threshold, with pre-threshold further divided into type 1 and type 2. Treatment is recommended for threshold and pre-threshold type 1 ROP.

1. Pre-threshold ROP:

   Type 1 pre-threshold ROP: Defined as zone I plus disease with any stage, zone I stage 3 with no plus, and zone II stage 2 or 3 with plus disease. It needS immediate treatment.

   Type 2 pre-threshold ROP: Defined as zone I stage 1 or 2 without plus disease and zone II stage 3 without plus disease. Close follow-up is recommended.
2. Threshold ROP: ROP of more than 5 contiguous or 8 cumulative clock hours of stage 3 with plus disease in zone I or zone II. It has risk of more than 50% to develop RD if untreated.

8.2.2 Aggressive Posterior ROP APROP

Extensive stage 3 neovascularization in zone I: It develops a flat network of neovascularization early on in the disease with severe plus disease in all four quadrants without the preexisting ridge. Typically, it does not progress through thc stages of ROP. APROP progresses rapidly, is often difficult to treat, and has a poor prognosis.

8.2.2.1 Follow-Up

Follow-up can be determined by assessing vascularization and ROP stage at each zone (Table 8.1).

Remember: Close follow-up after 1 week is mandatory for

1. Type 2 pre-threshold disease
2. Immature vascularization in zone I

8.2.2.2 When to Stop Acute Screening for ROP

Full retinal vascularization

Zone III retinal vascularization in the absence of prior ROP in zone I or II (until PMA is 37 weeks)

Zone III retinal vascularization with no type 1 ROP (stage 3 ROP in zone II, any ROP in zone I, or worse ROP (until 45 weeks))

If the patient has received anti-vascular endothelial growth factor (VEGF) injections in the past, continue screening until at least PMA = 65 weeks.

Make sure that there is no abnormal vascular tissue present that could reactivate and worsen as ROP has entirely regressed.

Long-term monitoring

Preterm infants should be followed up within 4–6 months of being discharged from acute ROP screening.

Treatment: Treatment can be provided using anti-VEGF intravitreal injection, laser photocoagulation, vitrectomy, and RD repair surgery for stages 4 and 5.

Treatment should be initiated within 3 days for threshold ROP or type 1 pre-threshold ROP.

Table 8.1 Follow-up exam according to retinopathy of prematurity (ROP) stage

	After 1 week	After 1–2 weeks	After 2 weeks	After 3 weeks
Immature vascularization	At Zone I	At zone II posterior	At zone II	–
ROP stage zone I	Stages 1 or 2	–	–	–
ROP stage zone II	Stage 3	Stage 2	Stage 1	
ROP stage zone III	–	–	–	Stage 1 or 2
Regressing ROP	–	Zone I	Zone II	Zone III

- The anti-VEGF treatment for ROP:
- This is usually for plus disease in zone I or posterior zone II with stage 1 or 2; it is given usually:
  1. Half adult dose (0.25 mg for ranibizumab) (0.65 mg for bevacizumab), aflibercept 0.4 mg
  2. Dependent on gestational age; can be half adult distance from limbus (~1–2 mm)

     The most important drawback is the higher recurrence rate than the laser, and it can be repeated after 1 month. The benefit is the continued growth in the avascular retina, whereas laser therapy led to permanent destruction of the peripheral retina.

8.2.2.3 Laser Treatment for ROP

This is usually for zone II anterior and zone III ROP with stage 3 and plus disease.

8.2.3 Prognosis

The onset of serious ROP correlates better with postmenstrual age (gestational age at birth plus chronologic age) rather than with postnatal age.

Spontaneous regression of retinopathy of prematurity (ROP) occurs in almost 75%.

Consequences of ROP development and treatment include:

1. Axial myopia: It is one of the most common sequelae of significant ROP, whether treated or spontaneously regressed, which may be severe.
2. Strabismus.
3. Glaucoma, with risk of angle closure that develops before the age of 10 years.
4. Retinal detachment.
5. Cataract.

8.2.3.1 Conditions That Mimic ROP

Familial exudative vitreoretinopathy (FEVR) is a group of inherited bilateral retinal disorders, typically following AD inheritance. These conditions are characterized by abnormal retinal angiogenesis leading to incomplete vascularization of the peripheral retina, which results in retinal ischemia. FEVR can mimic ROP but is distinct in several ways. Unlike ROP, FEVR occurs in full-term infants who do not have a history of supplemental oxygen use. The presence of bilateral avascular peripheral temporal retina, along with a progressive clinical course, helps differentiate FEVR from ROP. Proliferation in the temporal retina can cause dragging of the retina, increasing the risk of retinal breaks and rhegmatogenous retinal detachment (RRD). FEVR may also lead to exotropia.

Approaches to pediatric cataract

8.3 Pediatric Cataract

Pediatric cataract is one of the treatable causes of blindness in children (Khokhar et al. 2017). The incidence is 3:10,000. The causes of pediatric cataract are multifactorial.

8.3.1 Etiology

The laterality and morphology and the general condition of the child of the cataract may offer hints as to its cause and time of insult.

8.3.1.1 Unilateral or Bilateral Cataract

Bilateral Cataract

33–50% idiopathic

20–30%: inherited; AD in 75% of the cases, may be AR or XL

20–30%: associated with systemic disease as metabolic disease (galactosemia, Lowe syndrome, hypoparathyroidism, Fabry's disease), congenital infection (TORCH), chromosomal anomaly (trisomies 21, 18, 13), skeletal anomaly (Hallermann-Streiff syndrome, Nance-Horan syndrome), ocular anomaly (aniridia, anterior segment dysgenesis)

Unilateral Cataract

Mostly 90% are idiopathic, sporadic, isolated, non-syndromic, and associated with ocular anomaly as persistent fetal vasculature (PFV)

Table 8.2 Types of pediatric cataract and their characteristics

Anterior polar	Opacity at anterior capsule or it may have projection to anterior chamber (pyramidal cataract) Usually does not affect visual acuity May be dominant inheritance	Seen with Peters anomaly Associated with persistent pupillary membrane , aniridia, anterior segment dysgenesis
Anterior subcapsular	Sunflower Anterior lenticonus	Seen with Wilson disease Seen with Alport
Posterior polar	Posterior capsular plaque	Ocular associations, posterior lenticonus, persistent fetal vasculature
Coronary (supranuclear)	Crown-like opacity in deep cortex, surrounding the nucleus Usually does not affect vision Sporadic	
Cortical spoke-like		Systemic associations like Fabry's disease, mannosidosis
Sutural cataract	Opacity following Y suture anterior or posterior	
Blue dot cataract	Scattered blue dot cortical opacities common and innocuous	Associated with Down syndrome
Lamellar (zonular cataract) surrounding clear nucleus and overlaying the clear cortex may have rides extended to equator	The commonest developmental cataract. 50% of visual significant cataracts. Usually AD, bilateral asymmetrical	May be associated with hypovitaminosis D, hypocalcemia
Central (pulverulent)	Dominant inheritance, fetal and embryonal nucleus opacity with clear center. Nonprogressive, bilateral	
Total cataract	– Morgagnian cataract (uncommon), nucleus sink due to liquefaction of outer zone of the lens – Dense complete opacification	Seen with rubella syndrome
Membranous cataract (partially absorbed)	Cataract lens is absorbed with fusion anterior and posterior capsule	Seen in Hallermann-Streiff syndrome

8.3.1.2 Morphological Classification (Table 8.2)

According to the Location of Opacity:

Anterior: anterior polar, anterior subcapsular
Central: cortical, nuclear, lamellar, sutural
Posterior: posterior polar, posterior subcapsular
Total (diffuse): central total, partially absorbed

- General evaluation

  Preoperative evaluation is important to examine the eye and the child's general condition.

- History taking

  Presence of cataract would suggest a congenital origin or, if developed later, between infancy and adolescence, indicate a developmental onset. In addition, inquire about the mother's history of infections during the first trimester of pregnancy, as well as any family history of cataracts, as these can provide crucial clues to the etiology.

- Ocular examination
  1. Assess visual acuity by preferential looking test, if the child resists occlusion of one eye. Indicators of severe visual impairment: no fixation, nystagmus, and sensory strabismus.
  2. The morphology and density of cataract are important for several reasons; it can give a clue to the age of onset, visual prognosis, etiology, and heritability (Table 8.3).
  3. Fundus examination with indirect ophthalmoscope is essential to rule out any posterior segment pathology.

Table 8.3 Cataract morphology and its associated potential etiology

Oil droplet	Galactosemia
Blue dot	Congenital
Posterior subcapsular	Radiation, steroid induced
Sunflower	Wilson disease
Rossette	Blunt trauma
PSCC	Corticosteroid use, uveitis, retinal abnormalities, radiation exposure, and trauma
Anterior lenticonus	Alport syndrome

- Investigation:
  1. Screen newborns with red reflex test.
  2. Workup for bilateral cases without known hereditary basis.
     (a) Serology for intrauterine infection (TORCH screen)
     (b) Serum glucoses, calcium, phosphate
     (c) Urine: reducing substances (galactosemia), amino acids (Lowe syndrome), hematuria (Alport syndrome)

The visually significant cataract

8.3.1.3 Management

Nonsurgical Management:

– Non-visually significant cataract

It is used for partial cataract less than 3 mm, and paracentral, peripheral opacities (frequently after trauma) can be managed by refraction and prescription of appropriate correction.

Cyclopentolate once or twice daily may be used.

Amblyopia treatment with either patching or atropine penalization.

Surgical Management:

Mainly for bilateral or unilateral visually significant dense cataract

- Considerations regarding surgery
  1. Biometry: At birth, the keratometry is about 52 D, decreasing rapidly within the first 6 months and then gradually, reaching an adult value of around 44 D by 2–3 years of age.
  2. Axial length (AL): This can be measured using either contact or emersion methods, with the latter being more accurate. It is important to note that 1 mm error in AL measurement leads to an error of about 2.5 D in IOL power calculation.

     The preferred IOL formulas for children are SRK/T and Holladay 2, as they demonstrate the least predictive error. There are several IOL formulas, and we depend on the axial length to choose the best IOL formula (e.g., Hoffer Q preferred for AXL <20 mm).
  3. Target refraction: It is preferable to aim moderate hypermetropia, undercorrection, in the early postoperative period because children's eyes continue to grow, and every 1 mm growth in axial length will cause 3 diopters of myopia.
     – The IOL power implanted is intentionally reduced by a predetermined percentage (undercorrected) from the calculated IOL power.
- Surgical procedures:

Lensectomy + primary posterior capsulotomy (PCCC) + anterior vitrectomy.

8.3.1.4 Complications:

1. Visual axis opacification: the commonest late complication of pediatric cataract surgery. It occurs as a result of proliferation of lens epithelial cells from the equator to the anterior surface of the vitreous.

   An adequate posterior continuous curvilinear capsulorhexis (PCCC), with or without vitrectomy, is crucial to prevent VAO. VAO occurs in 30–40% cases of pediatric cataract, even after a primary posterior capsulorhexis, with higher rates in younger children. PCCC is recommended for children under 4–6 years and for children who may be uncooperative for YAG laser capsulotomy. Its incidence reaches 100% if posterior surgical capsulotomy was not done.

2. Glaucoma: The incidence of glaucoma is 10–25%, but its incidence increases to more than 90% if cataract surgery was completed before 4 weeks of age.
3. Postoperative inflammation: It is more common in children than adults due to increased tissue reactivity. Decreased surgery time, minimal manipulation during surgery, and in-bag IOL implantation reduce it.
4. IOL-related complication: IOL deposits, synechiae, IOL opacification, and decentration can be seen in the postoperative period.

- Postoperative follow-up

  Pediatric cataract surgery is the beginning of the journey of long-term follow-up.

We should follow up the child regularly.

1. Refraction and visual acuity

   Early visual rehabilitation stimulates binocularity and lowers strabismus and amblyopia incidence even in the child who had IOL implantation or left aphakia. All children should be followed up by refraction regularly because the eye's refractive state is susceptible to change due to the eye growth.
2. IOP

   Aphakic or pseudophakic children should be followed up with regular IOP measurements. Secondary glaucoma may be suspected by an excessive myopic shift in relation to axial length and enlarged corneal diameter.
3. Amblyopia screening

   With either patching or atropine penalization.
4. Lens-related factors such as visual axis clarity

Visual axis opacification needs to be cleared surgically or by laser to allow visual development.

8.3.1.5 Leukocoria

Remember Credit-p

C Congenital cataract, Coats disease, coloboma of optic nerve and choroid

R Retinoblastoma, retinopathy of prematurity

E Endophthalmitis

D Dysplasia of retina

I Inflammatory cyclitic membrane

T

P Toxocariasis

PFV

Most common: congenital cataract

Most dangerous: retinoblastoma

- Persistent fetal vasculature

  PFV is mostly unilateral (90%), leading to amblyopia in the affected eye.

  It is divided as anterior or posterior. Posterior PFV has poorer prognosis.

  The anterior subtype is marked by retrolental opacity and cataract, an elongated ciliary process with anteriorly displaced ciliary body, and a membranous transformation of the anterior vitreous face causing traction on the peripheral retina. It also features a shallow anterior chamber, which predisposes to angle closure, poor pupil dilation, and microphthalmos.

  The posterior subtype has been defined by:

  A stalk of tissue extending from the optic nerve to the retrolental area causing retinal folds, dysplasia, or detachment optic nerve dysplasia.

  Differential diagnosis is retinoblastoma, where calcification seen on imaging is suggestive of malignancy.
- Retinoblastoma:

  Almost 95% of newly diagnosed cases will have no family history of retinoblastoma. Most frequent age at diagnosis is 18 months, and 95% will be diagnosed by 3 years. In an affected child of healthy parents, parents' copies are probably normal. The following generalizations serve as guidelines:

1. Healthy parents with one affected child have a 6% chance of having additional affected children.
2. If two or more siblings are affected, it suggests a chromosomal defect in one parent, increasing the risk of each additional child inheriting the condition to 40%.

3. A parent with bilateral retinoblastoma has a 50% chance of passing the affected chromosome to their children. With 80% penetrance, 40% of the offspring will exhibit the condition phenotypically.

   Growth into the vitreous is referred to as endophytic (endo-, towards the inner retina), while growth towards the sclera is termed exophytic (exo-, towards the outer retina).

   Blood tests in retinoblastoma may reveal basophilia. Direct spread into the optic nerve and CNS is the most common site of metastasis.

   Although retinoma typically follows a benign course, the fellow eye may develop retinoblastoma, and the genetic implications are the same.

   In retinoblastoma, CT is generally avoided as an imaging modality in possible Rb cases to minimize exposure to radiation in these patients, who are at an increased risk of secondary malignancies. Lumbar puncture and bone marrow biopsy are not part of a routine initial evaluation unless there are other signs/symptoms to suggest systemic involvement.

   Over 90% of newly diagnosed cases are new mutations and have no family history. If this patient has a new germline Rb1 mutation, he has an 85% chance of bilateral disease. Fifteen percent of unilateral cases are germline and therefore transmissible. If the parent of this child has a germline Rb1 mutation, this patient has an 85% risk of bilateral disease.

- Coats disease

  It is a unilateral disease characterized by telangiectasia and aneurysm in the peripheral temporal retina with exudation posteriorly. It is more frequent in males (3:1) and in children less than 8 years of age. It has the most severe and worse prognosis in children less than 3 years of age.

Stages of Coats Disease:

Stage 1 includes temporal telangiectasia with focal exudation.

Stage 2 is associated with diffuse exudation.

Stage 3 includes exudative RD.

Stage 4 includes total RD.

Almost 50% may progress to stage 4, and 10% may develop neovascular glaucoma.

Leber's miliary aneurysm is a milder variant of the Coats disease and rarely progresses to exudative retinal detachment. Type 1 idiopathic macular telangiectasia is now regarded as the same condition as Coats disease (see retina chapter).

Coats disease is typically managed by focal laser performed to areas of leakage identified on FFA, and anti-VEGF injections can be considered. Vitrectomy can be considered in cases of RD.

The main DDx is retinoblastoma with the latter including calcium on imaging (Table 8.4).

Table 8.4 Comparison between Coats disease and retinoblastoma

Feature	Coats disease	Retinoblastoma
Presentation	Older patient, unilateral, male	Younger presentation, maybe bilateral, no sex predilection
Leukocoria	Gray to pink	White
Telangiectasia	Classic, vessels can be traced	With tumor infiltration, vessels dip into the mass
Vitreous seeding	Absent	Maybe present
Calcification	Not a feature	Can be seen on ultrasounds and CT scan
Intraocular mass	Not a feature	Seen in endophytic cases
FFA	Leaks with telangiectatic vessels	Double circulation

8.4 Congenital Infections

Maternal TORCH infections relatively common

Congenital rubella

Commonest in developing countries

15–20% have congenital cataract (bilateral in 80%). It is described as a white nuclear or total cataract (dense). Following cataract surgery, brisk uveitis can occur because of spread of virus particle, which leads to heavy inflammation, so postoperative cataract extraction in rubella syndrome is characterized by severe inflammation due to live virus retained within residual lens cortex.

Other ocular manifestations: The most common ocular manifestation is pigmentary retinopathy that occurs in 40% (salt and pepper), which is a benign nonprogressive retinitis. Visual fields and ERG are normal, and congenital glaucoma is seen in 10% of the cases. Other associations include cloudy cornea, miotic pupil, and hypermetropia.

The most common clinical finding in infants with congenital rubella syndrome is sensorineural hearing loss.

Although children with congenital rubella syndrome may develop either cataract or glaucoma, their coincidence in an infant is rare, and congenital cataract and glaucoma are unlikely to be found simultaneously.

Lens capsule forms in the fifth week of embryogenesis. Most of virus transmission to fetus occurs during the first 8 weeks of pregnancy.

8.4.1 Herpes Simplex Virus (HSV)

Herpes simplex (HSV-2 infection is commoner than HSV-1)

Perinatal infection after exposure to maternal herpetic infection is transmitted at the time of delivery by passage through an infected birth canal. Congenital HSV infection is usually symptomatic with vesicular dermatitis, keratoconjunctivitis, pneumonitis, or meningoencephalitis. Other ocular manifestations include retinitis and cataract.

8.4.2 CMV Intrauterine Infection

Congenital CMV infection is the most common congenital ocular infection in developed countries (2%), although it is mostly subclinical. Most cases occur by maternal viremia during pregnancy, and infection is silent and asymptomatic. Ocular findings include chorioretinitis which is the most common ocular manifestation presenting as a peripheral retinal lesion (atrophic and hyperpigmented). Other manifestations include microphthalmia, cataracts, and optic disc anomalies (atrophy).

8.4.3 Toxoplasmosis

Ocular manifestations include chorioretinitis, iridocyclitis, retinal detachment, nystagmus, and strabismus. Systemic features include microcephaly, hydrocephalus, cerebral calcification, psychomotor retardation, jaundice, and seizures.

Other intrauterine infections include varicella and syphilis.

Hutchinson's triad, considered diagnostic of congenital syphilis infection, includes peg-shaped teeth, eighth nerve deafness, and interstitial keratitis.

8.4.4 Neonatal Conjunctivitis

Ophthalmia neonatorum is conjunctivitis that occurs within the first 28 days of life. Etiology can be classified based on inflammation onset (Table 8.5).

Table 8.5 Differential for ophthalmia neonatorum according to onset

Onset	Organism	Treatment
Within 24 h of birth	Chemical	Observation
2–4 days	*Neisseria gonorrhoeae*	Systemic ceftriaxone
5–14 days	Chlamydia	Systemic erythromycin

8.4.4.1 Herpes Simplex Virus Can Be Present

Management of ophthalmia neonatorum always involves systemic treatment because of the risk of systemic involvement.

Chemical conjunctivitis from topical silver nitrate application typically begins within 24 h of birth. Conjunctival scraping in this case shows few to no polymorphonuclear neutrophils (PMNs).

Chlamydial conjunctivitis (aka inclusion conjunctivitis) may lead to pneumonia, so it is treated via oral erythromycin. Approximately 15% of newborns with conjunctivitis develop chlamydial pneumonitis.

Herpes keratitis may lead to encephalitis, hepatitis among others, treated via IV acyclovir.

Gonorrhoeae may be associated with corneal ulceration and endophthalmitis. So, it is treated via IV penicillin.

Gonococcal conjunctivitis requires invasive systemic antibiotic therapy, such as ceftriaxone, with topical therapy being secondary. Ocular irrigation can help remove infectious agents from the ocular surface. *Neisseria gonorrhoeae* is known for its ability to penetrate an intact corneal epithelium and cause corneal perforation.

Unilateral blepharitis can be a significant sign of herpes simplex infection in children.

Herpes simplex complex results from infection with herpes simplex viruses 1 and 2 (HSV-1 and HSV-2). Close personal contact with infected individuals is the main risk factor for herpes simplex. Diagnosis is primarily clinical, although the virus can be cultured from vesicles.

Herpes simplex type 2 is a notable cause of neonatal conjunctivitis with keratitis affecting the corneal epithelium. Untreated neonatal herpes keratitis can lead to corneal scarring and severe amblyopia. In infants with immature immune systems, the usual hyperacute purulent conjunctivitis might not be observed. Treatment requires both topical and IV antibiotics to address this severe infection.

Conflict of Interest None.

References

Cestari DM, Hunter DG (2012) Learning strabismus surgery: a case-based approach. Lippincott Williams & Wilkins

Dogra MR, Katoch D, Dogra M (2017) An update on retinopathy of prematurity (ROP). Indian J Pediatr 84:930–936

Khokhar SK, Pillay G, Dhull C, Agarwal E, Mahabir M, Aggarwal P (2017) Pediatric cataract. Indian J Ophthalmol 65(12):1340–1349

Nihalani BR, Hunter DG (2011) Adjustable suture strabismus surgery. Eye 25(10):1262–1276

Clinical Review of Eyelid and Oculoplasty: Part I

9

Taher Alshammari, Hisham Kamel,
Saif Aldeen Alryalat, and Osama H. Ababneh

Abstract

This chapter reviews oculoplastic disorders, starting with eyelid anatomy and its role in ocular health. It highlights meibomian gland dysfunction as a common cause of dry eye symptoms. The chapter discusses eyelid masses ranging from benign to malignant, emphasizing the importance of early detection and treatment, as well as congenital eyelid diseases that can impact visual development. It also evalutes ptosis and lid retraction, along with their correction strategies, and contrasts ectropion and entropion in terms of causes and surgical management. Overall, the chapter aims to enhance understanding in oculoplastic care.

Keywords

Oculoplastic · Eyelid anatomy · Eyelid masses · Inflammatory conditions · Lid retraction

9.1 Overview

In this chapter, we delve into the diverse aspects of oculoplastic disorders and their management, starting with an exploration of the intricate anatomy of the eyelid and its role in maintaining ocular health and function. Recognizing the critical structures and the interplay between them is paramount to understanding various eyelid pathologies, their presentations, and implications.

A key component of many inflammatory eyelid conditions is meibomian gland dysfunction, a common source of dry eye symptoms and ocular discomfort. We delve into the presentation, pathophysiology, and management approaches for this prevalent condition.

Understanding the approach to eyelid masses, from benign lumps and bumps to more worrisome malignancies, is critical for early detection, appropriate biopsy selection, and effective treatment strategies.

Our discussion extends to congenital eyelid diseases, elaborating on a variety of conditions present from birth that may not only affect the aesthetic appearance but can also pose significant

T. Alshammari
Department of Special Surgery, Prince Mohammed Medical City, Al-Jouf, Kingdom of Saudi Arabia

H. Kamel
Research Institute Ophthalmology, Cairo, Egypt

S. A. Alryalat
Department of Ophthalmology, The University of Jordan, Amman, Jordan

The University of Colorado Anschutz Medical Campus, CO, USA

O. H. Ababneh (✉)
Department of Ophthalmology, The University of Jordan, Amman, Jordan
e-mail: o.ababneh@ju.edu.jo

S. A. Alryalat (ed.), *Ophthalmology Board and FRCS Part 2 Exams*,
https://doi.org/10.1007/978-981-96-1517-9_9

threats to visual development if not promptly addressed.

Further sections tackle the common and impactful conditions of ptosis and lid retraction. These eyelid malpositions can significantly influence visual function and require a nuanced approach to their correction.

We then contrast ectropion and entropion, two conditions that constitute the outward and inward turning of the eyelid, respectively. Despite their divergent presentations, they share common threads in their causes, implications, and principles of surgical management.

In the realm of oculoplastic surgery, we explore a range of surgical techniques applied to address various functional and aesthetic conditions, highlighting the art and science that underlie this sub-specialty.

Finally, the chapter concludes with a potpourri of miscellaneous topics, touching on some additional diseases and syndromes, along with pertinent management considerations that an oculoplastic surgeon should be well versed with.

Throughout the chapter, the content is interlaced with illustrations, case scenarios, and tables to bolster understanding, highlight common pitfalls, and promote the application of this knowledge in the clinical context. Whether you are a trainee or a practicing clinician, this chapter serves as a comprehensive guide for various oculoplastic conditions.

9.2 Clinical Anatomy of the Eyelid

The eyelid, a complex structure crucial for protecting the eye and maintaining visual clarity, can be anatomically and functionally subdivided into various components. This section aims to delve into the intricacies of its anatomy that is relevant for clinical ophthalmology.

Orbital Septum: This membranous sheet extends from the periosteum around the orbital rim (arcus marginalis) to the eyelid margins, where it fuses with the levator aponeurosis in the upper eyelid and the lower eyelid retractors. Situated between the orbicularis oculi muscle (superficially) and the preaponeurotic orbital fat (deeply), the septum acts as a protective barrier against the spread of infections from the anterior to the posterior eyelid and orbit. The lacrimal gland and the orbital fat are located posterior to the septum, with the latter being commonly encountered during eyelid surgery.

Orbital Fat: It is divided into intraconal (central) and extraconal (peripheral) components; orbital fat is a frequent surgical landmark during eyelid procedures such as blepharoplasty. The upper eyelid contains two fat pads: a small medial fat pad and a larger central preaponeurotic fat pad, but it lacks a lateral fat pad due to the presence of the lacrimal gland. Conversely, the lower eyelid includes a small lateral fat pad and a larger medial fat pad, both separated by a fibrous septum extending from the capsulopalpebral fascia to the orbital septum. The main fat pad in the lower eyelid is divided by the inferior oblique muscle into middle and medial fat pads, with the medial pad being lighter in color. Notably, as the orbital septum ages, it may weaken, allowing these fat pads to bulge and form eyelid bags.

Lacrimal Gland Fossa: It is situated in the frontal bone in the anterior lateral orbit; this fossa accommodates the lacrimal gland, which is responsible for tear production.

Glands of the Eyelid: Eyelids are home to multiple gland types, each with distinct secretions and functions that play vital roles in eyelid health, tear production, and overall ocular surface maintenance. Here, we discuss three primary eyelid gland types: meibomian glands, glands of Zeis, and glands of Moll.

- **Meibomian Glands**: These modified sebaceous glands are characterized by their branching, holocrine nature. Embedded within the tarsal plates, they open posteriorly to the eyelashes and secrete the anterior, outermost lipid layer of the tear film. There are 30–40 meibomian glands in the upper lid and 20–30 in the lower lid, with **para**sympathetic nerves predominantly supplying them.

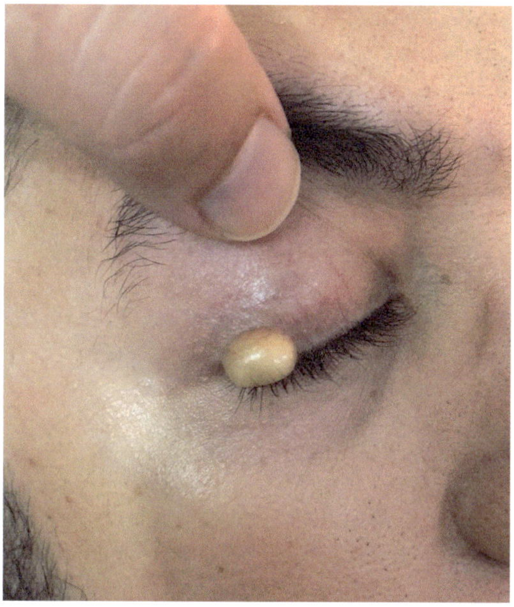

Fig. 9.1 Cyst of Zeis at the right upper lid (large opaque painless cyst)

- **Glands of Zeis:** Also among the modified sebaceous glands, the glands of Zeis open posterior to the eyelashes, with an average of two glands per follicle (Fig. 9.1).
- **Glands of Moll** (Ciliary Glands): As modified sweat glands, these structures also open posterior to the eyelashes and drain either into the gland of Zeis duct or directly into the follicle. Notably, these are the only glands that are more numerous in the lower lid compared to the upper lid.

There are also sebaceous glands located within the caruncle and eyebrow hairs. It is important to note that while all cutaneous tumors are more commonly found in the lower eyelid, sebaceous gland carcinoma is an exception and more often appears in the upper eyelid (more meibomian glands are found in the upper lid).

Two other noteworthy glands include the **glands of Wolfring** (peripheral tarsal border) and **Krause** (conjunctival fornix). Like the main lacrimal gland, these are eccrine in nature. On the other hand, the glands of Moll function in an apocrine manner, while goblet cells, similar to sebaceous glands, are holocrine.

Eyelashes: There are around 100 eyelashes in the upper eyelid compared to 50 in the lower eyelids forming 2–3 rows of eyelashes.

Arterial and Nerve Supply, Venous and Lymphatic Drainage: The eyelids receive their blood supply from various sources, featuring a complex network of veins and lymphatics, while nerve supply provides both sensory and motor control. Understanding these networks is crucial in surgical planning and postoperative care to prevent complications.

Arterial Supply: The eyelid has dual blood supply:

- Preseptal portion: This portion receives blood primarily from the superficial temporal artery and a few branches from the facial artery, which are both derived from the external carotid artery.

Postseptal portion: This portion receives its blood supply from two main arcades: the marginal arcade and the peripheral arcade. The marginal arcade is formed by branches of the ophthalmic artery, including the lateral palpebral arteries (from the lacrimal artery) and the medial palpebral arteries (directly from the ophthalmic artery). These arteries create the marginal arcade, which runs 2 mm from the eyelid margin, located in front of the tarsal plates and behind the orbicularis muscle. The peripheral arterial arcade is positioned above the superior tarsal border, between the levator aponeurosis and Müller's muscle, and is distinct from the marginal arcade, which lies on the tarsal surface of each eyelid margin.

An important feature of eyelid arterial supply is the presence of anastomoses between the facial artery (external carotid) and the palpebral arteries (internal carotid) at the lateral aspects of the eyelids.

Venous Drainage: The venous drainage of the eyelids can also be divided into preseptal, which primarily drains medially into the ophthalmic and angular veins and laterally into the superficial temporal vein, and postseptal, which drains into orbital veins. These vessels eventually drain into the cavernous sinus.

Lymphatic Drainage: This follows a divided pattern:

- The medial third of both eyelids drains into the submandibular nodes.
- The lateral two-thirds of both upper and lower eyelids drain into the superficial preauricular nodes and then into deeper cervical nodes.

Nerve Supply: The sensory innervation of the eyelids is supplied by divisions of the trigeminal nerve:

- The upper lid receives innervation from branches of the nasociliary nerve, a division of the ophthalmic nerve (V1).
- The lower lid receives innervation from the infratrochlear branch of the ophthalmic nerve (which also supplies the upper lid) and the infraorbital nerve, a branch of the maxillary division of the trigeminal nerve (V2).

High Yield: The blood supply to the upper eyelid consists of two arcades. The marginal arcade is located on the anterior tarsal surface, 2–3 mm from the lid margin, while the peripheral arcade is situated on the anterior surface of the Müller's muscle, just above the superior tarsal border. These arcades are formed by the anastomosis of the superior branch of the medial palpebral artery (a branch of the ophthalmic artery) and the superior branch of the lateral palpebral artery (a branch of the lacrimal artery). In the lower eyelid, the marginal arcade is positioned 2 mm from the lid margin. It is formed by the inferior palpebral artery (a branch from the ophthalmic artery) and the inferior branch of the lacrimal artery. Additionally, a branch of the maxillary artery also supplies the lower eyelid, instead of the peripheral arcade.

Orbital Muscles: The muscles of the eyelids and brow are crucial to the functioning of the eyelid, which protects the eye, and contributes to tear film distribution and drainage. These muscles can be broadly categorized into those that elevate the brow and eyelids and those that depress it.

Muscles that Elevate the Brow and Eyelids:

- **Levator Palpebrae Superioris**: Originating above the tendinous ring from the lesser wing of the sphenoid bone, this muscle extends forward above the superior rectus. At Whitnall's ligament, it transitions into the levator aponeurosis, with lateral and medial horns attaching to respective canthal tendons and the eyelid skin. This muscle elevates the upper eyelid by approximately 15 mm from downgaze to upgaze and assists the superior rectus in elevating the globe.
- **Müller's Muscle (Superior Tarsal Muscle)**: This smooth muscle arises from the undersurface of the levator aponeurosis and inserts into the upper tarsal plate. Its sympathetic innervation originates from the superior cervical ganglion. Approximately 15 mm long, Müller's muscle elevates the upper eyelid by 2 mm. A less developed muscle with similar innervation, the capsulopalpebral fascia (inferior tarsal muscle) is present in the lower lid.
- **Frontalis Muscle**: This muscle originates at the scalp and inserts into the eyelid, lifting the brow. Its lateral weakening can lead to a higher incidence of lateral ptosis in the elderly.

Muscles that Depress the Brow:

Orbicularis Oculi: This muscle originates from the second branchial arch and is innervated by the facial nerve. It functions to lowers the entire brow. The orbicularis oculi is divided into two portions: palpebral and orbital. The palpebral portion can be further divided into the pretarsal and preseptal sections (which lie anterior to the orbital septum) and extends from the medial to the lateral palpebral ligaments. This portion aids in reflex tearing and tear pumping. In contrast, the orbital portion allows for tight eye closure. Additionally, the muscle of Riolan, a distinct muscle, forms the gray line midway between the anterior and posterior lamella at the lid margin.

- **Corrugator Supercilii**: Originating at the frontal bone and inserting into the skin medially, this muscle pulls the eyebrow

downward and medially, leading to vertical forehead furrows.
- **Procerus Muscle**: This muscle originates at the nasal bone and inserts into the medial side of the frontalis, pulling the medial eyebrow downward and producing horizontal furrows over the nose bridge.
- **Occipitofrontalis**
- **Depressor Supercilii**

All these muscles receive facial nerve innervation, except for the levator palpebrae superioris, which is innervated by the oculomotor nerve, and Müller's muscle, which is innervated by sympathetic nerves carried by the oculomotor nerve. Notably, the fibers of the levator muscle extend superiorly to intermix with the frontalis muscle. The upper eyelid structure is divided into pretarsal and post-tarsal sections by the superior palpebral sulcus.

Eyelid Ligaments: Several ligaments contribute to eyelid structure and function.

- **Lockwood's Ligament**: This structure functions as a suspensory system for the globe and serves as the lower eyelid retractor system. It originates posteriorly from fibrous attachments to the inferior side of the inferior rectus muscle, extends anteriorly as the capsulopalpebral fascia, and attaches posterior to the lacrimal sac.
- **Whitnall's Ligament (Superior Transverse Ligament)**: This ligament originates from the levator muscle. Medially, it springs from the connective tissue of the trochlea, while laterally, it attaches to the capsule of the orbital lobe of the lacrimal gland and to the lateral orbital wall, approximately 10 mm above the lateral orbital tubercle.

9.3 Meibomian Gland Diseases

Meibomian gland dysfunction (MGD) is a chronic, widespread disorder affecting the meibomian glands, often marked by obstruction of the terminal duct and/or qualitative/quantitative changes of glandular secretion. This condition leads to alterations in the tear film, symptoms of eye irritation, visible inflammation, and ocular surface disease.

Assessment: The assessment of MGD often involves a test for tear film deficiency, which is indicative of a mucous or lipid abnormality. The tear breakup time test is a common diagnostic method. Recently, new devices are available that can evaluate the meibomian glands and their oily secretion as Meiboflow or LipiFlow. MGD, the etiology for 85% of dry eye syndrome, can be treated using oral antibiotics such as doxycycline or azithromycin. These antibiotics are used for their anti-inflammatory and oil-enhancing effects and to block staphylococcal lipase production, rather than for their antimicrobial effects.

Management: Doxycycline 100 mg taken twice daily for 2 weeks and then once daily for another 6–12 weeks is a common regimen. However, it can cause side effects such as cutaneous complications, urticaria, contraindications in pregnancy or breast-feeding women and children, and gastrointestinal upset. Oral doxycycline is particularly helpful in patients with posterior blepharitis as it can change the constitution and viscosity of lipids, therefore improving symptoms. Azithromycin is another option especially in children, typically taken 250 mg or 500 mg for 5 days. It is worth noting that conjunctival bacterial colonies are most effectively reduced by topical antibiotics. Other topical therapies include weak topical steroids and tear substitutes.

Associated conditions: Acne rosacea can manifest as MGD, in addition to its skin manifestations. Effective treatment typically involves oral tetracycline (250 mg twice daily) or oral doxycycline (100 mg twice daily), which has beneficial anti-inflammatory effects on sebaceous gland dysfunction in rosacea. These treatments can improve both the ocular and the skin manifestations of the disease. Additional therapy should include management of blepharoconjunctivitis, such as lid hygiene, judicious use of low-dose topical corticosteroids, and lifestyle modifications including limiting the intake of spicy foods, caffeine, and alcohol. Among various associations with MGD, the use of isotretinoin, a medication used primarily for severe acne, has been linked to the dysfunction of the meibomian glands.

Inflammatory conditions of the eyelid range from chronic, noninfectious inflammation to acute bacterial infections. Two commonly encountered conditions are the chalazion and hordeolum.

Chalazion: A chalazion is a sterile, painless, lipogranulomatous inflammatory lesion that forms within the tarsal plates of the eyelid due to obstruction of meibomian gland orifices and the consequent retention of sebaceous secretions. It is more common in the upper eyelid due to the higher number of glands. Patients with MGD or rosacea are at higher risk for developing multiple or recurrent chalazia.

Histopathological examination of a chalazion reveals lipogranulomatous inflammation, with lipids surrounded by various inflammatory cells, including foreign body multinucleated giant cells, epithelioid cells, lymphocytes, plasma cells, neutrophils, and eosinophils. A fibrous pseudocapsule may also form around the lesion.

There are different types of chalazia depending on which gland is affected:

* An internal or deep chalazion is caused by the blockage of meibomian glands.
* An external or superficial chalazion results from the blockage of the glands of Zeis and is located at the anterior lid margin and not within the tarsal plate (cyst of Zeis, Fig. 9.1).

It is important to note that recurrent chalazia may indicate an underlying malignancy. As such, a full-thickness diagnostic biopsy of the eyelid is recommended for recurring cases.

Hordeolum: A hordeolum is a painful acute infection of one of the sebaceous glands of the eyelid, typically caused by *Staphylococcus* bacteria. The infection may affect the external eyelid (glands of Zeis), the so-called external hordeolum (stye), or the inner eyelid (meibomian glands), the so-called internal hordeolum leading to painful, tender, red, swollen lesions.

9.4 Eyelid Masses

It can be broadly classified as benign masses and malignant ones (aka neoplasia).

9.4.1 Benign Lesions

Capillary hemangioma (strawberry nevus), the most common benign tumor in childhood (Fig. 9.2), usually presents within the first several weeks of life but is NOT present at birth. It is typically unilateral and more likely to involve the upper eyelid. The female-to-male ratio is 3:1. Its rapid growth during infancy is characteristic. Blanching with pressure can distinguish capillary hemangiomas from port-wine stains in patients with Sturge-Weber syndrome. Capillary hemangiomas may lead to amblyopia, resulting from either ptotic occlusion of the palpebral aperture or production of significant astigmatism due to corneal warpage. The first-line treatment for capillary hemangiomas is intralesional steroids, while oral propranolol is the treatment of choice when

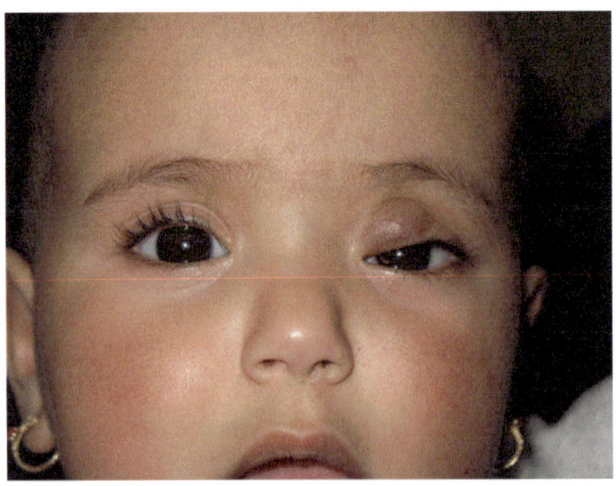

Fig. 9.2 Left supero-nasal swollen-reddish mass (capillary hemangioma) in a one-year-old child with significant mass effect on the cornea causing astigmatism

available. Oral steroids are also used when lesions are refractory to propranolol or in the absence of propranolol. Topical beta-blockers such as timolol maleate gel are less effective and generally considered only for smaller, non-amblyogenic, "cosmetic" lesions or as an adjunctive treatment for residual hemangiomas after other treatments. Capillary hemangiomas typically start to involute spontaneously by 12 months of age, with 40% of tumors completely regressing by age 4 and 70% by age 7. Kasabach-Merritt syndrome, a rare complication, involves platelet sequestration associated with multiple large capillary hemangiomas, leading to thrombocytopenia. In contrast, Maffucci syndrome is characterized by skin hemangiomas combined with enchondromata of the hands, feet, and long bones as well as bowing of the long bones.

Cavernous Hemangioma: Cavernous hemangioma consists of larger, dilated blood vessels compared to capillary hemangioma, with "caverns" between them filled with blood. High internal reflectivity with nonhomogeneous tissue (blood in caverns) can be observed on A-scan ultrasound. Presentation is in the third to fifth decades with slowly progressive, painless unilateral proptosis. Nevus flammeus (port-wine stain) is a type of cavernous hemangioma of the dermis. Unlike capillary hemangiomas, it does not blanch with pressure. It is usually permanent and can be a characteristic of certain syndromes, like Sturge-Weber syndrome.

Lymphangiomas are not connected to the orbital circulation. Unlike capillary hemangioma, they often appear at birth or during early childhood. While cavernous hemangioma is an encapsulated tumor, lymphangioma lacks a capsule. It can present acutely with hemorrhage, leading to ecchymosis and proptosis. It can increase in size with upper respiratory tract infection.

Papilloma (aka skin tag) is a benign growth composed of fibrovascular connective tissue covered by irregular, acanthotic, and hyperkeratotic stratified squamous epithelium. It is primarily caused by human papillomavirus (HPV) types 6 and 11, whereas HPV types 16 and 18 are associated with carcinogenic effects.

Dermolipomas are benign fatty tumors typically located in the superotemporal quadrant. These lesions are considered choristomas, which are normal tissue located in an abnormal location. Dermolipomas often contain other dermal elements such as hair follicles, sweat glands, or sebaceous glands. Clinically, they present as subconjunctival yellowish-pink masses that are often confused with epibulbar dermoids, although dermolipomas lack the latter's potential for malignant transformation. These lesions are usually asymptomatic but may cause discomfort due to associated ocular surface irritation or cosmetic concern due to their prominence. Surgical excision can be considered for symptomatic lesions, taking care to preserve the overlying conjunctiva.

Epidermoid cysts: They are uncommon and different from sebaceous cysts as they are lined by keratinized stratified squamous epithelium and contain keratin. They result from implantation of surface epidermis during trauma or surgery, while a minority are developmental along embryonic lines of closure (Fig. 9.3).

Molluscum contagiosum is a common skin infection caused by a human-specific DNA poxvirus. It typically affects otherwise healthy children with a peak incidence between 2 and 4 years (Fig. 9.4). The infection with usually

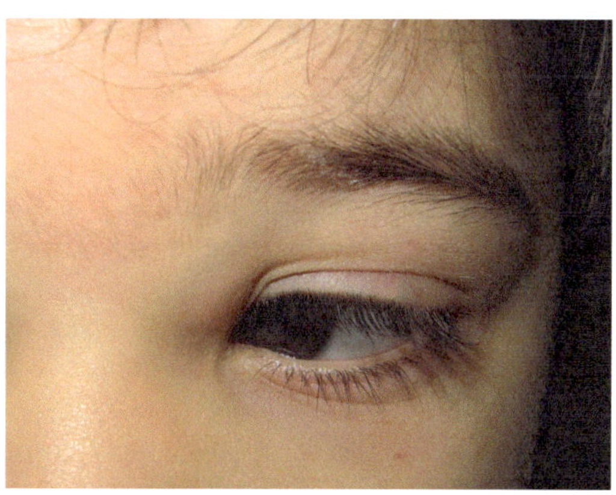

Fig. 9.3 Dermoid cyst (fullness) at the left superomedial angle in a 6 years-old child

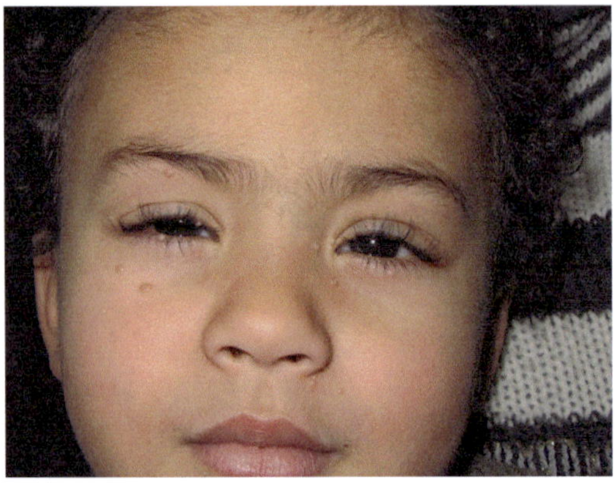

Fig. 9.4 Multiple Molluscum contagiousm in a young patient (small multiple white raised bumps around the eyes) with right follicular conjunctivitis and reddness

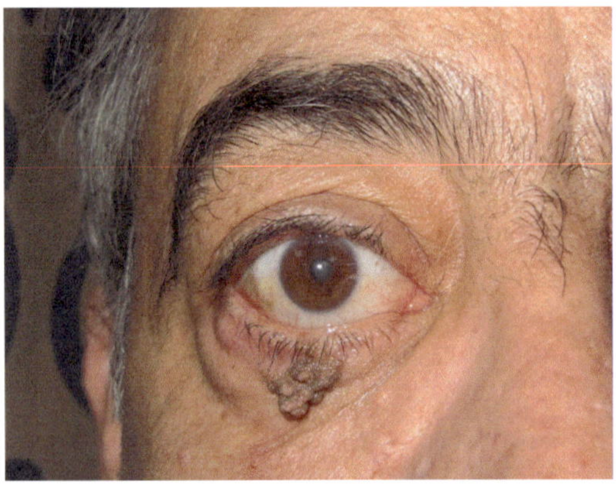

Fig. 9.5 Right lower lid seborrheic keratosis (irregularly shaped brownish growth) in a 60-years-male patient

spontaneous resolution generally occurs within a few months. Molluscum contagiosum is more prevalent in warm and humid climates or areas with poor hygiene. Treatment options include shave excision, curettage, or lesion destruction through cauterization, chemical ablation, cryotherapy, and pulsed-dye laser therapy.

Seborrheic keratosis (aka basal cell papilloma, seborrheic wart, or senile verruca) is a very common benign lesion that slowly grows and typically appears on the face, trunk, and extremities of elderly individuals. It presents as a discrete light- to dark-brown plaque with a friable, greasy, verrucous surface and has a characteristic "stuck-on" appearance (Fig. 9.5).

Actinic keratosis (aka solar or senile keratosis) is also a common and slowly growing lesion where histology shows dysplastic epidermis with hyperkeratosis, parakeratosis, and cutaneous horn formation. It occurs due to sun exposure in fair skin populations. Although low, it has a potential for malignant transformation. Treatment is done by excision or cryotherapy.

Congenital nevi present at birth as small pigmented macules and increase in size with aging. Generally, they have up to 5% risk for small and up to 20% risk of malignant transformation for giant nevi. They are classified according to their estimated adult size from small to giant (>20 cm). The risk of melanoma is directly related to the size of congenital nevi. Giant congenital nevi, those larger than 20 cm in diameter, have a 5–7% risk of transformation into melanoma by age 60. These nevi can lose color, increase in size, and develop irregular borders over time.

Acquired nevi generally present after birth and have **lower** malignant transformation risk. They include intradermal, junctional, and compound. Intradermal nevi are the most common with no malignant potential, while junctional and compound nevi have low malignant potential. To differentiate between them, junctional nevi are darker and generally flat (aka macular), while compound nevi are lighter and elevated.

Nevus of Ota (aka oculodermal melanocytosis) is composed of pigmented dendritic melanocytes present in the dermis. It is usually unilateral and congenital. It may undergo malignant degeneration, with the choroid being the most common site of involvement.

Syringomas are benign proliferations of eccrine sweat glands.

Pilomatricoma, also known as pilomatrixoma or calcifying epithelioma of Malherbe, orignates from germinal cells of the hair bulb and is the most common hair follicle proliferation encountered by ophthalmologists. It primarily affects children and is more common in females. The condition has almost no malignant potential. Calcification is frequently observed and is often accompanied by a foreign body giant cell reaction.

Pyogenic granuloma is a rapidly growing vascularized proliferation of granulation tissue at the site of prior surgery or trauma.

Plexiform neurofibromas typically present in childhood as a manifestation of neurofibromatosis type 1 with a characteristic S-shaped deformity of the upper eyelid.

Hemangiopericytoma is a type of soft tissue sarcoma that originates from pericytes in the walls of capillaries. It is best treated through complete surgical excision. If the excision is incomplete, the tumor may recur and has the potential to undergo malignant degeneration.

Sturge-Weber syndrome (encephalotrigeminal angiomatosis) is a congenital, sporadic phacomatosis manifesting as:

- Port-wine stain, a congenital malformation of vessels within the superficial dermis, appears as a sharply demarcated soft pink patch that does not blanch with pressure. It is typically distributed along one or more divisions of the trigeminal nerve (Fig. 9.6). About 10% of individuals with this condition have associated ocular or CNS involvement, including Sturge-Weber. Screening for glaucoma should begin in infancy. Cosmetic treatment can be performed using lasers, such as erbium laser.

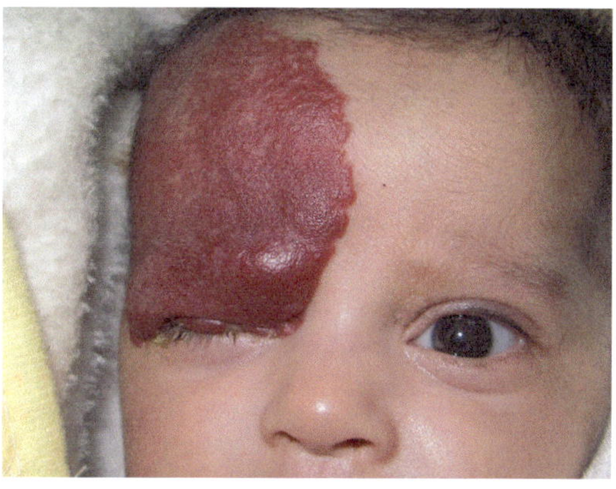

Fig. 9.6 Port-Wine stain in a few months baby involving the first branch of the trigeminal nerve with occlusion of the visual axis. The left eye is widely open

- Leptomeningeal hemangioma: This involves the ipsilateral parietal or occipital region and may cause contralateral focal or generalized seizures, hemiparesis, or hemianopia.
- Ocular features: These may include ipsilateral glaucoma, episcleral hemangioma, iris heterochromia, and diffuse choroidal hemangioma.

Xanthelasma is a common and frequently bilateral lesion occurring in middle-aged individuals at the medial upper (more commonly) or lower eyelids. They are flat, yellow skin lesions located in the dermis, histologically consisting of foamy histiocytes. While associated with hyperlipidemia in 30% of people, the majority of patients do not have an associated hyperlipidemic condition.

9.4.2 Congenital Anomalies Predisposing to Malignancy

Xeroderma pigmentosum is an AR characterized by skin damage on exposure to sunlight, leading to progressive cutaneous abnormalities, including multiple malignancies. It is most commonly associated with squamous cell carcinoma (SCC), but may also develop basal cell carcinoma (BCC) or melanoma.

Gorlin-Goltz syndrome, also known as nevoid basal cell carcinoma syndrome, is a rare autosomal dominant disorder that typically presents at puberty. It is characterized by the development of multiple basal cell carcinomas (BCCs). In addition to the multiple BCCs, individuals with this syndrome may experience jaw cysts, skeletal abnormalities, neurological abnormalities, endocrine disorders, and facial dysmorphism.

Muir–Torre syndrome is a rare AD condition characterized by the presence of sebaceous tumors (sebaceous adenoma, epithelioma or carcinoma, and/or keratoacanthoma) alongside visceral malignancies, with colorectal cancer being the most common. This syndrome increases the risk of both cutaneous and internal malignancies, including BCC and sebaceous gland carcinoma.

Bazex syndrome, also known as acrokeratosis paraneoplastica, is a dermatological condition commonly associated with the diagnosis of squamous cell carcinoma of the upper aerodigestive tract.

Cowden's disease consists of multiple hamartomas and breast cancer.

9.4.3 Eyelid Malignancies (Table 9.1)

- **Basal cell carcinoma** is the most common malignant tumor in clinical ophthalmology, accounting for more than 90% of malignant eyelid tumors. It is characterized by slow growth, local invasiveness, and a lack of metastasis. The tumor most commonly occurs on the lower eyelid, followed by the medial canthus (which has the highest recurrence rate), the upper eyelid, and lastly the lateral canthus. Nodular type and noduloulcerative (rodent ulcer) are the most common (Fig. 9.7), appearing with rolling edges and central ulceration. Histologically, islands or nests of basaloid cells occur, with palisading of the cells (i.e., a single layer of elongated cells) at the periphery of the islands.
- Morpheaform or fibrosing (sclerosing) basal cell carcinoma is a more aggressive and less common form of basal cell carcinoma (Fig. 9.8). Histopathologically, it infiltrates laterally beneath the epidermis as an indurated plaque, with tumor cells displaying hyperchromatic nuclei and relatively little, poorly defined cytoplasm. Radiation therapy is gen-

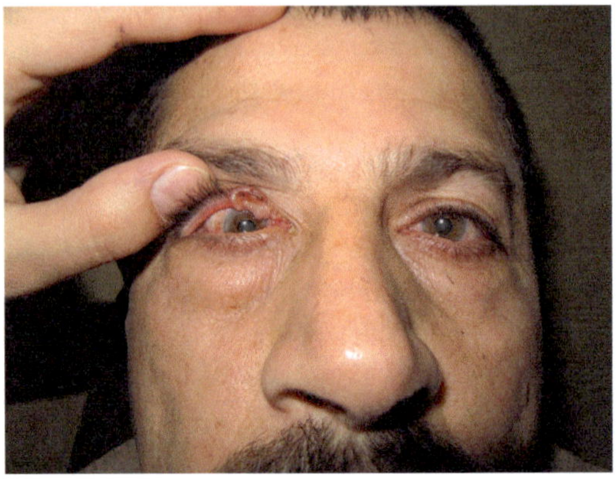

Fig. 9.7 Right upper lid medial basal cell carcinoma (Rodent Ulcer)

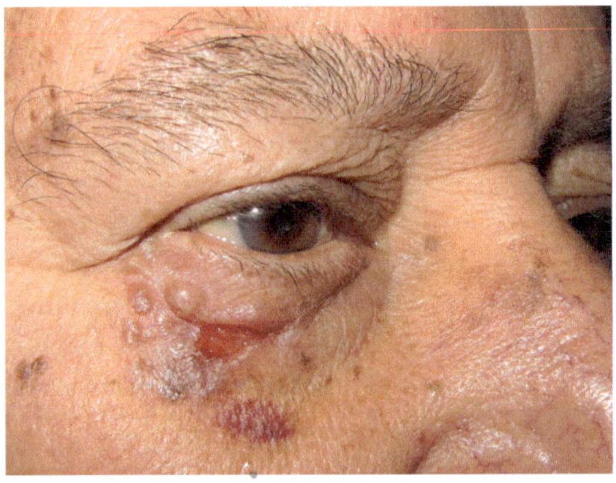

Fig. 9.8 Sclerosing basal cell carcinoma of the right lower lid showing multiple bumps, ulcerations and skin thickening

Table 9.1 Comparison between the three most common eyelid malignancies

	Basal CC	Squamous CC	Sebaceous CC
Most common site	Lower lid	Lower lid	Upper lid
Histology	Islands or nests of basaloid cells, with palisading of the cells	Pink (eosinophilic) cytoplasm, intercellular bridges, and keratin pearls	Skip areas and pagetoid intraepithelial spread
Poor prognostic factors	Morpheaform subtype, which has peripheral radiating cords without peripheral palisading	Spindle cell morphology	Duration of symptoms longer than 6 months, size >10 mm, an infiltrative growth pattern
Associated syndromes	Gorlin-Goltz syndrome; xeroderma pigmentosum; PTCH gene on chromosome 9	Xeroderma pigmentosum	Muir–Torre syndrome
Management	Staged excision with pathologic margin control (SEPMC)	Surgical excision	Surgical excision (radioresistant)

erally not recommended as the initial treatment of periocular basal cell carcinoma (BCC). The optimal surgical excision approach for treating eyelid BCC is staged excision with pathologic margin control (SEPMC), also known as staged excision.

Morpheaform lesions (peripheral radiating cords without peripheral palisading) and lesions on the medial canthus (more prone to invade the orbit and sinuses and more difficult to treat) have the poorest prognosis.

The following conditions predispose to BCC:

- Gorlin-Goltz syndrome (aka basal cell nevus syndrome)
- Xeroderma pigmentosum
- PTCH gene on chromosome 9

The patient's raised shiny pearly lesion with overlying telangiectatic vessels and madarosis is typical of nodular basal cell carcinoma.

Squamous cell carcinoma accounts for approximately 5% of all eyelid cancers (Fig. 9.9). It can spread via the lymphatic system to the preauricular lymph nodes from the upper lids and to the submandibular lymph nodes from the lower lids and medial areas in about 20% of patients. Individuals who are immunosuppressed, such as those with AIDS or renal transplants, are at increased risk. Favorable prognostic factors include the presence of pink cytoplasm, intercellular bridges, and keratin pearls. Conversely, spindle cell morphology indicates a more aggressive type of squamous cell carcinoma.

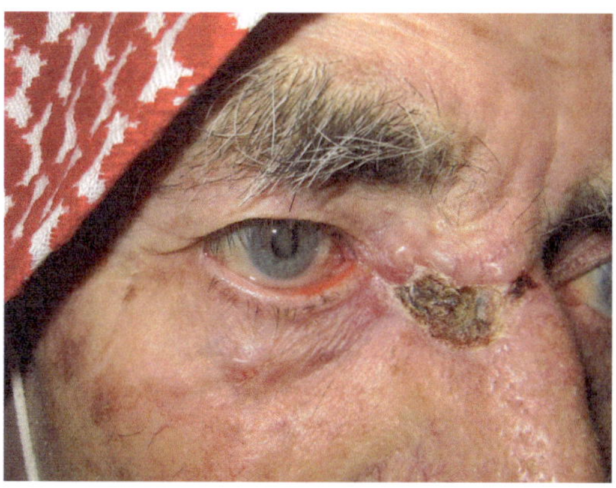

Fig. 9.9 Squamous cell carcinoma of right medial canthus and lower lid with cicatricial ectropion in an 85 years old patient showing skin lesion near the eye with redness and ulcerations covered with scabbings

Actinic keratosis is the premalignant form of SCC that develops in elderly in sun-exposed areas, but is not common on eyelids.

As shown in Fig. 9.10, ulcerative squamous cell carcinoma is a serious condition that often presents as an aggressive, ulcerative, and destructive lesion. It often has a characteristic raised, rolled border with a central ulceration. Chronic sun exposure, human papillomavirus (HPV), and immunosuppression are known risk factors. Urgent intervention is crucial due to the potential for orbital invasion and metastasis. A biopsy should be performed for any suspicious lesion, and treatment usually involves surgery excision.

Sebaceous gland carcinoma accounts for 1–5% of all eyelid cancers. These rare, slow-growing tumors often present as a unilateral chronic blepharitis (spreading or pagetoid type), most commonly from the **upper** lid due to its higher number of sebaceous glands. While usually originating in the meibomian gland (Fig. 9.11), it may also arise from the

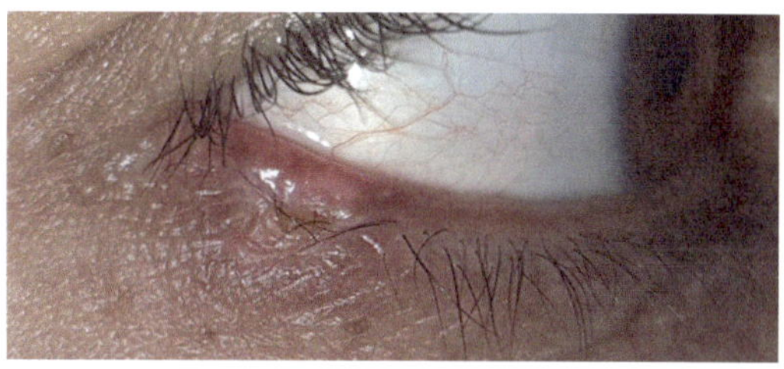

Fig. 9.10 Close-up image of an eye with a lesion on the lower eyelid. The lesion appears as a red, swollen bump near the eyelashes representing Ulverative sqaumous cell carcinoma with loss of eyelashes

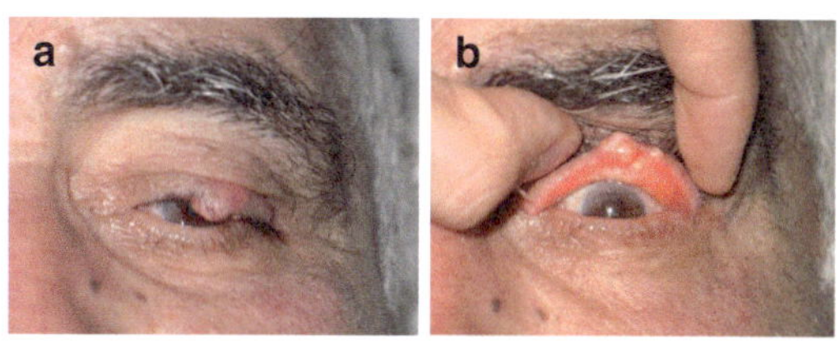

Fig. 9.11 External photo of a patient with Sebaceous carcinomas including view externally as in (**a**) and internally as in (**b**)

gland of Zeis or sebaceous glands of the eyelid skin. They show a female predominance. Histopathologically, they are characterized by skip areas and pagetoid intraepithelial spread of malignancy, meaning a negative margin does not guarantee complete excision. Therefore, wide surgical margins and map biopsies of the surrounding area are recommended. Poor prognostic factors include a symptom duration longer than 6 months, upper lid involvement, tumor size >10 mm, infiltrative growth pattern, moderate or poor differentiation, lymphatic or vascular invasion, orbital invasion, and multicentric growth. Sebaceous carcinomas may be seen in Muir–Torre syndrome in association with visceral malignancy. There may be simultaneous involvement of the lower and upper lid on one side (5%). Sebaceous cell carcinoma is relatively radioresistant, and surgical excision is the treatment of choice.

Note that ocular sebaceous carcinomas generally have a relatively benign course and rarely metastasize. In contrast, eyelid sebaceous carcinomas frequently exhibit metastasis and have a poor prognosis, with an overall mortality rate of around 5–10%.

Two clinical types of sebaceous gland carcinoma are known: nodular type; hard, discrete, immobile nodule with yellowish discoloration, and the spreading (pagetoid) type with diffuse thickening of the lid margin with loss of eyelashes.

Melanoma is rare, with 50% being nonpigmented. Lentigo maligna and nodular melanoma are the most common forms affecting the eyelid. Lentigo maligna, also known as Hutchinson freckle or intradermal melanoma, is a melanoma in situ and is managed by excision. It accounts for 90% of head and neck melanomas. Nodular melanoma represents approximately 10% of cutaneous melanomas. Lentigo maligna presents as a flat, irregularly shaped, unevenly pigmented lesion, which slowly enlarges and may progress to nodular lentigo maligna melanoma. Premalignant changes often extend beyond the clinically involved area. Cryotherapy can be used as an adjunctive treatment for conjunctival melanomas, but it is not recommended for cutaneous melanoma. Note that melanoma is the eyelid malignancy with the highest distant metastasis risk.

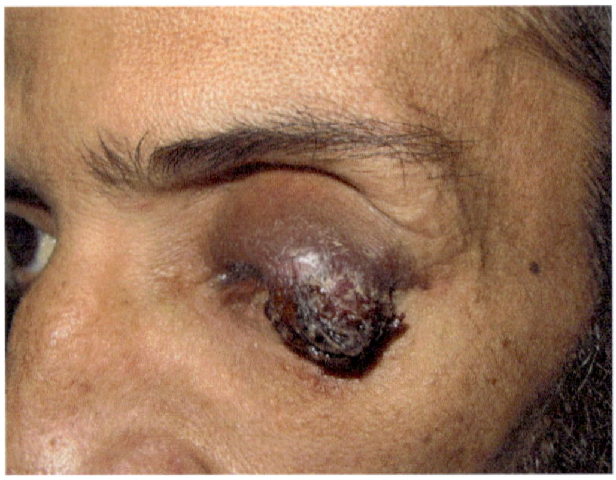

Fig. 9.12 Kaposi sarcoma of left upper lid

Kaposi sarcoma in HIV patients is a vascular tumor that appears as pink, red-violet to brown lesions mostly on conjunctiva or eyelid (Fig. 9.12), which may be mistaken for a hematoma or nevus.

*** When a patient has AIDS with eyelid tumor, think of either Kaposi or SCC.

Tumors of hair follicles are generally common in women. These include trichoepithelioma, trichilemmomas, and pilomatrixoma. Cowden's disease consists of multiple trichilemmomas and breast cancer. Pilomatrixoma is more common in children than in adults. Calcification is a feature. Malignant transformation is rare in pilomatrixoma.

9.4.3.1 High Yield Notes

Remember that neoplasia at the canthal region generally has a higher recurrence rate, which might be due to incomplete excision. So, deep delayed recurrence is not uncommon. During management of such lesions, where flap might be needed to replace the excised area, thick flaps (e.g., forehead) may hide recurrences and hence thinner flaps (e.g., harvested from the retroauricular area or upper eyelid) are a better option.

Medial canthal BCCs are generally deeply infiltrative than those from the eyelid margins with higher recurrence rates.

The most important prognostic predictor for lesions is mostly its thickness.

The abovementioned malignancies are more common than metastatic cancer of the eyelid.

9.4.4 Mimicking Lesions

Keratoacanthoma is a rapidly growing tumor (within weeks), which then remains static for 2–3 months but subsequently regresses (within months to a year) and usually occurs in fair-skinned individuals with a history of chronic sun exposure. It occurs mostly in lower lid. Surgical excision is the treatment of choice. Complete involution leaves an ugly scar. Doing irradiation alone is another option, however, with higher recurrence, complications, and failure rates. In keratoacanthoma, complete surgical excision with biopsy is recommended rather than observation. Keratoacanthoma has a central keratin-filled crater (aka keratotic) plug rather than cutaneous horns. Cutaneous horns occur in seborrheic and actinic keratosis and skin cancers. Cellular atypia may be present, so it might be considered a low-grade form of squamous cell carcinoma (SCC).

9.5 Congenital Eyelid Diseases

Epicanthic folds: These are bilateral vertical folds of skin extending from the upper or lower lids towards the medial canthi. They can be categorized into four varieties:

- **Epicanthus Tarsalis**: A normal racial structure in some Asian patients (Orientals), originating in the upper tarsal plate and terminating in the skin of the medial canthus. The fold is more prominent in the upper lid than in the lower lid.
- **Epicanthus Inversus**: Rare and often associated with congenital eyelid anomalies like blepharophimosis syndrome. The fold starts from the lower eyelid tarsal region and extends up to the medial canthus. The fold is broader below, in the lower lid, than in the upper lid (Fig. 9.13).
- **Epicanthus Palpebralis**: Equally distributed between the upper and lower lids, running from the upper eyelid tarsal region medially. It is the most common type in Caucasians.
- **Epicanthus Supraciliaris**: Originates in the eyebrow region and terminates over the lacrimal sac.

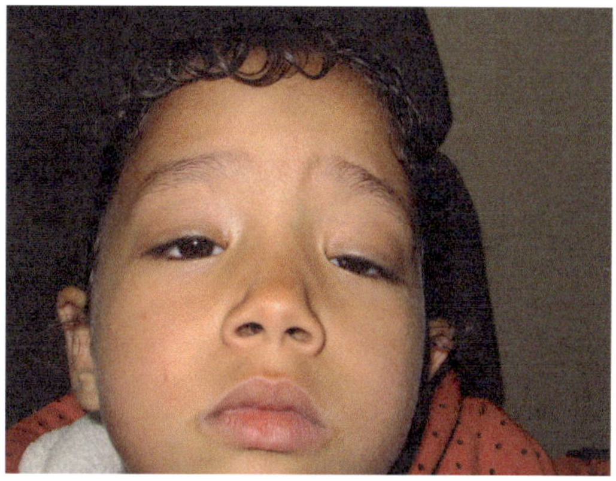

Fig. 9.13 Epicanthus Inversus, telecanthus and ptosis in a patient with Blepharophimosis syndrome

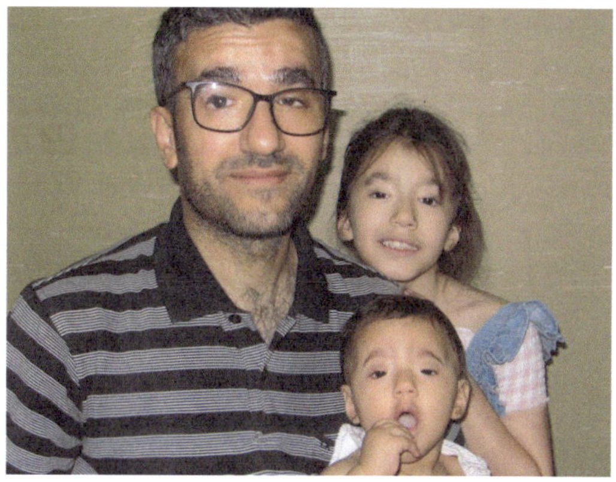

Fig. 9.14 Father and two daughters with Blepharophimosis syndrome

Treatment usually involves Y–V plasty for small folds or Mustarde double Z-plasty surgical techniques for larger folds.

Blepharophimosis, Ptosis, and Epicanthus Inversus Syndrome (BPES): BPES is an autosomal dominant congenital condition characterized by narrowing of the palpebral fissure (Fig. 9.14). It is invariably bilateral and can cause amblyopia in about 50% of patients. The syndrome is often associated with widened intercanthal distance (telecanthus), ptosis, and epicanthus inversus. Other less findings include lower eyelid ectropion, poor development of the orbital rims and nasal bones (nasal bridge hypoplasia), and hypertelorism. Systemically, it is commonly associated with primary amenorrhea (type 1). Gene location is on chromosome 3.

Epiblepharon: It is a condition where an extra fold of skin stretches horizontally across the anterior lid margin, typically found in individuals of Eastern Asian ethnicity. The condition usually resolves spontaneously with age in most children and does not require treatment. In cases where intervention is necessary, the Hotz procedure can be used.

Eyelid Coloboma: It is a congenital defect, typically found at the junction of the middle and inner thirds of the upper lids or the middle and outer thirds of the lower lids. Upper lid colobomas are often associated with conditions like cryptophthalmos, facial abnormalities, and Goldenhar syndrome, whereas lower lid colobomas are associated with Treacher Collins syndrome. Eyelid colobomas are more common in the upper eyelid and often carry a risk of exposure keratopathy. They can occur as isolated findings (Fig. 9.15) or in association with other congenital anomalies. Early closure of the eyelid defect is often required.

Euryblepharon: Increased vertical separation of the temporal aspect of the palpebral fissure, with associated lateral canthal malposition and lateral ectropion (Fig. 9.16).

Ankyloblepharon: Upper and lower eyelids are joined by thin skin tags.

Blepharochalasis: Characterized by recurrent bouts of upper eyelid non-pitting edema leading to thinning, stretching, and fine wrinkling of the involved skin, usually in younger patients.

Eyelid Imbrication Syndrome: Upper lid overlaps the lower lid on closure, causing lower lashes to irritate the superior marginal tarsal conjunctiva causing papillary conjunctivitis.

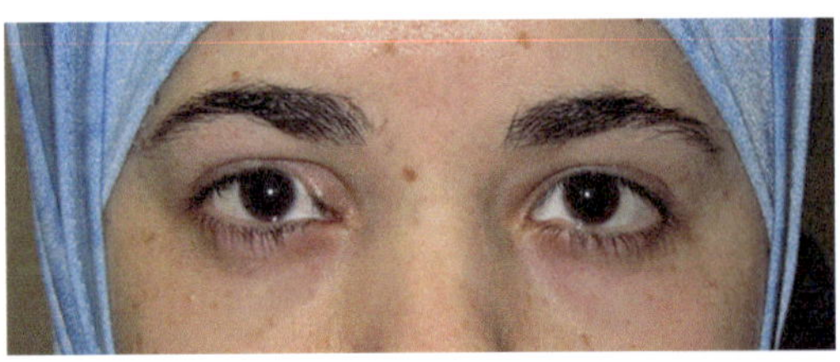

Fig. 9.15 Right upper lid isolated medial coloboma

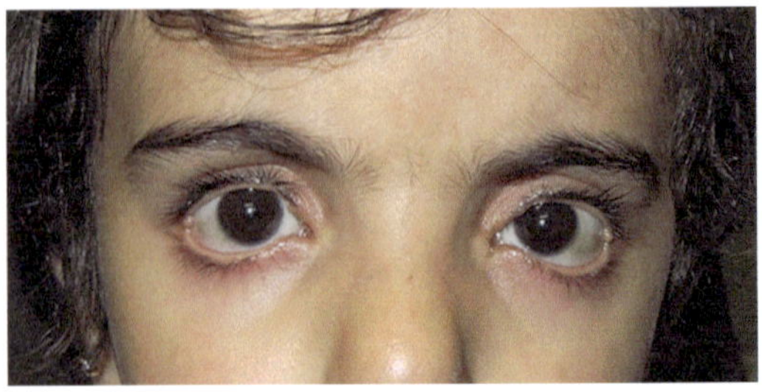

Fig. 9.16 Bilateral Euryblepharon (Lateral widening of the palpebral fissure)

Telecanthus: A wide intercanthal distance in the presence of a normal interpupillary distance (the intercanthal distance is more than half the interpupillary distance Fig. 9.13).

Hypertelorism (Telorbitism): Wider-than-normal separation of the bony medial orbital walls.

Exorbitism: An angle >90° between the lateral orbital walls, often associated with shallow orbital depth. This and hypertelorism typically refer to congenital abnormalities.

9.6 Ptosis and Eyelid retraction

Ptosis literally means organ prolapse (abnormal low position), and here we are talking about eyelid ptosis. Normally, the upper lid lies 1–2 mm below the superior limbus. Sometimes, the ptosis is not actually due to eyelid prolapse, a condition termed pseudo-ptosis, occurring in cases of contralateral lid retraction, ipsilateral hypotropia, dermatochalasis, and brow ptosis. After excluding pseudo-ptosis, consider the following etiologies:

Involutional (Aponeurotic) Ptosis: It is the most common cause of ptosis and affects both genders equally. It occurs with aging and is associated with good levator function. This condition may worsen towards the end of the day due to the weakness of the compensatory frontalis muscle, similar to ocular myasthenia gravis. It can also worsen in the reading (downgaze) position or following cataract sur-

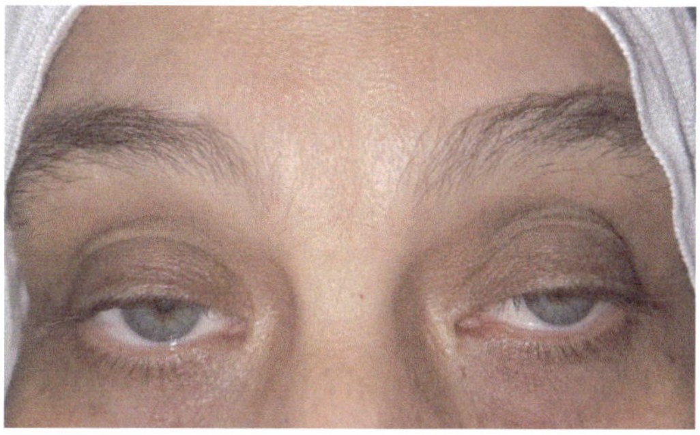

Fig. 9.17 Left more than right Involutional ptosis with bilateral high lid crease

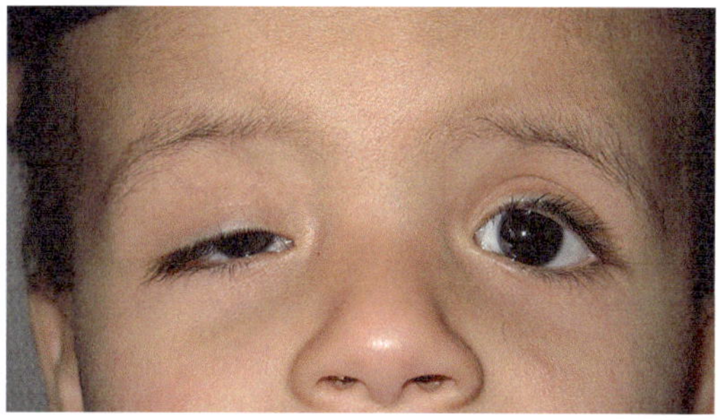

Fig. 9.18 Right congenital ptosis covering the visual axis while the left eye is open

gery. Often, the supratarsal tissues are thinned in this condition. Aponeurotic ptosis, depicted in Fig. 9.17, is one of the most common types of acquired ptosis. It typically occurs due to a disinsertion or dehiscence of the levator aponeurosis from its insertion on the tarsal plate, often associated with aging, contact lens wear, or ocular surgery. Clinically, aponeurotic ptosis presents with a high eyelid crease (above 12mm) and good levator function and a deep upper lid sulcus. The ptotic eye often shows an increased upper eyelid sulcus depth compared to the contralateral eye. Treatment usually involves surgical reattachment of the levator aponeurosis to the tarsal plate.

Aponeurotic ptosis can be a complication in 5–10% of cataract surgeries or may be caused by long-term hard contact lens wear. Acute postoperative cases can relate to edematous changes, but the chronic persistent form is the one requiring management. The causes of persistent or chronic ptosis usually involve damage (either chemical by anesthesia or mechanical) to the levator aponeurosis or scarring to the levator complex. Management options depend on the severity and include levator advancement, mullerectomy for mild cases, or levator resection for more severe cases. An abnormally high or indistinct upper eyelid crease characterizes this condition; however, levator function remains normal.

Congenital Ptosis: It arises due to maldevelopment of the levator muscle, which results in muscle fibers being replaced by fibrous tissue. This condition is characterized by poor levator function, an absent lid crease, and a higher eyelid on the affected side upon downgaze (Figs. 9.13 and 9.18). Congenital myopathic ptosis is unilateral in 70% of cases and may be accompanied by strabismus (primarily hypotropia) and anisometropia. Amblyopia is present in 20% of cases, generally due to anisometropia and strabismus, rather than occlusion. In downgaze, the ptosis is reduced or absent as the fibrotic levator muscle cannot stretch. Early surgery is indicated when the visual axis is obstructed; otherwise, treatment is typically delayed until the late preschool years. Figure 9.18 provides an example of congenital ptosis.

Myasthenia Gravis: Refer to the Neuro-Ophthalmology chapter for more information.

Horner Syndrome: Refer to the Neuro-Ophthalmology chapter for more information.

High Yield Note: Summary of characteristic findings in each etiology:

- Levator aponeurosis dehiscence: Abnormally high or indistinct upper eyelid crease, normal levator function.
- Congenital ptosis: Eyelid retraction on downgaze leading to an increase in the margin–reflex distance 1 (MRD1).
- Myasthenia gravis: Variability of ptosis along with other signs of myasthenia gravis.

Assessment:

- **Margin–reflex distance (MRD_1)** is the measurement from the upper lid margin to the corneal reflection of light held by the examiner while the patient fixates in the primary position. The normal MRD_1 is 4–5 mm.
- **Palpebral fissure height** refers to the distance between the upper and lower lid margins, measured at the center of the pupillary plane. This measurement is typically shorter in males (7–10 mm) compared to females (8–12 mm).
- **Levator function** (upper lid excursion) is assessed by placing a thumb firmly against the patient's brow to negate the action of the frontalis muscle, while the eyes are in downgaze. The patient is then asked to look up as far as possible, and the amount of excursion is measured with a ruler. The measurements are repeated 3–4 times, ensuring that the patient does not move their head or use the frontalis muscle, and the average excursion is taken. Levator function is graded as normal (15 mm or more), good (12–14 mm), fair (5–11 mm), and poor (4 mm or less).
- **Upper lid crease** is the vertical distance between the lid margin and the lid crease in downgaze. This measurement is typically around 10 mm in females and 8 mm in males. The skin crease is also used as a guide to the initial incision in some surgical procedures.
- **Pretarsal show** is the distance between the lid margin and the skin fold with the eyes in the primary position.

Note that the frontalis muscle action must be eliminated during exam.

The normal adult palpebral fissure is 27–30 mm horizontally and 8–11 mm vertically.

Supplementary Signs

- **The pupils** are affected in Horner and third CN palsy, but never in myasthenia gravis.
- **Motility**: Always check extraocular muscle motility in any case of ptosis or anisocoria.
- **Myasthenia** signs include fatigability (inability to maintain upgaze >60 s), Cogan's twitch (overshoot of the upper lid on saccade from downgaze to the primary position), positive ice test, and variability.
- **Marcus Gunn jaw-winking** phenomenon is lid retraction that occurs with mastication muscle activation, due to aberrant regeneration of mandibular branch of fifth with seventh CNs. It is mostly unilateral and does not improve with age.
- **Bell's phenomenon** up and temporal gaze upon blinking or forceful eyelid closure.

The main difference in the upper lid appearance is a low or absent skin crease in about 50% of Asians due to the low fusion of the orbital septum with the levator aponeurosis and insertion on anterior tarsal surface, close to the lashes.

In a child with new-onset ptosis, the next step is to look for anisocoria.

9.6.1 Surgical Repair

The levator aponeurosis merges with the orbital septum approximately 3–4 mm above the superior edge of the tarsal plate. Its posterior fibers attach to the upper third of the anterior surface of the tarsal plate, while Müller muscle inserts into the upper edge of the tarsal plate. Both structures can be accessed through either the skin or the conjunctiva. **Conjunctiva–Müller resection** can achieve a maximum eyelid elevation of 2–3 mm, making it suitable for cases of mild ptosis with good levator function (at least 10 mm), such as most instances of Horner syndrome and mild congenital ptosis. However, this procedure is ineffective and is contraindicated if there is no change in eyelid position after the application of topical phenylephrine.

Levator resection is typically employed when the levator function ranges between 5 and 10 mm. For cases of severe ptosis with droopiness >4 mm and very poor levator function (<4 mm), a brow (frontalis) sling suspension is recommended. This procedure is often indicated for conditions such as ptosis associated with third nerve palsy, severe congenital ptosis, or cases where previous ptosis surgery was unsatisfactory. Various materials can be used for the suspension including donor fascia lata, autogenous fascia lata, temporalis fascia, supramid, silicone, and Gore-Tex. Absorbable sutures like Vicryl are not effective for long-term eyelid suspension.

The most important test to decide on surgical management of ptosis is levator function; if levator function is <4 mm, frontalis suspension techniques are required. If levator function is >4 mm, levator resection can be tried.

MRD-1 can be used to determine the amount of resection where:

- If the levator function is >8 mm, one might resect 3–4 mm of levator for every millimeter of ptosis.
- If the levator function is 5–7 mm, one might need to resect more, 5–6 mm of levator for every millimeter of ptosis, since the levator is more dysfunctional.

The lid crease incision when performing a frontalis suspension with sling material fixation to the tarsal plate should be no higher than the upper edge of the tarsal plate.

Certain etiologies have specific surgical corrective options that are usually preferred:

- Horner ptosis is almost always corrected by Fasanella-Servat procedure, which is a corrective surgery to address moderate amount of ptosis with good levator function.
- Levator dehiscence is usually managed by levator advancement.
- Severe congenital ptosis (levator function <4 mm) is managed by frontalis sling suspension surgery.

Kearns-Sayre syndrome is a neuromuscular disorder characterized by ptosis and heart block, typically defined by a triad of features: onset of symptoms before the age of 20; pigmentary retinopathy (a "salt-and-pepper" appearance in the retina that can affect vision, though often leaving it intact); and chronic progressive external ophthalmoplegia (CPEO). While it is mostly sporadic, Kearns-Sayre syndrome can also be inherited as a mitochondrial disease.

9.6.2 Eyelid Retraction

Eyelid retraction is a condition in which the upper eyelid (less commonly the lower lid) is pulled up (or down) from the normal position. This can expose an abnormal amount of the eye's surface, potentially causing dryness and discomfort. Several conditions, both neurological and systemic, can cause eyelid retraction.

Upper lid retraction can be seen in a variety of conditions, including Graves' eye disease (most common cause), an eye with contralateral ptosis (Hering's law of equal innervation), hepatic failure, hydrocephalus in children (sunset sign), and Parinaud's syndrome (Fig. 9.19). In general, causes can be classified as follows:

- Neurogenic causes include tertiary syphilis, dorsal midbrain syndrome, palatal myoclonus, unopposed levator action due to facial palsy, third nerve misdirection, and impending tentorial herniation.
- Miscellaneous causes include Down syndrome, thyroid eye disease (Graves' ophthalmopathy), large globe, essential hypertension, hepatic cirrhosis, meningitis, uremia, sphenoid wing meningioma, and lymphoma in the superior cul-de-sac.

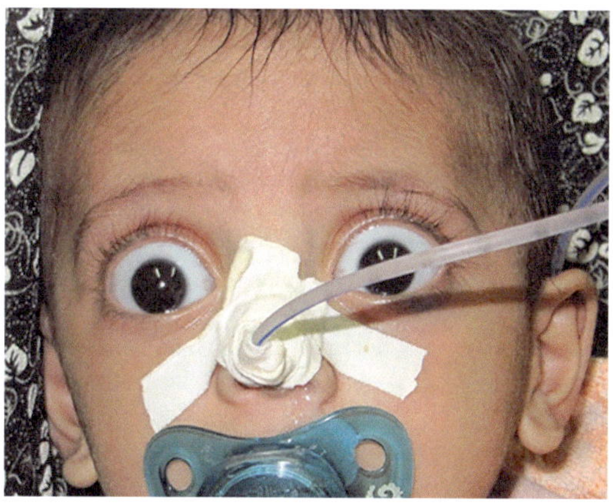

Fig. 9.19 Bilateral upperlid retraction in Parinaud's syndrome (Collier sign)

Signs in Eyelid Retraction:

- **Dalrymple Sign**: Lid retraction in primary gaze, usually associated with thyroid eye disease.
- **Kocher Sign:** A staring and frightened appearance of the eyes, particularly marked on attentive fixation. This is also typically seen in thyroid eye disease.
- **Von Graefe Sign**: Delayed descent of the upper lid on downgaze (also known as lid lag). This is most commonly found in thyroid eye disease, but less commonly in congenital ptosis.
- **Pseudo-Graefe Sign** (Pseudo-Lid Lag): Similar to von Graefe sign, but is due to aberrant regeneration of fibers of the oculomotor nerve (III) into the levator of the upper lid.
- **Collier Sign:** Neurogenic lid retraction that worsens with attempted upgaze. It can be unilateral or bilateral, and it is classically described as a component of the dorsal midbrain syndrome (Parinaud's syndrome).

Management of eyelid retraction: Eyelid retraction might be caused by medical diseases; therefore, these conditions need to be managed first before considering surgery. When necessary, surgical options for correcting eyelid retraction include levator muscle recession (i.e., weakening), which can involve either the levator muscle or Müller's muscle.

9.7 Ectropion and Entropion

Entropion and ectropion are two common eyelid malposition conditions that can cause significant discomfort and ocular morbidity. Entropion refers to the inward turning of the eyelid margin, often leading to corneal irritation or damage due to the lashes rubbing against the cornea. On the other hand, ectropion describes the outward turning or eversion of the eyelid margin. Table 9.2 provides a detailed comparison between entropion and ectropion, highlighting their key characteristics, associated symptoms, and commonly used methods of surgical repair.

9.7.1 Ectropion

Involutional (age related, senile) ectropion (Fig. 9.20) is demonstrated by the following:

- Horizontal lid laxity is indicated when the central part of the lid can be pulled 8 mm or more away from the globe, and the lid fails to snap back to its normal position upon release before the patient blinks.
- Lateral canthal tendon laxity is identified by the rounded appearance of the lateral canthus

Table 9.2 Comparison between ectropion and entropion

	Ectropion	Entropion
Definition	An outward turning (eversion) of the eyelid margin	An inward turning (inversion) of the eyelid margin
Muscular etiology	Often results from weakening in orbicularis oculi function as in facial nerve dysfunction	Usually due to weakening in eyelid retractor muscles, which are innervated by the oculomotor and sympathetic nerves
Method of surgical repair	Repair often involves tightening the lower lid to lateral orbital wall	Repair typically involves suturing the retractors to the tarsus to tighten the lid and prevent inversion and tightening the lower lid to lateral orbital wall
Prevalence of congenital form	Congenital form is rare, typically appearing with specific syndromes (e.g., blepharophimosis)	Congenital form is more common than in ectropion, but is still considered rare
Associated symptoms	Can lead to symptoms of dryness, tearing, and exposure keratopathy	Can cause corneal irritation or damage due to the lashes rubbing against the cornea, leading to symptoms such as tearing, foreign body sensation, and potentially reduced vision
Commonly associated conditions	Often associated with aging, facial nerve palsy, and skin scarring from trauma or previous surgeries	Often associated with aging, conjunctival scarring from trachoma, and spastic conditions like blepharospasm

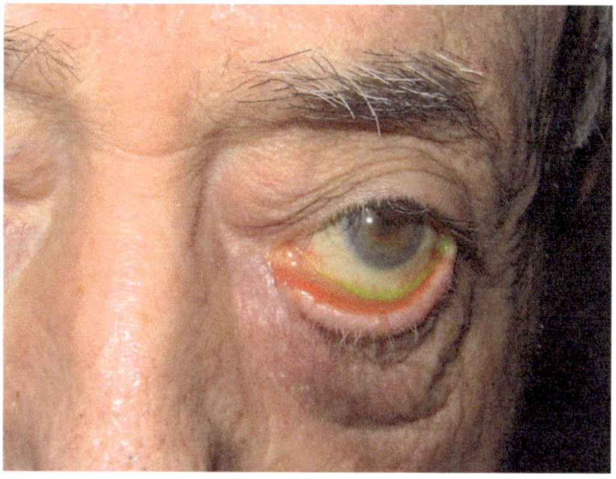

Fig. 9.20 Left lower lid involutional ectropion in an elderly person with exposed lower tarsal plate

and the ability to pull the lower lid medially by more than 2 mm.

- Medial canthal tendon laxity is demonstrated by pulling the lower lid laterally and observing the position of the inferior punctum. In a normal lid, the punctum should not be displaced more than 1–2 mm. Mild laxity allows the punctum to reach the limbus, while severe laxity may cause it to reach the pupil.
- The above changes also predispose to entropion. However, overriding of the pretarsal by the preseptal orbicularis muscle and disinsertion of lower lid retractors are specific for only entropion.

Ectropion after skin surgery is usually cicatricial and can be managed by incision and relaxation of the vertical traction; horizontal eyelid tightening; or vertical lengthening of anterior lamella.

9.7.2 Surgical Repair

- Lateral tarsal strip procedure, in which the lateral tarsus after shortening is tightened and reattached to the lateral orbital rim
- Horizontal lid shortening by excision of a full-thickness pentagon

9.7.3 Congenital Ectropion

It is typically caused by a vertical tissue loss in the anterior lamella of the lateral third of the lower eyelid, often accompanied by canthal tendon laxity. This condition is commonly associated with Down syndrome, blepharophimosis, and Möbius syndrome or lamellar ichthyosis. Isolated congenital ectropion due to horizontal lid laxity is a very rare occurrence.

9.7.4 Cicatricial Ectropion

It is caused by scarring and shortening of eyelid anterior lamellae (skin and underlying tissues).

- Mild localized cases can be managed by excising the offending scar tissue and performing a procedure like Z-plasty to address the vertical skin deficiency.
- For severe generalized cases, treatment involves the use of transposition flaps or free skin grafts. Potential sources for these grafts include the upper eyelids, posterior auricular area, preauricular region, and supraclavicular areas.

Preferred treatment for cicatricial ectropion is lateral tarsal strip plus skin graft (Fig. 9.21).

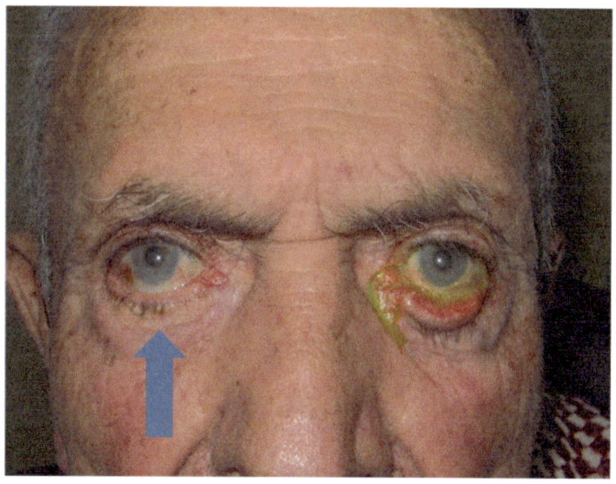

Fig. 9.21 Left Lower cicatricial ectropion. The right lower lid was treated with lateral tarsal strip and a full thickness skin graft (arrow) 2 years ago

9.7.5 Paralytic Ectropion (Fig. 9.22)

It is caused mostly by facial nerve palsy (CN VII). Temporary measures can be done to prevent exposure keratopathy; if no improvement after 6 months, permanent measures should be considered. Therapeutic measures typically target the cause of facial nerve palsy and may comprise eyelid-tightening surgeries or interim solutions like lubrication and taping the eyelid closed during sleep.

- Inducing ptosis by levator disinsertion or Botox.
- Lateral canthus strip procedure.
- Suturing the upper and lower lid margins medial to punctum (aka medial canthoplasty).
- In patients with lagophthalmos, either gold or platinum weights can be implanted into the upper lid.
- Lateral tarsorrhaphy.
- Brow ptosis repair.

Paralytic ectropion is often associated with failure of the lacrimal pump and resulting tearing. Even after successful correction of the eyelid malposition, the lacrimal pump function usually does not return, as the orbicularis muscle does not regain its normal tone.

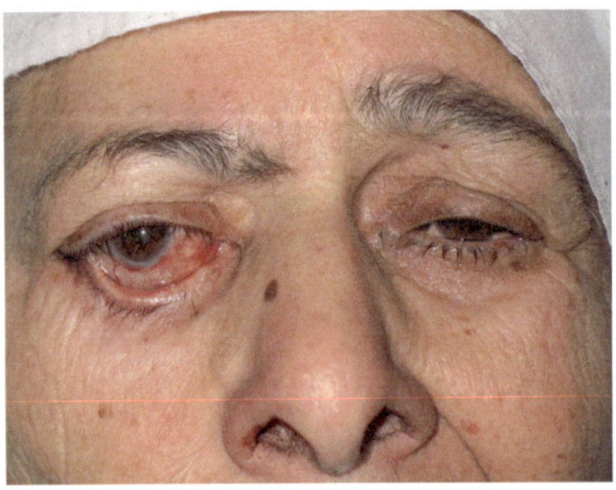

Fig. 9.22 Right paralytic ectropion and brow ptosis in a facial nerve palsy patient and red, irritated eye with significant right brow ptosis togerther with loss of nasolabial fold

9.7.6 Mechanical Ectropion

It is caused by a mass effect pulling the lower lid away from the globe.

9.7.6.1 High Yield Notes

Ectropion combined with alteration of eyelid anatomy, or loss of eyelashes, should suggest the possibility of malignancy and the need for a biopsy. Loss of lashes is not a typical involutional change.

While involutional is the most common form of ectropion, it is very rare to see ectropion at birth (congenital). So, congenital ectropion is the rarest form.

Paralytic ectropion occurs when there is interruption of the innervation to the orbicularis oculi as found in cranial nerve VII palsy or Bell's palsy.

Ectropion repair techniques: Encompass several procedures, including the lateral tarsal strip procedure, full-thickness wedge excision, medial canthal tendon resection, medial canthal tendon plication, and Z-plasty. The Kuhnt-Szymanowski procedure is a specific approach for ectropion correction that combines a blepharoplasty-type incision on the lower eyelid with a wedge resection of the lateral part of the posterior lamella of the lower eyelid.

9.7.7 Entropion

Involutional (age-related) entropion is demonstrated by the following:

Upper lid entropion is most commonly caused by cicatricial changes in the tarsal plate. A lower lid entropion is in many ways analogous to involutional blepharoptosis of the upper eyelid, as one of the mechanisms is believed to be related to dehiscence of lower lid retractors (aka capsulopalpebral fascia). Other mechanisms include medial and lateral canthal tendon laxity and override of the preseptal orbicularis pushing the lid margin inward. These additional mechanisms will further weaken the retractors, dominating the orbicularis action. In a similar concept, severe orbicularis contractions as in severe cases of essential blepharospasm may also result in entropion, which is managed by botulinum toxin in this case.

Associated features with involutional entropion are the following:

- Disinsertion of the lower lid retractors: this results in vertical lid instability and the lower eyelid typically positioned higher than normal and a decreased excursion (i.e., movement) of the lower lid in downgaze.
- Horizontal lid laxity.
- Overriding the pretarsal by the preseptal orbicularis during lid closure, the preseptal orbicularis muscle moves the lower border of the tarsal plate anteriorly away from the globe, and the upper border towards the globe, thus tipping the lid inwards.
- Medial and lateral canthal tendon laxity

Clinical clues to the disinsertion of the lower lid retractors include:

- White line below the tarsal border caused by the dehisced edge of the disinserted retractors
- Higher-than-normal lower eyelid position
- Decreased movement of the lower lid on downgaze
- Deepening on the inferior cul-de-sac of the inferior conjunctival fornix (rather than shrinking)

Surgical repair aims mainly to correct overriding preseptal muscle and laxity.

Entropion Repair Techniques: These include lid retractor reattachment, botulinum toxin injection of orbicularis oculi, Quickert-Rathbun sutures, and transverse everting sutures. Quickert-Rathbun rotational sutures can be done as a quick bedside procedure by placing several sutures in the eyelid, everting it. Optimally, reattaching the capsulopalpebral fascia to the tarsus would restore the normal anatomy. Other measures work on different mechanisms described above as follows:

- Transverse everting sutures prevent the overriding of the preseptal orbicularis. They are quick and easy to place, providing temporary correction that typically lasts several months. This method is useful in situations where a more complex procedure may not be feasible, such as with a confused patient.
- The Wies procedure offers a durable correction. It involves full-thickness horizontal lid splitting and insertion of everting sutures. The scar formed acts as a barrier between the preseptal and pretarsal orbicularis muscles, and the everting suture effectively shifts the pull of the lower lid retractors from the tarsal plate to the skin and orbicularis muscle.

Lower lid retractor reinsertion involves direct exposure and advancement of the retractors, which provides a more precise approach compared to the Wies procedure. The subciliary skin incision used, along with the retractor reinsertion, helps prevent overriding of the preseptal orbicularis muscle. This procedure can be used as a primary treatment or reserved for cases of recurrence. Quickert suture repair is considered a temporizing measure with a high recurrence rate and therefore is most appropriate for temporary conditions such as acute spastic entropion.

Management of horizontal lid laxity can also be done by lateral tarsal strip and can be done in association with entropion repair (everting sutures).

Overriding of the pretarsal orbicularis by the preseptal orbicularis can be done by excision of a strip of preseptal orbicularis or everting sutures.

Acknowledgments None.

Conflict of Interest None.

Financial Disclosure None.

Suggested Reading

American Academy of Ophthalmology (2017) Basic and clinical science course. Section 7. Orbit, Eyelids and Lacrimal System, San Francisco, USA

Chern KC, Wright KW (1997) Review questions in ophthalmology. A question and answer book. Lippincott Williams & Wilkins

Dutton J (2018) Atlas of oculoplastic and orbital surgery. Lippincott Williams & Wilkins

Kanski JJ. Kanski's clinical ophthalmology E-book: a systematic approach. 6th and 9th ed. Elsevier Health Sciences; 2019.

Kakizaki H, Malhotra R, Selva D (2009) Upper eyelid anatomy: an update. Ann Plastic Surg 63(3):336–343

Jager RD, Lamkin JC (2006) The Massachusetts eye and ear infirmary. Review manual for ophthalmology, 3rd edn. Lippincott Williams & Wilkins

Tyers AG, Collin JRO (2001) Colour Atlas of ophthalmic plastic surgery. Butterworth-Heinemann

Clinical Review of Eyelid and Oculoplasty: Part II

10

Taher Alshammari, Hisham Kamel,
Saif Aldeen Alryalat, and Osama H. Ababneh

Abstract

This chapter continues the exploration of oculoplastic disorders, focusing on various surgical interventions and their applications. It begins with a discussion of key procedures, including temporal artery biopsy, Hughes procedure, and blepharoplasty, detailing their indications, techniques, and expected outcomes. The chapter further examines eyelid trauma, addressing its causes, assessment, and management to restore function. Additionally, it covers miscellaneous surgeries and disorders, highlighting less common but significant conditions that may require surgical intervention. By providing a thorough overview of these surgical approaches, the chapter aims to increase the understanding of their roles in oculoplastic care and improve clinical outcomes for patients experiencing eyelid disorders and trauma.

T. Alshammari
Department of Special Surgery, Prince Mohammed Medical City, Al-Jouf, Kingdom of Saudi Arabia

H. Kamel
Research Institute Ophthalmology, Cairo, Egypt

S. A. Alryalat
Department of Ophthalmology, The University of Jordan, Amman, Jordan

The University of Colorado Anschutz Medical Campus, CO, USA

O. H. Ababneh (✉)
Department of Ophthalmology, The University of Jordan and Jordan University Hospital, Amman, Jordan

Keywords

Oculoplastic surgery · Eyelid trauma · Temporal artery biopsy · Surgical techniques · Miscellaneous surgeries

10.1 Plastic Surgeries

The following sections will continue previous ones in Chap. 9.

10.1.1 Temporal Artery Biopsy

A temporal artery biopsy (TAB) involves the surgical removal of a small piece of the temporal artery (2.5–3.0 cm), which is located on the side of the head above the ears (Osei et al. 2023; Hansen et al. 2023). This procedure is often performed when giant cell arteritis (GCA) is suspected. Temporal artery biopsy is the gold standard for diagnosing GCA. However, temporal artery ultrasound is a fast and noninvasive procedure which may provide a supplementary tool or an alternative to biopsy with slightly lower sensitivity and specificity.

S. A. Alryalat (ed.), *Ophthalmology Board and FRCS Part 2 Exams*,
https://doi.org/10.1007/978-981-96-1517-9_10

Either the frontal (anterior) or the parietal (posterior) branches of the superficial temporal artery can be harvested for the biopsy. The safest area to perform a TAB is of the frontal branch of the superficial temporal artery (STA) that is above the line between the ear tragus and 1.0 cm above the lateral brow and more than 3.5 cm lateral to the lateral canthus (Fig. 10.1).

Incisions within the "danger zone," which is located between the zygomatic arch and the brow vertically and from the lateral canthus to 3.5 cm lateral to it horizontally, might have complications. These complications include the following:

- Injury to the frontal branch of the facial nerve (also known as the temporal branch) which runs very superficially along the zygomatic arch
- Higher incidence of brow ptosis

The frontal (temporal) branch of the facial nerve is a motor nerve that innervates the frontalis and portions of the orbicularis oculi muscles. It is vulnerable to injury if a TAB is performed in the danger zone (below line A in Fig. 10.1).

The danger zone is the area where the temporal branch of the facial nerve and the frontal branch of the superficial temporal artery are separated only by the superficial temporal fascia. Here, the superficial temporal artery is located within the superficial temporal fascia, while the temporal branch of the facial nerve is situated deeper within the fascia's fibrofatty layer. In some cases, the temporal branch of the facial nerve may be positioned directly beneath the frontal branch of the superficial temporal artery, raising the risk of nerve injury during the procedure (for more details, refer to the article "Temporal artery biopsy: time for a rethink on training?").

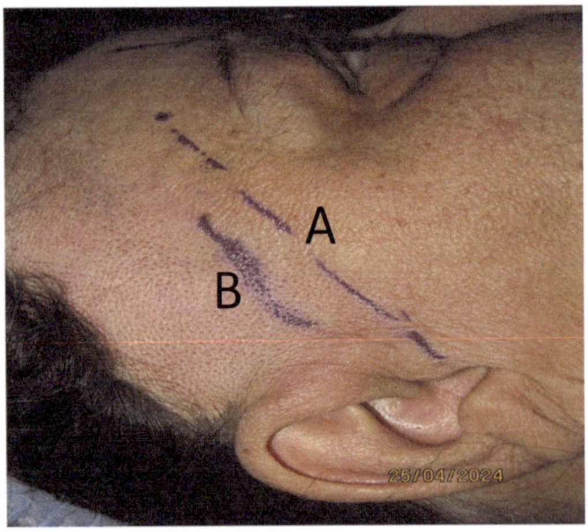

Fig. 10.1 Right Temporal artery biopsy. (**A**) The danger zone is the area under the line connecting the tragus to 1 cm above the lateral brow. (**B**) The site for TAB incision where the artery is palpated

10.1.2 Hughes Procedure

The Hughes procedure, or tarsoconjunctival flap advancement, is a surgical technique commonly used for the reconstruction of full-thickness lower eyelid defects that involve more than 50% and up to 100% of the lower eyelid margin. It is named after Wendell Hughes, an American ophthalmologist who first described it in 1937.

The Hughes procedure is typically a two-stage process:

- In the first stage, a tarsoconjunctival flap, also known as the "Hughes flap," is advanced from the upper to the lower eyelid to reconstruct the posterior lamella. The tarsoconjunctival flap is made up of tarsus (the dense connective tissue that forms the plate of the eyelid) and conjunctiva (the mucous membrane that covers the front of the eye and lines the inside of the eyelids). Concurrently, the anterior musculocutaneous lamella is reconstructed, often using a free or advancement full-thickness skin graft. This first stage helps to recreate the anatomical structure of the eyelid, maintaining its stability and functionality (Fig. 10.2 a–c).
- The second stage of the procedure typically takes place several (around 4) weeks later, after new vasculature has formed within and around the anterior graft and posterior flap. During this time, the affected eye remains covered by the blood-supplying flap pedicle. In the second stage, the flap pedicle is finally divided at the level of the new lower lid margin. This allows the new eyelid to function normally and provides the final cosmetic result (Fig. 10.2d).

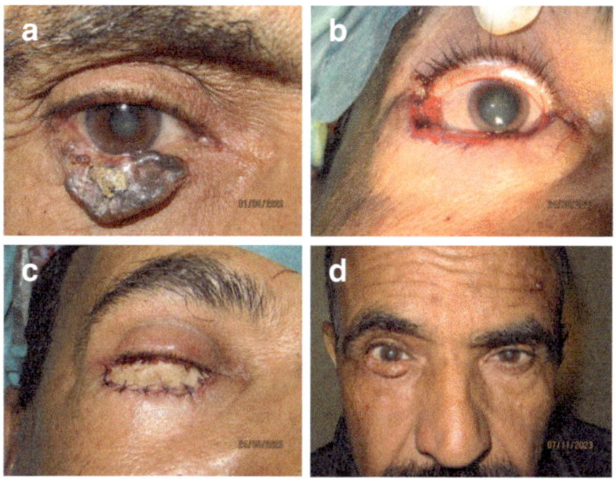

Fig. 10.2 (**a**) Hughes flap procedure. Right lower lid large Pigmented Basal Cell Carcinoma more than 50% of eyelid width. (**b**) Large lower lid defect more than 80% of the lid width. (**c**) First stage with tarsoconjunctival flap and a full thickness preauricular skin graft. (**d**) Two months after the first stage and one month after the second stage with viable right lower lid

Due to the prolonged period of time the eye must remain covered (patched) between the two stages of the Hughes procedure, it is generally not a good option for patients who only have vision in one eye (monocular patients). This procedure is known for providing excellent functional and cosmetic outcomes in the reconstruction of large lower eyelid defects, especially those resulting from trauma or tumor excision. However, like any surgical procedure, it carries some risk of complications, including infection, graft failure, and cosmetic dissatisfaction. As such, the patient's individual situation and overall health must be carefully considered before undertaking the procedure.

10.1.3 Blepharoplasty

Blepharoplasty is a surgical procedure performed to reshape the eyelids by removing and/or repositioning excess tissue as well as reinforcing the surrounding muscles and tendons. It is often undertaken to rejuvenate the eyes, typically in individuals aged 40–60 years. This procedure can be applied to both the upper and lower eyelids.

Procedure Details: Classically, blepharoplasty involves the removal of the pseudo-herniated fat pad that protrudes through a weakened orbital septum as well as removing a strip of skin. This fat pad, which normally cushions the eye, can bulge forward and create a "baggy" appearance.

Lower eyelid blepharoplasty can be performed through either a skin (transcutaneous) or a transconjunctival approach, while the upper eyelid is approached through the skin crease. The transconjunctival (retroblepharoplasty) technique is only utilized for lower eyelid blepharoplasty, offering the advantage of avoiding a visible scar on the skin of the eyelid. This method also has a lower incidence of postoperative eyelid retraction compared to the transcutaneous approach due to less skin excision. However, it does not allow for skin removal and thus cannot repair dermatochalasis (excessive eyelid skin).

Upper eyelid blepharoplasty is typically performed using an incision along the eyelid crease, allowing access to the necessary structures while leaving a minimally visible scar.

The peripheral arterial arcade, situated between the levator aponeurosis and Müller muscle just above the superior border of tarsus, serves as a crucial anatomical landmark in upper eyelid surgery. If it is unintentionally identified during an upper eyelid blepharoplasty, it may signal a dehiscence of the levator aponeurosis, which could result in postoperative ptosis. In such instances, reattachment of the levator to the tarsus might be necessary.

Complications: The most common complication of lower eyelid blepharoplasty is lower eyelid retraction or frank ectropion. Contributing factors include inadequate evaluation of lateral canthal laxity during preoperative assessment, overly aggressive removal of lower eyelid skin, and postoperative scarring of the anterior lamellae. Pyogenic granulomas may develop, especially with a transconjunctival approach, but they are neither frequent nor severe. Lash loss is rare, as surgical incisions are usually distant from the lash follicles. Infections are uncommon unless the patient is immunocompromised.

Contraindications: Patients with dry eye syndrome should avoid blepharoplasty, as the condition could be exacerbated by postoperative lagophthalmos. Anticoagulation and uncontrolled hypertension are also contraindications, as they may increase the risk of retrobulbar bleeding, thereby compromising vision.

Additional Procedures: When repairing blepharoptosis or entropion, an incision through the orbital septum is necessary to access the eyelid retractors and preaponeurotic fat pads, which can sometimes result in fat prolapse. Elevating the lower lid suborbicularis oculi fat (SOOF) can enhance the midface's youthful appearance and is typically performed through a transconjunctival or subciliary approach. The SOOF and retro-orbicularis oculi fat (ROOF) act as a buffer between mimetic muscles and the underlying periosteum, with their prolapse contributing to visible aging. Additionally, the temporal fat pad, located where the deep temporalis fascia divides over the zygomatic arch, plays a significant role in facial esthetics.

10.1.4 Canthal Tendon Surgeries

The medial canthal tendon consists of anterior and posterior portions. The anterior portion attaches to the frontal process of the maxillary bone (anterior lacrimal crest) and serves as the origin of the superficial head of the pretarsal orbicularis. The posterior portion inserts into the posterior lacrimal crest and fossa. The medial and lateral portion of the pretarsal muscle becomes the medial and lateral canthal tendon.

Medial canthal tendon avulsion requires reattachment of anterior and posterior crus to the lacrimal crest. The posterior attachment is crucial for achieving a natural eyelid appearance:

- Reattaching only the anterior crus to the anterior lacrimal crest may result in an anteriorly displaced, flat eyelid appearance, rather than a natural, convex contour.
- Proper attachment of the posterior crus to the posterior lacrimal crest is essential for restoring the normal eyelid contour at the medial canthus and ensuring a natural appearance. In cases of fracture, transnasal wiring or Y-shaped miniplate fixation may be necessary.

The lacrimal sac fundus is located in the lacrimal fossa between the anterior and posterior crus of the tendon. Placing sutures in this area can increase the risk of lacrimal sac injury, potentially leading to nasolacrimal obstruction. Medial canthal tendon injury, especially affecting the posterior crus, often results in unilateral rounding of the medial canthal tendon and acquired telecanthus.

The lateral canthal tendon needs to be attached to the periosteum inside the orbital rim toward Whitnall's tubercle. It should be attached 2mm higher than the medial canthal tendon.

10.1.5 Miscellaneous Surgeries

This section provides a concise overview of several miscellaneous plastic eye surgery procedures, outlining their primary aims and essential characteristics. Each surgical technique listed caters to a range of ocular conditions, from lid deformities such as entropion and ectropion to more complex disorders such as full-thickness eyelid defects and lagophthalmos. The procedures differ in their approach, whether through direct repair, tissue rearrangement, or use of implants, each addressing the unique needs of the individual oculoplastic patient. Table 10.1 serves as a quick reference for understanding the diversity and specialization within the field of oculoplastic surgery.

10.2 Eyelid Trauma

Traumatic ptosis is a condition that may arise following eye trauma due to dehiscence of the levator aponeurosis or edema resulting in blepharoptosis. In such cases, it is recommended that the ptosis should be observed for **6 months** prior to any surgical intervention, as it may resolve spontaneously, especially in younger patients where healing may plateau.

During the treatment of eyelid lacerations, if visible adipose tissue, specifically orbital fat, is noticed, this should raise concern for the potential of an injury to the globe. Additionally, when repairing a partial-thickness eyelid laceration, care should be taken not to inadvertently suture the orbital septum into the subcutaneous tissues as this can lead to lid retraction in downgaze. In cases of full-thickness eyelid defect repair, the most common complication tends to be eyelid rigidity, which manifests as ptosis and lagophthalmos. Care should also be undertaken to examine the lacrimal drainage system and to rule out punctal and/or canalicular lacerations. When planning the reconstruction, it is important to use any available tissue from the face, and particularly from the eyelids, even if they appear to be ischemic. Eyelid tissue is highly vascular, and replantation of convulsed eyelids can still be successful several hours after the trauma. In the case of full-thickness mucosal grafts, predominantly from the hard palate, they have been observed to maintain their original epithelium posttransplantation onto the ocular surface. However, it is important to understand that submucosal glands generally do not survive the process.

When treating injuries such as those resulting from canine bites, the surgical repair should proceed as with any other eyelid reconstruction and should be planned as soon after the injury as possible. In all cases, it is essential not to discard any tissue from the facial region, even if the tissue appears to be of poor quality. The face, including the eyelids, has an excellent blood supply, and avulsed tissue may heal successfully, even if it initially appears to be ischemic. For burn injuries, topical medications are generally not recommended during the acute phases of first- or second-degree burns. For full-thickness or third-degree burns, it is important to cover the affected tissue with appropriate treatments. Silver sulfadiazine 1% in a water-miscible base or a non-sensitizing antibiotic ointment, such as gentamicin in a water-miscible base, should be applied to the burn area.

Indirect traumatic optic neuropathy is usually the result of a blunt trauma to the frontal bone. In relation to zygomaticomaxillary complex (ZMC) fractures, it is worth noting that inferior rectus entrapment is the least likely associated complication. Lastly, assessing eyelid avulsion requires a specific approach. The only definitive, and therefore mandatory, method to determine whether there is an avulsion involves pulling directly on the eyelid, against the vector of the tendon.

Table 10.1 Overview of miscellaneous plastic eye surgery procedures

Surgery	Aim	Notes
Tarsoconjunctival flap advancement (Hughes procedure)	Repair of lower lid full-thickness defects greater than 50%	This procedure reconstructs the posterior lamella. Typically, it involves the use of a temporary bridge flap from the upper to the lower and a full-thickness skin graft or advancement. However, it is not advisable to take two flaps from the same eyelid as this will weaken the eyelid
Lower lid suborbicularis oculi fat (SOOF) elevation	Reduction of lower eyelid retraction or hollowness	This procedure uses the fat pads beneath the orbicularis oculi muscle to support the lower lid, thus improving its contour and position
Quickert-Rathbun sutures (everting suture)	Temporary repair of entropion	This bedside procedure involves placing several sutures (2–3) in the eyelid to evert it, providing relief from entropion, especially in patients not suitable for surgery
Hotz procedure	Management of epiblepharon and entropion in children	Involves the excision of a strip of skin and muscle from the lower eyelid and the fixation of the skin crease to the tarsal plate to correct the lid margin position
Y-plasty or Y-V plasty	Correction of epicanthal folds and mild telecanthus	This surgical technique involves creating a Y-shaped incision to rearrange tissues and reduce the prominence of the fold
Z-plasty	Correction of cicatricial ectropion	This procedure is used for tissue rearrangement in scar revision. It helps to relieve tension along the scar line and can improve both the function and appearance of the eyelid
Wies procedure	Entropion repair	Involves a full-thickness horizontal lid splitting and the insertion of everting sutures to correct the inversion of the lid margin
Gold weight implantation	Management of lagophthalmos	The gold weight implant is placed in a pretarsal location underneath the orbicularis oculi muscle. It provides additional weight to aid eyelid closure in cases of facial nerve palsy
Lower eyelid retractor repair	Entropion repair	This surgical procedure involves the repair or tightening of the lower eyelid retractors, an important component in the correction of entropion

10.3 Miscellaneous

Eyelash Disorders

- **Distichiasis**, or double-row eyelashes, is often a congenital condition and can be inherited in an autosomal dominant manner. Most patients with this condition also exhibit primary lymphedema of the legs, known as lymphedema–distichiasis syndrome. This hereditary form of distichiasis is linked to a mutation in the FOXC2 gene. In contrast, acquired distichiasis typically presents with nonpigmented, stunted cilia and is usually symptomatic. When a lash is removed, it generally regrows within approximately 8 weeks.
- **Poliosis**, or whitening of hair, usually eyelashes or eyebrows, can be caused by chronic inflammation (such as chronic blepharitis), melanocyte-directed diseases (like sympathetic ophthalmia or Vogt-Koyanagi-Harada disease), vitiligo, and Waardenburg syndrome. Aging does not typically cause poliosis.
- **Madarosis**: Loss of lashes.

Floppy eyelid syndrome: It is characterized by chronic papillary conjunctivitis, easily everted and flaccid upper eyelids, and nonspecific irritation. It is associated with conditions such as obesity, keratoconus, eyelid rubbing or mechanical pressure, obstructive sleep apnea, hyperglycemia, and eyelid imbrication syndrome. Symptoms and signs are often worsened by sleeping face down, as the pillow can evert the eyelids. The primary pathology of floppy eyelid syndrome is a reduction in tarsal elastin fibers.

Botulinum toxin: Type A acts by inhibiting acetylcholine release by binding to motor nerve terminal receptors. Botulinum toxin B, on the other hand, presents a higher diffusion rate and quicker action but offers shorter duration and more injection discomfort than its type A counterpart.

Ocular cicatricial pemphigoid (OCP), a type II hypersensitivity reaction, primarily affects the conjunctiva or the inferior fornix. Its classic histological feature is the binding of complement and immunoglobulins to the epithelial basement membrane, distinguishing it from pemphigus characterized by epithelial acantholysis and intraepithelial bullae. OCP's disease activity can increase postocular surgery, necessitating systemic treatment such as steroids to reduce cicatrization progression from 75% to approximately 10%. This approach differs from the usual first-line treatment for mild-to-moderate cases—dapsone—and for severe cases—potent immunosuppressives like cyclophosphamide.

Figure 10.3 shows a case of Limbal dermoid, which is a congenital lesion that typically appears on the ocular surface. Dermoids are choristomas, which are masses of normal tissue found in an abnormal location. These growths consist of keratinized stratified squamous epithelium and often include other elements such as hair follicles, sebaceous glands, sweat glands, and occasionally bone, cartilage, or fat. They are typically

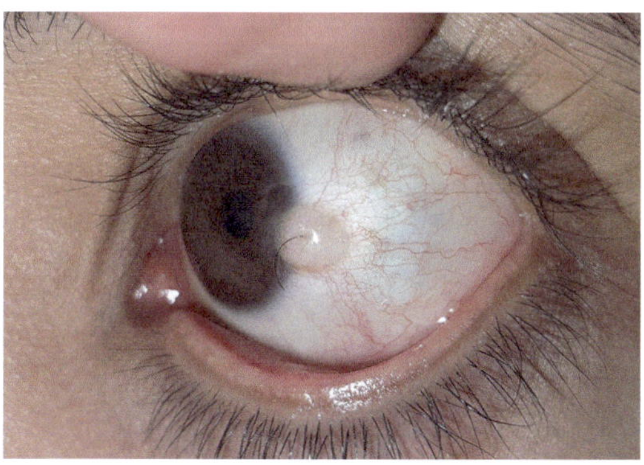

Fig. 10.3 Ocular limbal Dermoid. The growth is typically smooth, round or oval, and located at the limbus

slow growing, non-tender, and often found at the limbus or corneal surface. Although they can be managed conservatively if asymptomatic, surgical excision is usually considered if they cause vision impairment or cosmetic concerns.

Craniosynostosis refers to the partial or complete premature fusion of cranial sutures, typically presenting with ocular hypertelorism, proptosis, beaking of the nose, and midface hypoplasia. In contrast, patients with blepharophimosis are more likely to develop telecanthus and ectropion.

The normal ocular surface is predominantly colonized by *Staphylococcus epidermidis*, accounting for over 50% of its flora. This includes other organisms like *Staphylococcus aureus*, *Streptococcus* species, *Corynebacterium* spp., and *Moraxella catarrhalis*. Notably, *Escherichia coli* is a normal part of the infant ocular surface post-vaginal birth. However, Gram-negative organisms, including *Serratia* and *Fusarium* species, are pathogenic and not part of the normal ocular flora. Eyelid bacteria such as *Staphylococcus aureus* toxins can lead to secondary phenomena like phlyctenules, marginal keratitis, and chronic follicular reaction.

There are specific mites associated with the eyelid. *Demodex folliculorum*, a mite living in meibomian glands, is a common commensal in adults. "Sleeves" at the base of lashes indicate their presence. Contrarily, *Pthirus pubis* (crab louse), a pathological mite infesting pubic hair and eyelashes, causes itchiness and sometimes conjunctivitis. Treatment options include mechanical removal or application of bland ointments applied to the lids to suffocate adult lice.

Recurrent pterygium can be managed with topical mitomycin or 5-FU after excision, conjunctival autografting, or advancement of a conjunctival flap. Pingueculae, associated with actinic damage to subepithelial collagen, exhibits "elastosis," a non-true elastin staining.

Trifluridine, an anti-herpesvirus drug, can cause punctal stenosis and raised intraocular pressure, along with ocular irritation. Conjunctival intraepithelial neoplasia often develops on the bulbar conjunctiva. Basal cell carcinoma, particularly of the medial canthal location, carries the worst prognosis, especially the fibrotic type.

Other conditions include pilomatrixoma (a benign tumor of the hair follicle), syringoma (a sweat gland-derived growth), and nevi, whose pigmentation and growth increase around puberty but carry least potential for malignancy when they are subepithelial or dermal. Kaposi's sarcoma is aggressive in immunocompromised individuals, generally affecting the lower extremities of older men and being treatable through radiation therapy.

Acknowledgments None.

Conflict of Interest None.

Financial Disclosure None.

References

Osei G, Rainsbury P, Morris D, Haridas A (2023) Temporal artery biopsy: time for a rethink on training? Eye (Lond) 37(3):506–510. https://doi.org/10.1038/s41433-022-01963-1

Hansen MS, Terslev L, Jensen MR, Brittain JM, Døhn UM, Faber C, Heegaard S, Klefter ON, König EB, Subhi Y, Wiencke AK, Hamann S (2023) Comparison of temporal artery ultrasound versus biopsy in the diagnosis of giant cell arteritis. Eye (Lond) 37(2):344–349. https://doi.org/10.1038/s41433-022-01947-1

Further Reading

American Academy of Ophthalmology (2017) Basic and clinical science course. Section 7. Orbit, Eyelids and Lacrimal System, San Francisco, USA

Dutton J (2018) Atlas of oculoplastic and orbital surgery. Lippincott Williams & Wilkins

Kanski JJ. Kanski's clinical ophthalmology E-book: a systematic approach. 6th and 9th edn. Elsevier Health Sciences; 2019.

Chern KC, Wright KW (1997) Review questions in ophthalmology. A question and answer book. Lippincott Williams & Wilkins

Jager RD, Lamkin JC (2006) The Massachusetts eye and ear infirmary. In: Review manual for ophthalmology, 3rd edn. Lippincott Williams & Wilkins

Tyers AG, Collin JRO (2001) Colour Atlas of ophthalmic plastic surgery. Butterworth-Heinemann

Clinical Review of Sclera and Conjunctiva

11

Mohammed Aloqaily, Saif Aldeen Alryalat, and Mo'ath AlShawabkeh

Abstract

This chapter explores diseases of the sclera and conjunctiva, detailing their diverse presentations and causes, including infections, autoimmune disorders, drug reactions, and tumors. While many conditions are benign, some can threaten vision, highlighting the need for early diagnosis and management. Key conditions discussed include episcleritis, scleritis (and its subtypes), conjunctivitis, degenerative disorders, and neoplasms. Each condition is systematically presented, covering definition, risk factors, clinical manifestations, diagnostics, and management strategies. Comparative tables and high-yield notes enhance understanding. A further readings section provides references for readers interested in more detailed information, ensuring a comprehensive overview of scleral and conjunctival disorders.

M. Aloqaily
Hamad Medical Corporation, Al-Doha, Qatar

S. A. Alryalat
Department of Ophthalmology, The University of Jordan, Amman, Jordan

The University of Colorado Anschutz Medical Campus, CO, USA

M. AlShawabkeh (✉)
Department of Ophthalmology, The Hashemite University, Zarqa, Jordan

Keywords

Sclera · Conjunctiva · Conjunctivitis · Scleritis · Neoplastic conditions

11.1 Overview

Diseases affecting the sclera and conjunctiva are frequently encountered in medical practice with a broad range of presentations, underlying pathophysiology, and etiologies such as infections, autoimmune diseases, drug reactions, or tumors.

Despite the benign nature and mild presentation of many scleral and conjunctival pathologies, some can cause more catastrophic consequences and can threaten the vision, which mandates an early recognition, diagnosis, and management of such cases. Furthermore, clinical presentation and examination are considered the cornerstones in diagnosing scleral and conjunctival diseases, although some laboratory tests and imaging modalities can be helpful in diagnosing and confirming some entities.

This chapter discusses the various conditions affecting the sclera and the conjunctiva including episcleritis, scleritis (with its various subtypes), scleral discoloration-associated conditions, conjunctivitis (with its various subtypes), degenerative conjunctival disorders, and neoplastic conditions of the conjunctival. In addition, other less common conditions are highlighted in some

S. A. Alryalat (ed.), *Ophthalmology Board and FRCS Part 2 Exams*,
https://doi.org/10.1007/978-981-96-1517-9_11

sections such as in miscellaneous conjunctivitis. Moreover, each condition will be presented and elaborated in a systematic way that includes the definition, risk factors, etiology, presentation and clinical manifestations, diagnostic modalities, and management, in order to deliver the information comprehensively and understandably. Nevertheless, the chapter also includes both comparison and elaborating tables, information that was frequently noticed in exam books, in addition to high-yield notes to provide and deliver an integrated message in brief.

The references section will also include the multiple references that were utilized to write this chapter for the readers who are interested in seeking more detailed and specific knowledge about any condition specifically (AlRyalat 2022; Bowling 2015; Kaiser et al. 2014; Yanoff and Duker 2008; Basic Clinical Science Course (BCSC) of the American Academy of Ophthalmology 2021; Tagg and Kardon 2010; Watson and Young 2004).

11.2 Episcleritis

Episcleritis, which refers to inflammation of the episcleral tissue, is a frequently encountered disease. It is considered benign and self-limited with a predilection toward females (except for children) and the middle-aged population. In addition, etiology is idiopathic in most cases. However, it is associated with several ocular (more common) and systemic diseases such as dry eye, contact lens wearing, rheumatoid arthritis, inflammatory bowel disease, dermatological condition, infections, vasculitis, and medications. It can be divided into two separate entities, which are simple and nodular episcleritis.

11.2.1 Simple Episcleritis

This type accounts for the majority of episcleritis cases (75%). Patients present acutely, with bilateral eye redness, grittiness, and occasionally photophobia without the vision being affected. On examination, redness might take a specific, sectoral distribution (intrapalpebral, triangular-shaped, distribution) or even diffuse.

The diagnosis is mainly clinical, and the management is conservative with reassurance, as the disease will resolve over the next few days. Cool compressors and artificial tears can be used in mild cases. Topical steroids, topical NSAIDs, and oral NSAIDs can also be used if needed. Furthermore, underlying systemic diseases should be evaluated and managed, if present.

11.2.2 Nodular Episcleritis

In this type, patients will also present with eye redness and discomfort early in the morning after waking up. However, it is gradual in onset and will take several days to develop completely. On examination, a red, tender interpalpebral nodule will be noticed. Other findings such as elevated intraocular pressure and anterior chamber reaction are infrequently encountered.

The diagnosis is also clinical. And management is the same as the simple variant, although it is more frequently required.

High-Yield Notes

- The sclera remains spared in isolated episcleritis. If severe discomfort is present, scleritis should be ruled out.
- Episcleritis is associated with high risk of recurrence (around 66%).
- Use of topical phenylephrine 2.5% drops can help in the clinical differentiation between episcleritis and scleritis as the redness improves or disappears in the case of former only.
- Nodular variant tends to last longer than the simple variant, yet both are self-limited.
- Nodular type has a predilection toward the female gender while the simple type affects both genders equally.

11.2.3 Scleritis

Scleritis refers to the progressive inflammation of scleral tissue, which can be accompanied by episcleral inflammation. Although it is uncommon as compared to episcleritis, scleritis can extend further to involve the cornea, which makes it vision threatening. The patients usually present with a painful red eye, and it is frequently associated with underlying systemic and autoimmune diseases (in around 50% of cases) with rheumatoid arthritis being the most common. It can also arise following infection, trauma, or surgery, with pterygium excision surgery being the most common. In addition, it is more commonly encountered in females and during the fourth–sixth decades.

Eye pain usually develops over time (gradually), is described as dull, radiates to other areas (such as ear, face, and jaw), increases with eye movement, and might be worse at night. On examination, sectoral or diffuse redness, tenderness, and scleral edema with a bluish-violet hue will be noticed (Fig. 11.1). Complications such as keratitis, uveitis, cataract, glaucoma, or hypotony can be seen with anterior scleritis, while vitritis and retinal detachment are seen more with posterior scleritis.

Although the diagnosis of scleritis is clinical, investigations looking for underlying etiology or possible complications are done according to each case specifically. Furthermore, the mainstay of management resides in limiting and reducing inflammation and the associated ocular damage. Medical management can include the use of NSAIDs, corticosteroids, and immunosuppressive therapies; meanwhile, surgical treatment is of a more limited role (for scleral perforation or high risk of rupture, for example).

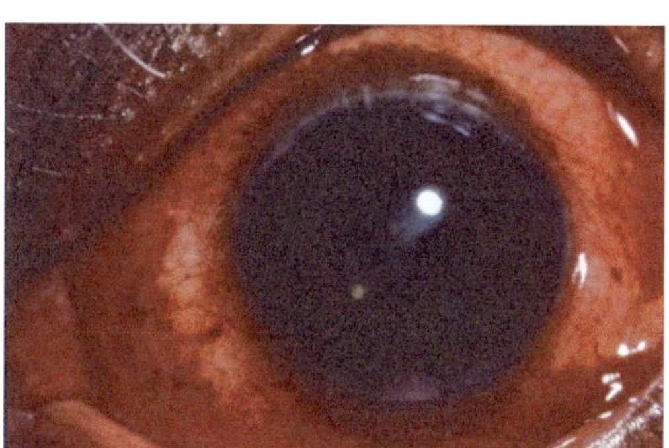

Fig. 11.1 Diffuse anterior scleritis. Courtesy to Retina Rocks®

Scleritis can be divided into immune-mediated scleritis (most common) and infectious scleritis. Furthermore, the immune-mediated form can be further divided into anterior and posterior scleritis.

11.2.3.1 Anterior Scleritis

Anterior scleritis, in which the inflammation is anterior to the rectus muscles, is considered the most common type and can be divided into necrotizing and non-necrotizing types. Medications used in the treatment of non-necrotizing types include topical steroids, systemic NSAIDs, periocular steroid injections, and systemic steroids for severe or refractory cases. Necrotizing forms are usually treated with systemic steroids along with immunosuppressive and biological agents for controlling underlying systemic illnesses. These medications are used in an escalating way according to responsiveness.

High-Yield Notes

- When scleritis recurs, it is usually of the same type; however, it can progress to more severe type in some cases.
- Non-necrotizing anterior scleritis can be diffuse or nodular. It can last for several years with several recurrences, but the overall prognosis of vision is satisfactory.
- Nodular scleritis patients are more likely to suffer from an old herpes zoster ophthalmicus in comparison to diffuse scleritis patients. Therefore, infectious etiologies (see below) should be ruled out.
- Necrotizing anterior type is considered the most aggressive with the worst prognosis, and if not managed appropriately, it may lead to several complications and even loss of vision.

11.2.3.2 Posterior Scleritis

Posterior scleritis, in which the inflammation extends posterior to the insertion of rectus muscles, is considered rare, yet it can lead to serious consequences such as serous retinal detachment and choroidal folds (Figs. 11.2 and 11.3). It can develop solely or with anterior scleritis with the same inflammatory changes that happen in anterior scleritis. In addition, myositis is frequently encountered with this condition and will lead to

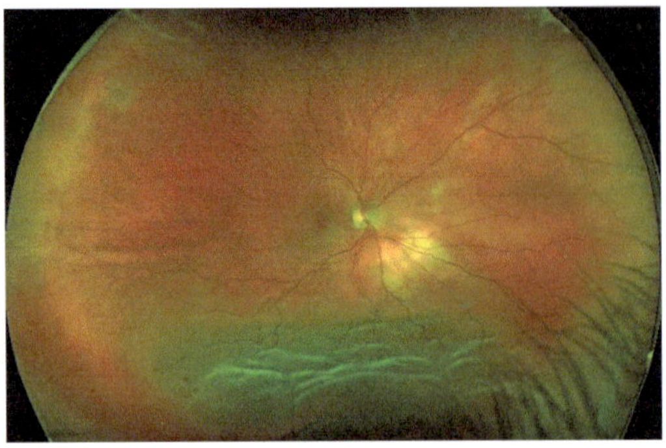

Fig. 11.2 Exudative retinal detachment in posterior scleritis. Courtesy to Retina Rocks®

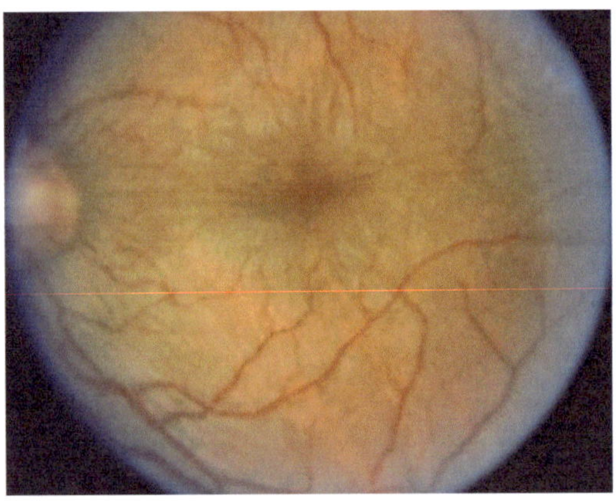

Fig. 11.3 Choroidal folds in posterior scleritis. Courtesy to Retina Rocks®

the experience of diplopia and painful eye movement, among others.

On detailed examination, several findings might be noted such as exudative retinal detachment, uveal effusion along with choroidal detachment, optic disc edema, and proptosis, among others. Several diagnostic modalities such as ultrasonography, CT, or even MRI can be indicated and will reveal the presence of several findings such as scleral thickening, optic disc edema, and retinal detachment.

11.2.3.3 Scleromalacia Perforans

This is a necrotizing scleritis without inflammation, a rare type of anterior scleritis in which scleral thinning occurs without inflammation. It usually develops in older females with long-lasting systemic illnesses (rheumatoid arthritis mainly) and is speculated to originate following type 3 hypersensitivity reaction due to immune complex accumulation. Patients present with general, nonspecific irritation symptoms without pain or vision change. However, despite the name "perforans," perforation actually occurs very rarely.

Several necrotic plaques might develop adjacent to the limbal region, enlarge, and even merge, which leads to scleral thinning. The scleral will appear as a thin, white, and avascular area. In addition, choroidal exposure and staphyloma development might happen. Management mainly focuses on treating the underlying disease along with treating and preventing complications.

Table 11.1 Systemic diseases commonly associated with scleritis and other ocular presentations

Disease	Ocular manifestations
Rheumatoid arthritis	Immune-mediated scleritis Episcleritis Dry eye disease (most common) Ulcerative keratitis
Granulomatosis with polyangiitis (Wegener granulomatosis)	Necrotizing scleritis Peripheral ulcerative keratitis Occlusive retinal vasculitis Nasolacrimal duct obstruction and dacryocystitis
Polyarteritis nodosa	Necrotizing scleritis Peripheral ulcerative keratitis Occlusive retinal periarteritis

11.2.4 Systemic Illnesses Associated with the Development of Scleritis

Several systemic pathologies have been associated with the development of scleritis and other ocular pathologies. Table 11.1 highlights some of the common diseases that are linked to such ocular manifestations.

11.3 Infectious Scleritis

This entity presents similarly to immune-mediated scleritis, although rare. It is more seen in male patients and can develop following eye

Table 11.2 Examples of organisms associated with infectious scleritis

Infectious organism	Characteristics
Herpes zoster virus	The most common cause of infectious scleritis Necrotizing scleritis (refractory)
Mycobacterium tuberculosis	Nodular or necrotizing scleritis
Mycobacterium leprae	Necrotizing scleritis Nodular form can occur with lepromatous leprosy subtype
Treponema pallidum	Diffuse anterior scleritis (with secondary syphilis) Nodular anterior scleritis (with tertiary syphilis)
Borrelia burgdorferi	Posterior scleritis

Table 11.3 Examples of diseases associated with apparent scleral discoloration

Disease	Associated ocular abnormalities
Alkaptonuria	Blue or black pigmentation of the sclera
Hemochromatosis	Brown (bronze) scleral and conjunctival discoloration
Osteogenesis imperfecta (type 1 and type 2A)	Blue sclera, megalocornea, corneal arcus, and shallow orbits
Ehlers-Danlos syndrome (type VI)	Blue and fragile sclera, microcornea, keratoconus, ectopia lentis, and retinal detachment

surgeries, traumas, or infection extension from adjacent structures such as the cornea. In addition, some treatments (mitomycin C injections and beta irradiation, for example) are associated with a higher risk. Several organisms have been associated with the development of infectious scleritis (Table 11.2).

11.4 Conditions Associated with a Scleral Discoloration

Several conditions may present with a change in the appearance of scleral color from normal white. The mechanism behind this change varies according to the specific pathophysiology of the disease. For instance, it can be due to the deposition of materials that cause pigmentation or due to an increase in scleral translucency due to an underlying pathology (Table 11.3).

11.5 Congenital Ocular Melanocytosis

It is a rare condition characterized by an increase in the number, size, and pigmentation of ocular melanocytes, which can also affect other tissue's melanocytes simultaneously. In fact, the oculo-dermal type, which affects both the eye and the dermis, is considered the most common type; meanwhile, isolated ocular melanocytosis is the least common one.

Oculo-dermal melanocytosis has a predilection toward dark-skinned people and presents with unilateral deep bluish or brownish pigmentation of the facial skin. However, ocular melanocytosis presents with grey pigmentation of the sclera and episclera.

Congenital ocular melanocytosis can be associated with several other ocular manifestations affecting the ipsilateral eye. For instance, it is associated with the appearance of iris hyperchromia and mammillations, fundus and trabecular hyperpigmentation, and uveal melanoma.

Although it is more commonly seen in darker races compared with whites, the risk of melanoma is higher in white individuals.

High-Yield Notes

- Episcleritis rarely progresses to scleritis. However, it is usually present along with scleritis.
- Simple episcleritis and non-necrotizing scleritis are considered non-granulomatous diseases, whereas nodular episcleritis and necrotizing scleritis are granulomatous.

- In auto-inflammatory sclerokeratitis, subtenon corticosteroid injections are relatively contraindicated due to the increased risk of perforation.
- Rheumatological disorders, connective tissue, or other autoimmune diseases are associated with around one-third of non-necrotizing anterior scleritis and around two-thirds of necrotizing anterior scleritis.
- Diffuse scleritis is composed of more than 40% of anterior scleritis (most common), followed by nodular form. Meanwhile, necrotizing scleritis is the least common form of anterior scleritis.
- Chlamydial infection is not associated with infectious scleritis.
- Although associated with a wide range of ocular manifestations, Behcet's disease is not associated with immune-mediated scleritis.

11.6 Infectious Conjunctivitis

In general, patients with conjunctival inflammation of any etiology present with nonspecific symptoms such as itching, redness, burning, and various forms of discharge (see Table 11.4). Conjunctival signs can help in determining the likely etiology (see Table 11.5).

High-Yield Notes

- Folliculosis is normal in children, and in the fornix and upper tarsal plate in adults.
- Follicular conjunctivitis is considered chronic if it lasts more than 4 weeks.

Table 11.4 Conjunctival discharge types and common associations

Discharged material	Associated disease
Watery	Acute viral or allergic conjunctivitis
Mucoid	Chronic allergic conjunctivitis and dry eye
Mucopurulent	Acute bacterial conjunctivitis, especially chlamydia
Moderately purulent	Acute bacterial conjunctivitis
Severely purulent	Gonococcal conjunctivitis

- The superior edge of superior tarsus has a small papilla, which hinders it as a suitable papillary reaction detection site.

11.6.1 Viral Conjunctivitis

Viral conjunctivitis is a common disease in all age groups. Several viruses can be responsible for this infection with adenovirus being the most commonly encountered. It is transmitted through respiratory and ocular secretions. The presentation of patients varies depending on the severity of infection, systemic involvement, and causative infectious agent (Table 11.6). In addition, several signs will be noticed on examination including eyelid edema, lymphadenopathy, follicles (prominent), and in severe cases conjunctival membranes and scarring. Nevertheless, inflammation is not necessarily limited to conjunctiva and may extend to cause keratitis or anterior uveitis in severe cases.

The diagnosis of viral conjunctivitis is usually clinical; however, investigations can be done if the diagnosis is suspicious or refractory for treatment (Table 11.7). Furthermore, the management depends on the speculated causative agent. For instance, adenovirus has no specific drug, and the disease usually self-resolves within 2–3 weeks; meanwhile, herpetic infections of the eye must be treated using topical preparations (acyclovir ointment or ganciclovir gel) or even oral formulations in vulnerable populations (immune-deficient children or severe disease). In the case of molluscum contagiosum, the management will depend on the patient's condition, waiting for self-resolution if immunocompetent or removal of the lesion in immunocompromised. Other management methods include precaution to reduce the risk of transmission, topical steroids, artificial tears, povidone-iodine (decrease infectivity of adenovirus), and compressors.

11.6.2 Bacterial Conjunctivitis

Infection of the conjunctiva via bacterial organisms is considered common but fortunately self-

Table 11.5 Review of conjunctival disease signs

Conjunctival signs	Most common association	Notes
Hyperemia	Nonspecific signs of conjunctival inflammation	–
Hemorrhages	Coxsackie A24 and enterovirus conjunctivitis	–
Chemosis	Hallmark of allergic conjunctivitis	–
Membranes	Sever viral and bacterial infections, Stevens-Johnson syndrome, *Corynebacterium diphtheria* and gonococcus	True membranes might bleed after stripping due to absence of underlying epithelium, in contrast to pseudomembranes which do not
Follicles	Viral conjunctivitis, chlamydial conjunctivitis, and hypersensitivity to topical medications (brimonidine or neomycin, for example)	Lesions resemble rice grains Most apparent at inferior fornix
Papillae	Allergic conjunctivitis, chronic blepharitis, and contact lens wear	Has a vascular core which gives it the appearance of red dots most apparent in the upper lid Classified into micropapillae, macropapillae (<1 mm), and giant papillae (>1 mm)
Cicatrization	Trachoma, chemical injuries, ocular cicatricial pemphigoid, and Stevens-Johnson syndrome	
Lymphadenopathy	The most common cause is viral and chlamydia	The preauricular area is the most commonly affected followed by submandibular nodes

Table 11.6 Viral conjunctivitis and their presentations

Disease	Causative agent	Presentation
Acute follicular conjunctivitis	Adenovirus (different serological variants) The most common form	Itching, redness, watery discharge with mild photophobia unilaterally The contralateral eye may be affected days after May be associated with mild systemic symptoms such as sore throat (mild)
Pharyngoconjunctival fever	Adenovirus (serotypes 3, 4, and 7)	Similar presentation to acute follicular conjunctivitis Sore throat is more noticeable May be associated with keratitis Preauricular lymphadenopathy (90% of cases)
Epidemic keratoconjunctivitis	Adenovirus (serotypes 8, 19, and 37) The most severe form	Photophobia is prominent Associated with membranes formation Associated more with keratitis (80%) and subepithelial opacities
Acute hemorrhagic conjunctivitis	Enterovirus (70), coxsackievirus (A24), and adenovirus (11)	Associated with conjunctival hemorrhage
Herpes simplex virus	Follicular conjunctivitis is more in primary infection	Associated with the presence of skin vesicles Usually unilateral
Molluscum contagiosum	Poxvirus	Presents with irritation and discharge (watery/mucoid) unilaterally Causing chronic follicular conjunctivitis Centrally umbilicated, dome-shaped nodules on examination of eyelid margin

limiting. *Streptococcus pneumoniae*, *Staphylococcus aureus*, *Haemophilus influenzae*, and *Moraxella catarrhalis* are considered among the most common causative agents. However, other less commonly encountered organisms such as *Neisseria gonorrhoeae* and *Chlamydia* must be considered, as missing them may lead to catastrophic consequences.

Table 11.7 Diagnostic tests that can be used in some cases of viral conjunctivitis

Diagnostic test	Findings and notes
Giemsa stain	Adenovirus: mononuclear cells Herpes simplex: multinucleated giant cells
Polymerase chain reaction (PCR)	Nucleic acid amplification Highly sensitive and specific
Viral culture	Highly specific but has many drawbacks such as cost and time
"Point-of-care" immunochromatography	Looking for adenovirus antigens in tears High sensitivity and specificity
Serology	Looking for IgM/IgG titers against adenovirus Rarely used in practice

Patients will present with the general symptoms of conjunctivitis such as redness and discharge with bilateral involvement of the eyes for the most part; eyelid crusting might be noticed upon waking up. Furthermore, in severe cases, systemic symptoms will develop, especially in susceptible individuals (such as children and immunocompromised). On examination, several signs of inflammation may be noticed such as redness, edema, discharge, superficial corneal punctate, and lymphadenopathy, among others, depending on the severity of infection.

The diagnosis is clinical in the majority of cases. Nevertheless, gram staining, special cultures (such as enriched media), and polymerase chain reaction may be used in severe or refractory cases to help in the management.

The management of such cases can vary as most of the cases may resolve spontaneously within days and depending on the speculated causative organism and severity of infection. For most cases, topical antibiotics (ointment, gels, drops), eye irrigation, hand washing, avoiding contact lenses, and home observation are used. In addition, systemic antibiotics along with other specialist advice (especially in pediatrics) may be required in special conditions such as gonococcal, meningococcal, and *Haemophilus influenzae* infections, and when the element of cellulitis is present.

High-Yield Notes

Staphylococcus aureus, *Moraxella lacunata* (especially common in chronic blepharoconjunctivitis), and enteric bacteria are considered the most common organisms in chronic conjunctivitis. Meanwhile, in the acute form, *Staphylococcus aureus* is the most common.

Gonococcal and meningococcal infections may develop peripheral corneal ulcerations that may progress to perforation.

- Topical antibiotics that can be used include chloramphenicol, aminoglycosides, quinolones, macrolides, polymyxin B, fusidic acid, and bacitracin. These are usually used four times/day up to 1 week.
- Treatment of gonococcal and meningococcal infection should be combined with appropriate systemic antibiotics if the risk of systemic involvement is high.
- *Haemophilus influenzae* conjunctivitis should be treated with systemic antibiotics due to the risk of other coexistent infections (such as otitis media).
- The role of topical steroids is not definitive but thought to reduce the risk of scarring in some cases.

11.6.3 Special Cases of Bacterial Conjunctivitis

11.6.3.1 Chlamydia Infection of the Eye

Chlamydial conjunctival infection can be divided into chlamydial inclusion conjunctivitis and trachoma depending on the serotype. Serotypes D–K are responsible for the former, while trachoma is caused by serotypes A, B, Ba, and C.

Adult chlamydial inclusion conjunctivitis is a disease that affects the eye and genital areas (oculo-genital) that transmit through genital secretions (seen more in young, sexually active adults) and to a lesser degree through eye-to-eye spread; it has around 1-week incubation period. In addition, patients will present with several signs and symptoms such as redness, discharge (watery to mucopurulent), and tender lymphadenopathy and can cause chronic follicular conjunctivitis. Furthermore, superficial punctate corneal inflammation is common, while conjunctival scarring and superior corneal pannus are not, and that is why this condition is not vision threatening. Nevertheless, while it is a self-limiting disease, it may progress to chronic stage if not managed.

The PCR test remains the test of choice. However, other tests such as Giemsa stain, direct immunofluorescence, and McCoy culture of the cells, among others, can also be used. The management of this disease should not be delayed once suspected clinically, and empirical treatment with azithromycin and doxycycline is the first choice for patients and their partners, and erythromycin, ciprofloxacin, and amoxicillin are alternatives. In addition to the systemic treatment, topical antibiotics (erythromycin or tetracycline ointments) may be used as adjuvants for faster relief of eye symptoms. Finally, precautions to decrease the risk of transmission and referral for follow-up and retesting should be taken. Comparison between adult inclusion conjunctivitis and the neonatal variant (see below) is shown in Table 11.8.

Trachoma is associated with low socioeconomic status, poverty, and bad hygiene. It is transmitted through fly as a vector but also through eye/nasal discharges. Furthermore, it is considered as the most common cause of irreversible, preventable loss of vision; this can be due to recurrent infections which will result in chronic inflammatory response and blindness as a consequence.

The presentation of trachoma patients depends on the stage they are presenting in either active or cicatricial (Table 11.9).

High-Yield Notes
- In inflammatory trachoma, papillary element is predominant in ages <2 years.
- Follicular conjunctivitis is more severe inferiorly than superiorly, except in trachoma, which is a disease of superior conjunctiva.
- The two stages are not exclusive; there is overlap between them.

Furthermore, the World Health Organization developed a grading system of five components for trachoma as follows: the trachomatous inflammation (follicular) (aka TF), trachomatous inflammation (intense) (aka TI), trachomatous conjunctival scarring (aka TS), trachomatous trichiasis (aka TT), and corneal opacity (CO). Each one has a specific definition.

The diagnosis is usually based on clinical suspicion with other diagnostic modalities of adult inclusion conjunctivitis such as dipstick enzyme immunoassay. Once the diagnosis is suspected or confirmed, the management will be according to the **SAFE strategy**.

In the **SAFE strategy**, trachoma is managed using **S**urgery (to relieve trichiasis and entropion), **A**ntibiotics (to patients and their families with azithromycin being the drug of choice; erythromycin and doxycycline can be used as alternatives), **F**acial cleanliness (a crucial preventive measure), and **E**nvironmental improvement (including good hygiene and sanitation).

11.6.3.2 Neonatal Conjunctivitis

Ophthalmia neonatorum, which is conjunctival inflammation during the first month of life, is considered the most common neonatal infection.

Table 11.8 Differences between adult and neonatal types of inclusion conjunctivitis

	Neonatal inclusion conjunctivitis	Adult inclusion conjunctivitis
Severity	More severe	Less severe
Discharge	More	Less
Inclusion bodies on histology	More	Less
Follicular response	Less	More
Membranes or pseudomembranes	Can present	Rare

Table 11.9 The characteristics of trachoma inflammatory and cicatricial stages

	Active (inflammatory) trachoma	Cicatricial (chronic) stage
Age	Preschool children	Middle age
Reaction	Mixed follicular papillary with mucopurulent discharge	The entire conjunctiva is affected, most notable on the upper tarsal plate
Others	Superior epithelial corneal inflammation (keratitis) Pannus formation	Healed limbal follicles turning into shallow depressions (Herbert pits) Broad confluent scars (Arlt line) Severe corneal opacification Trichiasis, distichiasis Corneal vascularization Cicatricial entropion

Table 11.10 Etiologies of neonatal conjunctivitis, associated organisms, and presentations

Cause	Possible associated organisms	Notes
Transmission during delivery	*Chlamydia trachomatis*	– Within 1st–3rd weeks – May present with systemic features such as pneumonitis and otitis media – Associated with mucopurulent discharge and pseudomembranes
	Neisseria gonorrhea	– During the first week – Associated with hyperpurulent discharge – May cause severe eyelid edema
	Herpes simplex virus (mostly HSV-2)	– Within 1st–2nd weeks – May be associated with the appearance of skin vesicles or encephalopathy
Other organisms (mostly at the end of the first week and associated with purulent discharge)	Staphylococci	More with mild cases
	Streptococci	
	H. influenzae	
	Several Gram-negative organisms	
Chemical conjunctivitis	Due to the use of topical agents	– Occurs within the first day – Associated with watery discharge

It may be associated with systematic manifestations in severe cases and frequently acquired during delivery (Table 11.10). In addition, several risk factors have been implicated in its development including maternal infections, microorganisms that present in birth canal, ocular trauma, and inadequate ocular prophylaxis. The diagnosis will depend on history, examination, as well as investigations.

The specific diagnosis of the cause will depend on the clinical presentation along with other laboratory tests. For instance, the results of sexually transmitted illnesses may reveal a specific pathogen, and the results of polymerized chain reaction (PCR) might reveal chlamydia, HSV, or gonococcal infections. Furthermore, several stains and cultures could be used (Table 11.11).

In light of above, prophylaxis of this disease is frequently done; several agents can be used such as povidone-iodine solution or erythromycin and tetracycline ointments. In addition, silver nitrate solution can be used in gonococcal endemic areas as adjunct.

High-Yield Notes

Povidone-iodine is considered one of the safest antiseptics with the lowest risk of conjunctival and corneal toxicities.

The treatment of such conditions will largely depend on the cause. In the case of chemical conjunctivitis, for example, artificial tears are sufficient. However, topical antibiotics (broad spectrum) should be used in mild cases, while the addition of systemic antibiotics (such as ceftriax-

Table 11.11 Specific investigations done for some neonatal conjunctivitis-associated organisms and their management

Causative organism	Investigation example	Antibiotics
Chlamydia trachomatis	Polymerized chain reaction (PCR)	Oral erythromycin (2 weeks) Erythromycin/tetracycline ointment adjunctly
Neisseria gonorrhoeae	PCR Chocolate agar or Thayer–Martin cultures	Third-generation cephalosporins Adjunct topical antibiotics can be used Adding drug to cover chlamydia can be done
HSV	PCR Gram stain (reveals multinucleated giant cells) Papanicolaou smear (reveals eosinophilic intranuclear inclusions) Viral cultures (from scraped tissue of vesicular fluid)	High-dose acyclovir (intravenous) Topical acyclovir may be used adjunctly

one) in moderate and severe cases as well as admission to hospital if needed, until specific sensitivities are revealed, and drugs are changed accordingly.

11.6.4 Parinaud Oculo-Glandular Syndrome

This rare disease is assumed to develop following infection via several pathogens of which *Bartonella henselae* (causing cat scratch disease) is the most common. It has been, also, linked to tularemia, sporotrichosis, tuberculosis, rickettsia, and acute *C. trachomatis* infections, among others. The patients will manifest with unilateral caseating granulomatous, follicular conjunctivitis, ipsilateral lymphadenopathy (preauricular), and low-grade fever. The management of this condition depends on the underlying cause.

11.7 Allergic Conjunctivitis

Allergic conjunctivitis, along with hay fever, asthma, and eczema, is considered part of atopy, which is the susceptibility to hypersensitivity reactions due to exposure to certain antigens. The reaction develops due to degranulation of mast cells following exposure to IgE (type 1, immediate hypersensitivity reaction) as a local reaction or part of more systemic one. In addition, it is usually associated with nonspecific papillary response.

11.7.1 Acute Allergic Conjunctivitis

This is a frequently seen condition that results after exposure to environmental allergens such as pollens. The patients usually present with noticeable chemosis along with itchiness and watery discharge, usually affecting both eyes. The diagnosis is based on the clinical picture, and there is no need for treatment in most cases as it is self-limiting.

High-Yield Notes
Anaphylactoid reaction develops following the use of topical preparations (such as penicillin or anesthetics) and presents rapidly with itching, chemosis, and conjunctival injection.

11.7.2 Seasonal and Perennial Allergic Conjunctivitis

Both of these entities are substantially common, presenting similarly (eye redness, itching, eye/nasal watery discharge, hyperemia, and chemosis of variant degrees). The diagnosis is based solely on presentation in most cases and no need to perform skin tests for specific allergy. Table 11.12 summarizes the differences between the two conditions.

Table 11.12 Comparison between seasonal and perennial allergic conjunctivitis

	Seasonal allergic conjunctivitis	Perennial allergic conjunctivitis
Frequency	More common	Less common, milder
Seasons' predominance	Worse in spring/summer	All around year, worse in autumn
Highly associated allergens	Pollens from tree and grass	Antigens from house dust mites, fungus, and animal dandruffs

The management is largely symptomatic. Patients can use artificial tears, mast cell stabilizers (e.g., cromolyn sodium, nedocromil sodium), antihistamines (e.g., emedastine, epinastine, levocabastine), and nonsteroidal anti-inflammatory drugs (NSAIDs). Drops that have combined mechanism of action are available; for example, azelastine and ketotifen work as both antihistamine and mast cell stabilizers.

11.7.3 Giant Papillary Conjunctivitis

This condition results when papillary conjunctivitis, that resulted from mechanical injury, exacerbates and results in the emergence of giant papillae on the tarsal conjunctiva. Several mechanisms are speculated by which mechanical injury develops including those associated with contact lens (most encountered, especially soft type), ocular prosthesis, and surgical sutures, among others.

The patients will present with several symptoms such as redness, itchiness, mucoid discharge, blurry vision, and foreign body sensation; these symptoms may increase when contact lens is removed. Furthermore, on examination, contact lens hypermobility and deposits, along with superior tarsal papillae, can be seen. Focal ulceration with white scarring area (on large papillae) and ptosis may develop.

The management largely depends on the removal of the offensive agents such as contact lens (discontinued and then replaced), sutures, and filtering bleb (partial removal), changing the type of the used lenses or prosthesis, along with changing the used preservatives and solutions and making sure of proper and adequate cleaning techniques. In addition, topical medications such as antihistamines and mast cell stabilizers (non-preserved type when used in patients wearing soft contact lenses) can be used as adjunct.

Mucous fissuring syndrome, in which mucus that results from other diseases is manually removed frequently, and vernal and atopic keratoconjunctivitis (see below) are other causes of giant papillary conjunctivitis.

11.7.4 Vernal Keratoconjunctivitis (VKC) and Atopic Keratoconjunctivitis (AKC)

These entities are considered as more severe forms of allergic conjunctivitis (Table 11.13).

High-Yield Notes

- Both VKC and AKC are bilateral conditions in which the diagnosis is based more on the clinical picture and investigations are not generally necessary.
- Horner–Trantas dots refer to a cluster of eosinophils and calcified degeneration at the limbus area.
- Retinal detachment is seen more in patients with AKC than with normal population.

The management of both conditions is similar to a large degree. Nevertheless, AKC is more severe and refractory and requires treatment for longer period. In general, precautious and supportive measures such as allergen avoidance, cold compressors, and eyelid hygiene should be used. In addition, further treatment can be divided into topical, systemic, and surgical treatment.

Topical medications include mast cell stabilizers, topical antihistamines, combined formulations (antihistamine with vasoconstrictors), NSAIDs, topical steroids (short but intensive regimen, for cases with severe conjunctivitis and

Table 11.13 Characteristics of vernal keratoconjunctivitis (VKC) and atopic keratoconjunctivitis (AKC)

	Vernal keratoconjunctivitis	Atopic keratoconjunctivitis
Age and gender	Young (starting around 5 years), mainly boys	Adult (30–50 years), no gender predilection
Associations	– Other atopic conditions – Seasonal, more noticed, and worse in late spring and summer	– Atopic conditions (especially eczema) are very common in those patients or in patients who had VKC in childhood – Often perennial and worse during winter
Conjunctival scraping	Eosinophils are more numerous	Eosinophils are less numerous
Conjunctival involvement	– Worse superiorly – Mucoid discharge – Papillae are larger – Horner–Trantas dots	– Inferior predilection – Watery discharge – Papillae are smaller – Cicatricial changes
Keratopathy	– Punctate epithelial erosions – Epithelial macro-erosions – Plaques and shield ulcers – Subepithelial scars – Pseudo-gerontoxon – Keratoconus/corneal ectasia	– Punctate epithelial erosions – Epithelial defects that may progress to perforation and descemetocele – Peripheral vascularization and stromal scarring – Vulnerability to secondary infections (fungal/bacterial/herpes simplex keratitis)
Eyelid disease	– Milder and less prominent	– Several skin changes such as dryness, erythema, scaliness, fissuring, among others – Hertoghe sign – Dennie–Morgan folds
Cataract		– Presenile, anterior/posterior cataracts are common; may be aggravated by long steroid therapy – Managed through surgery, which may increase the risk of endophthalmitis and retinal detachment
Natural history	Majority will have remission later; but some will progress to AKC	Low probability of remission

noticeable keratopathy), steroid ointment (applied on eyelids in AKC), topical antibiotics (for significant keratopathy), and mucolytics (acetylcysteine, in cases of VKC with mucoid discharge). Furthermore, topical preparation of immune modulators can be used; for instance, ciclosporin is used in cases refractory to or when steroids should be avoided. In addition, tacrolimus ointment can be used in severe eyelid involvement in AKC.

In regard to systemic management, oral antihistamines, antibiotics (doxycycline or azithromycin), and immunosuppressive agents (steroids, ciclosporin, tacrolimus, azathioprine, in refractory cases of AKC) should be considered according to the response of the patient.

Surgical procedures such as superficial keratectomy, surface maintenance/restoration surgery, or eyelid procedures are considered last resorts for refractory cases such as persistent ulceration or removal of plaques and shield ulcers, among others.

11.8 Immune-Mediated Conjunctivitis

11.8.1 Ocular Cicatricial Pemphigoid (Conjunctivitis Associated with Mucous Membrane Pemphigoid)

This is an autoimmune disease that results from type 2 hypersensitivity reaction against the basement membrane antigens. The type ocular cicatricial pemphigoid (OCP) has predilection toward the ocular membranes including the conjunctiva and will result in catastrophic consequences such as cicatrization. It is mainly diagnosed through immunohistofluorescence.

In contrast to other conjunctival diseases, systemic treatment is the cornerstone for the management of this condition. Dapsone is the drug of choice for mild/moderate cases and can be replaced by sulfasalazine if not well tolerated. Nevertheless, if dapsone is not suitable or effective for any cause, it can be replaced or used in adjunct with other antimetabolite drugs such as azathioprine and methotrexate, while cyclophosphamide is kept as a last resort for severe/refractory situations. Other systemic measures include steroids (prednisolone, for acute settings) and possible use of intravenous immunoglobulins with rituximab.

Local measures are of importance to be used along with the systemic treatment and include the use of artificial tears, topical immunosuppressants (steroid, tacrolimus, ciclosporin), lid hygiene, and other measures (antibiotics, retinoic acid (decreased keratinization), subconjunctival injections of mitomycin C, and contact lens) that can be used according to the specific presentation.

Finally, the role of surgery varies according to the case but must be considered once the disease is controlled. Surgical procedures include cataract surgery, limbal stem cell transfer, mucous membrane autografting, lateral tarsorrhaphy, keratoplasty, and keratoprosthetics, among others.

High-Yield Notes

In addition to OCP, other causes of cicatrization include Stevens-Johnson syndrome (see below), trachoma, trauma, and chemical injury, among others. Nevertheless, conjunctival pemphigoid is the most frequently encountered cause.

11.8.2 Stevens-Johnson Syndrome (SJS) and Toxic Epidermal Necrolysis (TEN or Lyell Syndrome)

SJS and TEN (the more severe form of SJS) are diseases that are speculated to result from delayed type 4 hypersensitivity reaction that develop following the use of some drugs most of the time but can also arise following infection with certain organisms (such as *Mycoplasma pneumoniae*).

The management of this disease largely depends on identifying and stopping the offending agents whether a drug or infection, along with supportive management with hydration, electrolytes, and nutrition control which is of high importance. In addition, prophylaxis with antibiotics may be considered. The use of steroids and immunosuppressive medications is debatable.

The management of the ocular features depends mostly on the presenting phase (acute or late) as well as the complications that developed. For instance, during the acute phase, topical lubricants, topical cycloplegics, corneal protection (via contact lenses or moisture chambers, for example), handling of symblepharon (lysis of already developing or scleral ring for prevention), and treating infection if present, among others, can be done according to the situation. Meanwhile, during later chronic stage, other methods can be done along with adequate lubrication such as the use of topical trans-retinoic acid (reverse keratinization), grafting of mucous membranes, and other different measures aiding in corneal recovery (such as lamellar corneal grafting, limbal stem cell transplantation, keratoprosthesis). Table 11.14 summarizes the characteristics of OCP and SJS.

High-Yield Notes

- The diagnosis of these blistering disorders is usually clinical, but supporting evidence can be found in biopsy results.
- Dry eye can develop due to destruction and occlusion of lacrimal ducts and goblet cells.
- Watery eye can develop because of lacrimal puncta fibrosis.
- In OCP, immunohistofluorescence can be done for diagnosis using a solution (such as Michel fixative; it does not fix the sample); the results will show immunoglobulins and complements attached to epithelial basement membrane.
- Various precipitating factors are speculated to develop SJS/TEN, including drugs (sulfonamides, trimethoprim, Dilantin, acetamino-

Table 11.14 Characteristics of conjunctivitis associated with blistering mucocutaneous diseases

	Mucous membrane pemphigoid	Stevens-Johnson syndrome
Hypersensitivity reaction	Type 2	Type 4
Specific predilections	Older ages, more in females	Adults
Systemic features	– Mucosal and skin lesions – Subepidermal blisters on mucosal surfaces, oral one mostly – Strictures in the esophagus and larynx – Tense blisters and erosions on the skin of the head, extremities, and groin areas	– Symptoms of mucosal involvement and general, flu-like symptoms that vary according to severity such as nasal pain/discharge, pain with eating, and shortness of breath, among others – Skin lesions, which vary in presentation (purpuric, hemorrhagic, etc.) – Sloughing of wide area of skin may occur
Conjunctival findings	– Papillary conjunctivitis with accompanying edema and hyperemia – Fine subconjunctival fibrosis along with inferior fornix shortening – Symblepharon formation – Plica flattening – Caruncle keratinization – If severe enough, necrosis may ensue	– Papillary conjunctivitis of various intensity; membrane and pseudomembrane development along with the accompanying hyperemia, hemorrhages, and blisters (acute) – Cicatrization (late) – Forniceal shortening and symblepharon (late) – Keratinization and plaque development (late)
Eyelid findings	– Trichiasis – Chronic blepharitis – Ankyloblepharon	– Lid margins' hemorrhagic crusting (acute) – Cicatricial entropion and ectropion (late) – Trichiasis and metaplastic lashes (late) – Ankyloblepharon (late)
Corneal findings	– Dryness – Infiltration – Peripheral vascularization – Keratinization of conjunctiva – Conjunctivalization of the cornea – Corneal opacification	– Varies from small erosions to large defects and even perforation – Bacterial keratitis (acute) – Keratinization (late) – Vascularization and scarring (late)

phen, anticonvulsants, among others), infections (*Mycoplasma pneumoniae* and herpes simplex virus), and some cancers.

11.9 Miscellaneous Conjunctivitis

11.9.1 Superior Limbic Keratoconjunctivitis (SLK)

SLK is a chronic disease that can last for years and has a predilection for middle-aged women, especially if they have thyroid dysfunction (most commonly hyperthyroidism). It is assumed to develop due to the trauma (between upper lid and superior bulbar conjunctiva) resulting from recurrent blinking, which is attributed in many cases to decrease tearing and laxity of conjunctiva, and the inflammation that will develop as a consequence. In addition, contact lenses, eye surgery, or previous eye trauma are risk factors.

Patients present with episodes of eye burning, foreign body sensation, and mucoid discharge that are associated with frequent blinking, usually bilateral. On examination, papillary hypertrophy of the superior tarsal plate and of the limbal area, redundant conjunctiva on upper limbal area (on downward pressure), petechial hemorrhages, and hyperemia of the superior bulbar area (radial band, stained positive with rose Bengal) might be seen. Meanwhile, the corneal involvement may include punctate corneal erosions, filamentary keratitis, and mild pannus formation (late), all of which occur superiorly. It is worth mentioning that keratoconjunctivitis sicca will develop in around half of patients.

After performing thyroid function test, and perhaps a biopsy or cytology (looking for keratinization of superior bulbar area), the management will consist of topical lubricants (frequent and regular use), topical acetylcysteine, and mast cell stabilizers. In addition, topical steroids are spared for severe cases, and retinoic acid and topical cyclosporine can be used as an adjunct.

Other measures that can be used include soft contact lens wearing, steroid injections (supratarsal, relieve inflammation), and resection of the superior limbal conjunctiva (refractory cases), among others.

High-Yield Notes
- SLK is a superior conjunctival and limbal disease.
- Management of underlying thyroid disease, if present, usually improves SLK.
- Topical rebamipide has shown promising results.

11.9.2 Ligneous Conjunctivitis

This is a rare, life-threatening disease that affects multiple organs including the respiratory tracts, kidneys, middle ear, and eyes, among others. It occurs most commonly in childhood, and once it affects the eyes, patients will present with bilateral granulomatous conjunctivitis along with pseudomembranes (fibrin rich) on the tarsal area. On examination, enlarging conjunctival mass (lobular shaped, red-white colored, covered by mucoid discharge), along with corneal vascularization, scarring, or infection, can be seen. In addition, patients in whom plasmin-mediated fibrinolysis is affected are at higher risk, and several factors may activate the episodes such as fever, use of antifibrinolytic therapies, or even minor traumas.

Unfortunately, there is a low chance of spontaneous resolution, and the management may not be effective. The management is composed of surgical removal of the lesion (using meticulous diathermy) followed by topical application of heparin and steroids frequently (decrease inflammation until recovery). Furthermore, topical use of ciclosporin and steroids may delay reappearance. Other measures that can be used include plasminogen, amniotic membrane transplantation (after surgery), and prophylactic heparin (before surgery). Pulmonary involvement can result in death in severe cases.

11.10 Congenital Anomalies of the Conjunctiva

11.10.1 Limbal Dermoid

This refers to the appearance of yellow, soft mass that contains dermal elements in subconjunctival area with projecting hair. Most of the time, it arises in the inferior-temporal area of limbus during childhood, and the symptoms depend on the size of the mass. Management of such lesions depends on the symptoms and the size of the mass, with small masses removed by simple excision while larger ones may require lamellar kerato-sclerectomy.

High-Yield Notes
- Limbal dermoids are considered choristoma, that is, the appearance of normal tissue in an abnormal location.
- Limbal dermoid is associated with several systemic syndromes such as Goldenhar syndrome, Treacher Collins syndrome, and linear nevus sebaceus syndrome.

11.10.2 Dermo-Lipoma

It is similar to the limbal dermoid as it is a yellow, soft subconjunctival mass containing a dermoid component, and it may present with hair. However, it is more common in adults, containing fat tissue, and appears, mostly, near the outer canthus area (superior-temporal area, in contrast to limbal dermoid which presents inferotemporally mostly). The management is conservative, and surgical debulking (rather than complete excision) is spared for symptomatic lesions or for cosmetic causes. Dermo-lipoma can also present with systemic syndromes as in limbal dermoids.

11.11 Degenerative Conjunctival Disorder

11.11.1 Pterygium

It is a triangular shape degeneration of bulbar conjunctiva tissue that extends toward the limbus and cornea. It is more commonly bilateral and nasal. It is more noticed in males, and several factors have been implicated in its development including ultraviolet light (the most significant), hot climates, and dryness, among others. Patients present with varying symptoms depending on the size of the lesion and can range from being asymptomatic to nonspecific symptoms such as irritation and inflammatory symptoms to even change in vision and limiting eye movement. On examination, a triangular lesion invading the corneal area will be seen. In addition, stocker line (iron line at the head of the lesion) and Fuchs islets can be seen.

Management depends on the speed and degree of growth; for instance, rapidly growing lesions should be excised. Different procedures can be done such as simple excision (high recurrence rate), autografting of conjunctiva or amniotic membrane, and peripheral lamellar keratoplasty (in case of deep lesions), among others. Meanwhile, medical management role is largely symptomatic such as the use of lubricants and measures to reduce ultraviolet light exposure. It is worth mentioning that the use of topical mitomycin C and beta-radiation (using strontium 90) might reduce the risk of recurrence after autografting; however, it has some serious side effects that may even affect the vision.

11.11.2 Pinguecula

It is a common disease that also results from the degeneration of conjunctiva, leading to the appearance (growth) of yellow or white collections adjacent to the limbus (also bilateral, more on the nasal side); the etiology is similar to pterygium; however, it does not cross the limbus to cornea (does not invade Bowman's membrane). Most patients present asymptomatically. Nevertheless, inflammation can develop or in some cases it may progress to become a pterygium. The diagnosis is clinical, and the mainstay of management is symptomatic such as topical lubricants. In contrast to pterygium, surgeries play no role in most cases unless for cosmetic reasons or disturbing symptoms with negligible recurrence rate.

11.11.3 Conjunctivochalasis

Conjunctivochalasis occurs when part of the conjunctiva becomes redundant as a result of the aging process; it appears to develop more in patients with eye dryness and inflammation. The redundant conjunctiva will prolapse over the lower lid margin. Most patients describe general symptoms such as tearing, discomfort, or foreign body sensation. The diagnosis is clinical, and the management is symptomatic. In mild cases, topical medications such as lubricants, antihistamines, or steroids can be used, while in more severe and refractory cases, surgical resection can be done.

High-Yield Notes

- Elastotic degeneration in pterygium and pinguecula is considered the most specific histological finding and can be seen through stains such as Verhoeff–van Gieson. It tends to have diffuse and patchy pattern in pterygium and a nodular pattern in pinguecula.
- Pterygium and pinguecula are considered benign lesions with no risk of malignant transformation.
- Trauma, corneal ulcers, cicatrizing conjunctivitis, and other diseases can result in the development of pseudo-pterygium. It can be discriminated from true ones by its location and attachment degree to the cornea (usually firm at its apex).

11.12 Conjunctival Tumors

11.12.1 Benign Tumors

11.12.1.1 Conjunctival Nevus

This is a benign disease that arises from the conjunctival melanocytes. It is considered the most common tumor to arise from these cells. The nevus develops around 1st–2nd decades and is mostly asymptomatic; it can be inflamed in some cases. On examination, a lesion of variable size and pigmentation will be noticed, mostly close to the limbus.

Since these lesions have a low risk of malignant transformation, the management can be based on a routine follow-up. However, excision should be done once signs of malignant transformation are encountered or sometimes for cosmetic reasons.

High-Yield Notes

- Conjunctival nevi are divided into compound, subepithelial, and junctional based on the location histologically.
- Amelanotic nevus characterized by absence of pigmentation is quite common.
- Signs of malignant transformation include change in size or pigmentation, appearance at older ages, and uncommon locations (such as fornix and caruncle), among others.

11.12.1.2 Conjunctival Papilloma

These lesions resemble a proliferation of squamous epithelium. They are more commonly present in young adults, which can be attributed to the strong association with human papillomavirus (especially, serotypes 6 and 11). Most of the time, they arise in the juxta-limbal, fornix, or caruncle areas.

Conjunctival papilloma can be further characterized according to the affected patient age group. For instance, serotypes 16 and 18 affect adults more and mostly present juxta-limbal. It has the potential to become malignant. In contrast, serotypes 6 and 11 present more in pediatric age groups, affecting the caruncle area mostly, and are of benign nature. It can be classified according to the gross histology into sessile and pedunculated lesions.

Patients present asymptomatically. However, if the lesion is large, it can cause symptoms such as irritation. Reassurances along with observation are the mainstay of treatment as they may regress spontaneously. For larger or worrying lesions, excision or cryotherapy can be done.

11.12.1.3 Benign Melanosis

In this condition, several flat, brown pigmented patches start to develop early in life (first years), affecting bilateral eyes in asymmetrical fashion (more juxta-limbal). It is seen more in darker-skinned people and is speculated to play a protective role against neoplasia.

High-Yield Notes

In contrast to malignancies, benign melanosis is characterized by normal melanocyte number. Melanosis also tends to increase in size as the patient gets older.

11.12.2 Malignant Tumors

11.12.2.1 Primary Acquired Melanosis (PAM)

In this condition, golden-yellow to darker chocolate brown, irregular, flat areas of pigmentation appear on the conjunctiva, mostly unilateral and involving the limbal and bulbar areas. It is associated with female gender and white populations in the middle age or older. It arises due to melanocyte hyperplasia, abnormal increase in meaning production, or both; this is in contrast to benign melanosis. Furthermore, it can be classified according to the degree of atypia, with more atypia increasing the risk of malignancy transformation.

Careful observation along with biopsies (for histological and immunohistochemical analysis) is done for this condition. In addition, excision of the lesions or cryotherapy along with follow-up can be done in cases with high risk or containing large lesions.

High-Yield Notes

- Change of lesions from flat to more nodular appearance (nodular thickening) and the involvement of more than two clock hours should raise the suspicion of malignant potential.
- Pagetoid spread is considered the most important predictor for progression to melanoma.
- Causes of secondary acquired melanosis of the conjunctiva include pregnancy, radiation, Addison disease, and topical epinephrine drops.

11.12.2.2 Conjunctival Melanoma

Melanoma is considered a rare condition in the eye. It develops in older ages (sixth decade) with high risk of metastasis (mainly to lymph nodes, lungs, brain) and mortality rate (although with better prognosis than cutaneous melanoma). It originates from already existing PAM (most commonly) and nevi or can arise fresh (de novo). Patients mostly present with newly developed painless lesion, most commonly on the bulbar conjunctiva.

The diagnosis depends on ocular exam (including slit lamp and fundus exam, ultrasonography, etc.), histological findings, and looking if the lesion has metastasized. The management of conjunctival melanoma is done through surgical excision with wide safety margin as a cornerstone. In addition, other adjunct therapies, such as radiotherapy, cryotherapy, and vemurafenib (in metastatic cases), can be done, along with observation and follow-up for recurrence.

Factors associated with worse prognosis in melanoma include location (palpebral worse than bulbar, for example), pagetoid spread, and thickness of more than 2 mm.

11.12.2.3 Conjunctival Lymphoma and Lymphoproliferative Lesions

This entity includes several conditions with reactive lymphoid hyperplasia being the most common. However, special attention should be given to conjunctival lymphoma due to the risk behind it. It can develop newly (de novo), as extension from orbital lymphoma, or as part of systemic one. Lymphoma presents frequently as a painless, salmon-colored pathology on the bulbar area. However, reactive lymphoid cells and amelanotic nevi could also present with a salmon-colored lesion.

Biopsies are the mainstay of diagnosis (done bilaterally). Other investigations should be done according to the case (looking for systemic involvement, more common if affected bilaterally). The management is largely variant and formulated according to each case, with several measures and medications under consideration such as excision, radiotherapy, chemotherapy, cryotherapy, and systemic treatment, among others. As conjunctival lymphoma can be the presentation of another underlying systemic disease, patients should be evaluated by the oncologist.

Conflict of Interest None.

References

AlRyalat SAS (2022) Eye yield ophthalmology basics for board and FRCS part 1 exams

Basic Clinical Science Course (BCSC) of the American Academy of Ophthalmology. Section 8: External disease and cornea. 2021–2022

Bowling B (2015) Kanski's clinical ophthalmology, 8th edn. W B Saunders

Kaiser, Peter K., Neil J. Friedman, Pineda II PK. The Massachusetts eye and ear infirmary illustrated manual of ophthalmology E-book. Elsevier Health Sciences, 2014.

Tagg NT, Kardon RH (2010) Scleritis. In: Ocular disease: mechanisms and management expert consult. Elsevier, pp 642–653. https://doi.org/10.1016/B978-0-7020-2983-7.00082-6

Watson PG, Young RD (2004) Scleral structure, organisation and disease. A review. Exp Eye Res 78(3):609–623. https://doi.org/10.1016/s0014-4835(03)00212-4

Yanoff, Myron, Jay S. Duker (2008) Ophthalmology E. Elsevier Health Sciences.

Clinical Review of Orbit and Lacrimal System: Part I

12

Osama H. Ababneh, Rhoda Hijazi, Lna Malkawi, and Saif Aldeen Alryalat

Abstract

This chapter provides an overview of orbital diseases, highlighting the orbit's role in housing the eye and its appendages. It covers common conditions like thyroid eye disease and inflammatory disorders, detailing their clinical presentations, diagnostics, and management strategies. The chapter also examines cystic and vascular lesions, neural tumors, and implications of trauma and infection, emphasizing effective emergency treatment protocols. In the neoplasm section, both benign and malignant tumors are analyzed, along with their pathophysiology and modern management approaches. Surgical interventions such as evisceration, enucleation, and exenteration are discussed, including indications and complications. Finally, the chapter emphasizes the importance of imaging modalities in diagnosing and managing orbital conditions.

Keywords

Orbit · Orbital diseases · Trauma · Infection · Tumors

12.1 Overview

The orbit and lacrimal systems are integral components of the ophthalmological domain; their complex anatomy and vast array of pathologies present unique challenges to even the seasoned clinician. This chapter is designed to provide an in-depth understanding of these areas, thereby equipping readers with the knowledge and skills needed to navigate this complex landscape.

A thorough understanding of the orbit is crucial, given its role as the housing structure for the eye and its appendages. Pathologies within this small anatomical space often have far-reaching consequences, affecting vision and other ocular functions. We delve into the various aspects of orbital diseases, starting with the most common,

O. H. Ababneh (✉)
Department of Ophthalmology, The University of Jordan, Amman, Jordan

R. Hijazi
Sam Houston State University, College of Osteopathic Medicine, Huntsville, TX, USA
e-mail: rxh086@SHSU.EDU

L. Malkawi
Department of Radiology, The University of Jordan, Amman, Jordan

Department of Radiology, University of Colorado Anschutz Medical Campus, Aurora, CO, USA

S. A. Alryalat
Department of Ophthalmology, The University of Jordan, Amman, Jordan

The University of Colorado Anschutz Medical Campus, CO, USA

S. A. Alryalat (ed.), *Ophthalmology Board and FRCS Part 2 Exams*,
https://doi.org/10.1007/978-981-96-1517-9_12

such as thyroid eye disease and inflammatory conditions. We explore the clinical presentations, diagnostic criteria, and latest management strategies that are pivotal in modern ophthalmological practice. This chapter also investigates the diverse array of cystic and vascular lesions that can present within the orbit, along with a detailed study of neural tumors. These conditions, though less common, demand a high level of clinical acumen for timely diagnosis and effective management. The section on trauma and infection offers an understanding of the immediate and long-term implications of these conditions and highlights effective treatment protocols, which are invaluable in an emergency clinical setting.

In the section dedicated to neoplasms, we emphasize both benign and malignant tumors, dissecting their pathophysiology, clinical implications, and state-of-the-art management strategies currently employed. Furthermore, we delve into surgical interventions such as evisceration, enucleation, and exenteration, discussing their indications, procedures, complications. As we explore the orbit's labyrinth, it becomes evident that understanding the imaging modalities used to visualize these structures is paramount. In the Imaging Revision section, we revisit various imaging techniques, emphasizing their interpretation and effective utilization in diagnosis and management.

The forthcoming section on the lacrimal system will provide a comprehensive understanding of the anatomy, physiology, pathological conditions, and management strategies associated with this critical system. As tears play a crucial role in maintaining ocular health, understanding the lacrimal system's functioning and potential issues is essential for effective clinical practice.

By the end of this chapter, readers will have a comprehensive understanding of the complex and diverse pathologies that can affect the orbit and lacrimal system. This knowledge will undoubtedly serve as an indispensable tool in preparing for the Ophthalmology Board and FRCS Part 2 Exams, and, more importantly, it will prove invaluable in day-to-day clinical practice.

Before digging deeper into the chapter, here are some terminologies related to orbital conditions that you need to understand:

- Proptosis: Forward protrusion of the globe
- Exophthalmos: Proptosis specific to thyroid eye disease
- Dystopia: Vertical displacement of the globe in the coronal plane
- Enophthalmos: Retrodisplacement of the globe back into the orbit

Terminologies related to orbital tissue and tumor classifications:

- Choristoma: Normal tissue located at an abnormal site, derived from one or two embryonic germ layers.
- Teratoma: Normal tissue in an abnormal location, formed from all three embryonic germ layers.
- Hamartoma: Overgrowth or increased growth rate of tissue, with one element predominating, for example, a hemangioma.
- Dermoid: A cyst that contains dermal appendages (pilosebaceous units) lined with keratinized squamous epithelium.
- Epidermoid: A cyst wall that does not have adnexal structures.

References used in this chapter include the following (Allen 2014; Ali 2018; AlRyalat 2021; American Academy of Ophthalmology n.d.; Denniston and Murray 2014; Hollsten 1992; Kanski 2019; Nagendran et al. 2020; Ababneh et al. 2015; Al-Ryalat et al. 2016; Rose and Wright 1992; Salmon, 2019; Shields et al. 2004; Wright et al. 1992; Ababneh and Msallam 2014; Bartalena et al. 2021; Dickinson and Perros 2001; Dolman 2018; Mourits et al. 1997).

12.2 Thyroid Eye Disease (TED)

It is also known as Graves' ophthalmopathy or thyroid-associated orbitopathy.

Etiology: Autoimmune mediated (not hormonal). Due to similar antigenicity between orbital tissue (namely orbital fibroblasts) and thyroid tissue, the antibodies attacking the thyroid also attack the orbit. These antibodies include thyroid-stimulating hormone antibodies (anti-TSH) as the most common, thyroglobulin antibodies, and thyroperoxidase antibodies.

TED is the most common extra-thyroid manifestation of Graves' disease. It can occur in hyper-, eu-, and hypothyroid status, but most commonly with Graves' hyperthyroidism (90% of patients).

Associations: Approximately 5% of patients with myasthenia gravis (MG) have an associated TED, while 1% of thyroid eye disease patients have associated MG, which is considered a common disease association. The most common eyelid feature of TED is lid retraction, whereas ptosis is more typical in ocular MG. Therefore, patients with ocular MG presenting with lid retraction or those with TED presenting with ptosis or **exotropia** should be evaluated for the possibility of having both disorders.

Cigarette smoking is the strongest modifiable risk factor for TED with an odds ratio of 7.7 among smokers compared to nonsmokers. The risk increases proportionally with the number of cigarettes smoked daily.

TED is 5–8X more common in females.

It is characterized by 2–3 years of active inflammation, followed by fibrosis (Rundle curve).

The median age at the time of diagnosis is 43 years, with a range of 8–88 years.

12.2.1 Manifestations

- Upper and lower lid retraction (Fig. 12.1) is the most common clinical feature of TED; it can be unilateral or bilateral and/or asymmetrical (90% of cases).
- Proptosis (60% of cases).
- Exposure keratopathy (Fig. 12.2) and ocular surface disease (injection mostly epibulbar at the site of muscle insertion).

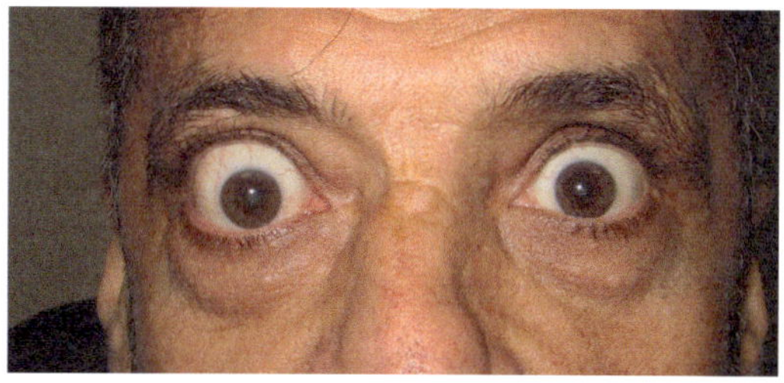

Fig. 12.1 Bilateral, asymmetrical, right more than left upper eyelid retraction in TED patient giving a startled expression

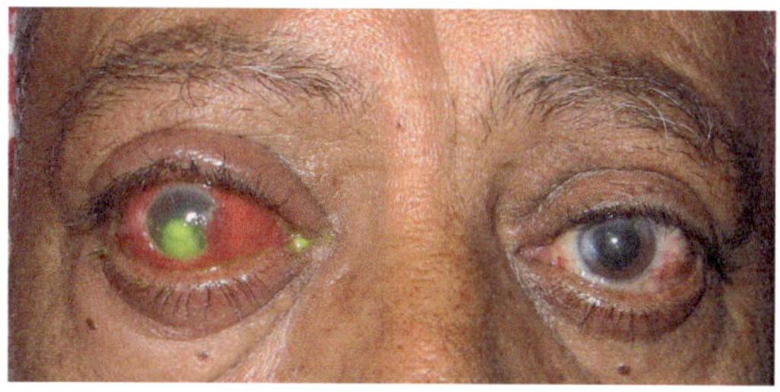

Fig. 12.2 Right Exposure Keratopathy with inferior keratitis and injection in a patient with TED

- Diplopia from restrictive myopathy (40% of cases) initially from inflammation and then from fibrosis (Fig. 12.3), with hypotropia being the most common.
- Optic neuropathy due to compression of optic vessels by swelling muscles (5% of cases). They have a characteristic inferior visual field defect that might be related to superior rectus size.

12.2.2 Signs

Most common eyelid signs are lid retraction, followed by Von Graefe's sign (lid lag), and then lagophthalmos.

Von Graefe's sign (lid Lag) refers to the delayed downward movement of the upper eyelid when the eye moves downward, making it a dynamic sign. In contrast, lid retraction is a static sign and can

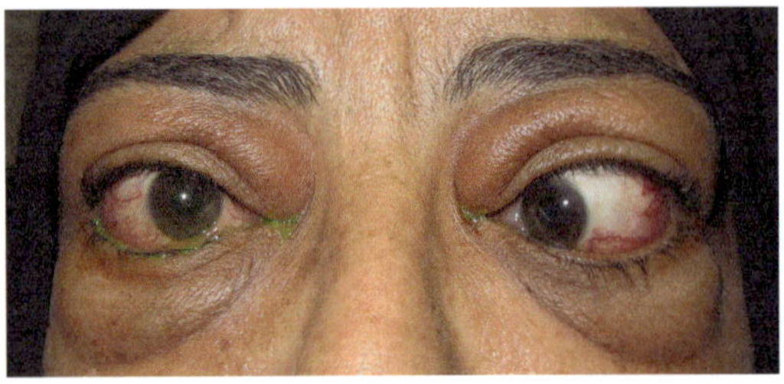

Fig. 12.3 Limitation of extraocular muscle movements with esotropia, diplopia, injection over both lateral recti muscles, bilateral eyelid swelling in a patient with acute TED

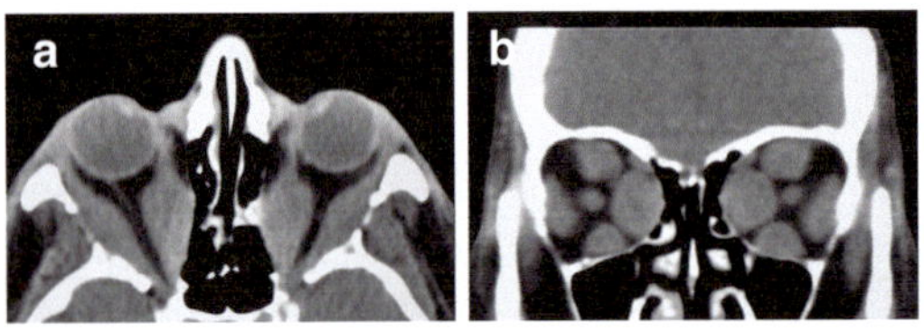

Fig. 12.4 Thyroid eye disease (TED). (**a**) Axial CT scan without contrast of the orbits demonstrates bilateral extraocular muscle hypertrophy with tendon sparing involving medial and lateral rectus muscles. This patient's clinical photograph is provided in Fig. 12.3. The Intraocular lenses in both eyes demonstrates an esotropic apperance. (**b**) A coronal CT image from the same patient exhibits diffuse hypertrophy of the four recti muscles bilaterally with slight involvement of the superior oblique muscles. The enlargement is most pronounced in the medial and inferior rectus muscles bilaterally

also be observed in cases of cicatricial eyelid retraction or congenital ptosis in downgaze.

Extraocular muscles are frequently involved in TED, becoming thickened and fibrotic (Fig. 12.4); this causes restrictive strabismus. The most commonly affected muscle in TED is the inferior rectus, followed in decreasing order by the medial rectus, superior rectus, lateral rectus, and oblique (the mnemonic I aM SLOW). Given this order of frequency with extraocular muscle involvement, TED patients most commonly present with a hypotropia (restricted inferior rectus) or esotropia (restricted medial rectus) or both.

When reviewing radiographic studies (CT or MRI) of the orbit and extraocular muscles, one should look for thickened extraocular muscles **without** involvement of the tendon insertion at the globe. The muscle volume is increased in all extraocular muscles except possibly the inferior oblique. It is also associated with higher fat content on imaging.

Muscle is involved as a fusiform muscle enlargement with sparing of tendons (usually patients older than 40 years of age) and increased fat content (usually patients younger than 40 years of age).

Bell's phenomenon occurs with forced closure of eyelid, where the globe rotates 15 degrees above the horizontal plane. It is absent in 10% and is reduced in thyroid orbitopathy (enlarged inferior rectus muscle).

Of patients with TED, 90% have hyperthyroidism, 6% euthyroid, 3% autoimmune thyroiditis, and 1% primary hypothyroidism.

When assessing thyroid eye disease, we need to assess disease activity, mostly with clinical activity score (CAS) and severity as follows:

12.2.3 Clinical Activity Scales

A clinical activity score (CAS) is obtained by assessing two symptoms (Mourits et al. 1997):

- Orbital ache: periorbital or retro-orbital pain
- Gaze-evoked pain

Five Signs:

- Conjunctival redness: Any redness is graded according to the area affected (trace, <50%, >50%). Dilated vessels over the insertions of these muscles are common and almost pathognomonic.
- Eyelid erythema.
- Eyelid edema: Fullness and skin thickening.
- Chemosis: Differentiated from conjunctivochalasis.
- Swelling of the plica or caruncle: The plica is the fold of conjunctiva lying adjacent to the caruncle.

A score of above 3 (4 and above) is considered indicative of active thyroid, with a positive predictive value (PPV) of over 80% (Dickinson and Perros 2001).

The Bahn-Gorman scale is used to grade diplopia in TED: Grade I represents intermittent diplopia that occurs only when the patient is fatigued; grade II involves inconstant diplopia that is present only on lateral or upward gaze; grade III is characterized by constant diplopia that occurs when looking straight ahead and level gaze, but can be corrected with prisms; and grade IV describes constant diplopia that cannot be corrected by prisms.

12.2.4 Severity Scale (Dolman 2018)

1. Mild TED: This stage has a minor impact on daily life and typically does not warrant immunomodulation or surgical treatment. Patients usually have one or more of the following:
   - Minor lid retraction (<2 mm)
   - Mild involvement of soft tissue
   - Exophthalmos <3 mm above the normal range for race and gender
   - No or intermittent diplopia, with corneal exposure that responds well to lubricants
2. Moderate-to-severe TED: Patients without sight-threatening TED whose eye disease has sufficient impact on daily life to justify the risks of immunosuppression (if active) or surgical intervention (if inactive). They usually have two or more of the following:
   - Lid retraction ≥2 mm
   - Moderate-to-severe involvement of soft tissue
   - Exophthalmos of 3 mm or more above the normal range for race and gender (18–21 mm Caucasians, 21–23 mm African-Americans)
   - Inconstant or constant diplopia
3. Sight-threatening (very severe) TED: This is the most severe form, where patients are at risk of dysthyroid optic neuropathy and/or corneal breakdown.

Eyelid Assessment:

- MRD1 is the distance between the center of the pupil and upper lid margin in primary gaze (normally, the upper lid covers 1-2 mm of the iris, leaving 4-5 mm distance from the margin to reflex (MRD1)).
- MRD2 is the distance between the center of the pupil and lower lid margin in primary gaze (normally, the lower lid at the tip of the iris, leaving 5 mm distance from the margin to reflex (MRD2)).
- Levator function measures the movement of upper lid from down to up (normally >10 mm).

12.2.5 Management

Depends on stage: Patients usually have a stage of active inflammation (2–3 years), followed by a stage of fibrosis.

Depends on grade: Mild in minimal ocular surface disease, severe when visual acuity is affected by optic neuropathy or exposure keratopathy, and moderate in other manifestations.

A. In active inflammation stage:

Mild disease, only lubrication ± low-dose topical steroid, selenium supplements, smoking cessation, salt restriction, head elevation, sunglasses

For moderate and severe (EUGOGO protocol) (Bartalena et al. 2021):

- No compressive optic neuropathy: 60–80 mg oral prednisolone daily OR IV methylprednisolone 0.5 g/week for 6 weeks and then 0.25 g/week for another 6 weeks. Check for liver, kidney functions, and blood pressure.
- With compressive optic neuropathy: 1 g/day methylprednisolone for 3 days and then 40 mg/day oral prednisolone. Consider surgical orbital decompression if no response or cortisone is contraindicated.

  Radiotherapy has a delayed effect and is not superior to steroids, so it is never given alone for optic neuropathy.

  Orbital steroids (peribulbar) have inferior efficacy to systemic but also lower systemic side effects.

Consider immunosuppressive therapy for active disease with 3 or more (7) score in EUGOGO score.

B. In chronic fibrotic stage:

Post-inflammatory complications occurring due to tissue fibrosis, usually surgically managed 6–12 months after subsided inflammation when healing plateau and stable condition. Multiple pathologies usually result, including proptosis, diplopia, and lid retraction. As the surgical management of one pathology affects the others, the surgical order to be followed is conventional orbital decompression followed by strabismus surgery followed by lid surgery. Always follow this order in management. Before undertaking surgical correction, the angle of deviation should be stable for 6 months.

- Proptosis: managed by orbital decompression when the difference between both eyes is >3 mm or bilateral proptosis is >21 mm. Start with the lateral wall (reduce protrusion by 3 mm) and then lateral and medial walls (3–7 mm reduction). Then add an inferior wall (reduce protrusion by 6–10 mm for three walls). Finally, the roof can be removed.
- Diplopia: Only recession of recti, usually the inferior and medial. Aim for no diplopia at primary and reading gaze, rather than all gazes.
- Lid retraction: Levator aponeurosis disinsertion or recession (blepharotomy).

Orbital Decompression

– Lateral orbitotomy: This approach offers the most direct access to the lateral orbit, situated between the optic nerve and the lateral rectus muscle.

Medial wall decompression: The frontoethmoidal suture line marks the boundary between the orbit and the sinuses below and the anterior cranial fossa above. This suture line is the highest point reached on the medial orbital wall during decompression surgery, as it is where the anterior and posterior ethmoidal arteries pass. Orbital floor decompression: To minimize the risk of diplopia and dystopia, surgeons often preserve the inferomedial orbital strut (IOS), which lies between the medial wall and the orbital floor. This strut acts as a support structure, and its preservation helps maintain the integrity of the orbital architecture. The inferomedial orbital strut (IOS) is the thin bony junction of the orbital medial wall and floor. Its fracture is common and leads to serious complications, including enophthalmos, globe dystopia (hypoglobus), and diplopia. Note that you can think of the IOS as the Achilles tendon for the orbit.

Medial incisions such as the transcaruncular, transconjunctival, and medial orbitotomy would lead to the medial orbit.

A transnasal endoscopic approach is particularly beneficial for addressing conditions in the medial orbit. It is frequently employed for the removal of the lamina papyracea during medial orbital wall decompression, especially in cases of thyroid eye disease.

Postoperative care following orbitotomy generally includes the administration of systemic corticosteroids to manage and reduce edema. These steroids, whether given intravenously or orally, are commonly prescribed in the immediate postoperative period to manage edema in the hope of minimizing optic neuropathy. However, it is important to note that there is no conclusive evidence proving the necessity or efficacy of corticosteroids or antibiotics in every orbitotomy case. During extubation, pressure patching can be helpful, but the patch should be removed as soon as the patient is alert enough for a clinical examination. This is crucial to ensure that there is no iatrogenic optic neuropathy and the patient is allowed to monitor their visual function during the postoperative period. Remember that TED-associated lid retraction for upper and lower lid might compromise superior conjunctival trabeculectomy.

Fundus images may depict chorioretinal folds, which can be caused by globe compression from the enlarged extraocular muscles of TED.

Radioactive iodine (RAI) treatment for the thyroid gland might exacerbate TED, so either choose other modalities for treatment (e.g., drugs or surgical) or give steroids before and after radioactive iodine.

Indication for Steroid in TED:

Active inflammation (redness, hotness, swelling, and pain)
Optic nerve compression
Exposure keratopathy
Before radiation treatment

Orbital Radiotherapy: It can be used in patients who cannot tolerate high doses of corticosteroids, but it carries the risk of ocular and retinal complications, mainly exacerbating diabetic retinopathy.

12.2.6 Dysthyroid Optic Neuropathy (DON)

Abnormality with any of the optic nerve functions in TED patients, including visual acuity, color vision, afferent pupillary reflex, and visual field.

Almost 70% of DONs have 20/20 vision, so central normal vision will not exclude DON.

Inferior visual field loss is the most common VF loss in DON.

Older males are more likely to develop DON (unlike TED in general).

Management: Pulse steroid (0.5–1 g IV methylprednisolone) for 3 days and then oral tapering; repeat the regimen after 1 week in mild cases, and consider urgent decompression if no/poor improvement.

12.3 Inflammatory Disease

Idiopathic orbital inflammation is characterized by a pleomorphic cellular infiltrate consisting of lymphocytes, plasma cells, and eosinophils with variable degrees of reactive fibrosis (Table 12.1).

When orbital inflammatory disease is accompanied with cavernous sinus involvement (multiple cranial nerve paresis), then it is called Tolosa-Hunt syndrome.

Systemic steroid is the mainstay management option (Fig. 12.5). Radiotherapy is an effective treatment for acute symptomatic improvement when no adequate response to steroids, and long-term control of orbital pseudotumor.

Idiopathic orbital inflammation (orbital pseudotumor) can affect any ocular structure except cornea (i.e., no keratitis).

Isolated enlargement of a single rectus muscle would be typical of myositis.

12.3.1 Pseudotumor vs. Thyroid Eye Disease Myopathy

In pseudotumor, the muscle and the tendon are involved resulting in painful eye movement.

In thyroid eye disease, tendons are spared, retraction of upper eyelid is seen (appearance of superior limbus), and there is typical involvement of inferior, then medial, and then superior followed by lateral recti muscles (mnemonic: I aM SLOW).

In Tolosa-Hunt syndrome commonly present with painful ophthalmoplegia, the most common cranial nerve affected is the sixth CN. Optic nerve involvement is rare, but might be involved as optic neuritis.

Orbital apex syndrome is similar to superior orbital fissure syndrome in every aspect except that in orbital apex syndrome, the optic nerve is involved, so visual acuity is affected more commonly.

Eye involvement occurs in up to 50% of patients with **granulomatosis with polyangiitis** (formerly known as Wegener granulomatosis). The c-ANCA test has been recognized as the most sensitive and specific diagnostic tool for **granulomatosis with polyangiitis**.

The lacrimal gland is the most common orbital structure affected in sarcoidosis, with the lung being the most commonly involved organ. Extraocular muscles and optic nerve are very rarely affected.

Table 12.1 Comparison between different orbital inflammatory diseases

	Idiopathic orbital inflammatory disease (IOID) (aka orbital pseudotumor)	Orbital myositis	Acute dacryoadenitis	Tolosa–Hunt syndrome	Granulomatosis with polyangiitis (GPA) (formerly known as Wegener granulomatosis)
Pathophysiology	Space-occupying pleomorphic inflammation, cellular infiltration followed by reactive fibrosis	Nonspecific inflammation of one or more extraocular muscles	Idiopathic, viral (e.g., mumps, Epstein–Barr virus, cytomegalovirus), or bacterial	Granulomatous inflammation of the cavernous sinus, superior orbital fissure, and/or orbital apex	Granulomatous idiopathic multisystem inflammation, small-vessel vasculitis, tissue necrosis
Unilaterality	Unilateral (children may be bilateral)	Unilateral	Unilateral	Unilateral	Often bilateral
Symptoms	Mild proptosis, periocular redness, swelling, and pain. Systemic involvement is common in children. Ophthalmoplegia, optic neuropathy	Mild proptosis, acute pain, exacerbated by eye movement, and diplopia. Lid edema, ptosis, and chemosis	Swelling of the lateral aspect of the eyelid leading to S-shaped ptosis. Downward and inward dystopia. Conjunctival injection and chemosis	Periorbital or hemicranial pain, diplopia, with pupillary and eyelid involvement (CN III). Mild proptosis if any (unlike others)	Proptosis, sinus involvement with bone erosions, scleritis, nasolacrimal duct obstruction (inflammatory or bone erosions), ophthalmoplegia
Association	Rare sinus or cranial involvement	Muscle belly involvement with or without tendons	Preauricular lymph node enlargement	The patient may be pyrexial	Spread from the paranasal sinuses or nasopharynx. Glomerulonephritis

Remember that the involvement of multiple cranial nerves (i.e., two or more) and then the pathology are mostly at the cavernous sinus.

Orbital pseudotumor in children generally have higher recurrence rate (almost a third of cases) compared to adults. Pediatrics mostly present bilaterally compared to adults. Pediatrics also have more uveitis, optic disc edema, and eosinophilia.

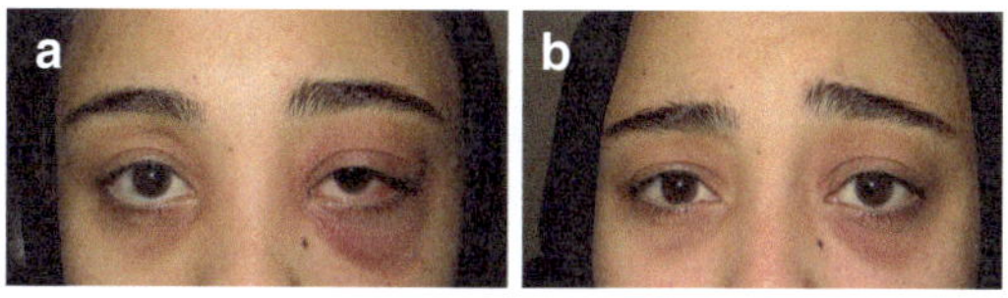

Fig. 12.5 21 years old female with left Idiopathic orbital inflammation (**a**), 3 days after treatment with IV methylprednisolone with significant improvement in eyelid swelling and redness (**b**)

12.4 Cystic Lesions

Various cystic lesions can present in the orbit, as detailed in Table 12.2.

Incomplete dermoid excision or rupture of the capsule may result in recurrence of the cyst with inflammation. Dermoids are lined with squamous epithelium and filled with keratinized material. As dermoids are filled by keratin, rupturing the wall during excision may leak keratin which causes severe granulomatous inflammation and foreign body reaction. Dermoid cysts are often adherent to suture lines, mostly the frontozygomatic suture laterally (Fig. 12.6).

The key difference between a dermoid cyst and an epidermoid cyst lies in the presence of adnexal appendages like hair follicles, sweat glands, and sebaceous glands. A dermoid cyst contains these structures, whereas an epidermoid

Table 12.2 Differential and characteristics of cystic orbital lesions

	Dacryops	Dermoid cyst	Sinus mucocele	Encephalocele
Pathophysiology	Obstructed lacrimal gland duct	Choristoma derived from ectoderm. Lined by keratinized squamous epithelium and surrounded by fibrous capsule. Contains dermal appendages (unlike epidermoid). But not blood vessels, so never bleed	Obstruction of paranasal sinus drainage	A congenital bony defect herniating meninges with or without brain tissue
Unilaterality/site	Frequently bilateral at superior fornix	Unilateral, usually superotemporal, occasionally superonasal	Unilateral, mostly from ethmoidal and frontal sinuses (rare from maxillary)	Unilateral, superomedial in infancy
Symptoms	Cosmetic in adults	Superficial, in infancy, anterior to orbital septum. Deep, in adolescents, posterior to orbital septum. Astigmatism with the flattest meridian adjacent to the dermoid. Proptosis, cosmetic	Proptosis and dystopia Diplopia in adults	Anterior (fronto-ethmoidal) causes lateral dystopia, while posterior (sphenoidal) causes inferior dystopia
Association	No association	Goldenhar syndrome (limbal dermoid). Deep dermoid might cause bony defects. No malignant potential	Bone erosion or thinning on CT scan	Pulsating proptosis present (due to CSF communication), but NO bruit or thrill, large bony defect, neurofibromatosis-1

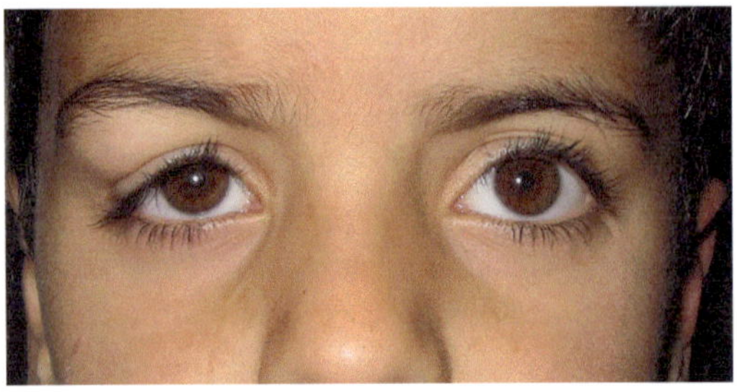

Fig. 12.6 Superior lateral orbital dermoid with lateral ptosis

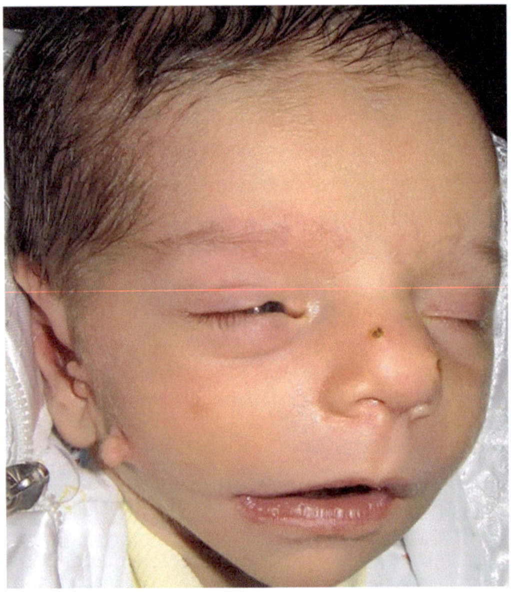

Fig. 12.7 Goldenhar's syndrome with right upperlid medial coloboma, limbal dermoid, facial hypoplasis and preauricular and facial skin tags

cyst is lined with keratinized stratified squamous epithelium, similar to the epidermis, but lacks skin adnexal structures such as hair follicles or glands. Both types of cysts can elicit a mixed inflammatory response if they rupture.

Goldenhar syndrome (oculo-auricular-vertebral spectrum) is a sporadic or autosomal dominant inherited syndrome of the first branchial arch (Fig. 12.7). It consists of a triad: 1- epibulbar dermoids; 2- facial anomalies, including facial hypoplasia, upper eyelid colobomas, preauricular skin tags, and aural fistulas; and 3- skeletal anomalies (hemivertebrae).

12.5 Vascular Abnormalities, Tumors, and Malformations

12.5.1 Vascular Abnormality

12.5.1.1 Carotid-Cavernous-Sinus Fistula (CCF)

When carotid-cavernous fistula occurs, the pressure within the cavernous sinus increases, manifesting as superior ophthalmic vein enlargement (as it drains into the cavernous sinus). This vein will transmit the increased pressure into the orbit. This transmitted pressure appears as cork-screw conjunctival vessels (arterialization of veins).

The classical manifestation includes the triad of pulsatile proptosis, conjunctival chemosis, and whooshing noise in the head (Fig. 12.8).

Complications include the following:

- Increased IOP: The most common cause of visual disability is increased IOP with progressive optic nerve damage (i.e., secondary glaucoma). Unfortunately, this form of secondary glaucoma does not respond well to the traditional medical and surgical therapy and is an indication for neuroradiological intervention.
- Ischemic oculopathy from stagnated blood (arterial and venous) and decreased venous drainage, manifesting as iris and posterior segment neovascularization, corneal edema, aqueous cells, and flare.
- Rapidly progressive cataract.
- Pulsatile proptosis.
- Central retinal vein occlusion.

*As the two cavernous sinuses are interconnected, unilateral fistula can cause contralateral proptosis, so a bilateral proptosis can be due to only one-side fistula.

The presence of ptosis may be helpful in differentiation from acute thyroid eye disease.

Carotid-cavernous fistula can be generally classified as direct or indirect:

- Direct fistula between internal carotid artery and cavernous sinus, where trauma (basal skull fracture) and ruptured intracavernous carotid aneurysm are common etiologies. All signs are stronger here except pulsation.
- Indirect through meningeal arteries, where atherosclerosis is a common etiology. Pulsation can be detected even on slit lamps.

Carotid-cavernous arteriovenous fistulas affecting the orbit frequently occur as a result of a basal skull fracture. The sixth cranial nerve (CN VI) is the most commonly affected nerve in carotid-cavernous fistulas due to its central position within the cavernous sinus. When CT and MRI results are inconclusive or when preparing for treatment, conventional angiography is employed as the diagnostic test for carotid-cavernous fistulas. Posttraumatic direct fistula has the poorest prognosis and is not likely to spontaneously close because of higher blood flow. For indirect fistulas, spontaneous closure occurs in 50% of cases, so mostly require observation (Table 12.3).

Imaging of dural-sinus (indirect) fistula is likely to show diffuse enlargement of the extraocular muscles resulting from venous engorgement and a characteristically enlarged superior ophthalmic vein; arteries are not usually distended due to their strong walls.

Contrast imaging is used to differentiate between the two types of fistula, with most common neuroimaging signs including proptosis, enlargement of the superior ophthalmic veins, and extraocular muscle enlargement.

Cavernous sinus thrombosis: The etiology is mostly posterior spread of infection from the orbit or sinuses. Mortality can reach 100% if untreated and 20% if treated.

Cavernous sinus thrombosis can occur in septic or aseptic individuals. Signs include ipsilateral ophthalmoplegia, rapid progression of proptosis, anesthesia in both the first and second divisions of the trigeminal nerve, and orbital congestion with treatment being antibiotics, anticoagulants, and surgery.

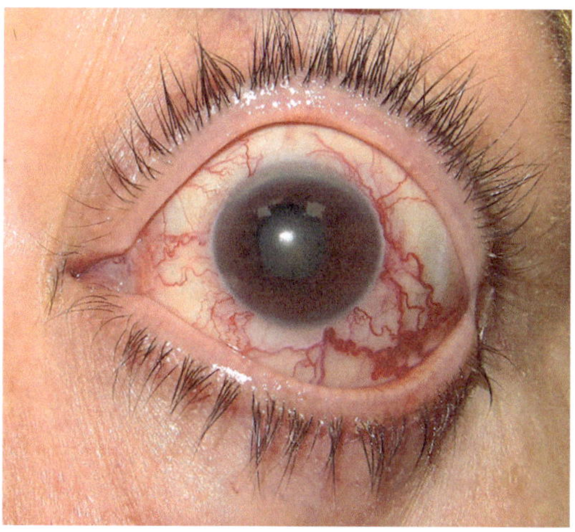

Fig. 12.8 Left carotid cavernous fistula featuring Corkscrew vessels with mild proptosis

12.5.2 Vascular Tumors and Malformations

Capillary hemangioma is the most common tumor of the orbit and periorbital area in childhood, with 5% incidence (Table 12.4) and (Fig. 12.9).

Table 12.3 Comparison between direct and indirect carotid cavernous fistula (CCF)

	Direct CCF (high flow)	Indirect CCF (low flow)
Etiology	Mostly after trauma including basal skull fracture	Mostly spontaneous in old, postmenopausal, hypertensive women presenting with conjunctival injection
Pathophysiology	Connection between the cavernous segment of the internal carotid artery (ICA) and the cavernous sinus	Connection between meningeal branches of the ICA and/or external carotid artery (ECA) and the cavernous sinus
Differentiating signs	Orbital bruits present mostly More sudden and severe signs	Orbital bruits absent mostly Gradual onset and subtle signs
Management	Endovascular repair	Observation

Table 12.4 Differential for vascular tumors in the orbit

	Varices	Lymphangioma	Capillary hemangioma	Cavernous hemangioma
Pathophysiology	Hamartomatous, congenital, or acquired after trauma, weakened segments of the orbital venous system	Hamartomatous Benign vascular malformation	Hamartomatous, endothelial proliferation	Vascular malformation
Unilaterality/site	Unilateral, superonasal	Unilateral, superonasal	Unilateral, superonasal	Unilateral, retrobulbar
Symptoms	Non-pulsatile, intermittent proptosis, visible eyelid lesions, phleboliths 20%	Soft bluish masses, early childhood, proptosis, spontaneous hemorrhage may occur (chocolate cysts) leading to acute presentation (unlike gradual for other vascular ones)	Girls 3X more. Rapid growth phase 3–6 m (oral b-blocker effective here), followed by resolution. 30% resolve by 3 years, 70% by 7 years. Laser if <2 mm thickness	70% in women, middle age Axial proptosis
Association	Eyelid and conjunctival varices, acute hemorrhage, and thrombosis	Not capsulated. Intracranial in addition to eyelid and conjunctival components, oropharynx involvement	PHACE syndrome. Eyelid and conjunctival hemangioma. Visceral hemangiomas Kasabach-Merritt syndrome (blood) Maffucci syndrome (bone)	Well circumscribed, encapsulated, and easy to remove

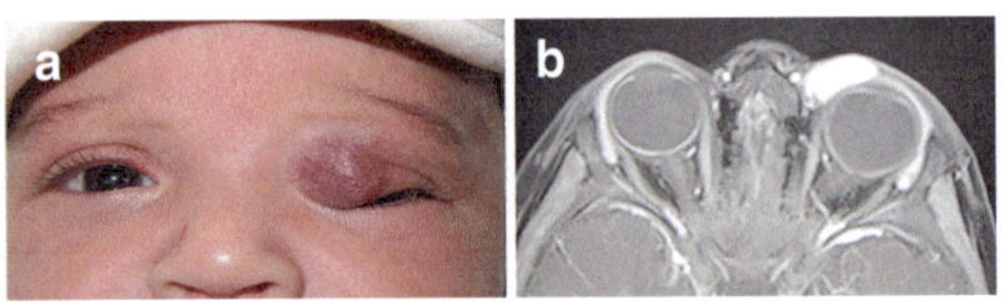

Fig. 12.9 Capillary hemangioma. (**a**) Clinical photograph of an infant demonstrating a capillary hemangioma located at the nasal aspect of the left eyelid, causing obscuration of the visual axis. (**b**) Axial contrast-enhanced T1-weighted orbital MRI of the same patient reveals a homogeneously enhancing extraconal lesion located medially in the left eyelid. There is no evidence of intra-orbital or intracranial involvement

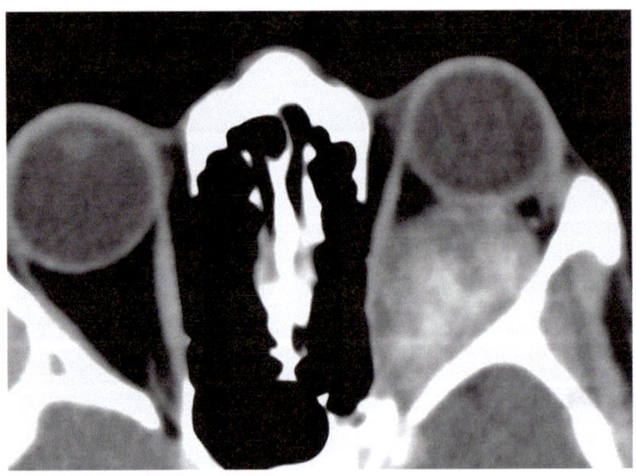

Fig. 12.10 Cavernous hemangioma. Axial contrast-enhanced CT of the orbits demonstrates a sizable intraconal lesion, which shows partial contrast enhancement, with mass effect on the posterior aspect of the eye globe and slight stretching of the extraocular muscles. Not shown in this figure are the delayed contrast images which display complete contrast filling

Cavernous hemangioma is the most common orbital tumor in adults.

Female preponderance is seen in almost all cases.

Majority of vascular tumors are hamartomatous and superonasal (causing dystopia), except cavernous hemangioma, which is vascular malformation within the muscle cone behind the globe causing axial proptosis (Fig. 12.10).

Capillary hemangioma may change in color and size during crying and straining.

Hamartoma is a disorganized overgrowth of mature tissues normally present in the involved area.

Mucocele and encephalocele can erode the bone, while vascular lesions cannot.

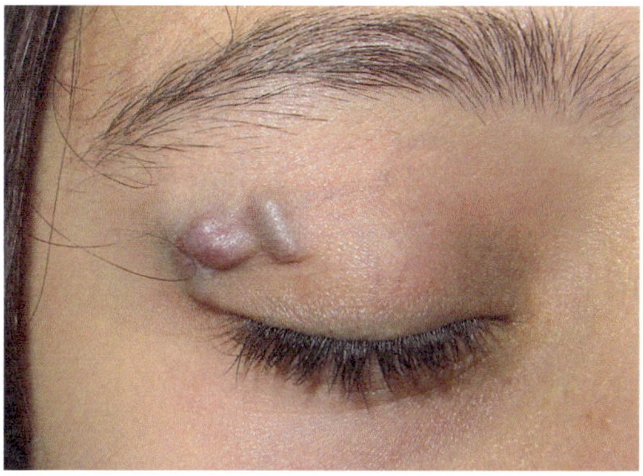

Fig. 12.11 Orbital varix (Reddish-purple, swollen bump) of right upper eyelid

Cavernous hemangioma is the only encapsulated vascular tumor in the orbit, and it does not respond to valsalva (a differentiating sign).

Vascular tumors generally have symptoms accentuated by valsalva and dependent positions, namely orbital varices and capillary hemangioma.

For vision-threatening periocular hemangiomas, oral propranolol is now preferred for the treatment. While topical timolol can be effective for superficial hemangiomas, it is not suitable for orbital lesions. Note that both dermoid and cavernous hemangioma are circumscribed, encapsulated lesions.

Orbital expansion with Valsalva along with phleboliths (small blood clots in a vein) is characteristic of an orbital varix where there is dilation of preexisting venous channels (Fig. 12.11).

Alternating exophthalmos and enophthalmos is a feature of orbital varix.

12.6 Neural Tumors

Glioma and meningioma arise from the optic nerve and its sheath, respectively, while neurofibroma and schwannoma arise from peripheral nerves rather than the optic nerve (Table 12.5).

CT and MRI of optic nerve gliomas typically reveal fusiform enlargement of the optic nerve, with MRI sometimes showing cystic degeneration. Optic nerve gliomas confined to the orbital optic nerve can be monitored, especially if vision remains good. Radiation therapy is employed if the tumor is unresectable due to involvement of the chiasm or tract and if symptoms are worsening. Chemotherapy is effective for progressive chiasmal or hypothalamic gliomas and can help avoid the complications associated with radiation. Surgery may be considered for progressive lesions expanding toward the chiasm.

Meningiomas generally do not destroy bone, but they do hyperostotic changes chronically. Hyperostosis of the sphenoid bone is characteristic of sphenoid wing meningiomas, which are the most common tumor of the intracranial space to spread to the orbit.

A progressively symptomatic optic nerve sheath meningioma that does not extend outside the orbit can also be managed by fractionated stereotactic radiation therapy (gamma knife). Optic nerve sheath meningioma confined to the orbit and with progressive visual loss should be managed by radiation therapy.

Foster Kennedy syndrome is characteristically caused by frontal lobe meningioma (classically olfactory meningioma), characterized by disc swelling on one side and optic atrophy on the other side.

Pseudo-foster Kennedy syndrome found with anterior ischemic optic neuropathy (AION).

Psammoma bodies are a microscopic finding representing a round collection of calcium, which can present in meningioma.

Meningiomas with ophthalmic manifestations include:

- Sphenoid wing meningioma causing proptosis
- Olfactory meningioma causing foster Kennedy syndrome
- Suprasellar meningioma compressing on optic chiasm leading to visual field defects
- Large intracranial meningioma causing increased intracranial pressure

Plexiform neurofibroma grows along sensory nerves and is considered invasive (Fig. 12.12).

Table 12.5 Neural tumors in the orbit and their characteristics

	Optic nerve glioma	Optic nerve sheath meningioma	Plexiform neurofibroma	Isolated neurofibroma
Pathophysiology	Pilocytic astrocytoma	Meningothelial cells of the arachnoid villi around intraorbital optic nerve	MC peripheral neural tumor of orbit	Peripheral neural tumor of orbit
Unilaterality/site	Unilateral Children Girls more than boys	Unilateral Middle-aged female	Early childhood	Middle age Third–fourth decades
Symptoms	Slowly progressive visual loss + dystopia	The classic (Hoyt–Spencer) triad consists of progressive visual loss, optic atrophy, and optociliary shunt vessels	Mechanical ptosis with a "bag of worm" mass Characteristic S-shaped deformity	Insidious mildly painful proptosis
Association	30% NF-1 (best prognosis)	NF-2. Psammoma bodies and calcifications	Almost exclusively in NF-1	10% NF-1 well circumscribed and relatively avascular

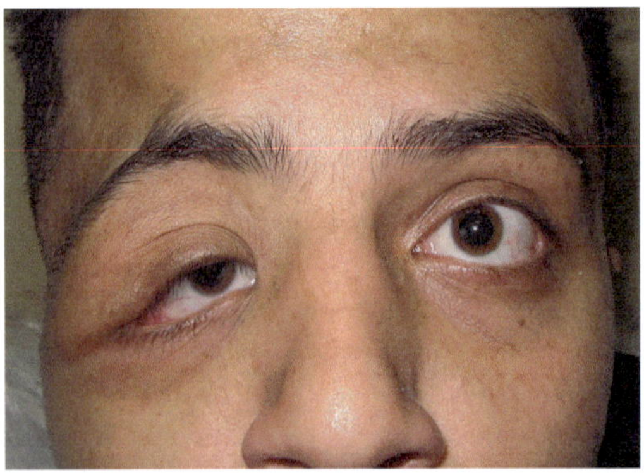

Fig. 12.12 A plexiform neurofibroma in a Neurofibromatosis patients causing right upper lid lateral S-shape deformity with inferior globe dystopia

Neurofibromatosis presents with pulsating proptosis of long duration mostly representing sphenoidal wing dysplasia.

12.7 Neoplasms

Orbital metastasis in children is mostly from sarcomas, while carcinoma is more common in adults.

The most common primary orbital malignancy in children is rhabdomyosarcoma. The most common metastatic tumor in children is neuroblastoma, and it may be bilateral.

Remember that lymphoma and leukemia have the same cellular origin.

The commonest leukemia involving orbit is acute lymphoblastic leukemia (ALL).

Lymphoma can occur in the ocular adnexa, primarily affecting the lacrimal gland, though conjunctival lymphoma tends to have the best prognosis. They are mostly non-Hodgkin B-cell marginal lymphomas and generally affect older adults. For localized lesions, radiotherapy is the treatment of choice, while chemotherapy is used for disseminated disease and certain subtypes.

The lacrimal gland is the most common site of lymphoma in the orbit, often presenting as painless downward proptosis (Fig. 12.13). Anterior orbital lesions may feel rubbery to the touch.

Rhabdomyosarcoma (RMS) is the most common soft tissue sarcoma in children, with 90% of cases occurring in those under 16 years old, with a mean age of 7 years. About 40% of RMS cases develop in the head and neck, making it the most common primary orbital malignancy in children, although it remains a rare condition. RMS classically presents as downward and lateral displacement of the globe (Fig. 12.14). It originates from undifferentiated mesenchymal cells, and mutations in the RB1 gene can increase susceptibility to this tumor. RMS often presents with rapid unilateral pro-

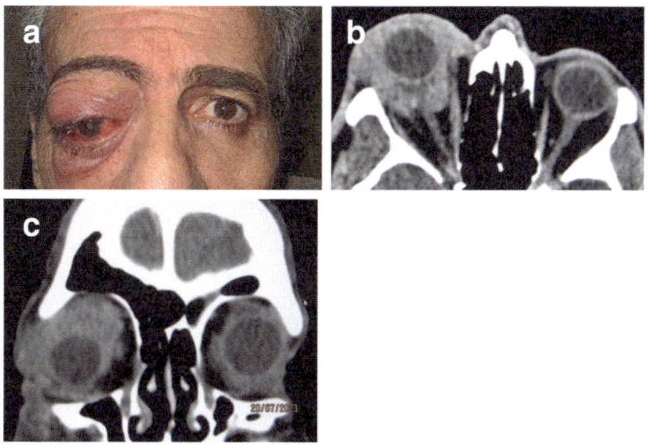

Fig. 12.13 Orbital Lymphoma. (**a**) Clinical photograph exhibits downward proptosis. (**b** and **c**) Contrast-enhanced axial and coronal CT scans of the orbit reveal a large, moderately and homogenously enhancing right retro-orbital soft tissue mass with both intraconal and extraconal components. The mass contours to the globe's outline and shows similar enhancement to the extraocular muscles. There is also marked right proptosis

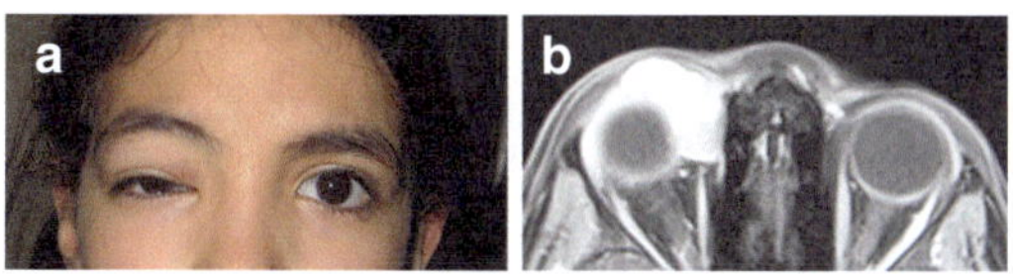

Fig. 12.14 Orbital Rhabdomyosarcoma. (**a**) Clinical photograph of a child with evident right upper eyelid swelling and ptosis. (**b**) Axial contrast-enhanced orbital MRI scan revealing two adjacent homogeneously enhancing superomedial anterior orbital lesions, which are exerting mass effect upon the right globe

ptosis and redness of the overlying skin, though it typically does not cause increased warmth. Bony destruction may be observed. Diagnostic workup should include prompt excisional biopsy with possible frozen section diagnosis, as well as bone marrow biopsy, and lumbar puncture. Treatment of primary orbital rhabdomyosarcoma generally involves radiation therapy and systemic chemotherapy. Exenteration is considered only in cases of treatment failure and recurrence.

The more the differentiated, the better the prognosis. Rhabdomyosarcoma's 5-year survival rate is 95%. The most common sites of metastases are lung and bone.

Differential diagnosis of rhabdomyosarcoma: orbital cellulitis, metastatic tumors (neuroblastoma, myeloid sarcoma).

Rhabdomyosarcoma Subtypes:

- Embryonal: most common type, accounting for more than 80% of total cases, more common superonasally. Cells may show light microscopic features of striated muscle differentiation.
- Alveolar: worst prognosis and has a predilection for the inferior orbit.
- Pleomorphic: best prognosis.

12.7.1 Metastasis

12.7.1.1 Adult

Orbital metastasis is less common than choroidal metastasis. Most commonly from breast (70%), lung, and prostate and then skin melanoma, GI tract, and kidney. Can present with a mass causing proptosis/dystopia (Most common), and enophthalmos with scirrhous tumors and chronic orbital inflammation.

They are usually not encapsulated and can erode the bone.

Radiotherapy is the mainstay of treatment. Prognosis for life is poor.

12.7.1.2 Children

Neuroblastoma often presents with the abrupt onset of proptosis, which is accompanied by a superior orbital mass and lid ecchymosis, typically around the age of 2 years. This tumor originates from neural crest-derived tissue of the sympathetic nervous system, and most commonly in the abdomen. Bilateral metastases can also occur in neuroblastoma cases.

Myeloid (granulocytic) sarcoma is a solid tumor composed of malignant cells of myeloid origin. It may exhibit a green color, often referred to as **chloroma**. This type of sarcoma can occur as a manifestation of established myeloid leukemia. In children around the age of 7 years, it typically presents with a rapid onset of proptosis, which can be bilateral, and may be associated with ecchymosis and lid edema.

Langerhans cell granulomatosis (histiocytosis) is characterized by clonal proliferations of histiocytes. When it involves the orbit, it typically presents as unilateral or bilateral osteolytic lesions and soft tissue involvement, often found in the superotemporal quadrant. Patients with solitary lesions, commonly eosinophilic granuloma, generally experience a more benign course.

Ecchymosis or eyelid redness with proptosis in a child can be due to a malignant process:

- Around 2 years of age, think of neuroblastoma, where ocular manifestations are due to metastasis from a primary, usually in the sympathetic paraganglion chain in the abdomen. These patients have increased urine levels of vanillylmandelic acid (VMA). Treatment of this metastatic orbital disease is a combination of radiation and chemotherapy.
- Around 7 years of age, think of rhabdomyosarcoma, a primary soft tissue tumor in the eye.

Leukemia can lead to orbital involvement, which typically presents with proptosis but usually without ecchymosis. Acute lymphoblastic leukemia is the most common form of leukemia to metastasize to the orbit. Often, orbital lesions are detected before any signs of leukemia in the blood or bone marrow appear.

Common Etiologies of Pulsatile Proptosis Include:

- Carotid-cavernous fistula
- Vascular orbital tumors

Transmitted intracranial pulsations through osseous orbital defects, which may be congenital (such as in neurofibromatosis type I) or occur following cranial surgery or large orbital roof fractures (not associated with bruit).

A common sign of a malignant lymphoproliferative lesion includes firm nodularity.

Breast cancer is the most common primary source of metastases to the orbit in women. Extraocular involvement is more common than bony involvement. The majority of patients with metastatic breast cancer present with proptosis except for scirrhous type (enophthalmos is characteristically seen with metastatic scirrhous carcinoma of the breast in adult women).

Orbital metastasis in men is mostly pulmonary in origin.

12.8 Trauma

Orbital fractures are categorized based on their location: the roof, the floor, the medial wall, and the lateral wall. The prevalence of these fractures differs based on age. In younger children (under 8 years old), fractures most commonly occur in the orbital roof. In older patients (over 8 years old), the fractures tend to occur in the orbital floor.

There are two primary reasons why orbital roof fractures occur more frequently in children. First, in young children, the frontal sinuses have not developed yet. These structures typically absorb the force of a frontal impact in adults, but in their absence, the force is transferred directly to the orbital roof, leading to fractures. Second, the proportion of the cranial vault to the face in children is greater (8:1) compared to adults (2:1), making the forehead more prominent and prone to injury.

Orbital floor fractures often impact the infraorbital nerve, a thin bony encasement in the orbital floor, leading to decreased sensation in the midface. These fractures can result from a blowout, a type of fracture where the orbital floor is broken but the inferior orbital rim remains intact. It is usually caused by a sudden increase in orbital pressure from an impact by a large object (over 5 cm in diameter).

The impact and subsequent fracture can lead to symptoms such as numbness in the cheek, upper lip, and teeth on the affected side, due to injury or swelling around the infraorbital nerve. Patients may also experience restrictive strabismus (misalignment of the eyes due to limited movement), seen in 40–63% of cases, and enophthalmos (retraction of the eyeball into the orbit), which may occur immediately or develop over time due to post-traumatic orbital fibrosis (Fig. 12.15). In cases where the inferior rectus muscle is trapped or swelled, there may be restricted upward gaze.

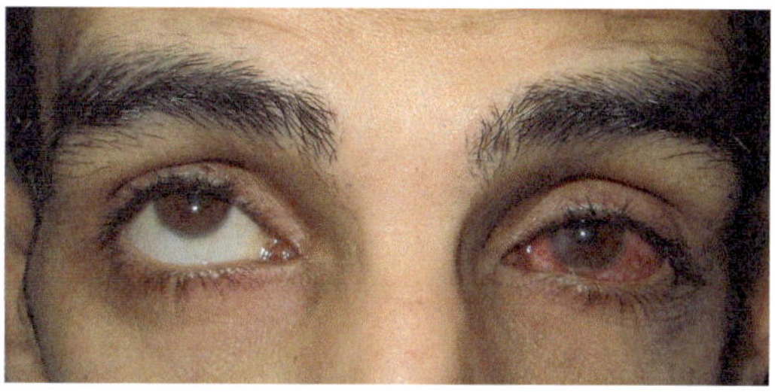

Fig. 12.15 Left enophthalmos, restricted upward movements, keratitis and Hypopyon following trauma and orbital floor fracture with trapped inferior rectus muscle

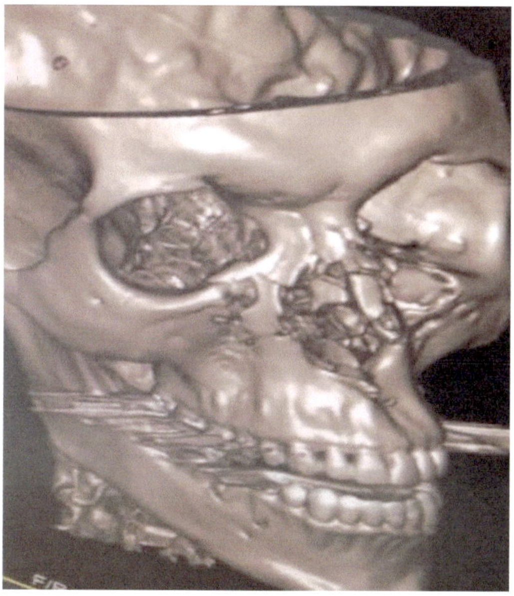

Fig. 12.16 LeFort type II fracture demonstrated through a three-dimensional (3D) CT scan of the facial bones, depicting multiple fractures involving the nasal bone and inferior rim of the right orbit

Management of orbital roof fractures primarily involves ruling out intracranial injury. Surgical repair is typically delayed until the swelling has subsided. Patients are given antibiotics and advised not to blow their nose to prevent the development of subcutaneous emphysema and the risk of forcing infected sinus contents into the orbit. Surgical repair of orbital floor fractures is optimally performed 2 weeks post-injury.

A particular type of orbital fracture known as a "white-eyed blowout fracture" (WEBOF) is more common in children and young adults. Despite minimal external signs, it involves small fractures, restrictive strabismus, and double vision. Early surgical intervention is necessary to avoid permanent damage to the inferior rectus muscle and its associated nerve. In patients younger than 18, small trapdoor floor fractures may trap orbital tissues, leading to rapid infarction and permanent extraocular muscle restriction.

Tenderness over the zygomaticofrontal suture is often associated with a zygomaticomaxillary (tripod) fracture.

Medial wall fractures are often accompanied by orbital floor fractures. Repair is typically necessary if the medial rectus muscle is entrapped. If both globe rupture and symptomatic blowout fracture are present, the globe rupture is prioritized for repair. Repair of both injuries simultaneously is not recommended due to the risk of worsening anterior or posterior segment injuries.

Trauma can also lead to retrobulbar hemorrhage, which is bleeding behind the eye. This condition requires immediate attention, often treated with lateral canthotomy and cantholysis, procedures to cut the lateral canthal tendon to relieve the pressure in the orbit. Lastly, Le Fort fractures are specific to the midface, involving the separation of the midface from the skull base, and must involve the pterygoid plates (Fig. 12.16). Among the three types of Le Fort fractures, only Le Fort I does not involve the orbit.

12.9 Infection

Infections in the orbital area can present differently and require different treatments based on their location, severity, and the patient's age. Children under the age of 9 with isolated ethmoid sinusitis that results in inferior or medial subperiosteal orbital abscesses typically respond well to medical treatment. These cases are characterized by intact vision and moderate proptosis. In other situations, surgical drainage through the ethmoidal sinus may be required.

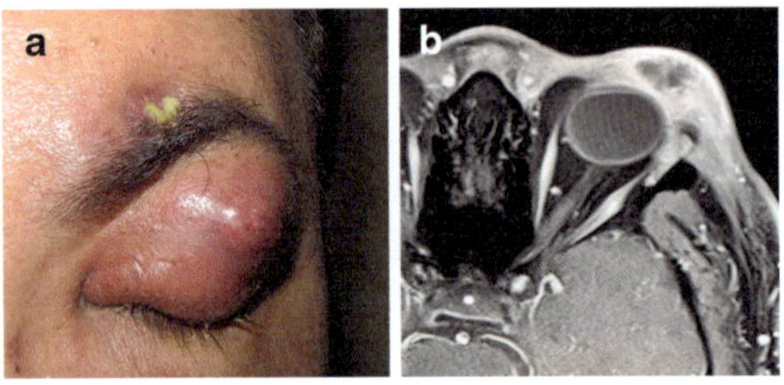

Fig. 12.17 Preseptal orbital abscess. (**a**) Clinical photograph capturing marked redness, swelling, and purulent discharge of the left upper eyelid and above the eyebrow at the site of previous sling ptosis repair surgery. (**b**) Axial T1 MRI with contrast of the left orbit revealing left preseptal swelling and a thick-walled abscess located within the left upper eyelid. Notably, there is no evidence of post-septal extension

However, there are certain scenarios where a more cautious or conservative approach should not be taken. These include instances of superior or lateral orbital involvement, acute optic nerve or retinal compromise, or frontal sinusitis. These guidelines are based on the work of Garcia and Harris, who emphasized the need for prompt and aggressive intervention in these high-risk situations.

Preseptal cellulitis, an infection of the eyelid and portions of skin around the eye, often occurs as a result of recent skin trauma. This is considered the most common risk factor for this type of infection (Fig. 12.17). This condition can be effectively managed with appropriate antibiotics and careful monitoring for potential complications. The timely treatment of preseptal cellulitis is crucial to prevent the infection from spreading into the orbit, which could lead to a more serious condition known as orbital cellulitis.

12.10 Evisceration, Enucleation, and Exenteration

These surgical procedures are conducted for severe ocular conditions. Evisceration involves the removal of all the eye's contents while preserving the sclera and the extraocular muscles. In contrast, enucleation implies the complete removal of the eye globe (Table 12.6). Exenteration is even more comprehensive, removing all orbital contents, including the eye globe and soft tissues. Evisceration generally has fewer complications and better implant motility, but it is contraindicated for intraocular tumors and for small eyes or those with a thinned-out sclera (phthisis bulbi).

Table 12.6 Comparison between enucleation and evisceration

	Evisceration	Enucleation
Clinical outcome	Better	Worse
Motility	Better	Worse
Pathology analysis	Worse	Better
Risk of post-op enophthalmos	Lower	Higher
Risk of infection extension	Lower	Higher
Most common indication	Blind, painful eye	Choroidal melanoma
Surgical difficulty	Easier and quicker	More difficult

Both enucleation and evisceration may cause ptosis due to disruption of the superior rectus muscle function and changes in the ocular pulley system. Anophthalmic socket infection, a common complication, can be treated with oral antibiotics.

12.10.1 Anophthalmic Socket Reconstruction Options

Dermis Fat Graft (DFG): A DFG fills an anophthalmic socket using a graft from the patient's own body. It is sourced from various areas such as the abdominal, gluteal, hip, groin, or thigh regions. DFG can be conducted as a primary procedure after enucleation or a secondary procedure for extrusion or migration of an orbital implant. A significant drawback is the unpredictable rate of fat atrophy, especially in adults. DFG is mainly indicated for extrusion or large exposure of an orbital socket implant and tends to grow with the orbit in children but shows unpredictable fat resorption in adults. Hydroxyapatite implant placement in an anophthalmic orbit can lead to complications of exposure and extrusion, with rates as high as 10–12%.

Conformer: A conformer is a clear acrylic or synthetic shell fitted post-enucleation or evisceration if the final artificial eye is not available. It maintains the eye socket's shape and allows eyelids to blink without rubbing the suture line. Worn for 6–8 weeks after surgery, the conformer shell holds the shape until the wound heals and the artificial eye is ready.

PEG System: This system improves prosthetic eye motility in porous hydroxyapatite implant. A drill hole is made in the implant, and after a follow-up period of 3–4 months, a PEG implant is inserted.

Hard Palate Graft: In eyelid socket reconstruction, a hard palate graft is commonly used, particularly for the lower eyelid. Full-thickness mucosal grafts such as those taken from the buccal mucosa typically maintain some degree of keratinization after being transplanted to the ocular surface, which aids in maintaining a stable and functional eyelid.

12.10.2 Complications and Precautions

The most common postoperative complication of enucleation is superior sulcus deformity due to inadequate volume replacement. Nonporous implants have a lower extrusion rate and are a cost-effective choice for patients not requiring implant integration. However, porous implants provide better motility but carry a higher risk of complications.

Chronic mucus discharge from an anophthalmic socket is usually due to papillary conjunctivitis.

The cornea can be preserved or removed during evisceration, as per the surgeon's preference. If preserved, the corneal endothelium should be removed. Unlike transplanted tissues, the body cannot reject a hydroxyapatite orbital implant.

Interestingly, a "phantom limb" pain syndrome secondary to a severed optic nerve is not reported after exenteration surgery.

An important advantage of enucleation over evisceration is that it does not expose or disseminate an occult intraocular malignancy. Consequently, all removed tissue and the enucleated globe should be sent for histopathological examination to ensure thorough evaluation. Evisceration, on the other hand, should only be performed after a preoperative B-scan ultrasound to rule out the presence of an intraocular mass, as neither CT nor MRI is as sensitive for detecting such masses.

12.11 Orbital Imaging

Radiological investigations play a crucial role in diagnosing and managing orbital conditions. A comprehensive understanding of these modalities is vital not just for identifying pathological changes, but also for discerning normal anatomical variations. The diverse array of imaging techniques, each with its unique strengths and limitations, contributes valuable information to our diagnostic arsenal.

This section begins with an overview of the most commonly used imaging modalities in the orbit—computed tomography (CT) and magnetic resonance imaging (MRI). We delve into the fundamental principles behind these technologies, their uses, and their limitations. This segment also emphasizes the significance of the Hounsfield scale in CT scans and the T1 and T2 weighting concept in MRI, elucidating their relevance in diagnosing different orbital conditions.

12.11.1 Computed Tomography (CT) Orbital Imaging

Computed tomography (CT) has become an essential tool in ophthalmology for diagnosing and managing orbital diseases due to its superior resolution of bony structures, ease of access, and shorter scanning time compared to other imaging modalities. CT scanning uses X-ray beams that rotate around the patient to generate cross-sectional images or "slices" of the body. These images can be reconstructed to form a three-dimensional view of the area of interest (Fig. 12.16), providing valuable insights into the anatomical structures and potential pathologies. The resulting images are measured in Hounsfield units (HUs), a quantitative scale that represents the radiodensity of tissues. This is crucial when assessing the nature of lesions within the orbit. In CT imaging, different tissues have different appearances based on their radiodensity. For instance, air is black (approximately −1000 HU), fat appears dark grey (−50 to −100 HU), fluid or muscle appears as a lighter grey (+20 to +40 HU), and bone appears white (+700 to +3000 HU). Understanding these characteristic appearances will help differentiate between normal and pathological tissues.

In evaluating CT scans, the ophthalmologist must be methodical. One approach is to start by assessing the bony orbit for fractures, deformities, or signs of bone remodeling. Then, evaluate soft tissues including the extraocular muscles, lacrimal gland, and optic nerve, looking for enlargement, infiltration, or displacement. Look at the intraconal and extraconal fat for signs of stranding or infiltration, and the globe for any signs of pathology. Finally, evaluate the sinuses and the cranial cavity for any abnormalities. CT scans can be performed with or without contrast. Contrast can be beneficial when trying to differentiate between tumors, inflammation, and vascular lesions, as it can highlight areas with increased vascular flow. However, contrast is typically not needed for bony lesions, trauma, or when evaluating the extent of sinus disease. Notably, CT scans provide excellent detail of calcifications, bony changes, and foreign bodies, making it particularly useful in cases of trauma, suspected foreign bodies, bony lesions, and sinus disease. However, due to the radiation exposure associated with CT, it should be used judiciously, especially in younger patients and pregnant women.

12.11.2 Magnetic Resonance Imaging (MRI) Orbital Imaging

Magnetic resonance imaging (MRI) is a crucial tool for diagnosing and managing orbital diseases, primarily due to its excellent soft tissue contrast and the ability to image in multiple planes without ionizing radiation. In MRI, tissues are characterized by their signal intensity: high-signal-intensity areas appear bright (white) on the image, while low-signal-intensity areas appear dark (black). This signal intensity is primarily dictated by the tissue's water and fat content. Fat and water generally produce high signal intensity on T1-weighted and T2-weighted images, respectively, while bone and air appear dark on both.

When interpreting MRI scans, a systematic approach is recommended. Begin by assessing the bony orbit for any deformities or lesions. Then, evaluate the extraocular muscles, optic nerve, lacrimal gland, and other soft tissues for signs of enlargement, infiltration, or displacement. Carefully examine the intraconal and extraconal fat for abnormalities, and review the globe for any signs of pathology. Lastly, evaluate adjacent structures such as the paranasal sinuses and brain. MRI can be performed with or without contrast. Gadolinium, the most commonly used contrast agent, can help differentiate between various lesions, as it enhances areas with increased blood flow or a disrupted blood-brain barrier. It is particularly useful in cases of inflammatory or neoplastic processes.

While MRI is more time consuming and expensive than CT, it provides superior soft tissue resolution. It does not involve ionizing radiation, making it more suitable for certain patient populations, such as pregnant women and children (Table 12.7). MRI is particularly beneficial in evaluating soft tissue lesions, optic nerve pathologies, vascular lesions, and intracranial extension of orbital diseases. In T1 MRI, both the vitreous and CSF appear black.

Table 12.7 Comparison between computed tomography (CT) and magnetic resonance imaging (MRI) in orbital imaging

	Computed tomography (CT)	Magnetic resonance imaging (MRI)
Uses	Ideal for visualizing the bony anatomy of the orbit, calcified structures, trauma, fractures, and sinus disease	Superior for soft tissue evaluation (including the brain, optic nerves, muscles, and globe), vascular lesions, optic nerve pathologies, and intracranial extension of orbital diseases
Terms used to describe images	Density: Measured in Hounsfield units (HUs). High-density structures (like bone) appear white, while low-density structures (like air) appear black	Intensity: High-signal-intensity areas appear white, and low-signal-intensity areas appear black. Tissue intensity depends on its water and fat content
Color of landmark structures	Bone (white), air (black), fat (grey), soft tissue/muscles (grey), fluids (dark grey)	Fat (white on T1), water (white on T2), bone (black), air (black), soft tissue/muscles (grey on T1, brighter on T2)
Advantages	Quick, widely available, cheaper, superior for bony details, better at imaging calcified structures, no issues with claustrophobia	Superior soft tissue contrast, multiplanar imaging without ionizing radiation, better for vascular imaging, optimal for evaluating optic nerve pathologies, superior in detecting intracranial extension of orbital diseases
Disadvantages	Ionizing radiation exposure, less detail in soft tissues, not as good for vascular imaging, may have artifacts from dental fillings	More time consuming, more expensive, potential claustrophobia, not as good at imaging calcified structures or bony details, cannot be used with certain implants (like pacemakers)

12.12 Miscellaneous

Endoscopic Dacryocystorhinostomy (DCR): Endonasal DCR is preferred as it can be done in less time, especially in elderly people, with better visualization through the endoscope, and less facial scarring. However, it has a lower success rate compared to external DCR depending on surgeons' experience (Table 12.8).

Crouzon's, Apert's, and Pfeiffer's syndromes are classified as craniofacial synostosis syndromes, which arise from the premature closure of one or more cranial sutures. These conditions often lead to various forms of horizontal strabismus, with V-pattern exotropia being the most prevalent. Common ocular findings associated with these syndromes include hypertelorism and proptosis. Apert's syndrome is notably characterized by a significant degree of syndactyly, setting it apart from the other syndromes.

Treacher Collins syndrome and Goldenhar syndrome are classified as craniofacial cleft syndromes. Goldenhar syndrome involves abnormalities of the first and second branchial arches and can result in eyelid colobomas, lipodermoids, Duane syndrome, and facial hypoplasia.

The manifestation of an acquired, proptotic, or "bulging" eye can generally be classified into six main categories:

1. Inflammatory: Includes conditions such as thyroid eye disease, idiopathic orbital inflammatory syndrome, sarcoidosis, and granulomatosis with polyangiitis (previously known as Wegener granulomatosis)
2. Infectious: Encompasses bacterial or fungal infections, notably mucormycosis leading to orbital cellulitis
3. Neoplastic: Involves benign or malignant tumors, which could be primary, such as a cavernous hemangioma in adults, or secondary arising from metastasis of a primary malignancy (like prostate, breast, lung cancers), or extension from adjacent structures, as seen in a sinus mucocele or intracranial meningioma
4. Trauma: As the result of an injury to the eye or orbit
5. Vascular: Related to blood vessel abnormalities or diseases
6. Hematologic: Including lymphoproliferative disorders and lymphoma

Table 12.8 Comparison between endoscopic (endonasal) and external dacryocystorhinostomy (DCR)

	Endonasal	External
Success rate	Lower	Higher
Operative time	Lower	Higher
Aesthetic outcome	Better	Worse with facial scar
Blood	Less	More
Disruption of gland pump function	No	Yes, due to orbicularis incision

The annulus of Zinn is made up of superior and inferior orbital tendons. The superior tendon forms the entire superior rectus muscle and portions of the lateral and medial rectus muscles. Conversely, the inferior tendon forms the entire inferior rectus muscle and parts of the medial and lateral rectus muscles.

Silent sinus syndrome (SSS) leads to enophthalmos or hypoglobus due to orbital floor collapse in the presence of asymptomatic chronic maxillary sinusitis, caused by negative pressure in the maxillary sinus. The syndrome is most frequently associated with underlying aberrant nasal anatomy. The preferred management of SSS is endoscopic antrostomy, with or without uncinectomy, to restore normal sinus aeration, combined with orbital floor reconstruction.

For children aged between 6 and 9 years, any new mass growth should be assumed to be malignant until proven otherwise, with rhabdomyosarcoma being the most common.

In optociliary shunt, collateral vessels are retinochoroidal vessels. These may be linked to conditions such as vein occlusion, optic disc drusen, hemangioma, chronic papilledema, diabetes, or tumor formation.

Pulsatile lesions in the orbit may be due to vascular lesions (like hemangioma), a carotid cavernous fistula, or transmitted pulsation in the absence of the sphenoid wing or orbital roof.

Proptosis on a CT scan is typically diagnosed when 1/3rd or more of the globe lies anterior to the inter-zygomatic process line.

Phthisis bulbi is characterized by the atrophy, shrinkage, and disorganization of the eye and intraocular contents, which can lead to osseous metaplasia of the retinal pigment epithelium (RPE).

Enophthalmos, or the inward displacement of the eye, can be caused by various factors, including silent sinus syndrome, orbital varix, orbital wall fracture, scirrhous breast carcinoma, and chronic conditions leading to fat atrophy, such as malnutrition.

In fibrous dysplasia, most orbital lesions are monostotic, with the frontal bone being the most frequently affected. Among sinus lesions, a mucocele is the most common to invade the orbit. The most common neoplasm to invade the orbit is squamous cell carcinoma, while the most common mesenchymal tumor found in the orbit is fibrous histiocytoma.

Mucormycosis: It is postulated that patients with diabetes do better than other immunocompromised patients with mucormycosis. Debridement of all devitalized tissue, until free bleeding tissue is encountered, is extremely important; it may include almost any structure. Exenteration is reserved for potentially lethal disease that is progressing unresponsive to other forms of treatment or as a palliative treatment for severe pain. It has been demonstrated that the more extensive the debridement, the better the prognosis. Since the addition of treatment with amphotericin B, survival rates have jumped from <5% to >70%. Early diagnosis with local excision, systemic stabilization, and IV amphotericin give mucormycosis patients the best chance for survival.

Hyperostosis can be seen in meningioma, metastatic prostate cancer, or fibrous dysplasia.

Doxorubicin does not cause canalicular obstruction despite being excreted in the tear.

The eye is the most common site for extracutaneous involvement of juvenile xanthogranuloma, and intraocular lesions rarely regress spontaneously.

Retrobulbar hemorrhage can be managed by lateral canthotomy and cantholysis, mannitol, and aqueous suppressants; however, steroids may worsen the condition acutely.

The trochlea is the sole cartilaginous structure within the normal orbit. Rituximab is a monoclonal antibody that targets the B-cell CD20 receptor.

The facial nerve moves from a position deep to the superficial musculoaponeurotic system (SMAS) beneath the zygoma to a more superficial location above the zygoma. Dissection in these areas must be performed with caution.

MALT lymphomas can spontaneously remit in 5–15% of cases. They may also transform into a higher-grade lesion, typically a large-cell type, in 15–20% of cases. MALT lymphomas are not always benign or aggressive; at least 50% of patients may develop systemic disease within 10 years.

Endoscopic sinus surgery may inadvertently lead to damage of nasolacrimal duct, an extraocular muscle, or optic nerve or even penetrate the globe. A sensitive finding in direct naso-orbital-ethmoid fracture is telecanthus (Allen 2014).

Acknowledgments None.

Conflict of Interest None.

References

Ababneh OH, Msallam MM (2014) Bilateral simultaneous pyogenic granuloma after perforated punctal plug insertion. Ophthalmic Plast Reconstr Surg 30(5):e113–e115. https://doi.org/10.1097/IOP.0b013e3182a5ba6b

Ababneh OH, AboTaleb EA, Abu Ameerh MA, Yousef YA (2015) Enucleation and evisceration at a tertiary care hospital in a developing country. BMC Ophthalmol. 15:120. https://doi.org/10.1186/s12886-015-0108-x

Ali MJ (ed) (2018) Principles and practice of lacrimal surgery. Springer

Allen R (2014) Hereditary disorders affecting the lacrimal system. Curr Opin Ophthalmol:25. https://doi.org/10.1097/ICU.0000000000000092

AlRyalat SA (2021) Basics of lacrimal system for ophthalmology board exams. Springer. https://doi.org/10.1007/978-981-16-2968-6_4

Al-Ryalat NT, Ezzat JW, Ababneh OH, AlRyalat SA, Al-Hadidy AM (2016) Isolated bilateral lacrimal gland agenesis. J Pediatr Ophthalmol Strabismus 53:e35–e38. https://doi.org/10.3928/01913913-20160719-01

American Academy of Ophthalmology (n.d.) Basic and clinical science course. Section 7. Orbit, Eyelids and Lacrimal System, San Francisco, USA

Bartalena L et al (2021) The 2021 European Group on Graves' orbitopathy (EUGOGO) clinical practice guidelines for the medical management of Graves' orbitopathy. Eur J Endocrinol 185(4):G43–G67. https://doi.org/10.1530/EJE-21-0479

Denniston A, Murray P (eds) (2014) Oxford handbook of ophthalmology. Oxford University Press

Dickinson AJ, Perros P (2001) Controversies in the clinical evaluation of active thyroid-associated orbitopathy: use of a detailed protocol with comparative photographs for objective assessment. Clin Endocrinol 55(3):283–303. https://doi.org/10.1046/j.1365-2265.2001.01349.x

Dolman PJ (2018) Grading severity and activity in thyroid eye disease. Ophthal Plastic Reconstruct Surg 34(4S):S34. https://doi.org/10.1097/IOP.0000000000001150

Hollsten LD (1992) Complications of lacrimal surgery. Int Ophthalmol Clin 32(4):49–66

Kanski JJ (2019) Kanski's clinical ophthalmology E-book: a systematic approach. 6th and 9th ed. Elsevier Health Sciences

Mourits MP et al (1997) Clinical activity score as a guide in the management of patients with Graves' ophthalmopathy. Clin Endocrinol 47(1):9–14. https://doi.org/10.1046/j.1365-2265.1997.2331047.x

Nagendran S, Alsamnan M, Strianese D, Malhotra R (2020) Ectopic lacrimal gland tissue: a systematic review. Ophthalmic Plast Reconstr Surg. 36(6):540–544

Rose GE, Wright JE (1992) Pleomorphic adenoma of the lacrimal gland. Br J Ophthalmol. 76:395–400

Salmon JF (2019) Kanski's clinical ophthalmology E-book: a systematic approach. Elsevier Health Sciences

Shields JA, Shields CL, Epstein JA et al (2004) Primary epithelial malignancies of the lacrimal gland. The 2003 Ramon L. Font Lecture. Ophthalmic Plast Reconstr Surg 20:10–21

Wright JE, Rose GE, Garner A (1992) Primary malignant neoplasms of the lacrimal gland. Br J Ophthalmol 76:401–407

13 Clinical Review of Orbit and Lacrimal System: Part II

Osama H. Ababneh, Rhoda Hijazi, Lna Malkawi, and Saif Aldeen Alryalat

Abstract

This chapter examines the lacrimal system, detailing its anatomy, physiology, and pathological conditions. It highlights the essential role of tears in ocular health and the importance of understanding the lacrimal system for effective clinical practice. Key topics include lacrimal production and drainage systems, lacrimal gland tumors, congenital disorders, and acquired drainage obstructions. The chapter also addresses inflammation, dysfunction, and trauma of the lacrimal gland, along with surgical management strategies for various conditions. By the end, readers will gain a comprehensive understanding of the diverse pathologies affecting the lacrimal system, which will be invaluable for the daily clinical practice.

Keywords

Lacrimal system · Lacrimal gland tumors · Congenital disorders · Ocular health · Surgical management

O. H. Ababneh (✉)
Department of Ophthalmology, The University of Jordan, Amman, Jordan

R. Hijazi
Sam Houston State University, College of Osteopathic Medicine, Huntsville, TX, USA
e-mail: rxh086@SHSU.EDU

L. Malkawi
Department of Radiology, The University of Jordan, Amman, Jordan

Department of Radiology, University of Colorado Anschutz Medical Campus, Aurora, CO, USA

S. A. Alryalat
Department of Ophthalmology, The University of Jordan, Amman, Jordan

The University of Colorado Anschutz Medical Campus, CO, USA

13.1 Anatomy and Physiology

The nasolacrimal apparatus includes the lacrimal gland, the excretory lacrimal ducts, lacrimal punctae and canaliculi, the lacrimal sac, and the nasolacrimal duct (Fig. 13.1). The lacrimal gland is located on the superolateral surface of the orbit and is divided into two sections: the small palpebral portion and the larger orbital portion, where each have six and four ducts, respectively. These portions are separated by the levator palpebrae superioris aponeurosis. The lacrimal caruncle is found in the inner corner of the eye and can be seen superficially.

These ducts are combined when fluid is secreted onto the eye's surface. The lacrimal canaliculi (8.0 mm long) are divided into the supe-

S. A. Alryalat (ed.), *Ophthalmology Board and FRCS Part 2 Exams*,
https://doi.org/10.1007/978-981-96-1517-9_13

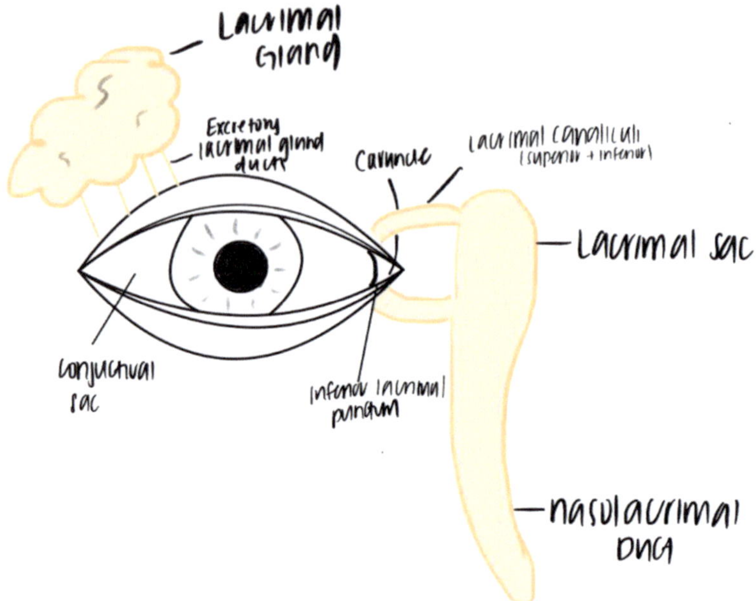

Fig. 13.1 The nasolacrimal apparatus

rior and inferior ducts within each eyelid, forming a common canaliculus in around 80% of patients. The common canaliculus connects to the lacrimal sac (12–15 mm long), which begins on the lateral aspect of the nose and drains directly into the nasolacrimal duct (15–18mm) and out into the nose. The valve of Hasner is a mucosal fold at the distal end of the nasolacrimal duct which prevents reflux into the nasolacrimal duct.

*Canaliculi—stratified columnar epithelium with goblet cells
*Lacrimal sac—stratified columnar epithelium with goblet cells
*Nasolacrimal duct—stratified columnar epithelium

> High yield note: Biopsy of the palpebral portion can impair tear production because it contains secretory ducts for itself and the orbital portion.

Accessory lacrimal glands—Krause's, Wolfring's, and Popov's glands are structurally and histologically similar to the lacrimal gland and surrounded by myoepithelial cells.

- Krause's gland: inside stoma of conjunctival fornix, 20–40 in upper fornix, and 6–8 in lower fornix
- Wolfring's gland: 2–5 located on superior border of the tarsal plate
- Popov's gland: located within the caruncle

Meibomian glands are sebaceous glands that produce the superficial oily layer of the tear film

Tears function: lubricant for eye and for protection and nurishment of the cornea

Tears to prevent bacterial growth—contain lysozyme which breaks down bacteria cell walls making them more susceptible to our immune defenses. Tears also contain high levels of IgA. Salt content within tears also contributes to the dehydration of most non-halophilic bacteria. (Salmon 2019)

Innervation: The lacrimal gland has sensory, parasympathetic, and sympathetic innervations (Fig. 13.2). Sensory innervation is provided by the lacrimal nerve, a branch of the ophthalmic nerve (CN V1) of the trigeminal nerve.

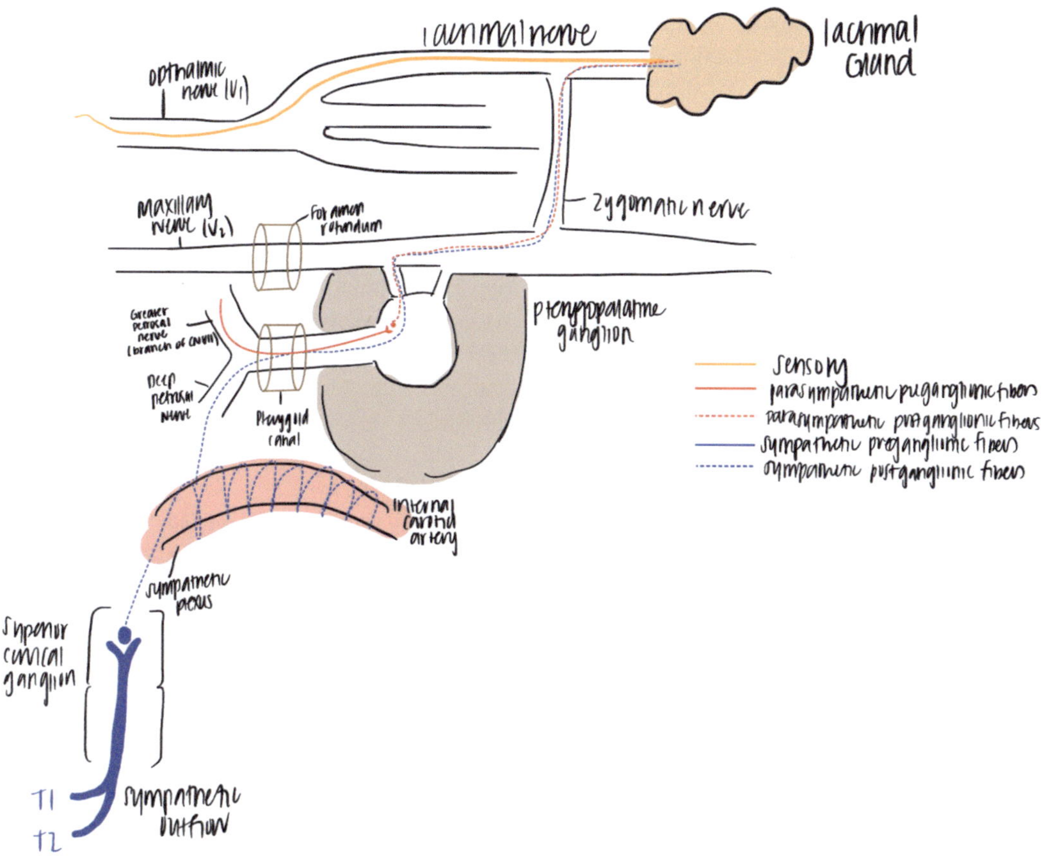

Fig. 13.2 Innervation of the lacrimal system including sensory, parasympathetic, and sympathetic innervation

- Postganglionic sympathetic fibers stem from the superior cervical ganglion and travel superiorly to wrap around the internal carotid artery to form the internal carotid plexus to enter the pterygoid canal as the deep petrosal nerve.
- Combining with parasympathetic preganglionic fibers of the greater superficial petrosal nerve stemming from the superior salivary nucleus of the facial nerve (CN VII) in the pons, the two travel along the same path on the superior zygomatic branch of the maxillary nerve (CN V2) to supply the gland via the anastomoses between the zygomaticotemporal and lacrimal nerves.
- Sympathetic innervation is thought to reduce tear production via vasoconstriction.
- Parasympathetic innervation leads to reflex tearing.

13.1.1 Nerve Palsies/Dysfunctions

- Seventh nerve palsies will lead to decreased lacrimation and dry eye symptoms.
- Electroneurography (ENog) and electromyography (EMG) are used for facial nerve testing.

- Systemic parasympathetic dysfunction will lead to decreased tear production and dry eye symptoms.
- Schirmer's test and tear breakup time are most commonly used to evaluate tear production and determine etiology of dry eye symptoms.
  - Schirmer's test: Filter paper is placed under the lower eyelid to evaluate the amount of wetting; decreased wetting may indicate decreased tear production.
  - Tear breakup time: Measures time for a tear film to break up on the eye surface; decreased time may indicate reduced tear production (Gordin et al. 2015; Rahman et al. 2012; Korn et al. 2021).

Arterial Supply

- Lacrimal artery, a branch of the ophthalmic artery from the internal carotid
- Infraorbital artery, a branch of the maxillary artery from the external carotid
- Drained by the ophthalmic vein
- Lymphatic drain into the superficial parotid nodes

> High-yield note: Parasympathetic preganglionic fibers of the greater superficial petrosal nerve from CN VII synapse in the pterygopalatine ganglion before supplying the lacrimal gland. The sympathetic fibers from the internal carotid plexus are postganglionic, synapsing at the superior cervical ganglion.

13.2 Lacrimal Production System

A lacrimal apparatus is a group of structures responsible for generating tears (Fig. 13.1). The excretory lacrimal ducts drain tears from the lacrimal gland into the eye (AlRyalat 2021). This process serves various crucial purposes like providing nutrients and oxygen to the avascular cornea and eliminating debris and foreign particles while moisturizing the eyes. The preocular tear film comprises outermost lipid, middle aqueous, and inner mucus components (Paulsen et al. 2003).

- Lipid component secreted by meibomian glands in the eyelids.
- Aqueous component is secreted by the main lacrimal gland, Krause's, and Wolfring's glands.
- Mucus component is secreted by the conjunctival goblet cells, (epithelial, acinar cells) and excretory duct cells of the lacrimal gland (Paulsen et al. 2003).

The lacrimal gland produces tears in the upper outer corner of each eye at a rate 1.5 microliter/minute (Fig. 13.1). The parasympathetic nervous system controls the gland and has two types of tears: basal and reflex. Basal tears are continuously produced slowly and steadily to keep the eye's surface moist and prevent it from drying out. Reflex tears, on the other hand, are produced in response to irritation or emotion and are produced in larger quantities than basal tears.

Once tears are produced by the lacrimal gland, they spread across the surface of the eye with each blink of the eyelids. The tears then enter the

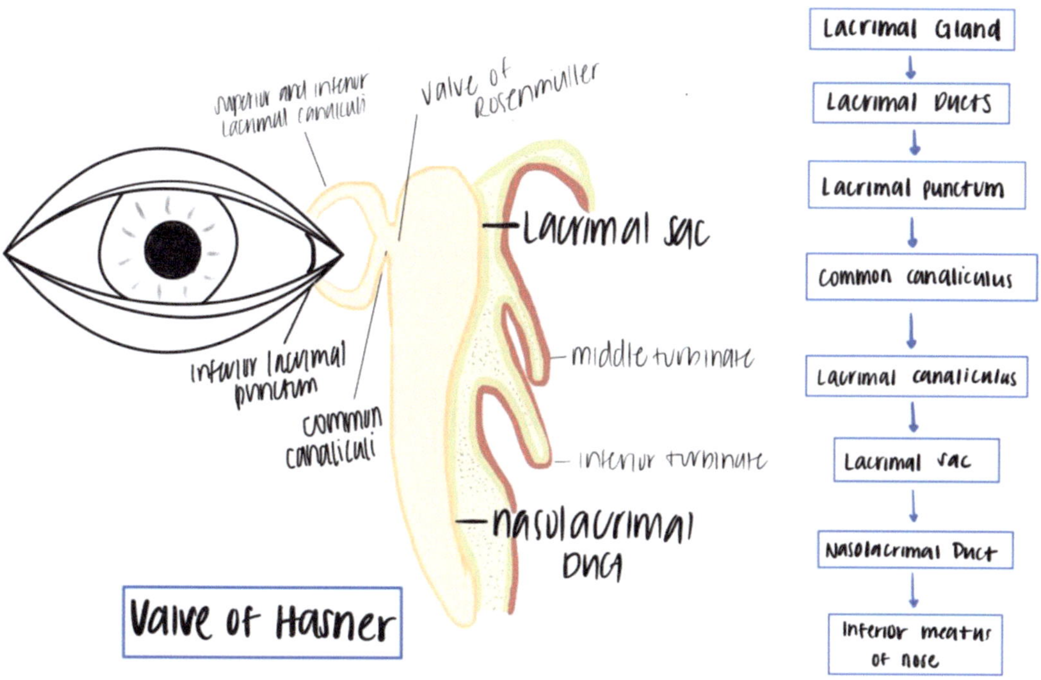

Fig. 13.3 The nasolacrimal apparatus and sequential steps of drainage

lacrimal drainage system, which directs them into the nasal cavity, where they are either absorbed by the lining of the nose or blown out through the nose. As a whole, the intricate mechanism of tear creation is crucial in preserving ocular well-being and operation. These tears are fundamental sources of nourishment, shielding the cornea while simultaneously eradicating impurities that would otherwise accumulate on its surface (Korn et al. 2021).

Recent findings: It was previously thought that the main lacrimal gland was producing tears by reflex, and the accessory glands were basal secretion. However, recent evidence shows that they all function as a reflex (Conrady et al. 2016)

13.3 Lacrimal Drainage System

An intricate network of components makes up the path for tears to be drawn from the eye's surface and into the nasal passage. This is called the **lacrimal drainage system** (Fig. 13.3), which facilitates a process wherein tears produced by the lacrimal gland are dispersed across the eyes' surface as they cleanse away impurities while providing lubrication that counters dryness. The base station for this cycle lies at the upper outer corner of one's orbital bony structure, where a sensitive tear-making gland is.

The lacrimal drainage system begins at the lacrimal punctae on the medial aspect of both upper and lower eyelids. The lower punctum is responsible for around 60–70% of the drainage. Their primary function is collecting tears from eye surfaces that later channel through canaliculi—two vertical channels on each eyelid's inner side

- The lower canaliculi (10 mm) is longer than the upper canaliculi (8 mm), and both have a diameter of 0.5 mm.
- The two canaliculi converge to form the common canaliculi. The common canaliculus opens into a broader passageway at the valve of Rosenmuller known as the lacrimal sac (12–15 mm), which sits in a lacrimal fossa (formed by lacrimal bone and frontal process of maxilla) near the medial edge of one's eye. This sac serves as reservoir for tears before they travel down into another channel called the nasolacrimal duct (15–18 mm long), an extended pipeline joining this sac with our nasal cavity, and sits in the osseous nasolacrimal canal, a groove in the maxillary bone.
- Fascia surrounds the lacrimal sac, except for below the medial canthal tendon, making this section more vulnerable to extension.
- The venous plexus is situated between the fascia and sac, and the angular vein is anterior to the sac.
- The nasolacrimal duct has thicker epithelium than the lacrimal sac.

The nasolacrimal duct ultimately empties the tears into the inferior nasal meatus through the valve of Hasner, where it may be absorbed or eliminated through exhalation when air passes out from the nose. The mechanism operates in a manner that enables eliminating excessive tear accumulation on the eye surface, which can lead to uncomfortable sensations and unclear vision problems. The valve of Hasner is a mucosal fold located at the distal end of the nasolacrimal duct. It functions to prevent air from entering into the lacrimal sac during expectoration.

> High-yield point: The most common place of acquired obstruction in the lacrimal drainage system is at the nasolacrimal duct. The most common place of congenital obstruction is at the valve of Hasner.

Upper and lower canaliculi = Lined with pseudostratified and stratified columnar epithelium, surrounded by a dense ring of connective tissue and muscle fibers from the lacrimal portion of the orbicularis oculi

Lacrimal sac and nasolacrimal duct = Composed of a double-layered epithelium with a superficial and a deep, flattened layer of cells

Metastases are very rare because there are no lymph nodes in the lacrimal gland.

13.4 Lacrimal Gland tumors

Table 13.1 provides overview of lacrimal gland tumors and their characteristics

> High-yield point: 50% of lacrimal gland tumors are epithelial and 50% are non-epithelial. Pleomorphic adenomas make up 50% of epithelial tumors, with the other 50% being malignant carcinomas; 50% of malignant carcinomas are adenoid cystic carcinomas and 50% of the adenoid cystic carcinomas are basaloid variant.
>
> ***This is called the "Rule of 50"***
>
> High-yield point: The highest risks for lacrimal gland tumors are age, history of lymphoma, and incomplete removal of a benign tumor.
>
> Some lesions can be confused with lacrimal gland tumors when they are found near the superolateral orbit. These include epidermoid or dermoid cysts, prolapsed orbital fat, and dermolipoma (Mueller 2022)

Table 13.1 Lacrimal gland tumors and their characteristics

Epithelial tumors: benign	Description	Demographic	Effect on surrounding bone	Calcifications	Histology	Management
Pleomorphic adenoma **Most common** epithelial tumor of lacrimal gland (Fig. 13.4)	Slowly progressive proptosis (months-years, average = 2 yrs.) Acceleration of symptoms indicates malignancy (20%) and can transform into pleomorphic adenocarcinoma	2nd–5th decade Slightly more common in men, painless, firm mass	Extensive bone invasion is rare because it is usually slow-growing. It may indent the bone or globe , but will not erode	Often associated with calcific degeneration	Pseudoencapsulated glandular tissue, epithelial and myoepithelial proliferation with keratin and myxoid tissue formation	Complete excision with upper lid crease approach, but varies based on location, Incomplete removal is associated with recurrence Biopsy with pseudo-capsule can increase risk of recurrence due to rupture
Epithelial tumors: malignant, rare						
1. Adenoid cystic carcinoma (**most common** malignant) COD: Intracranial neural invasion through superior orbital fissure	Solid areas of malignant epithelial cells Perineural invasion is common Aggressive and painful symptoms show in less than a year Most malignant epithelial neoplasm Abnormalities in MYB or MYB-NFIB between chromosome 6q22–23 and chromosome 9pq23–24 (Persson et al. 2009)	Middle-aged (40–50s), Slightly more common in women	Bone involvement through intracranial invasion via distant metastasis or large tumors (Khatib et al. 2021)	Rare but common in large tumors (Khatib et al. 2021)	Unencapsulated "Swiss-cheese" pattern in basaloid cells with multiple mitoses, Can identify neurofilaments via immunohistochemical staining to confirm perineural invasion	Complete resection with radiotherapy and chemotherapy Tumor debulking followed by external beam radiation (Rose and Wright 1992)

(continued)

Table 13.1 (continued)

Epithelial tumors: benign	Description	Demographic	Effect on surrounding bone	Calcifications	Histology	Management
2. Mucoepidermoid carcinoma	Characterized as low-, intermediate-, and high-grade tumors, with only high-grade tumors having poor survival Translocation of chromosome 11 and 19: t(11:19) (q21;p13) leading to fusion of oncogene CRTC1-MAML2 (Daniel et al. 2014)	> 60 years old, Even among male and females	Bony scalloping can invade adjacent structures	Yes (von Holstein et al. 2013)	Varies in number of mucous, epidermoid, and intermediate cells Generally contains a **cystic** component	Complete resection radiation and chemotherapy
3. Squamous cell carcinoma	Symptoms include diplopia, proptosis, and eyelid edema, Rapid progression and painful Pain may be associated with periocular invasion (Hotta et al. 2005)	Very rare	Bony destruction can occur	None	Proliferating keratinization	Local resection and radiotherapy

Non-epithelial tumors						
Lymphoma	Symptoms include diplopia, dry eye, and limited ocular motility, 25% of cases are bilateral, 14% have history of lymphoma, 34% present with systemic lymphoma at time of diagnosis (Jenkins et al. 2003) Majority are non-Hodgkin's B cell lymphomas, Most common subtype is extranodal marginal zone lymphoma (EMZL, MALT lymphoma) Translocations between chromosomes 14 and 18 or between 3 and 14 for EMZL Other etiologies include Ig-G4 related disease, Sjogren's syndrome, and gastric *H. pylori* infection (Vest et al. 2020)	>60 years' old More commonly female (Andreoli et al. 2015)	None	None	Small cells diffusely infiltrating with abundant cytoplasms Homogenous	Local radiotherapy when localized in orbit, Chemotherapy and rituximab when widespread

13.5 Congenital Disorders

13.5.1 Lacrimo-Auriculo-Dento-Digital (LADD) Syndrome AKA Levy-Hollister Syndrome or Ohdo-Bleph

LADD syndrome is an autosomal dominant disorder caused by mutations in the fibroblast growth factor receptor 2 (FGFR2) and its ligand, FGF10. FGFR2 is a tyrosine kinase receptor, and mutations in this receptor lead to decreased tyrosine phosphorylation and reduced ligand recruitment. Various tissues in the body are under the direction of the FGFR1-4 proteins involved in development and maintenance. This syndrome is characterized by aplasia of the lacrimal and salivary glands, along with other features such as small, cup-shaped, low-set ears, hypo and microdontia, hearing loss, and malformation digits. It may be confused with other lacrimal and salivary gland syndrome due to overlapping symptoms related to aplasia. (Lew et al. 2007)

13.5.2 Congenital Nasolacrimal Duct Obstruction

This condition is relatively common, affecting about 5–20% of newborns. It occurs due to incomplete canalization at the distal end of the nasolacrimal duct, leading to the formation of an imperforate membrane at the valve of Hasner (Fig. 13.4). This blockage in the nasolacrimal duct system results in excessive tearing and mucoid discharge (Perez et al. 2023; Vagge et al. 2018).

13.5.3 Congenital Accessory Canaliculi

Congenital canalicular duplication occurs in rare cases due to additional epithelial bud development from the upper lacrimal cord between the 18th and 24th week of embryological development. This condition is frequently asymptomatic, requiring no treatment. However, symptomatic cases may require surgical excision of the accessory canaliculi with direct suture closure.

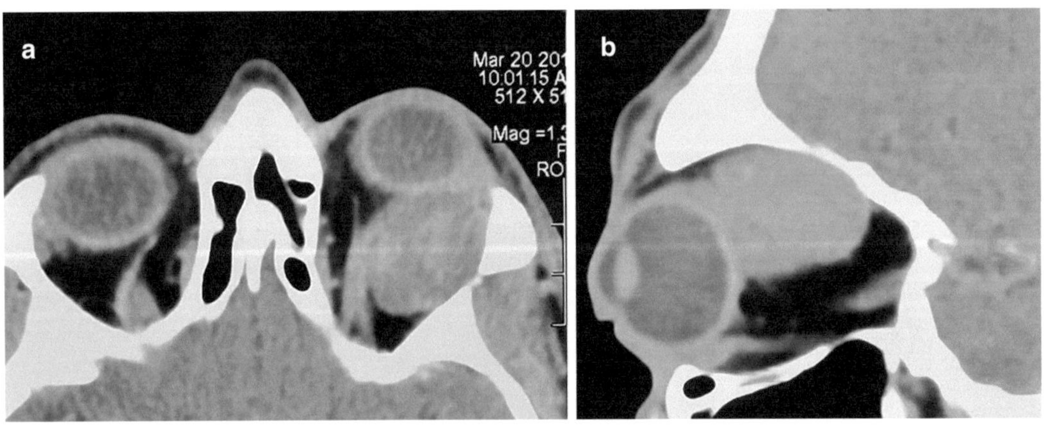

Fig. 13.4 Pleomorphic adenoma of the lacrimal gland. (**a**) Axial orbital CT with contrast, and (**b**) Sagittal contrast CT of the left orbit demonstrate a well-defined, moderately enhancing solid lesion occupying the left lacrimal gland fossa. The lesion exerts significant mass effect on the posterior globe, leading to proptosis. Additionally, the tumor is causing medial displacement of the optic nerve. There is associated bony remodeling

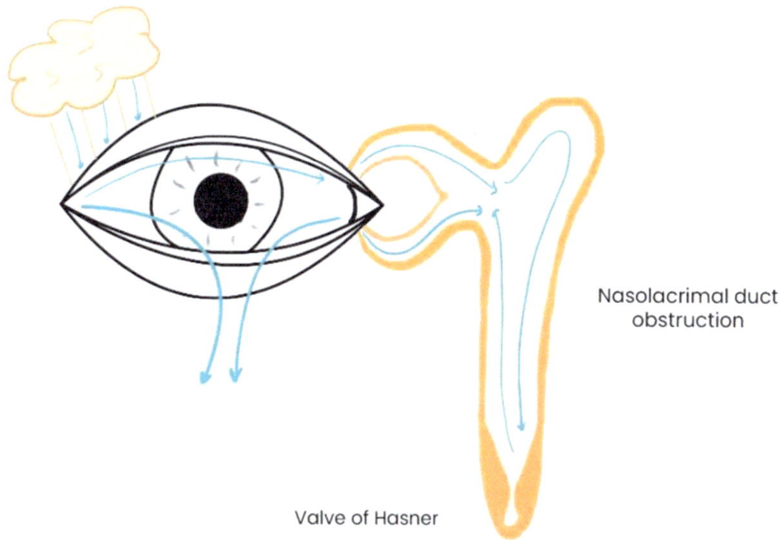

Fig. 13.5 Congenital nasolacrimal duct obstruction effect on drainage system

13.5.4 Congenital Lacrimal-Cutaneous Fistula

The formation of a rare fistula from the lacrimal sac to the medial canthus is termed a congenital lacrimal cutaneous fistula. This condition may present asymptomatically if the underlying canalicular system and lacrimal sac are intact and normally functioning. However, a third of patients with congenital lacrimal-cutaneous fistulae are present with an associated nasolacrimal duct obstruction which is often characterized by chronic mucopurulent discharge and onto the skin (Fig 13.5). These cases may require surgical excision and primary closure.

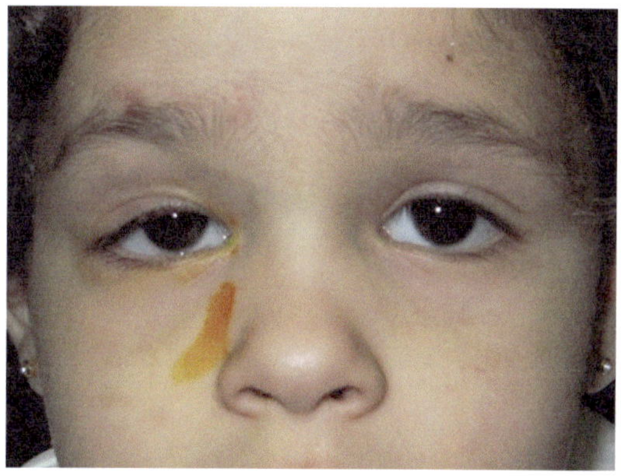

Fig. 13.6 A close-up photo of a young girl showing right upper lid mild ptosis, right increased lacrimal lake compared to left eye and leakage of fluorescein from a skin fistula from the lacrimal sac due to congenital nasolacrimal duct obstruction

13.5.5 Dacryocystocele

Dacryocystocele is a type of mucocele that occurs within the lacrimal sac with or without extension into nasal cavity secondary to congenital nasolacrimal duct obstruction. This condition typically presents at birth or between 1 and 4 weeks and occurs via the trapping of lacrimal sac goblet cell secreted mucus at the distal end of the nasolacrimal duct (valve of Hasner obstruction) as well as a functional obstruction of the valve of Rosenmüller (Fig. 13.6). Extension of the intranasal cystic portion commonly extends below the inferior nasal turbinate; thus, bilateral presentation warrants prompt examination and treatment due to the potential for airway obstruction resulting in difficulties with nasal breathing and breast feeding as newborns are preferential nasal breathers.

Conservative treatment involves prophylactic topical antibiotics and digital compression. However, probing and irrigation with possible inferior turbinate infracture may be required if infection occurs or symptoms fail to resolve. For recurrent cases, intubation with a lacrimal stent, balloon dacryoplasty, or dacryorhinostomy may be performed.

It is important to note that in the occurrence of swelling superior to the medial canthal tendon, consideration should be given to alternate diagnoses, such as meningoencephalocele or dermoid cysts, which should be evaluated appropriately with CT or MRI studies.

13.5.6 Lacrimal Gland Agenesis

Agenesis or aplasia of the lacrimal gland is rare and may occur alongside congenital abnormality of the salivary glands. It has been reported to be inherited in an autosomal dominant fashion. Treatment with occluded punctal plugs and lubricant is typically well tolerated.

13.6 Acquired Lacrimal Drainage Obstruction

Excessive tearing can be either:

- Hypersecretion (lacrimation)
- Impairment or obstruction of drainage (epiphora)

There is a wide differential, as detailed in Table 13.2.

Table 13.2 Acquired lacrimal drainage etiologies and their characteristics

Causes	Predisposing factors	Etiologies	Diagnosis	Clinical features	Management
Pseudoepiphora	Prior facial nerve injury or surgery Prior parotid gland surgery or inflammation	Aberrant nerve regeneration following damage to facial nerve or branches leading to abnormal connections between lacrimal and salivary glands Allergic conjunctivitis Irritant conjunctivitis Infection Anticholinergic or antidepressants	Evaluation of corneal and conjunctival epithelium Schirmer test, past medical history	Excessive tearing in response to gustatory or emotional stimuli Normal or increased tear production with no evidence of tear obstruction Absence of structural abnormalities in lacrimal system Absence of any symptoms suggestive of dry eye	Botulinum toxin injections to lacrimal gland Artificial tears in reflex tearing
Nasolacrimal duct obstruction (NLD)	Age History of facial trauma/surgery Anatomical abnormalities	Chronic inflammation Tumors, Trauma Stones Scarring	Diagnostic imaging (dacryocystography, dacryoscintillography), Syringing test	Epiphora Mucus discharge Recurrent infections (dacryocystitis) Pain, swelling, or tenderness over lacrimal sac Regurgitation upon pressure or syringing test	Topical antibiotics Surgical intervention dacryocystorhinostomy (DCR) Endoscopic dacryocystorhinostomy
Canalicular obstruction	Age History of facial trauma/surgery Anatomical abnormalities, Topical eye drops	Dislodged lacrimal plugs Tumor Stones Inflammation Trauma Systemic chemotherapeutic agents	Diagnostic probing Syringing test Partial obstruction may be discovered during lacrimal system irrigation	Epiphora Mucus discharge Recurrent infections Pain, swelling, or tenderness along the medial canthal region Regurgitation upon syringing test from same punctum	Canalicular stenting Reconstruction, canalicular dacryocystorhinostomy Conjunctival dacryocystorhinostomy (Lester Jones tube placement)

(continued)

Table 13.2 (continued)

Causes	Predisposing factors	Etiologies	Diagnosis	Clinical features	Management
Lacrimal sac tumor	Age Gender (more common in females) History of chronic inflammation Genetic factors	Benign or malignant tumors	Biopsy Diagnostic imaging	Epiphora Recurrent infections Pain, swelling, or telangiectasia over lacrimal sac Palpable mass over the lacrimal sac, bloody reflux upon syringing	Surgical excision Radiation therapy Systemic chemotherapy
Punctal disorders	Age History of inflammation or infection or prior irrigation	Scarring inflammation (Steven-Johnson syndrome) Infectious diseases Glaucoma medication Prior lacrimal plugs or cautery	Increased tear meniscus height, punctal occlusion on slit lamp, Delayed Fluorescein dye disappearance test	Epiphora, Ocular irritation, Punctal stenosis or abnormally large puncta	Punctal dilation, punctoplasty, punctal perporated plugs, or self-retaining bicanailcular intubation

13.7 Lacrimal System Inflammation

There are different causes of lacrimal gland or drainage system inflammation, as detailed in Table 13.3.

Table 13.3 Lacrimal gland or drainage system inflammation characteristics

Causes	Predisposing factors	Etiologies	Diagnosis	Clinical features	Management
Dacryocystitis	Previous history of chronic/ recurrent infections and obstruction	Obstruction of the nasolacrimal duct which leads to tear stasis and subsequent infection of the lacrimal sac	Clinical examination, swelling, pain and redness in the medial canthus area	Tearing, redness, swelling, pain, and tenderness over the lacrimal sac Purulent discharge with or without Fever	Oral and/or topical antibiotics, warm compresses, dacryocystorhinostomy (DCR) if conservative treatment fails
Canaliculitis	Previous history of chronic/ recurrent infections	Infection of the canaliculi, often secondary to obstruction or trauma	Clinical examination, microbiological tests	Tearing, redness, swelling, pain, and tenderness over the affected canaliculus Purulent discharge, punctal pouting	Topical and/or systemic antibiotics, Removal of any foreign bodies or concretions in the canaliculus Incision and curettage Canaliculoplasty or canaliculotomy if conservative treatment fails
Dacryoadenitis	Previous history of chronic/ recurrent infections, connective tissue disorders	Infection of the lacrimal gland Pathogenic etiologies Bacterial: *Staphylococcus aureus, Streptococcus pneumoniae, Haemophilus influenzae* Viral: *Adenovirus, Epstein–Barr, Cytomegalovirus* Fungal: *Aspergillus species, Candida species, Mucor species*	Clinical examination, imaging tests (CT, MRI)	Pain and tenderness, S-shaped ptosis, redness Fever, upper eyelid swelling mainly laterally, reduced lacrimal secretions	Treatment depends on underlying cause Oral and/or topical antibiotics Systemic steroids, Antivirals Antifungals Biopsy for recurrent cases, supportive treatment for idiopathic cases

(continued)

Table 13.3 (continued)

Causes	Predisposing factors	Etiologies	Diagnosis	Clinical features	Management
Sarcoidosis	History of sarcoidosis or systemic disease	Non-caseating Granulomatous Inflammatory disease of unknown etiology that affects multiple organs, including the lacrimal gland	Clinical examination imaging tests (CT, MRI), lacrimal gland biopsy	Tearing pain, swelling, and redness Fever, upper eyelid swelling Systemic symptoms such as fatigue, fever, weight loss, and joint pain	Systemic steroids Immunosuppressive therapy
Granulomatosis with polyangiitis (Wegener's granulomatosis)	History of Wegener's granulomatosis or systemic disease	Necrotizing granulomatous vasculitis that affects multiple organs, including the lacrimal gland, sinuses and kidneys	Clinical examination Blood testing Imaging tests (CT, MRI), Sinusitis Biopsy	Tearing pain, swelling, and redness Fever, upper eyelid swelling Systemic symptoms such as fatigue, fever, weight loss, and joint pain	Systemic steroids Immunosuppressive therapy
Orbital pseudotumor	Unknown, mostly isolated	Inflammatory disorder that affects the orbit, including the lacrimal gland	Clinical examination Imaging tests (CT, MRI)	Tearing pain, swelling, and redness, Fever, proptosis, diplopia and restriction of eye movements	Depends on the severity and duration of symptoms Systemic steroids, immunosuppressive therapy, radiation therapy

13.8 Lacrimal Gland Dysfunction

There are different causes of lacrimal gland dysfunction, as detailed in Table 13.4.

Table 13.4 Lacrimal gland dysfunction and their characteristics

Causes	Predisposing factors	Etiologies	Diagnosis	Clinical features	Management
Aqueous tear deficiency	Aging, systemic autoimmune diseases, hormonal changes, environmental factors	Medications (antihistamines, antidepressants, beta-blockers, diuretics, anticholinergics, isotretinoin)	Schirmer's test, tear breakup time test, fluorescein staining	Dryness, burning sensations, itching, redness, blurred vision, photophobia, gritty sensation	Artificial tears, punctal occlusion, anti-inflammatory therapy
Hypersecretory disorders	Neurological disorders	Medications (cholinergics, prostaglandin analogs, topical corticosteroids, topical NSAIDs, systemic medications), idiopathic	Clinical examination, patient history	Overproduction of tears, watery eyes, blurred vision	Surgery, botox injections
Sjogren's syndrome	Genetic predisposition, autoimmune disorders	Lymphocytic infiltration of the lacrimal and salivary glands Presence of autoantibodies, anti-SSA, and anti-SSB	Schirmer's test Biopsy of salivary gland Patient history	Dryness, burning sensations, itching, redness, blurred vision, photophobia systemic, symptoms such as fatigue, fever, weight loss and joint pain	Artificial tears Punctal occlusion Systemic immunosuppressive therapy
Non-Sjogren's syndrome	Systemic autoimmune diseases (RA, SLE, scleroderma, etc.) Environmental factors	Infection Lymphocytic infiltration of the lacrimal glands	Biopsy of the lacrimal gland Patient history	Dryness, burning sensations, itching, redness, blurred vision, photophobia	Artificial tears Punctal occlusion Systemic immunosuppressive therapy
Graft-versus-host disease	Allogeneic, hematopoietic stem cell transplantation	Immune reaction of donor cells against the recipient's tissue	Clinical history and examination Biopsy of lacrimal gland	Dryness, burning sensations, itching, redness, blurred vision, photophobia	Artificial tears Systemic immunosuppressive therapy Autologous serum eye drops
Neurogenic keratoconjunctivitis	Neurological disorders (MS, Parkinson's disease, trigeminal neuralgia), Horner's syndrome, Herpes zoster ophthalmicus Diabetes	Medications (anticholinergic, antidepressants, antipsychotics, antihistamines, anti-seizures medications, Parkinson's disease medications), idiopathic	Schirmer's test, fluorescein staining, patient history	Dryness, burning sensations, itching, redness, blurred vision, photophobia	Address underlying condition Artificial tears Punctal occlusion Anti-inflammatory therapy

13.9 Lacrimal Gland Trauma

Direct: blunt force trauma to the upper outer aspect of the orbit

- Pain, swelling, and tenderness over the gland
- Decreased tear production
- Visual disturbances secondary to tear insufficiency

Indirect: eyelid is forcefully closed when there is a sudden increase in intraorbital pressure, such as a motor vehicle accident

- Pain, swelling, and tearing
- Ecchymosis around the eyelid

Iatrogenic: may occur as a complication of surgical procedures in the orbit or upper eyelid, such as blepharoplasty or orbital decompression

- Pain and swelling
- Decreased tear production
- Abnormal positioning or shape of the gland

13.10 Surgical Management

Surgical management of lacrimal drainage system obstruction is detailed in Table 13.5.

Table 13.5 Surgical management of lacrimal drainage system obstruction

Surgical management	Description	Indications	Potential complications
Probing and irrigation	A procedure in which the lacrimal drainage system is flushed with saline or water solution using a small probe and special cannula inserted into the puncta	Congenital nasolacrimal duct obstruction, acquired nasolacrimal duct obstruction due to stenosis or chronic inflammation	Minor complications include bleeding, infection, major complications such as damage to the punctae and/or canaliculus with secondary stenosis, or obstruction. Rarely, canalicular or lacrimal sac perforation can occur or false passage creation
Intubation	A silicone tube is inserted into the lacrimal drainage system to help keep the system patent and promote drainage	Epiphora due to punctal or canalicular stenosis, nasolacrimal duct obstruction, failed previous probing	Minor complications include tube displacement, infection, and tube extrusion (conjunctival prolapse)
Balloon dacryoplasty	A small balloon catheter is inserted into the nasolacrimal duct and inflated to dilate the narrow segment of the duct	Congenital nasolacrimal duct obstruction due to stenosis, failed previous probing	Minor complications include bleeding, infection. Rarely, major complications such as damage to the punctae, canalicular laceration, or lacrimal sac perforation can occur
Turbinate infracture	The inferior turbinate is infractured to create more space in the nasal cavity and facilitate nasolacrimal duct drainage	Nasolacrimal duct obstruction due to nasal mucosal swelling, congenital nasolacrimal duct obstruction	Minor complications include bleeding, infection, and nasal crusting

(continued)

Table 13.5 (continued)

Surgical management	Description	Indications	Potential complications
Dacryocystorhinostomy (DCR)	A surgical procedure that connects the lacrimal sac directly into the nasal cavity to bypass the obstructed nasolacrimal duct	Chronic dacryocystitis, nasolacrimal duct obstruction refractory to other treatments, dacryocystocele	Minor complications include bleeding, infection, and damage to surrounding structures such as the medial canthal tendon, nasal mucosa, or septum. Rarely, major complications such as cerebrospinal fluid leak or injury to the orbit can occur. Minimal skin scar
Endoscopic DCR	A minimally invasive DCR procedure that uses an endoscope to visualize nasal cavity and access the lacrimal sac	Chronic dacryocystitis, nasolacrimal duct obstruction Absence of skin scar	Minor complications include bleeding, infection, and damage to surrounding structures such as the medial canthal tendon or the nasal mucosa. Rarely, major complications such as cerebrospinal fluid leak or injury to the orbit can occur
Conjunctivodacryocystorhinostomy (C-DCR)	A modification of the DCR procedure with complete bypass of the lacrimal drainage system in which the canalicular system can't be used or reconstructed. A Jones tube is placed through the osteotomy directly into the middle nasal meatus	Symptomatic patients with complete absence of the punctae and/or one or both of the canalicular system	Tube obstruction with mucous, tube migration, periodic tube cleaning, chronic foreign body sensation, pyogenic granuloma formation
Canaliculodacryocystorhinostomy	The obstructed area of common canaliculus is removed and patent canalicular directly anastomosed to lateral nasal wall mucosa using silicone stent	Obstructed common canaliculus or sclerotic lacrimal sac	High failure rate, need for Jones tube placement later on
Lacrimal punctal	Silicone plugs are inserted into the puncta to block the lacrimal drainage system and increase tear retention (occluded plug), or to increase drainage in cases of punctal stenosis (perforated plugs)	Aqueous tear deficiency (occluded plug), epiphora due to punctual stenosis (perforated plugs)	Discomfort, epiphora and plug extrusion or migration, foreign body sensation, pyogenic granuloma formation

Acknowledgment None.

Conflict of Interest None.

Further Reading

Ababneh OH, Msallam MM (2014) Bilateral simultaneous pyogenic granuloma after perforated punctal plug insertion. Ophthal Plast Reconstr Surg 30(5):e113–e115. https://doi.org/10.1097/IOP.0b013e3182a5ba6b

Ababneh OH, AboTaleb EA, Abu Ameerh MA, Yousef YA (2015) Enucleation and evisceration at a tertiary care hospital in a developing country. BMC Ophthalmol 15:120. https://doi.org/10.1186/s12886-015-0108-x

Allen R (2014) Hereditary disorders affecting the lacrimal system. Curr Opin Ophthalmol:25. https://doi.org/10.1097/ICU.0000000000000092

Ali MJ (ed) (2018) Principles and practice of lacrimal surgery. Springer

Al-Ryalat NT, Ezzat JW, Ababneh OH, AlRyalat SA, Al-Hadidy AM (2016) Isolated bilateral lacrimal gland agenesis. J Pediatr Ophthalmol Strabismus 53:e35–e38. https://doi.org/10.3928/01913913-20160719-01

AlRyalat SA (2021) Basics of lacrimal system for ophthalmology board exams. Springer. https://doi.org/10.1007/978-981-16-2968-6_4

American Academy of Ophthalmology (2023) Basic and clinical science course. Section 7. Orbit, Eyelids and Lacrimal System, San Francisco, United States of America

Conrady CD, Joos ZP, Patel BC (2016) Review: the lacrimal gland and its role in dry eye. J Ophthalmol 2016:7542929

Daniel L, Rao S, Muthusamy R, Yerramsetti D (2014) Mucoepidermoid carcinoma ex pleomorphic adenoma of the lacrimal gland: a rare presentation. Indian J Ophthalmol 62(6):743

Dickinson AJ, Perros P (2001) Controversies in the clinical evaluation of active thyroid-associated orbitopathy: use of a detailed protocol with comparative photographs for objective assessment. Clin Endocrinol (Oxf) 55(3):283–303. https://doi.org/10.1046/j.1365-2265.2001.01349.x

Denniston A, Murray P (eds) (2014) Oxford handbook of ophthalmology. Oxford University Press

Dolman PJ (2018) 'Grading severity and activity in thyroid eye disease. Ophthal Plast Reconstr Surg 34(4S):S34. https://doi.org/10.1097/IOP.0000000000001150

Gordin E, Lee TS, Ducic Y, Arnaoutakis D (2015) Facial nerve trauma: evaluation and considerations in management. Craniomaxillofac Trauma Reconstr 8(1):1–13

Hollsten LD (1992) Complications of lacrimal surgery. Int Ophthalmol Clin 32(4):49–66

Hotta K, Arisawa T, Mito H, Narita M (2005) Primary squamous cell carcinoma of the lacrimal gland. Clin Exp Ophthalmol 33:534–536. https://doi.org/10.1111/j.1442-9071.2005.01043.x

Jenkins C et al (2003) Clinical features associated with survival of patients with lymphoma of the ocular adnexa. Eye (Lond) 17(7):809–820

Kanski JJ (2019) Kanski's clinical ophthalmology E-book: a systematic approach. 6th and 9th ed. Elsevier Health Sciences

Khatib N, Ionescu IC, Briscoe D, Saeed P (2021) Adenoid cystic carcinoma of the lacrimal gland. Adv Ophthalmol Optom 6:147–158

Korn BS, Setabutr P, Burkat CN, Steele EA, Carter KD, Vagefi MR, Perry JD (2021) Basic and clinical science course, Section 7: oculofacial plastic and orbital surgery. American Academy of Ophthalmology

Lew ED, Bae JH, Rohmann E, Wollnik B, Schlessinger J (2007) Structural basis for reduced FGFR2 activity in LADD syndrome: implications for FGFR autoinhibition and activation. Proc Natl Acad Sci 104(50):19802–19807

Nagendran S, Alsamnan M, Strianese D, Malhotra R (2020) Ectopic lacrimal gland tissue: a systematic review. Ophthal Plast Reconstr Surg 36(6):540–544

Paulsen F, Schaudig U, Thale AB (2003) Drainage of tears: impact on the ocular surface and lacrimal system. Ocul Surf 1(4):180–191

Perez Y, Patel BC, Mendez MD (2023) Nasolacrimal duct obstruction. In: StatPearls. Treasure Island. StatPearls Publishing, (FL)

Persson M, Andren Y, Mark J, Horlings HM, Persson F, Stenman G (2009) Recurrent fusion of MYB and NFIB transcription factor genes in carcinomas of the breast and head and neck. Proc Natl Acad Sci U S A 106:18740–18744

Rahman A, Yahya K, Fasih U, Waqar-ul-Huda SA (2012) Comparison of Schirmer's test and tear film breakup time test to detect tear. Int J Ophthalmol 5(2):163–166

Rose GE, Wright JE (1992) Pleomorphic adenoma of the lacrimal gland. Br J Ophthalmol 76:395–400

Salmon JF (2019) Kanski's clinical ophthalmology E-book: a systematic approach. Elsevier Health Sciences

Shields JA, Shields CL, Epstein JA et al (2004) Primary epithelial malignancies of the lacrimal gland. The 2003 Ramon L. Font lecture. Ophthal Plast Reconstr Surg 20:10–21

Vagge A, Ferro Desideri L, Nucci P, Serafino M, Giannaccare G, Lembo A, Traverso CE (2018) Congenital Nasolacrimal Duct Obstruction (CNLDO): a review. Diseases 6(4):96

Vest SD, Mikkelsen LH, Holm F, Rasmussen PK, Hindso TG, Knudsen MK et al (2020) Lymphoma of the lacrimal gland—an international multicenter retrospective study. Am J Ophthalmol 219:107–120

von Holstein SL, Coupland SE, Briscoe D, Le Tourneau C, Heegaard S (2013) Epithelial tumours of the lacrimal gland: a clinical, histopathological, surgical and oncological survey. Acta Ophthalmol 91(3):195–206

Wright JE, Rose GE, Garner A (1992) Primary malignant neoplasms of the lacrimal gland. Br J Ophthalmol 76:401–407

Clinical Review of Cornea: Part I

14

Muawyah Al Bdour, Ahmed Alsaadi, Amna Almaazmi, and Saif Aldeen Alryalat

Abstract

This chapter provides a foundational overview of the cornea, emphasizing its role and importance in ophthalmology. It explores benign corneal changes and depositions, helping readers differentiate between natural variations and potential underlying issues. The discussion extends to congenital corneal anomalies and degenerative diseases, focusing on inherited conditions, their etiology, manifestations, and treatment options. Special attention is given to corneal dystrophies and ectasia, which present unique challenges for diagnosis and management. The chapter also highlights the significance of corneal tomography as a vital diagnostic tool, emphasizing its role in modern ophthalmological practice. By the end, readers will be well-equipped to diagnose and manage various corneal conditions effectively, ensuring timely and appropriate treatment.

Keywords

Cornea · Degenerative corneal disease · Ectasia · Corneal tomography · Inherited conditions

M. Al Bdour
Department of Ophthalmology, The University of Jordan, Amman, Jordan

A. Alsaadi
Zayed Military Hospital, Abu Dhabi, United Arab Emirates

Shaikh Khalifa Medical City, Abu Dhabi, United Arab Emirates

Sharjah University, Sharjah, United Arab Emirates

A. Almaazmi
Zayed Military Hospital, Abu Dhabi, United Arab Emirates

Sharjah University, Sharjah, United Arab Emirates

S. A. Alryalat (✉)
Department of Ophthalmology, The University of Jordan, Amman, Jordan

The University of Colorado Anschutz Medical Campus, CO, USA
e-mail: s.alryalat@ju.edu.jo

14.1 Overview

This chapter is a comprehensive guide dedicated to offering an in-depth understanding of various aspects related to the cornea, a key structure in ocular health and vision. As an ophthalmologist or an ophthalmology trainee, gaining a robust knowledge about the intricacies of the cornea and its pathologies is indispensable for effectively diagnosing and treating a wide range of conditions that could impact a patient's vision. This chapter is meticulously crafted to meet this requirement, providing detailed insights into every facet of the cornea, from benign changes to complex disorders.

S. A. Alryalat (ed.), *Ophthalmology Board and FRCS Part 2 Exams*,
https://doi.org/10.1007/978-981-96-1517-9_14

Clinical ophthalmology questions pertaining to this chapter's content are likely to be distributed across various areas of examination such as multiple choice questions (MCQs), structured oral examinations (SOEs), and objective structured clinical examinations (OSCEs). In the written section, often comprising MCQs, you can expect to encounter questions on corneal anatomy, congenital anomalies, degenerative diseases, dystrophies, ectasia, and the various types of keratitis. The questions often test knowledge of etiology, clinical presentation, diagnostic techniques including corneal tomography, and management strategies. This section often carries a considerable mark weight, around 15–20%, due to the broad range of topics covered. During the SOEs, examiners will evaluate your theoretical knowledge and understanding the clinical application. You may be presented with a clinical scenario such as a patient presenting with symptoms of infectious keratitis or corneal dystrophy, and be asked to discuss potential diagnoses, investigations, and treatment options. This can represent around 10–15% of the total mark weight. OSCEs typically test your practical skills, such as interpreting corneal tomography images or demonstrating how to educate a patient about post-keratoplasty care. You may also be asked to explain procedures such as different types of keratoplasty or corneal refractive approaches. This component usually carries a similar mark weight to the SOE, about 10–15%.

Starting with a concise overview, the chapter lays a solid foundation to familiarize readers with the basics of the cornea's role, function, and importance in ophthalmology. We then delve into the subtle yet critical benign corneal changes, and corneal depositions, help the readers to understand the difference between natural variations and symptoms of underlying issues.

Congenital corneal anomalies and degenerative corneal diseases sections delve into the world of inherited and progressive conditions, highlighting their etiology, manifestation, and potential treatment options. Special attention is given to corneal dystrophies and ectasia, and common disorders that present unique challenges to ophthalmologists. A thorough understanding of these sections will equip readers to diagnose these conditions accurately, enabling timely and effective treatment.

The chapter further emphasizes corneal tomography, a vital diagnostic tool that aids in visualizing and examining the cornea. With advancements in technology, its knowledge becomes even more crucial in modern ophthalmology practice. Following this, we delve into infectious and interstitial keratitis, two serious corneal conditions that can lead to severe vision loss if not treated promptly and effectively.

The Peripheral Ulcerative Keratopathy (PUK) section provides detailed insights into this less common, but potentially severe corneal disease primarily associated with systemic conditions. The chapter then moves onto a discussion about metabolic syndromes that affect the cornea, exploring the genetic and biochemical causes behind these disorders.

Keratoplasty, a significant surgical intervention involving the cornea, is discussed extensively, presenting its types, indications, techniques, and key considerations for successful outcomes. Lastly, we cover a range of miscellaneous topics that are crucial to a well-rounded understanding of the cornea and its related conditions.

In essence, this chapter serves as an exhaustive resource for anyone aiming to gain a deeper knowledge about the cornea, improving their proficiency in managing corneal conditions and contributing to better patient care in ophthalmology.

14.2 Benign Corneal Changes

The cornea undergoes various changes as we age, affecting different layers including the Descemet's and Bowman's membranes, the stroma, and the endothelial cells. The thickness of Descemet's and Bowman's membranes gradually increases with age, while the stroma generally remains constant. The corneal endothelium has a higher concentration of cells at the periphery, which naturally declines with age at a reported rate of around 0.6% annually.

Moreover, the cornea can exhibit a 5% increase in thickness during sleep or with the use of carbonic anhydrase inhibitors. An interesting transformation in astigmatism is observed as one ages, where with-the-rule astigmatism tends to convert to against-the-rule astigmatism. This phenomenon is primarily attributed to the continuous growth of the lens throughout life.

Several normal age-related changes occur in different corneal layers:

- *Epithelium*: The Hudson-Stahli line is a product of iron deposition in the epithelial cell cytoplasm. This is more concentrated in the basal cells and produces a horizontal pigmented line.
- *Bowman's layer*: The Limbal Girdle of Vogt appears as a yellowish opacity at 3 and 9 o'clock positions, indicative of elastotic degeneration of Bowman's layer, which may include calcium deposits.
- *Stroma*: Cornea farinata is an asymptomatic fine deposit located centrally in the deep stroma (near Descemet). It is best viewed by retro illumination.
- *Descemet*: Hassall-Henle bodies are outgrowths at the posterior surface of Descemet's membrane that occur peripherally as part of the aging process, and centrally in Fuchs' endothelial dystrophy cases. They also appear as corneal guttata, indicative of endothelial dysfunction, where the endothelium is displaced posteriorly.

Arcus senilis (Fig. 14.1), also known as cornea senilis, are lipid deposits forming rings in the cornea's outer region. These deposits are typically gray or white and often denser in the superior and inferior regions. Over time, they may expand and eventually form a complete ring around the cornea. This condition is nearly universal in patients over the age of 80. If similar findings appear in younger individuals, it is referred to as arcus juvenilis, and hyperlipidemia should be considered.

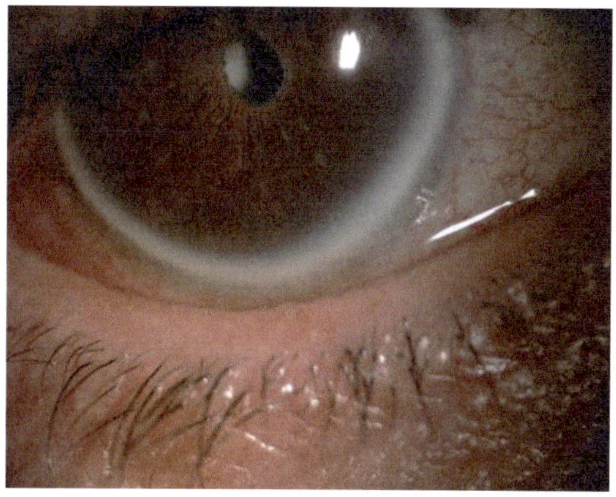

Fig. 14.1 A colored photograph showing arcus senilis

14.3 Corneal Depositions

Deposition in the corneal epithelium by either *crystal* (crystalline keratopathy) or *other materials* (vorticella keratopathy) has been described as follows. On the other hand, metals, among other *materials* (copper, gold, iron, silver, antacid, phenothiazines, and retinoid depositions) have been described to cause Bowman and stromal deposition. Almost all of them are not visually significant.

Crystalline keratopathy: crystals are deposited in the corneal epithelium and/or anterior stroma.

- Strep. viridans (alpha-hemolytic Streptococcus species) is the most common infectious cause.
- Dystrophy: Schnyder crystalline corneal dystrophy and Bietti crystalline corneo-retinal dystrophy.
- Cystinosis and tyrosinemia.
- Systemic paraproteinemia, such as multiple myeloma.
- Drugs: Topical fluoroquinolone, mainly ciprofloxacin. Systemic Tamoxifen in rare case reports.

Cornea verticillate (vortex keratopathy) is caused by deposits at the level of the basal epithelium forming a faint golden-brown whorl pattern. Most commonly associated with amiodarone.

They are generally visually insignificant so that they can be observed. Potential causes include:

- Medications (including amiodarone, indomethacin, chloroquine/hydroxychloroquine, chlorpromazine, naproxen, and tamoxifen).
- Fabry disease (X-linked alpha-galactosidase deficiency), vortex found in 90% of cases.
- Multiple myeloma
- Neurotrophic keratitis
- Lisch corneal dystrophy
- Epidemic keratoconjunctivitis
- Iron deposition (i.e., after radial keratotomy)

Amiodarone causes vortex keratopathy, characterized by deposits in the corneal epithelium. Even when these deposits are dense, they rarely lead to vision loss. The deposits can appear as early as 2 weeks after starting the drug and are likely to occur in most patients after 4 months of treatment. Although it may take up to a year for the deposits to clear, the changes are generally reversible once the drug is stopped. However, discontinuation of the drug is not required, and there is no need for epithelial debridement.

Note: Chlorpromazine is also associated with pigmentary retinopathy.

In cystinosis, the cystine deposits begin centrally within the anterior stroma and progress to involve the entire cornea.

Band keratopathy is bilateral calcium deposition mainly on Bowman's membrane.

It is also important to know the layer affected in each of the following conditions:

- Amiodarone keratopathy → affects the epithelium (vortex)
- Chlorpromazine → affects the epithelium (vortex)
- Chloroquine → affects epithelium (vortex)
- Band keratopathy, calcium → affects Bowman's membrane
- Chrysiasis → affects deep corneal stroma (Gold deposition)
- Wilson disease, copper → affects Descemet's membrane

Kaye dots are white punctate epithelial opacities anterior to a corneal graft suture line (Fig. 14.2). The dots represent epithelial cells in various stages of degeneration, and it has been hypothesized that they may result from an epithelial response to the area of tissue angulation. They are visually insignificant.

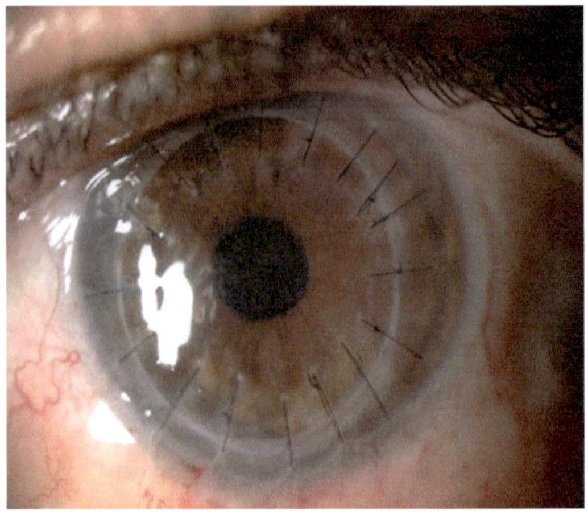

Fig. 14.2 Colored photograph showing Kaye dots around keratoplasty sutures

Other Materials

- Copper:

  In Wilson disease, copper accumulates in the peripheral Descemet's membrane of the cornea, forming a *Kayser–Fleischer ring*. This ring appears as a golden brown, ruby red, or green pigment, initially starting at the superior cornea and gradually spreading to meet deposits at the inferior cornea. There is no visible copper accumulation in the epithelium, Bowman's layer, or stroma. The Kayser–Fleischer ring typically disappears with appropriate treatment, making it a useful marker for monitoring therapy.
- Gold:

  Gold usage can lead to a condition known as *chrysiasis*, characterized by gold deposits in the deep stroma of the cornea, usually located in the periphery.
- Iron:

  Iron deposition in the corneal epithelium typically occurs during chronic inflammatory processes, appearing as a yellowish-to-brown line. This process is associated with several distinct formations:

- When the deposition occurs at the edge of a pterygium, it is known as Stocker's line.
- When observed around the keratoconus, the line is called Fleischer's ring.
- The line is referred to as Ferry's line at the edge of a trabeculectomy bleb.
- In the corneas of elderly individuals, this phenomenon manifests as the Hudson-Stahli line.

14.4 Congenital Corneal Anomalies

14.4.1 Posterior Keratoconus

Posterior keratoconus is typically unilateral (unlike KC), sporadic conditions are more common in women and present from birth.

Unlike keratoconus, it involves localized thinning of the posterior cornea without protrusion of the anterior corneal surface (intact Bowman, holding the anterior cornea intact). Posterior excavation may occur in multiple areas, often central or paracentral, with a generalized form potentially involving much of the cornea again, mostly central area. Thinning of the cornea can reduce stromal substance to one-third of its normal thickness. While the ectasia is usually stable, gradual progression can occur. The condition is associated with localized endothelial damage, corneal opacity, and focal deposits of pigment and guttae at the margins of the affected areas. Subtle irregularities in the anterior corneal over the area of posterior involvement can cause irregular astigmatism and amblyopia.

A congenital form of posterior keratoconus, inherited in autosomal recessive pattern, is believed to be part of anterior segment dysgenesis. This form is associated with bilateral corneal changes, short stature, intellectual disability, cleft lip and palate, and vertebral anomalies. Acquired posterior keratoconus can also occur, typically following trauma.

Posterior keratoconus may be a variant of Peters anomaly, but these conditions can be distinguished by the presence of Descemet's membrane, which is absent in Peters anomaly. Peters anomaly is marked a central or paracentral corneal opacity (leukoma) present at birth, resulting from the localized absence of the corneal endothelium and Descemet's membrane is beneath the area of opacity.

14.4.2 Sclerocornea

It is a nonprogressive, noninflammatory condition characterized by bilateral scleralization of the cornea. This scleralization may be limited to the corneal periphery or the entire cornea. The limbus is usually ill defined, with superficial vessels, extensions of normal scleral, episcleral, and conjunctival vessels crossing the cornea. While sclerocornea is usually sporadic, both autosomal dominant and recessive inheritance patterns have been reported, with no evident sex predilection. Only 10% of cases are unilateral.

The most common associated ocular finding is cornea plana, occuring in 80% of cases. Angle structures are also frequently malformed, and the condition is often associated with multiple systemic anomalies.

14.4.3 Congenital Anterior Staphyloma

This is a unilateral, sporadic condition characterized by an opaque cornea due to the absence of the endothelium and Descemet's membrane. The posterior cornea is lined by a thin layer of uveal tissue, and the anterior segment is usually markedly abnormal. Common abnormalities include iridocorneal adhesions, iris hypoplasia, and lens opacity. Exposure can lead to corneal scarring and keratinization, though inflammation is markedly absent. Unlike Peter's anomaly, congenital anterior staphyloma is usually unilateral, though the contralateral eye often shows some form of anterior segment abnormality. Cases are typically sporadic, with no familial or systemic association.

Post-natal keratectasia differs from congenital anterior staphyloma in that it lacks the thin layer of uveal tissue lining the posterior cornea.

Table 14.1 Comparison between different congenital corneal anomalies

	Microcornea	Megalocornea	Simple microphthalmia (anophthalmia)	Complex microphthalmia	Anophthalmia
Inheritance	AD	X-lined (90% males) mostly, or AD	Sporadic	Sporadic	Sporadic
Criteria[a]	Horizontal diameter <9 mm if <2 years OR <10 mm if >2 years	Horizontal diameter >13 mm for >2 years, >12 mm for <2 years	2SD below the mean for age	2SD below the mean for age	Complete absence globe, with remnant present
Ocular abnormality	Hypermetropia with shallow AC	High myopia with deep AC + astigmatism	Normal eye, but the lens is large Relative to the size of the eye, hypermetropia	Abnormal eye	Absence of extraocular muscles, short conjunctival sac, and microblepharon
Ocular association	Glaucoma, congenital cataract, leukoma, coloboma, aniridia	Lens subluxation, pigment dispersion, but normal IOP (compared to buphthalmos)	Uveal effusions associated with thickened sclera, glaucoma (especially angle-closure)	Dysgenesis, coloboma, orbital cyst	–
Systemic association		Down, Marfan, and Alport syndromes, craniosynostosis, and facial hemiatrophy	–	CNS abnormalities. Intrauterine infections, fetal alcohol syndrome	–
Notes	Associated with higher incidences of glaucoma following cataract surgery in children	Bilateral, non-progressive. Normal corrected VA	Usually bilateral	Even if unilateral, the other eye will be abnormal	–

[a]Normal corneal horizontal diameter is 10 mm <2 years and 12 mm >2 years

Keratectasia is thought to result from intrauterine keratitis or vitamin deficiency, leading to subsequent corneal perforation rather than an abnormal development process.

The visual prognosis for both congenital anterior staphyloma and post-natal keratectasia is poor due to the severe damage to the anterior segment associated with these conditions. Treatment options like penetrating keratoplasty and sclerokeratoplasty may help preserve the globe and improve cosmetic appearance. However, enucleation may be necessary for managing a painful, blind glaucomatous eye.

Other causes of congenital corneal anomalies are listed in Table 14.1.

14.5 Degenerative Diseases

Epithelial basement membrane dystrophy (EBMD): Approximately 50% of patients with recurrent corneal erosions are believed to have underlying EBMD, although only 10% of patients with EBMD will develop recurrent corneal erosions. Patterns of corneal epithelial findings evident on slit-lamp examination in eyes with EBMD include fingerprint lines, maps, dots, and a bleb pattern.

Superior limbic keratoconjunctivitis (SLK) is a bilateral chronic inflammation of the superior limbus and superior bulbar and tarsal conjunctivae. It is mostly idiopathic, and it is related to mechanical exposure of superior limbus, so it is associated with thyroid and collagen vascular diseases. Findings include giant papillary reaction in the upper tarsal conjunctiva (NOT follicular), and filamentary keratitis may develop.

Approximately half of the patients with SLK have some form of thyroid disease. But treating the thyroid condition typically has little impact on SLK itself.

Salzmann's nodular degeneration is characterized by scarring of the anterior stroma, often following trauma or recurrent infections, and is most commonly seen in middle-aged females. The nodules appear gray-white or blue-white, are elevated, and may be associated with recurrent erosions. Histologically, these nodules are composed of hyaline and fibrillar material replacing Bowman's layer. Amyloid degeneration, which can also result from corneal inflammation, or trauma, manifests as raised yellow-pink nodular masses in the cornea.

Patient typically reports a gradual loss of vision months after trauma, dry eye, trachoma infection, or surgery. Treatment may involve using an excimer laser following mechanical keratectomy to remove the anterior stromal scarring. Since Salzmann's nodular degeneration involves only partial thickness anterior stromal opacity, a full-thickness corneal transplant is not typically necessary.

Corneal keloids develop as a reaction to corneal perforation or injury and appear as white, protuberant masses, often resembling dermoids.

Lipid keratopathy occurs following prolonged corneal inflammation, characterized by yellow or cream-colored in areas of vascularized scarring.

Spheroidal degeneration (Actinic keratopathy) involves proteinaceous deposits (rather than lipid) as golden yellow spherules at the superficial corneal stroma and Bowman's membrane. The main etiology is sunlight exposure. It is usually bilateral and is more common in men. Stains with elastin stain.

On slit-lamp, aggregates of translucent, golden-brown globular deposits are noted in the interpalpebral superficial cornea in both eyes. Comparison between corneal depositions provided in Table 14.2.

Bullous keratopathy is a frequent consequence of corneal endothelial dysfunction, stemming from various causes. The most common types include pseudophakic bullous keratopathy, aphakic bullous keratopathy, and Fuchs endothelial dystrophy. Prior to diagnosing bullous keratopathy, it is important to rule out herpetic infection and high intraocular pressure (IOP), as these conditions can also cause reversible corneal edema.

In cases of painful bullous keratopathy in eyes with no visual potential, cauterization of Bowman's membrane and the anterior stroma may be considered. Diathermy is used to apply heat to the anterior stroma, creating a barrier that reduces fluid movement from the stroma to the epithelium, and thereby decreases bullae formation. This procedure can also help the epithelium adhere more securely to the stroma, reducing blister formation. If stromal cauterization does not provide relief, a conjunctival flap may be performed.

However, a conjunctival flap may lead to complications such as a less cosmetically pleasing appearance, reduced visibility of the anterior segment, and decreased effectiveness of topical ophthalmic medications in penetrating the anterior segment.

Thygeson superficial punctate keratitis is a bilateral, though sometimes asymmetrical, idiopathic condition characterized by punctate keratitis without an accompanying conjunctivitis. It commonly affects women in their 20 s and30s. Corneal sensation remains normal. The condition is highly responsive to topical corticosteroids, but

Table 14.2 Comparison between different degenerative corneal depositions

	Spheroidal degeneration	Lipid keratopathy	Salzmann's nodules
Appearance	Golden yellow spherules	Yellow or creamy scars	Nodules are gray-white
Deposition	Proteinaceous (elastnin)	Lipid	Amyloid
Etiology	Sun exposure (actinic)	Neovascularization	After trauma or infection

these may increase the risk of recurrence. Topical cyclosporine can also be beneficial. Individuals with the HLA-DR3 histocompatibility antigen have a 5.65 times greater relative risk of developing this condition. The disease is marked by recurrent episodes of corneal intraepithelial round opacities. Typically, about 20 oopacities are present in each eye, though up to 50 lesions have been reported. These lesions generally resolve within 4–6 weeks without leaving a trace but tend to recur frequently. The condition usually resolves after a few years, around 4 years, and is often asymptomatic between attacks.

Recurrent corneal erosions (RCE) of either dystrophic or traumatic origin can be treated with lubrication, application of hypertonic sodium chloride, therapeutic bandage lenses, pressure patching, anterior stromal puncture, or phototherapeutic keratectomy (PTK).

For eyes with post-traumatic recurrent erosions that do not involve the axial cornea or entrance pupil, anterior stromal micropuncture can be an effective treatment. This procedure promotes a firm adhesion between the corneal epithelium and the underlying stroma. However, it can cause visually significant scarring, so it should be used cautiously when the central or axial cornea is affected.

RCE usually usually manifests as sharp, unilateral pain upon awakening and is often linked to underlying conditions such as basement membrane dystrophy, previous ocular trauma, stromal dystrophy (most commonly Reis–Buckler dystrophy), or past eye surgeries like those for refractive errors, cataracts, or corneal transplantation. Management involves using preservative-free lubricating drops to maintain moisture in the cornea, along with topical cycloplegics, oral analgesics to control pain, in addition to topical corticosteroids, therapeutic bandage contact lenses. Other treatments include oral matrix metalloproteinase inhibitors to support epithelial repair, blood-derived eye drops for growth factors, amniotic membrane grafts to promote epithelial healing, and hypertonic saline solution or ointment to decrease corneal edema.

Surgical procedures include punctal occlusion with plugs which increases the tear film volume, epithelial debridement with diamond burr polishing, anterior stromal puncture, alcohol delamination, or excimer PTK.

Descemet's membrane tears:

- Curvilinear tears or horizontal ones → primary congenital glaucoma (Haab striae).
- Linear tears that are mostly vertical or oblique → forceps injury sustained during delivery.
- Linear vertical tears in adults → Vogt striae of KC.

The residual corneal changes can result in anisometropia, and the main cause of vision loss after such an injury is anisometropic amblyopia.

In pterygium, Bowman's layer always shows fragmentation.

14.6 Corneal Dystrophies

Mostly inherited corneal diseases are typically bilateral, symmetric, and slowly progressive (Soh et al. 2020; Weiss et al. 2015).

Inherited vs *familial*: If a disease is well known to be transmitted by family members, then it is familial. If the gene transmitted is identified, then it is termed inherited.

The first step in molecular testing is single gene sequencing directed to the known gene (e.g., CHST6 in macular dystrophy). If a gene is negative, a genetic panel would be the second step. Whole genome sequencing is left as a last resort, as this will sequence the all known genome.

Known genes and their respective dystrophy: TGFBI gene is the most commonly mutated gene in corneal dystrophy, located on chromosome 5, and follows autosomal dominant inheritance. It encodes a protein that binds to collagen 1,2,4 and inhibits cell adhesion. Found in Reis–Buckler, Thiel–Behnke, granular types 1 and 2, and lattice.

Meesman is due to mutation in KRT3, KRT12.

Macular dystrophy is due to CHST6 gene mutation.

14.6.1 Anterior Dystrophies

1. *Epithelial basement membrane dystrophy (EBMD)*

   Also known as Cogan dystrophy or map-dot-fingerprint.

   It is the most common anterior corneal dystrophy. Of an adult onset, where there is a defect in hemi-desmosomes that connect the basement with epithelium.

   Characterized by islands of basement membrane thickening and extension to epithelium, but the Bowman's membrane is intact.

   EBMD on exam represents four different components of corneal opacity include intraepithelial dot opacities (Cogan cysts) underlying map-like figures, and multiple crowded blebs.

   EBMD can be asymptomatic. It can manifest as recurrent bilateral epithelial erosions and/or may cause decreased vision by inducing mild irregular astigmatism. Irregular astigmatism results from irregular corneal contour from unevenly thickened basement membrane.

2. *Franceschetti corneal dystrophy (FRCD)*

   FRCD is characterized by recurrent epithelial corneal erosions that typically occur during the first few decades of life and can last from 1 to 7 days. During periods without pain,, the cornea appears normal under the microscope. By mid-life, individuals may develop diffuse central subepithelial opacities resulting from recurrent erosions, which can impair vision, along with subepithelial fibrosis or protruding keloid-like formations. As individuals reach their 30s to 40s, the frequency of painful erosive episodes generally decreases gradually.

3. *Meesmann corneal dystrophy (MECD)*

   MECD is an autosomal dominant disorder, caused by mutations in the KRT3, KRT12 (i.e., keratin genes). It is characterized by numerous tiny intraepithelial vesicles that extend to the limbus. Unlike epithelial basement membrane dystrophy (EBMD), which typically presents with both microcysts and lines extending to the limbus, Meesmann dystrophy is identified by clear microcysts alone and occurs earlier in childhood. The condition generally causes mild visual reduction or no symptoms, although some patients may experience foreign body sensation or tearing that can progress to painful recurrent epithelial erosions. The Bowman's layer and stroma remain normal.

4. *Lisch epithelial corneal dystrophy (LECD)*

   LECD is an X-chromosomal dominant disorder. Asymptomatic or blurred vision if the pupillary axis is involved.

   Compared to EBMD, Lisch consists of the lines without scattered microcysts.

   Signs: A and B, Diffuse grayish epithelial opacities form radial patterns. C, Opacification consists of crowded, transparent microcysts in retroillumination

5. *Gelatinous drop-like corneal dystrophy (GDLD)*

   GDLD is an autosomal recessive disorder (the severest epithelial dystrophy), recognized as one of the most severe epithelial dystrophies, and typically manifests in early childhood.

   It is characterized by amyloid deposits in the subepithelial and stromal layers of the cornea, which can be identified with Congo red staining. The symptoms are significant decrease in vision, photophobia, irritation, redness, and tearing.

   Signs: Initially, the lesions may appear similar to band-shaped keratopathy or present as clusters of small nodules in mulberry configuration. Superficial vascularization is often observed. As the condition progresses, patients may develop stromal opacification or larger nodular lesions with a kumquat-like lesions.

While trauma is the most common cause of recurrent corneal erosion syndrome, Reis–Buckler dystrophy is the most common dystrophy associated with recurrent corneal erosion syndrome.

14.6.2 Epithelial–Stromal Dystrophies

These dystrophies typically begin at childhood and are inherited in an autosomal dominant pattern due to mutations in the TGFBI gene. They primarily affect Bowman's membrane and the superficial stroma, while sparing the deep stroma and Descemet's membrane.

Main symptoms include: decreased vision with age as the central visual axis becomes involved and photophobia. Pain often accompanies epithelial erosions.

1. *Reis–Bücklers corneal dystrophy (RBCD)*
   Characterized by a sheet-like layer of granular deposits replacing Bowman's layer, which extends into the superficial stroma and may reach the limbus. The deposits can be stained with Masson's trichrome.
2. *Thiel–Behnke corneal dystrophy (TBCD)*
   Features scattered fleck opacities at the level of the Bowman's layer, followed by symmetrical honeycomb-like opacities in the subepithelial region, with peripheral cornea usually remaining clear. It is less severe compared to RBCD.

***RBCD and TBCD can be difficult to differentiate, especially in the first two decades of life. In the early stages, RBCD presents with more irregular, diffuse opacities with clear interruptions, whereas TBCD shows multiple flecks with a reticular pattern. RBCD tends to have more aggressive course compared to TBCD.

14.6.3 Stromal Dystrophies

1. *Lattice corneal dystrophy*
   Amyloid deposition (stain with Congo red) in the corneal stroma. Central superficial fleck-like opacities on direct illumination with isolated peripheral lattice lines in retroillumination. Thin branching develop by the end of the first decade, associated with diffuse subepithelial ground-glass haze of the central and paracentral cornea, sparing the periphery.
   The far peripheral stroma, Descemet's membrane, and the endothelium are not involved.
   Development of diffuse central haze in the second to third decade may reduce vision sufficiently to necessitate surgical intervention by fourth decade.
   Type II lattice corneal dystrophy, known as (Meretoja's syndrome), represents a systemic deposition of amyloid throughout the body, with manifestations that include multiple cranial (mostly well known to be transmitted seventh) and peripheral nerve palsies, characteristic facial appearance, and dry lax skin.
2. *Granular corneal dystrophy, type 1 (GCD1)*
   GCD1 is an autosomal dominant disorder characterized by the presence of hyaline deposits, which can be identified histologically using Masson's trichrome staining. They deposits may extend deeply toward Descemet's membrane, but do not reach the limbus. In children, a vortex pattern of brownish granules can be seen superficial to the Bowman's layer. As the patient ages, well-defined granules appear white on direct illumination, with clear stroma in between. Over time, the granules increase in size and number, eventually creating a snowflake appearance.
3. *Granular corneal dystrophy, type 2 (GCD2) (Avellino dystrophy)*
   Features a combination of granular and lattice dystrophies, characterized by both hyaline and amyloid deposits.
   Early signs include subtle, superficial stromal whitish dots that often develop small spokes or thorns. As the condition progresses, all affected eyes exhibit superficial whitish patches and spiky, spider-shaped deposits that appear partially translucent when viewed with retroillumination. ***Patients with GCD2 have fewer stromal opacities than those with GCD1.
4. *Macular corneal dystrophy (MCD)*
   MCD is an autosomal recessive disease caused by mutation in CHST6 gene which is present during childhood. Corneal thinning

and ectasia are important clinical features of MCD, resembling KC.

MCD is caused by mucopolysaccharides deposition (Alcain blue stain and colloidal iron).

In the early stages, MCD presents with central, superficial, irregular whitish fleck-like opacities, similar to those seen in GCD1. However, unlike GCD1, these opacities in MCD extend to the limbus and involve the deep stroma down to Descemet's membrane. As the disease progresses, a diffuse haze spreads throughout the entire corneal stroma, leading to significant corneal thinning. The epithelium generally remains smooth, although corneal erosions may occasionally develop. The cornea is much thinner than normal. As the condition advances, Descemet's membrane becomes grayer and may develop guttata excrescences, although endothelial decompensation is uncommon.

Patients with MCD typically experience severe visual impairment between the ages of 10 and 30. Corneal sensitivity is often reduced, and while photophobia and painful recurrent erosions can rarely occur.

5. *Schnyder corneal dystrophy (SCD)*

   SCD is also known as crystalline corneal dystrophy; however, crystalline are only 50%.

   It is caused by abnormal deposition of phospholipids and cholesterol in the basal epithelial cells, the Bowman's layer, and stroma. Corneal crystals often form at the limbus. As the disease progresses, patients experience a decrease in visual acuity and an increase in glare sensitivity, which typically worsens with age. The corneal changes in SCD are age dependent. Patients 23 years or younger generally presents with a disc-like central corneal opacity and/or central crowded comma-shaped subepithelial crystals. Between the ages of 23 and 38, additional signs include arcus lipoids. After the age of 38, midperipheral panstromal haze also develops, in a hazy appearance of the entire cornea.

6. *Central cloudy dystrophy of François (CCDF)*

   CCDF is an autosomal dominant condition that appears phenotypically identical to Crocodile shagreen. It is typically discovered incidentally and is characterized by cloudy central polygonal or rounded stromal opacities. These opacities gradually fade as they extend toward the anterior and peripheral areas and are surrounded by clear corneal tissue (Fig. 14.3).

7. *Congenital stromal corneal dystrophy (CSCD)*

   CSCD is an autosomal dominant disease characterized by moderate to severe visual loss.

   It presents with diffuse, bilateral corneal clouding and flake-like whitish stromal opacities distributed throughout the stroma. Unlike macular corneal dystrophy, pachymetry in CSCD typically shows increased stromal thickness.

8. *Fleck corneal dystrophy (FCD)*

   FCD is an autosomal dominant disease present within the first years of life.

   It is characterized by subtle, small, dandruff-like opacities that are sparsely scattered sparsely throughout any level of the otherwise clear stroma. These flecks can extend to the limbus and are best visualized by slit beam or retroillumination. The epithe-

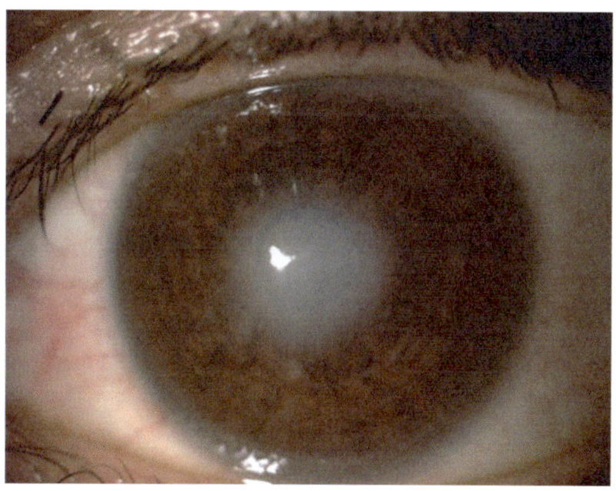

Fig. 14.3 Francois dystrophy

lium, Bowman's layer, Descemet's membrane, and endothelium remain unaffected. Corneal involvement may be asymmetric or even unilateral. Most patients are asymptomatic, although some may experience slight photophobia or decreased corneal sensitivity.

9. *Posterior amorphous corneal dystrophy (PACD)*

   PACD is an autosomal dominant disorder resents early in life. It is characterized by diffuse gray-white sheet-like opacities that can affect any layer of the stroma, although they are most prominent in the posterior stroma. Transparent stromal breaks are often observed. The cornea is typically thinner than normal, leading to hyperopia. Unlike posterior polymorphous corneal dystrophy, PACD is not associated with glaucoma.

10. *Pre-Descemet corneal dystrophy (PDCD) C1*

    Focal, fine, polymorphic gray opacities that may be central, annular, or diffuse are located in the deep stroma immediately anterior to Descemet's membrane.

14.6.4 Endothelial Dystrophies

14.6.4.1 All Develop Stromal Edema

1. *Fuchs endothelial corneal dystrophy (FECD)*

   FECD is characterized by an accelerated age-related loss of corneal endothelial cells.

   The condition typically begins with the formation of cornea guttata, which starts centrally and spreads peripherally (stage 1). While some patients may have guttata without further progression, others may advance to endothelial decompensation and stromal edema (stage 2). The Descemet's membrane becomes thickened as the disease progresses. Stromal edema may extend to the epithelium, leading to intraepithelial and interepithelial edema, including the formation of epithelial bullae; eventually resulting in bullous keratopathy (stage 3). In long-standing cases (stage 4), chronic edema can cause subepithelial fibrosis, scarring, and peripheral superficial vascularization. Patients often experience worse visual acuity worse in the morning due to increased stromal/epithelial edema after overnight eye closure. Additionally, pain, photophobia, and epiphora can occur as a result of epithelial erosions.

   FECD is also associated with glaucoma.

2. *Posterior polymorphous corneal dystrophy (PPCD)*

   PPCD is an autosomal dominant disorder and characterized by vesicular changes in the corneal endothelium. It features multilayered endothelial cells that exhibit epithelial cell-like behavior. The dystrophy often presents asymmetrically and is marked by distinctive opacities of the Descemet's membrane and endothelium, including geographic gray opacities and vesicular lesions. These lesions may be either single or grouped, often surrounded by gray circular opacities and can include parallel gray-white endothelial bands with white "flaky" material resembling railroad tracks that may extend across the corneal edema may develop, with around 20–25% of affected individuals requiring corneal transplantation.. Additionally, peripheral iridocorneal adhesions occur in about 25% of cases, and elevated intraocular pressure is seen in approximately 15% of cases.

3. *Congenital hereditary endothelial dystrophy (CHED)*

   Degeneration in endothelium during fifth gestation month due to abnormality at chromosome 20, leading to marked corneal thickening and opacity. Bilateral, often asymmetric. Corneal clouding ranging from diffuse haze to ground-glass milky appearance with occasional focal gray spots. Thickening of the cornea (can be 2–3 times the normal thickness). Corneal clouding with blurred vision often accompanied by nystagmus. Minimal to no tearing or photophobia (which are in the AD type). If associated with deafness, then termed Harboyan syndrome.

14.6.4.2 High-Yield Notes

The following dystrophies are high yield, along with their deposition and stains:

Macular dystrophy → Mucopolysaccharide deposits → Alcian blue stain
Granular dystrophy → Hyaline deposits → Masson trichrome stain
Lattice dystrophy → Amyloid deposits → Congo red stain

Table 14.3 lists common corneal dystrophies, their inheritance, pathology, and appearance.

The most common anterior corneal dystrophy is map-dot-fingerprint dystrophy.

Among the common corneal stromal dystrophies (granular, lattice, and macular), recurrent corneal erosions can be seen most frequently in lattice dystrophy and least common in granular.

In anterior membrane dystrophy, dots represent calcification of epithelial debris. Successful treatment can be via epithelial removal or stimulation (debridement or puncture of cornea) or occlusion therapy (patching, contact lenses, lubrication).

Dystrophies sparing the periphery:

- Thiel–Behnke corneal dystrophy
- Lattice corneal dystrophy
- Granular corneal dystrophy, type 1

Dystrophies containing amyloid (Stein with Congo red, crystal violet, Thioflavin T, Birefringence):

- Gelatinous
- Lattice
- Granular type 2 (Avellino)

Dystrophies with hyaline (stain with Masson trichrome):

- Granular 1
- Granular 2 (Avellino)

*Reis–Buckler also stain with Masson trichrome

Dystrophies with mucopolysacharides (stain with Prussian or Alcian blue, Colloidal iron):

Macular dystrophy: To differentiate macular dystrophy from others, especially when it has a granular opacity pattern, is tomography imaging, showing thinning in the cornea.

Most common stromal dystrophy is Lattice.

In granular corneal dystrophy, recurrent erosions can occur but are generally less frequent compared to anterior dystrophies or lattice dystrophy.

Central crystalline dystrophy of Schnyder is characterized by the accumulation of cholesterol crystals within the stroma. Similar to xanthelasma and corneal arcus, a small proportion of patients may have systemic hyperlipidemia. Fleck dystrophy is associated with keratoconus, atopy, or pseudoxanthoma elasticum.

Table 14.3 Comparison between several corneal dystrophy types

	Inheritance	Main pathology	Appearance	Notes
Epithelial basement membrane dystrophy	AD	Defect in hemidesmosomes leading to recurrent erosions	Intraepithelial dot opacities (Cogan cysts) underlying map-like figures, and multiple crowded blebs (Bron)	Most common
Epithelial recurrent erosion dystrophies	AD	Recurrent epithelial corneal erosions present in the first decades of life lasting 1–7 days	Central, subepithelial opacity and fibrosis	Normal between attacks
Meesmann corneal dystrophy	AD	Mutation in KRT3, KRT12 (i.e., keratin genes)	Intraepithelial vesicles extend to the limbus	The Bowman's layer and stroma remain normal
Lisch epithelial corneal dystrophy	X-linked	–	Lines without scattered microcysts	
Gelatinous drop-like corneal dystrophy	AR	Subepithelial and stromal amyloid deposits	Progressive epithelial erosion and stromal opacification	Superficial vascularization

Specular microscopy in Fuch's vs posterior polymorphous:

- Fuch's: pleomorphism, polymegathism, and a disruption of the endothelial monolayer by Descemet's membrane excrescences.
- Posterior polymorphous: vesicular endothelial changes. Presence of multilayer endothelial cells that look and behave like epithelial cells.

Symptoms of Fuchs' dystrophy are typically worse in the morning, when the corneal epithelium is more hydrated.

CHED has two forms:

- Recessive inheritance: present at birth, corneal edema, non-progressive, nystagmus.
- Dominant inheritance: occurs in the first or second year of life, decompensation, progressive nystagmus is NOT a feature.
- There are no known ocular or systemic associations of CHED.
- CHED presents like congenital glaucoma, except the corneal diameters and IOP are normal.
- Posterior polymorphous dystrophy present similar to ICE but with bilateral involvement.
- Dystrophies associated with glaucoma: Fuch's and posterior polymorphous.

Granular 2 (Avellino) dystrophy has the highest recurrence rate after keratoplasty, while macular dystrophy has the lowest rate of recurrence after keratoplasty. Least to reccur after keratoplasty are endothelial dystrophies including Fuch's and posterior polymorphous.

Fastest recurrence after penetrating keratoplasty occurs in Reis-Buckler dystrophy while Schnyder's and macular tend to recur slowly over 10 years.

14.7 Ectasia

Ectasia is a group of non-inflammatory, mostly bilateral corneal conditions characterized by corneal thinning, protrusion, and possible scarring. They affect men and women equally. Can be localized inferiorly as in keratoconus (KC) and pellucid marginal degeneration (PMD), or generalized as in keratoglobus (Table 14.4) (Gomes 2015; Moshirfar et al. 2019; Cornea Donor Study Investigator Group 2008).

Keratoconus presents with progressive myopia and astigmatism that develops around puberty. Patients have progressive irregular astigmatism as part of the disease process. Progression is highest in the second and third decades and tends to stabilize thereafter.

Forme Fruste keratoconus (FFK) can be defined as a cornea that has no abnormal findings by both slit-lamp examinations and placido-based corneal tomography, with the fellow eye diagnosed with keratoconus.

Diseases associated with keratoconus

- Keratoconus is associated with several conditions, including connective tissue disorders like Ehlers–Danlos syndrome; atopic eye conditions such as atopic keratoconjunctivitis; and Down's syndrome.

Leber congenital amaurosis has been associated with keratoconus, potentially due to eye rubbing associated with the oculo-digital sign, which may arise from poor vision. Note: In Marfan, despite being a connective tissue disease, the cornea is flatter than normal populations, so they do not actually predisposed to KC (Marfan-KC paradox).

Early signs of KC:

Table 14.4 Comparison between different ectasia types

	Keratoconus	Pellucid marginal degeneration	Keratoglobus
Incidence	Most common	Second	Least common
Thinning site	Central	Inferior	Generalized
Descemet's breaks	In between	Very rare	Common
Onset	Around puberty	20–50 years	Since birth

- Scissoring of the red reflex on retinoscopy, which can be one of the earliest indicators of keratoconus, potentially preceding noticeable changes in corneal curvature and thickness.
- Asymmetric refractive error with high or progressive astigmatism.
- Keratometry showing high astigmatism and irregularity, with the axis not aligning to 180°.
- Rizutti sign: characterized by a conical reflection on the nasal cornea when a penlight is shone from the temporal side.
- Fleischer ring: an iron deposit within the epithelium around the cone's base appearing brown and best visualized and best visualized with a cobalt blue filter.

Vogt's striae: fine, roughly vertically parallel striations in the pre-Descemet's stroma, which generally disappear with firm pressure applied to the eyeball.

Late signs include:

- Munson's sign: V-shaped indentation in the lower lid when the patient gazes downward.
- Acute hydrops: a condition where a break in Descemet's membrane allows aqueous fluid to enter the stroma, leading to severe corneal thickening, decreased vision, light sensitivity, tearing, and pain.

Stromal scarring following the resolution of acute hydrops can paradoxically improve vision in some cases by altering corneal curvature and reducing irregular astigmatism. Because of the location of the displaced cone, vertical coma is the most common high order aberration (HOA) found in patients with keratoconus.

Spectacles are useful in mild cases. Rigid gas-permeable contact-lens fitting is a low cost and highly effective initial management for irregular astigmatism resulting from keratoconus.

Corneal collagen cross linking can stop progression of the disease in around 80% of cases especially in the early stages of the disease.

Hydrops usually resolves on its own over several weeks. Once healed, some patients may experience improved vision as the corneal scarring that follows can flatten the cornea. Treatment is generally conservative and includes the use of topical hypertonic agents, patching or a soft contact lens, and occasionally cycloplegia to manage ciliary pain.

In KC, the same-size bed donor buttons help to neutralize part of the high myopia seen in eyes with keratoconus. Anterior lamellar keratoplasty has lower rejection rate than penetrating keratoplasty.

Pellucid Marginal Degeneration (PMD) is the second most common non-inflammatory corneal thinning disorder after keratoconus. It is characterized by bilateral, non-hereditary corneal ectasia with bilateral, clear, inferior (typically 4 o'clock to 8 o'clock), clear thinning of the inferior peripheral corneal stroma, typically between the 4 o'clock and 8 o'clock positions, with thinning approaching 20%. Unlike keratoconus, there are no breaks in Descemet's membrane, and the central cornea remains of normal thickness. The most ectatic area of the cornea is situated just above the region of thinning, leading to protrusion of the cornea in this area. This differs from keratoconus, where the corneal protrusion occurs at the site of maximal thinning.

In PMD, against the rule astigmatism is common, iron deposition on the cornea is rare, acute hydrop secondary to Descemet's membrane break has been reported in few cases. Contact lens fitting is usually most challenging for patients with pellucid marginal degeneration.

Keratoglobus is characterized by diffuse thinning of the cornea rather than a focal abnormality. It is associated with breaks in Descemet's membrane, similar to those seen in advanced keratoconus. Unlike Keratoglobus, which typically develops over time, keratoglobus is primarily considered a congenital condition present from birth. It has been linked to several systemic disorders, including Ehlers–Danlos syndrome, blue sclera, Marfan syndrome, and Leber's congenital amaurosis. This contrasts with cornea plana, which is characterized by a flat cornea often associated with hyperopia.

14.8 Diagnostics

14.8.1 Corneal Tomography

14.8.1.1 Overview

Corneal tomography imaging is mainly used in refractive surgery planning and ectasia diagnosis.

14.8.1.2 Topography and Tomography

Topography: Based on Placido disc principle: the reflection of concentric rings (aka. Mires) represent sleepiness, widely spaced rings represent flatter, and closely spaced rings represent steeper surfaces.

Used to map:

- Anterior corneal surface
- Anterior corneal curvatures

Tomography: Corneal tomography is a more advanced technique of capturing 3D corneal images based on a rotating Scheimpflug camera, where corneal thickness and posterior surface can additionally be acquired.

The shape of a normal cornea can be described as a prolate ellipse.

Before reading a tomography and accepting the tomography, make sure that the patient:

- Nonpregnant
- After delivery by 6 months
- If still lactating, 6 weeks after lactation cessation
- Off-contact lens wear for the past 2 weeks
- No dryness

The following is an example of a tomography, where reading it require the following steps:

1. Check patient identifiers (e.g., name, age)
2. Check numeric indices
3. Check the maps

14.8.2 Numeric Parameters

1. Quality of the image: OK mean all data points were collected correctly
2. Kmax: The maximum keratometry. Normally below 47 D (KC staging based on Kmax: mild <48 D, Moderate 48–54 D, Severe >54 D). Also the difference between both eyes should be below 2 D.
3. Thinnest location: Normally >500 μm, suspicious 450–500 μm
4. Location of thinnest Y coordinate: Normally <−0.50
5. Topographic astigmatism and its axis: Normally <1 D with axis <15. Compare with manifest astigmatism (where a large difference in dioptric power of axis might represent lenticular astigmatism) and check the axis looking for irregular astigmatism.
6. Q value (asphericity value) quantified indicator of the aspherical degree is defined as radial change from center to peripheral. Reflects the slope of the cornea: Normally from −1.0 (in myopes) to +0.5 (in hyperopes). It can be altered in refractive laser surgery, where it can be around +2.0 after myopia correction, and −2.0 in hyperopia correction. Reference: https://bmcophthalmol.biomedcentral.com/articles/10.1186/1471-2415-12-15
7. K1 power at the flat meridian, normally >34 D
8. K2 power at the steep meridian, normally <49 D, and should not differ by >1 D compared to K max*
9. K mean: should be between 40 and 46 D
10. Maps

*K2 represents the power and axis of the steepest meridian, while Kmax represent the power and axis of the steepest point. They difference should not exceed 1 D. Larger difference might suggest a point or a group of points that are conning and becoming steeper.

Always check that the dotted circle in the center is 5 mm.

**Remember to always check both eyes, as there might be a KC in the other eye, and the eye of interest is a Forme Fruste.

***Remember that the posterior map is very important in judging the presence of KC.

14.8.3 Maps

14.8.3.1 Back Elevation Map (Most Important)

On Pentacam rotating Scheimpflug camera maps, posterior elevation is measured as the maximum value above the best fit sphere (BFS) within the central 5 mm of the posterior cornea (Fig. 14.4).

Elevations above 15 μm are considered suspicious, with higher values indicating a greater likelihood of ectasia. Specific cutoff points are 35 μm for keratoconus and 29 μm for subclinical keratoconus. Sensitivity and specificity for detecting keratoconus are 97.3% and 96.9%, respectively, while for subclinical keratoconus, sensitivity and specificity are 68% and 90.8%, respectively.

The posterior elevation map is often a more reliable indicator of corneal instability due to disease, healing, or ectasia than the magnitude of the irregularity alone.

***Back elevation maps and values by Orbscan II topography are usually higher, so higher cut-off values should be considered (by around 10 μm).

14.8.3.2 Sagittal Map

Shows the astigmatism contributed at each point in the cornea (Fig. 14.5).

Display the shape with color codes (red for steep, and blue for flat). Different shapes can be categorized into symmetrical, asymmetric, skewed shapes, and special shapes.

The best are symmetric shapes (image below), considering that the K max <47.2 D:

For numerical data, the most important is the central 5 mm of the map.

The difference between the superior and inferior 5 mm margins (i.e., second circle) should be <2.5 D.

OR

The difference between the inferior and superior 5 mm margins should be <1.5 D. This makes you more sensitive to lower steep cornea.

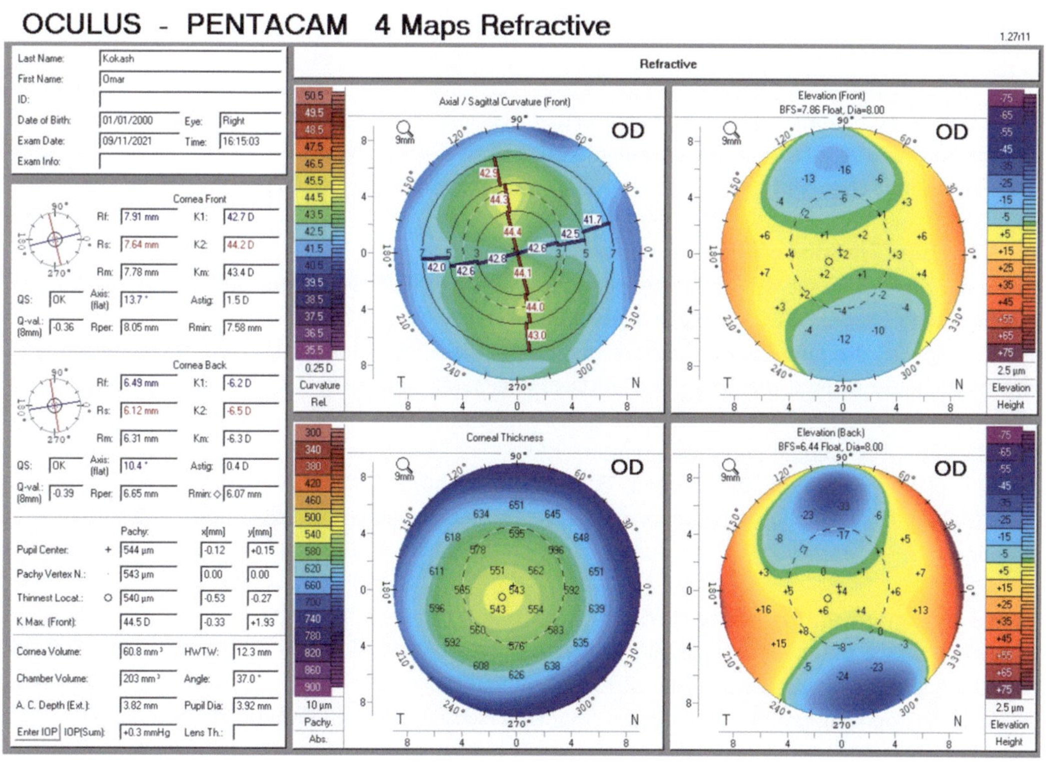

Fig. 14.4 The four maps of a normal Pentacam® tomography

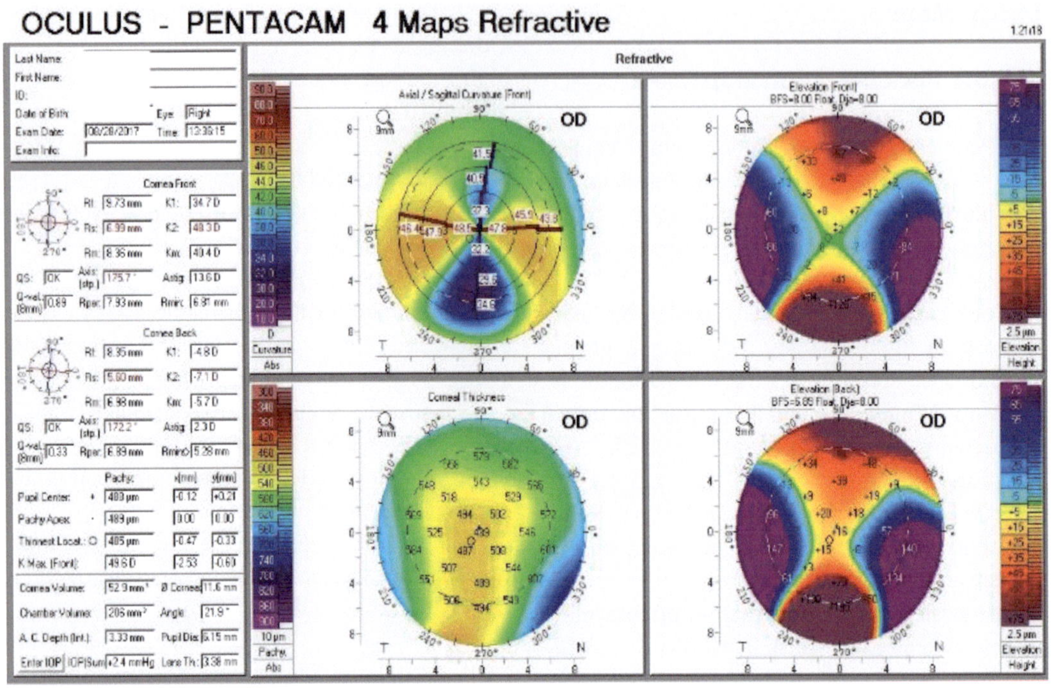

Fig. 14.5 An example of symmetric bow tie

***If sleepiness is more superior, then go for superior-inferior, while if sleepiness is more inferior, then go for inferior-superior.

- In KC, astigmatism progresses from a symmetrical bow-tie pattern, through an asymmetrical appearance to an inferio-temporally displaced steep-sided cone (Fig. 14.6).

14.8.3.3 Best Fit Sphere Elevation Maps

Elevation maps show the difference between the current image from the BFS (usually depend on patient's spherical equivalence): Anterior elevation map should show a maximum elevation of 15 μm within the central 5 mm, while the posterior elevation map should show a maximum of 20 μm elevation within the central 5 mm (Fig. 14.7). The shape should be symmetrical as in hourglass.

14.8.3.4 Pachymetry Thickness Map

To see where the thinnest location and the general thickness of the cornea: The difference between the opposing points at the central 5 mm should be <30 μm:

Progression map, when sequential images are available.

Spatial map: Spatial profile shows the progression from thinnest location toward the periphery of the cornea. The progression line (Red curve) should be within the normal slope and an average of <1.1.

14.8.4 Keratoconus on Tomography

In 2015, the Global consensus on KC provided a general definition for ectasia, and hence, for keratoconus:

- Abnormal posterior ectasia
- Abnormal corneal thickness distribution
- Clinical noninflammatory corneal thinning

While these are mandatory findings to diagnose keratoconus, the exact values for any parameter will vary based on the machine being used. Posterior corneal elevation abnormalities must be present to diagnose mild or subclinical keratoconus.

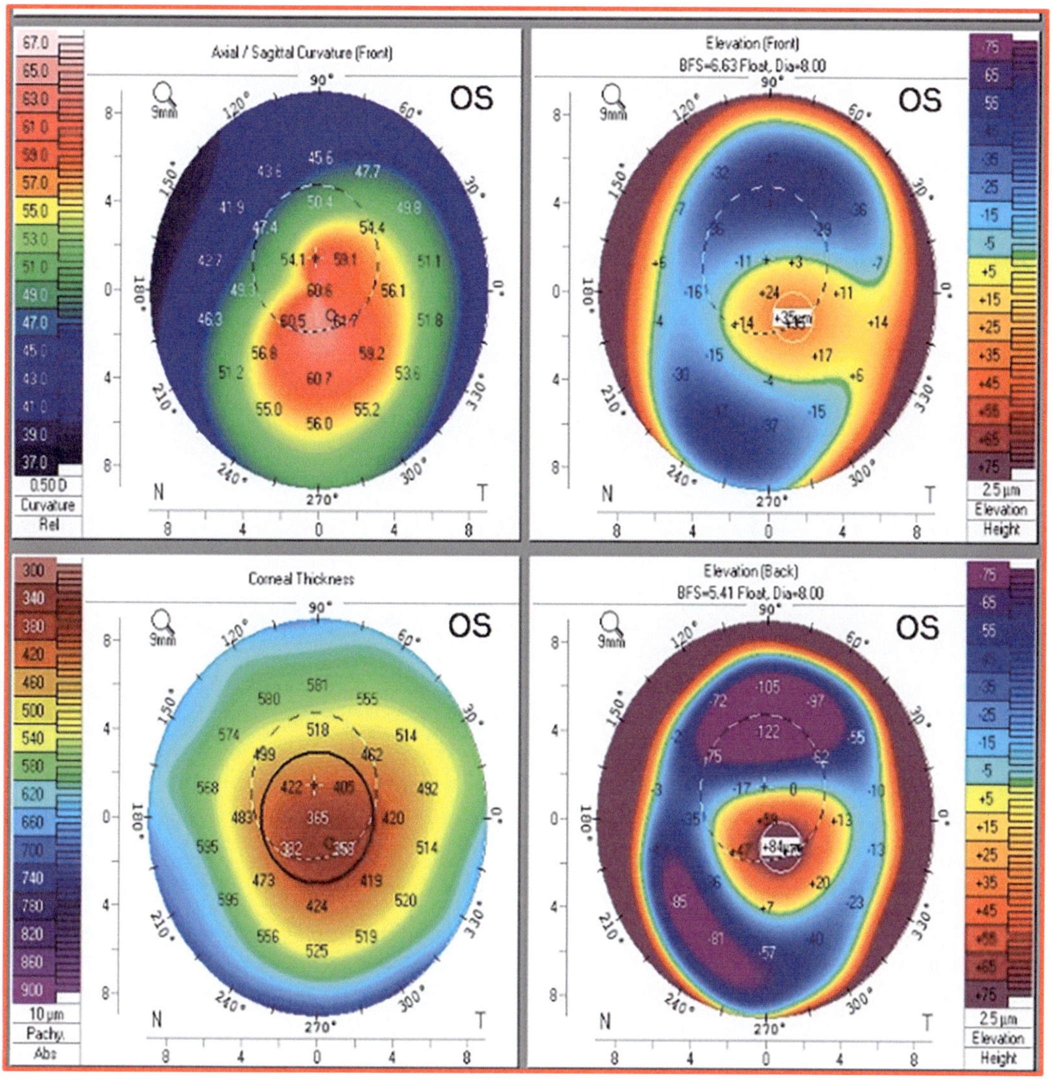

Fig. 14.6 Pentacam® tomography showing characteristics of keratoconus

As opposed to a "thinning disorder," keratoconus, pellucid marginal degeneration (PMD), keratoglobus, and post-refractive surgery corneal ectasia should be categorized as "ectatic diseases."

In contrast, conditions such as terrien marginal degeneration, dellen, and inflammatory melts are not considered ectatic diseases. Secondary changes, such as those occurring post-trauma, where no inherent ectatic propensity is present, are classified as "thinning disorder" rather than primary ectatic disease. It is also agreed that "keratoglobus and keratoconus" are different clinical entities, and "true unilateral keratoconus" is not recognized as a valid diagnosis.

The group considered central pachymetry the least reliable indicator (or determinant) for diagnosing keratoconus because keratoconus can be present in a cornea of normal central thickness.

If evidence suggestive of KC found, then:

First: Manage any pre-existing allergic eye diseases and prevent rubbing. It is important to note that there is no direct relationship between keratoconus and dry eye.

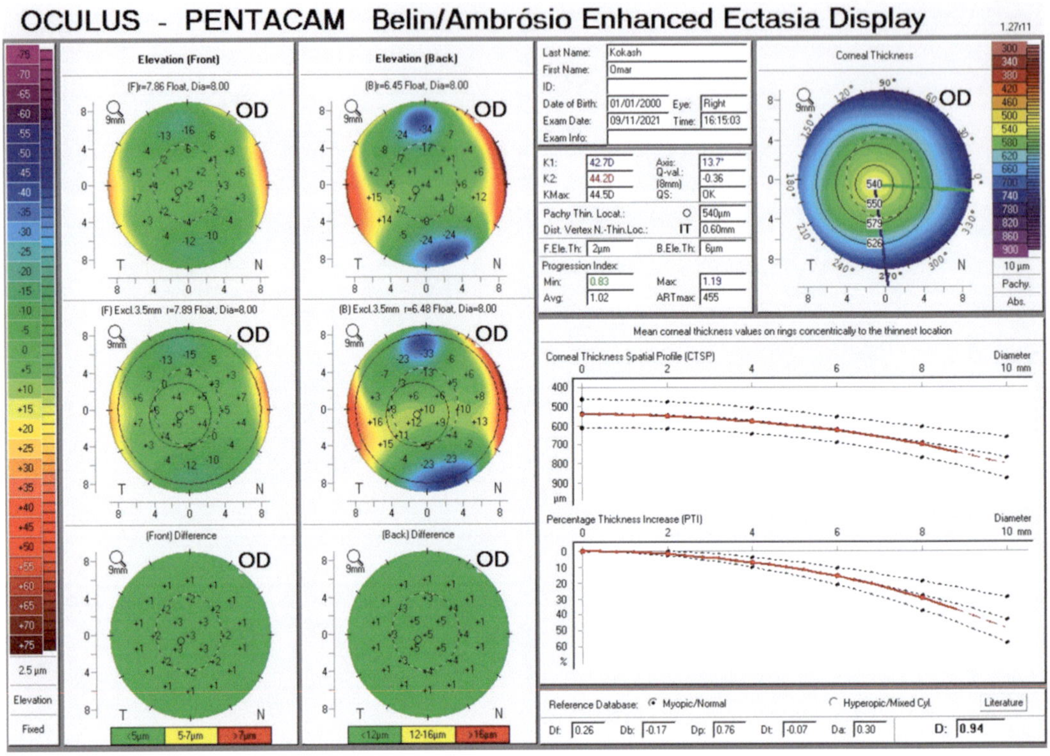

Fig. 14.7 Pentacam® tomography showing normal curvature

Second: anyone with progressive ectasia should undergo CXL no matter what age.

While evidence of progression has been a requirement to go for CXL, a group of patients with the following risk factors may under CXL without progression risk (as they are deemed as of high progression risk):

- Age of <17 years
- Kmax of >55 at presentation

These patients are at higher risk of having Kmax progressing >1.5 D/year. Middle eastern patients are also at higher risk of progression.

Signs of Ectasia Progression "Ectasia progression" is defined by a consistent change in at least two of the following parameters where the magnitude of the change is above the normal noise of the testing system:

1. Steepening of the anterior corneal surface
2. Steepening of the posterior corneal surface
3. Thinning and/or an increase in the rate of corneal thickness change from the periphery to the thinnest point.

Although progression is often accompanied by a decrease in best spectacle-corrected visual acuity (BSCVA), a change in both uncorrected visual acuity and BSCVA is not required to document progression.

Specific indices commonly used to document progression in 6 months:

Kmax (most commonly used) increase >1 D (or >1.5 D/year)
Kmean >0.75 D
CCT drop >2%

Conflict of Interest None.

References

Cornea Donor Study Investigator Group, gal RL, Dontchev M, Beck RW, Mannis MJ, Holland EJ, Kollman C, Dunn SP, Heck EL, Lass JH, Montoya MM, Schultze RL, Stulting RD, Sugar A, Sugar J, Tennant B, Verdier DD (2008) The effect of donor age on corneal transplantation outcome results of the cornea donor study. Ophthalmology 115(4):620–626.e6. https://doi.org/10.1016/j.ophtha.2008.01.003

Gomes JA, Tan D, Rapuano CJ, Belin MW, Ambrósio R Jr, Guell JL, Malecaze F, Nishida K, Sangwan VS, Group of Panelists for the Global Delphi Panel of Keratoconus and Ectatic Diseases (2015) Global consensus on keratoconus and ectatic diseases. Cornea 34(4):359–369. https://doi.org/10.1097/ICO.0000000000000408

Moshirfar M, Hopping GC, Vaidyanathan U, Liu H, Somani AN, Ronquillo YC, Hoopes PC (2019) Biological staining and culturing in infectious keratitis: controversy in clinical utility. Med Hypothesis Discov Innov Ophthalmol 8(3):145

Soh YQ, Kocaba V, Weiss JS, Jurkunas UV, Kinoshita S, Aldave AJ, Mehta JS (2020) Corneal dystrophies. Nat Rev Dis Primers 6(1):46

Weiss JS, Møller HU, Aldave AJ, Seitz B, Bredrup C, Kivelä T, Munier FL, Rapuano CJ, Nischal KK, Kim EK, Sutphin J (2015) IC3D classification of corneal dystrophies—edition 2. Cornea 34(2):117–159

15 Clinical Review of Cornea: Part II

Muawyah Al Bdour, Ahmed Alsaadi,
Amna Almaazmi, and Saif Aldeen Alryalat

Abstract

This chapter explores critical corneal conditions, focusing on infectious and interstitial keratitis, which pose a risk of severe vision loss if not treated promptly. It provides detailed insights into peripheral ulcerative keratitis (PUK), a serious corneal disease linked to systemic conditions, and examines metabolic syndromes that impact the cornea, highlighting their genetic and biochemical origins. Keratoplasty, an essential surgical intervention for corneal issues, is discussed in depth, covering its types, indications, techniques, and considerations for successful outcomes. The chapter also addresses various miscellaneous topics that contribute to a comprehensive understanding of the cornea and its associated conditions. This chapter serves as a valuable resource for enhancing knowledge of corneal pathologies and ultimately promoting better patient care in ophthalmology.

Keywords

Infectious keratitis · Interstitial keratitis · Metabolic syndrome · Keratoplasty · Miscellaneous

M. Al Bdour
Department of Ophthalmology, The University of Jordan, Amman, Jordan

A. Alsaadi
Zayed Military Hospital, Abu Dhabi, United Arab Emirates

Shaikh Khalifa Medical City, Abu Dhabi, United Arab Emirates

Sharjah University, Sharjah, United Arab Emirates

A. Almaazmi
Zayed Military Hospital, Abu Dhabi, United Arab Emirates

Sharjah University, Sharjah, United Arab Emirates

S. A. Alryalat (✉)
Department of Ophthalmology, The University of Jordan, Amman, Jordan

The University of Colorado Anschutz Medical Campus, CO, USA
e-mail: s.alryalat@ju.edu.jo

15.1 Infectious Keratitis

Infectious keratitis involves inflammation of the cornea by microbial invasion, typically resulting in stromal loss and disruption of the epithelium. Guidelines for diagnosing and treating infectious keratitis are outlined (Table 15.1) (Austin et al. 2017; Cabrera-Aguas et al. 2022).

Calcofluor white and acridine orange are effective stains for detecting Acanthamoeba and fungi. Gram stain and acridine orange are useful for identifying both aerobic and anaerobic bacteria, while mycobacteria can be visualized using Gram stain, acid-fast and lectin staining.

S. A. Alryalat (ed.), *Ophthalmology Board and FRCS Part 2 Exams*,
https://doi.org/10.1007/978-981-96-1517-9_15

Table 15.1 Diagnostic and therapeutic guidelines for infectious keratitis

	Staining		Culture		
Causative agent	Type	Sensitivity[a]	Type	Sensitivity[a]	Treatment
Bacterial	Gram Giemsa	57–67%	Blood agar Chocolate agar Thioglycolate broth Mannitol salt agar	58%	Fluoroquinolones *or* Aminoglycoside + Cephalosporins *or* Aminoglycoside + Vancomycin
Viral i. HSV1 ii. VZV iii. CMV	N/A	N/A	i. Vero cell line ii. MRC-5 cell line iii. MRC-5 cell line	i. 21% ii. 46%	i. Acyclovir (oral) + Trifluridine (topical) acyclovir (topical) Valganciclovir ii. Acyclovir (oral) Famciclovir (oral) Valacyclovir (oral) Acyclovir (topical) iii. Valganciclovir (oral) Valganciclovir (topical)
Fungal	KOH PAS GMS	68–99%	Sabouraud dextrose agar Blood agar Chocolate agar	25–59%	Natamycin Amphotericin Clotrimazole Fluconazole Itraconazole Voriconazole
Acanthamoeba	KOH PAS Calcofluor white	84%	Buffered charcoal yeast extract, *E. coli*-seeded non-nutrient agar	33%	Chlorhexidine + PHMB (topical) *or* Chlorhexidine + Brolene (topical) *or* Neomycin (topical)

Abbreviations: *KOH* potassium hydroxide, *HSV1* herpes simplex virus type 1, *VZV* varicella-zoster virus, *CMV* cytomegalovirus, *N/A* not available, *MRC-5* human lung embryonated cells, *PHMB* polyhexamethylene biguanide hydrochloride, *GMS* Gomori methenamine silver

[a]Specificity not included as these methods are considered the gold standard for the diagnosis of infectious keratitis and theoretically should be 100% in the absence of contamination

The American Academy of Ophthalmology Practice Recommendations

- The majority of community-acquired cases of bacterial keratitis resolve with empiric therapy and are managed without smears or cultures. Smears and/or cultures are specifically indicated in the following circumstances:
- If corneal ulcer is either central or large (>2 mm) or associated with significant deep stromal involvement.
- If the infection is chronic in nature or unresponsive to broad-spectrum antibiotic therapy (stop the antibiotic for 12 h before culture).
- History of corneal surgery.
- Atypical clinical features suggestive of fungal, amoebic, or mycobacterial keratitis (Fig. 15.1).
- *Do Not* scrape a descemetocele in order to avoid iatrogenic rupture.
- Topical antibiotics should be prescribed to prevent acute bacterial keratitis in patients presenting with a contact lens related to corneal abrasion.
- Patching the eye in a patient who wears contact lenses and has a corneal abrasion is not recommended due to the increased risk of bacterial keratitis, though the use of bandage contact lenses for managing epithelial defects remains controversial.

Cycloplegic agent, often-overlooked, can be helpful in reducing pain and preventing synechiae formation in bacterial keratitis, particularly when substantial anterior chamber inflammation is present. Corticosteroids may be considered after 24–48 h if the causative organism has been identified and/or the infection is responding to treatment. However, corticosteroids should be avoided in infections caused by *Acanthamoeba, Nocardia*, and fungi to prevent the risk of early corneal perforation.

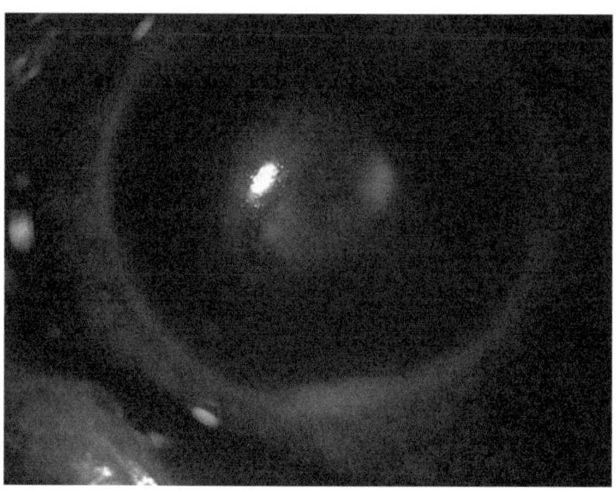

Fig. 15.1 Hypopyon secondary to keratitis

15.1.1 Bacterial Keratitis

Most important signs: ciliary injection, superficial stromal infiltrates, and ulcer.

Microbiology:

- Organisms capable of penetrating the cornea without prior epithelial defects include Corynebacterium Diphtheria, Haemophilus influenzae, Neisseria gonnorhoeae, and Listeria species (CHNL).
- *Pseudomonas aeruginosa* is the leading cause for contact lens keratitis, accounting for 60% of cases. It adheres to the cornea by binding to surface receptors exposed on injured epithelial cells.
- *Streptococcal viridans* is the primary pathogen responsible for infectious crystalline keratopathy. This condition is often associated with long-term topical steroid use and is commonly observed in patients who have had undergone penetrating keratoplasty. Treatment usually requires an extended course of both topical and oral antibiotics.

Streptococcal pneumonia (Pneumococcus) is the commonest cause of hypopyon corneal ulcer.

Management:

- Fourth-generation fluoroquinolones monotherapy (e.g., moxifloxacin or gatifloxacin) is the best initial regimen for small ulcers and might be combined with aminoglycoside.
- Dual fortified therapy (vancomycin and ceftazidime (third-generation cephalosporin)) is the best initial regimen for large aggressive disease. In case of cephalosporin allergy, Amikacin can be used.

- A significant corneal ulcer should be managed with broad-spectrum fortified antibiotics until the infectious microorganism is identified. Non-fortified antibiotics such as moxifloxacin 0.5%, tobramycin 0.3%, and ofloxacin 0.3% are not inadequate for treating severe cases particularly when dealing with a paracentral infiltrate that could potentially spread to involve the visual axis. Fortified antibiotics like vancomycin 5% and cefazolin 5% are preferred, although they primarily cover gram-positive organisms. Sub-conjunctival antibiotics are used for non-compliant patients (not superior to topical).
- Systemic antibiotics is considered in severe thinning, systemic involvement and in scleral involvement.
- If there is no improvement within 48 h, review antibiotic regimen. If there is no improvement in the following 48 h, consider re-scraping the corneal biopsy.
- Chlorhexidine and other regimens should be reserved for resistant cases, where acanthamoeba is suspected.
- Keratoplasty is reserved for unresponsive cases.

15.1.2 Fungal (Mycotic) Keratitis

Points of differentiation from bacterial keratitis:

- Fungal keratitis often follows trauma involving vegetative material.
- Typical fungal ulcers present with feathery or indistinct borders, unlike the more defined borders seen in bacterial ulcers.
- Satellite lesions and endothelial plaques are more frequently associated with fungal infections. In fungal keratitis, the corneal stroma, outside the area of cellular infiltration tends to be less edematous compared to bacterial ulcers.
- Hypopyon is more common in fungal keratitis which often has a fibrinous appearance, distinguishing it from the hypopyon seen in bacterial infections.

Yeasts, unlike molds, tend to produce a smoother and occasionally gelatinous appearing infiltration. Table 15.2 provides a detailed comparison between filamentous and non-filamentous keratitis.

Diagnostic Approach:

- Identification of fungal cells in specimens obtained from corneal scraping and tissue often makes use of specific stains such as KOH, Gomori's methenamine silver (GMS), or periodic acid-Schiff (PAS) stains.
- PCR also can be used with a sensitivity reaching 80%; however, no primers available to specify the type of fungus, so a high false positive rate is expected.
- Fungi can be cultured in Sabouraud dextrose, blood, and chocolate agars.
- Do biopsy if there is no improvement. Filamentous fungi tend to grow near the

Table 15.2 Comparison between filamentous and non-filamentous keratitis

	Yeast (e.g., candida) or non-filamentous	Filamentous (e.g., Fusarium[a] and Aspergillus)
Cellularity	Unicellular	Multicellular
Settings	Associated with dry eyes or chronic bandage contact-lens wear	Follows ocular trauma with vegetative matter
Area and temperature	Temperate climate. Cool environment	Tropical areas. Warm, humid environments
Appearance	Densely white suppurative ulcer	Fluffy margin and satellite ulcer
Aggressiveness	Less aggressive	More aggressive
First choice anti-fungal	Amphotericin B 0.15% Or Voriconazole 1%	Natamycin 5% or Voriconazole 1%

[a]Fusarium is the most common cause of fungal keratitis

Descemet, so the biopsy should be deep stromal. Confocal microscopy can visualize it.

Management:
- Voriconazole 1% (Anazole class of antifungals).
- Amphotericin B (Polyene-type antifungals), drug of choice for yeast.
- Natamycin 5% (Polyene-type antifungals), the only FDA-approved topical treatment for fungal keratitis.

The most appropriate initial therapy for fungal keratitis from the list of options is Amphotericin B, due to its broad spectrum activity against both yeast and filamentous molds. Although natamycin is effective against filamentous molds and has some anti-yeast activity, Amphotericin B provides broader coverage and is generally preferred as the initial treatment.

Regimen: One drop hourly while until re-epithelialization, followed by four times daily for the next 3 weeks. The frequent application is mainly due to their poor corneal penetration.

The use of steroids will lead to worse visual outcomes at any stage.

Major Clinical Trials:
- **Mycotic Ulcer Treatment Trial 1**: Compared topical natamycin versus topical voriconazole in treatment for fungal corneal ulcers. The study found that natamycin was superior in terms of visual improvement, particularly for ulcers caused by Fusarium. For non-Fusarium ulcers, there was no difference in visual acuity between the two treatments.
- **Mycotic Ulcer Treatment Trial 2**: Evaluated the impact of oral voriconazole (which has generally good bioavailability at cornea and AC) on the rate of corneal perforation in severe fungal keratitis. The study concluded that adding oral voriconazole to topical antifungals did not provide additional therapeutic benefits in advanced cases of filamentous fungal ulcers.

Cross-linking for infectious corneal ulcers, also known as photo activated chromophore for keratitis-corneal cross-linking (PACK-CxL) typically involves corneal de-epithelialization, application of topical 0.1% riboflavin for 30 min, followed by UVA light (365 nm) treatment for 30 min. While PACK-CxL shows promise for treating fungal and bacterial keratitis, it is contraindicated for viral keratitis.

15.1.3 Herpetic Keratitis

Herpetic keratitis is caused by either herpes simplex virus (HSV-1) or herpes zoster virus (also known as HSV-3).

HSV-1 causes facial while HSV-2 causes genital infections (so not relevant to the eye). Latent type 1 HSV (responsible for recurrent facial infection) generally resides in sensory ganglia, which is the Gasserian ganglion for HSV-1. The vast majority of the population are exposed to the herpes simplex virus during childhood and carry antibodies.

Primary herpetic infection is characterized by follicular reaction, vesicular blepharitis, and lymphadenopathy, findings that are not found in secondary infection. Vesicular blepharitis may occur in recurrent HSV infection, while dendrites are fleeting in primary infection. Primary infection generally affects pediatric population, and what is more important in ophthalmology is the secondary reactivation.

Secondary reactivation is the one responsible for keratitis and may occur with stress and immunosuppression. It is important to note that treating the primary infection does not lower the risk of reactivation. After one episode, the risk is about 10% at 1 year and 50% at 10 years. The higher the number of previous attacks the greater the risk of recurrence.

15.1.3.1 Herpes Simplex

Can cause epithelial, stromal (necrotizing and non-necrotizing), and disciform (endothelial) keratitis (Table 15.3).

Progression chances from epithelial keratitis to stromal keratitis/iritis are 10% (Not reduced by anti-viral).

HSV epithelial keratitis can be treated by:

Table 15.3 Comparison between epithelial, stromal, and endothelial keratitis

	Epithelial keratitis	Stromal keratitis	Disciform (endothelial) keratitis
Pathophysiology	Viral replication	Viral replication leading to immune-mediated destruction	Mostly a hypersensitivity to viral antigens
Corneal manifestation	Branching with bulbs, uptake with fluorescent lights. No AC reaction	Stromal necrosis ± melting. AC reaction with KPs underlying the area of active stromal infiltration. Epithelial defects may occur (but not as typical epithelial)	Central opacity with corneal edema (manifesting as halos), AC reaction, large granulomatous KPs (not fine ones). A surrounding (Wessely) immune ring of deep stromal haze representing antigen and immune complex deposition. Epithelial defect may occur (but not as typical epithelial)
Treatment	Topical Acyclovir ointment *5 for around 2 weeks. Epithelial debridement (i.e., scraping) for resistant cases 2 mm beyond ulcer. Oral is indicated for immunodeficient children and significant ocular surface disease and resistant cases.	Topical steroids (oral if severe) + topical antiviral (both for at least 4 weeks)	Topical steroids (oral if severe) + topical antiviral (both at least 4 weeks)
Prophylaxis	Acyclovir 400 mg*2 reduced recurrence by 50% (from 40% to 20%)	Acyclovir 400 mg*2 reduced recurrence by 50% (from 40% to 20%)	None

- Debridement
- Topical treatment with:
  - Acyclovir 3% ophthalmic ointment five times/day or
  - Trifluridine (Viroptic) drops nine times/day or
  - Vidarabine 3% ophthalmic ointment five times/day

Herpetic stromal keratitis (Fig. 15.2): Topical steroids are effective in reducing the persistence or progression of stromal keratitis compared with placebo. Recurrences after tapering steroid often respond well to a more gradual reduction in dosage. In contrast, a significant large proportion of patients treated with trifluridine and placebo experienced notable progression of herpetic inflammation, indicating that trifluridine alone does not provide substantial benefit for managing stromal keratitis.

Iridocyclitis: Causes raised IOP from trabeculitis. It occurs with or without keratitis, patchy iris atrophy provides a clue for diagnosis. Treatment is with topical steroid and oral acyclovir.

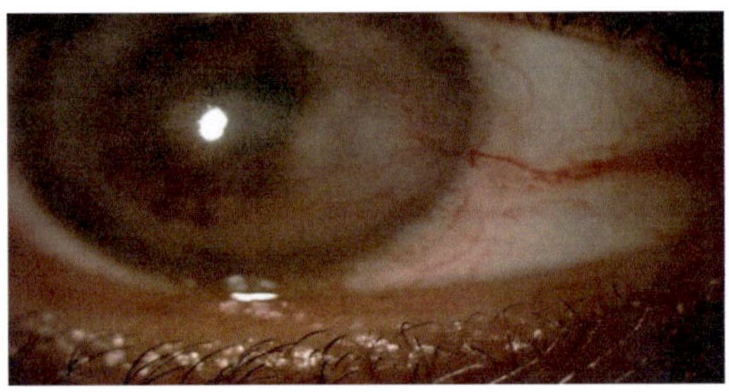

Fig. 15.2 Colored photograph showing stromal keratitis

Peripheral disciform keratitis lesions without significant neovascularization may be best untreated. When treatment is necessary, the lowest effective topical steroid dose is used, and most agree that a dose of prednisolone acetate 1% used more than once a day should be accompanied by a topical antiviral agent drop for drop.

Topical **interferon alpha-2a** appears to be an effective treatment adjunct for refractory herpes simplex keratitis in patients with cell-mediated immune dysfunction and subsequent lack of endogenous interferon.

Metaherpetic keratitis is the most severe form of HSV involvement of the cornea. Recurrent attacks of HSV, superficial bullae, stromal involvement, endotheliitis, and anterior uveitis can all be part of the metaherpetic phase of HSV. Factors that may be important in the pathogenesis of this finding include underlying stromal inflammation, overuse of prescribed topical antivirals, and impaired corneal sensation. However, active intraepithelial virus replication is not a risk factor.

Complications of keratitis:

- Neurotrophic keratopathy: failure of re-epithelialization with underlying stromal fibrosis (grayish), resulting from excessive corneal anesthesia, steroid should be restricted to minimum.
- Corneal neovascularization and lipid keratopathy are possible chronic complications.

According to HEDS (Herpetic Eye Disease Studies), oral acyclovir has no impact on the development of stromal keratitis or iritis in the following year when administered during active herpes simplex keratitis. However, oral acyclovir can decrease the likelihood of recurrent stromal disease in patients with a history of active herpes simplex keratitis. Stopping oral acyclovir does not lead to rebound of herpes simplex disease, but it is beneficial in treating herpes simplex iritis. HEDS shows that topical steroid effectively reduces the severity and the duration of herpes simplex stromal disease. However, there is no significant difference in visual outcome between patients treated with topical steroids and those receiving a placebo. The use of topical steroids does not increase the incidence of epithelial disease during treatment. The study did not specifically evaluate necrotizing stromal keratitis.

15.1.3.2 Herpes Zoster

An infection that include a complete dermatome with involvement of the eye and requires systemic treatment. The eye can be involved from ophthalmic division involvement, rarely from maxillary and almost never with mandibular. It has 3–5 days prodromal phase, followed by erythema, vesicles, crusting, and then pigmentation. Epithelial keratitis is seen in 50% of cases (if so, topical antiviral can be given).

The active viral replication leads to the sloughing of epithelial cells in HSV, whereas in HZV, the epithelial cells become swollen and heaped up. In HSV infections, the epithelial cells surrounding dendritic lesions are devitalized, heavily laden with virus, and stain well with rose bengal. This is in contrast with the pseudodendritic lesions seen in herpes zoster, which stain poorly with rose bengal. In addition, herpes zoster "dendrites" (pseudodendrites) are typically smaller and have less branching compared to the dendrites seen in herpes simplex infections (Table 15.4).

Nummular keratitis: Develops in 1/3 of cases at the site of epithelial lesions about 10 days after the onset of the rash. It represents the presence of anterior stromal granular infiltrates. Stromal keratitis develops 3 weeks after rash.

Endothelial (disciform) keratitis is less common than simplex, but is more severe and can lead to decompensation. In contrast, the number and density of the granulomatous KPs are less than simplex.

Anterior uveitis leads to sectorial iris atrophy with associated trabeculitis.

Table 15.4 Comparison between herpes simplex and herpes zoster keratitis

	Herpes simplex	Herpes zoster
Virus	HSV-1 (mostly), HSV-2	HSV-3
Clinically	Cross midline, milder pain, branching dendritic ulcer with bulbs	Respect midline, severer pain, finer dendritic lesions without the bulbs
Epithelium	Sloughed, so staining well with rose bengal	Swollen, poorly staining with rose bengal
First line	Topical acyclovir 3% *5 2 weeks	Oral acyclovir 800 mg *5 7–10 days
Severe cases	Oral acyclovir 400 mg *3–5	IV 5–10 mg/kg *3

No correlation between severity of skin rash and ocular involvement severity.

Post-herpetic neuralgia is defined as pain for more than 1 month after the rash has healed.

Initiating oral therapy with acyclovir within 3 days or when the rash is still vesicles (no crusting yet), reduces the severity/duration of acute episode and risk of post-herpetic neuralgia and also reduces the duration of the skin lesions.

Systemic steroids, although controversial, can be used as a treatment option in conjunction with acyclovir, potentially reducing the incidence of post-herpetic neuralgia when started early in the disease course. Newer oral antiviral agents like valacyclovir (Valtrex) and famciclovir (Famvir) offer improved gastrointestinal absorption, leading to higher blood levels and enhanced efficacy.

15.1.4 Acanthamoeba Keratitis

A parasitic infection commonly found in contact lens wearers with poor hygiene practices is characterized by pain that is disproportionate to clinical findings.

Early symptoms include epithelial irregularities, epithelial or subepithelial infiltrates, and pseudodendrites. A distinctive early sign is radial perineuritis which are seen within the first few weeks as thickened corneal nerves with ragged edges, arranged in a linear, radial pattern within the anterior or mid-stroma.

As the infection progress, later signs include stromal infiltrates (which can be ring-shaped, disciform, or nummular), satellite lesions, epithelial defects, scleritis, and anterior uveitis, with the possibility of hypopyon. In the early stage of pain (95% of the times) with clinical suspicion, corneal scrape culture should be obtained. It grows best on non-nutrient agar overlaid with *Escherichia coli* or Enterococcus. Various stains (e.g., Giemsa) may allow identification with light microscopy, and confocal microscopy can be used to visualize the organisms in vivo. Serological techniques are of no diagnostic value in Acanthamoeba keratitis diagnosis.

In early stages, simple mechanical débridement can be effective if the infection is limited to the corneal epithelium.

Treatment involves an hourly application of antiseptics such as PHMB, chlorhexidine, or a combination of both for 1–2 weeks. Chlorhexidine is the preferred treatment for Acanthamoeba keratitis because it targets both trophozoites and cysts. Due to resistance of the cystic phase, antimicrobials generally have limited effectiveness, as they are mainly active against the trophozoite phase. Antifungal drugs, such as voriconazole, may also be considered.

Even with early diagnosis, treatment usually lasts 3–4 months, and in cases of late diagnosis, treatment may extend up to 1 year. Melting in Acanthamoeba keratitis occurs at the periphery of the ulcer, rather than the center.

Topical steroids in Acanthamoeba keratitis might be started after 2 weeks of proper treatment, almost never initially.

Ring infiltrate can also be seen in topical anesthesia abuse. It is important to recognize that topical anesthetic abuse may resemble infections with herpes simplex, herpes zoster, Acanthamoeba, or pseudomonas.

15.2 Interstitial Keratitis

Interstitial keratitis is characterized by a non-ulcerative and non-suppurative inflammation that affects the corneal stroma while leaving Bowman's and Descemet's membranes typically intact. The inflammatory corneal lesions often result from the host's response to antigens stemming from bacterial, viral (accounting for 40% of cases), or parasitic infections or from autoimmune response (a cause in about 1% of cases). However, it is important to note that no active corneal infection is present.

The progression of this disease can be divided into two phases: the acute phase and the cicatricial or scarring phase.

The term interstitial keratitis often refers to the latter. In its chronic phase, the disease typically presents with feathery mid-stromal scarring accompanied by ghost vessels. In the active phase, symptoms include anterior uveitis, a cloudy cornea, and potential refilling of the ghost vessels. While congenital syphilis is often referred to as the "classic" cause of interstitial keratitis, the herpes virus is now the most common causative agent. Interstitial keratitis resulting from congenital syphilis is a bilateral condition that may not present until the patient is between 10 and 20 years of age, making it the most prevalent cause of bilateral interstitial keratitis. For children suffering from untreated congenital syphilis, the typical onset of interstitial keratitis is between 6 and 12 years of age, and the condition is not present at birth.

Cogan syndrome (CS) is a unique form of interstitial keratitis, characterized as an idiopathic autoimmune disease leading to inflammation in the eyes and the inner ears. This condition manifests as vestibule-auditory dysfunction and interstitial keratitis, with both organs having nearly equal chances of displaying the initial symptoms. Early corneal indications of CS consist of faint white subepithelial infiltrates in the periphery bilaterally. As the disease progresses, multifocal nodular infiltrates may develop later on in the posterior cornea. The average age of CS presentation is around 23 years. The disease typically progresses over a period ranging from 3 to 90 days and often responds positively to steroid treatment. Systemic vasculitis, most frequently polyarteritis nodosa (PAN), is a common association, with aortitis occurring in about 10% of cases.

15.3 Peripheral Ulcerative Keratitis (PUK)

A group of diseases begin by peripheral corneal ulceration and thinning. Intact epithelium and endothelium are the general rule (Table 15.5).

Rheumatoid arthritis (RA) is the main cause.

Differentials to consider in PUK include RA, collagen vascular diseases (ANCA-associated vasculitis, polyarteritis nodosa, and relapsing polychondritis), Mooren's ulcer, and infections such as tuberculosis and syphilis.

Rheumatoid arthritis can affect the eyes in various ways, including dry eye, scleritis, stromal keratitis, PUK, and paracentral keratolysis. Both type III and IV hypersensitivity reactions have, as well as vasculitis with inflammatory cell infiltration, have been implicated. Paracentral keratolysis, also known as a sterile melt, can occur even in relatively quiet eyes and may progress rapidly to descemetocele and perforation if not promptly treated. Management includes protecting the ocular surface from drying and exposure, using adjuncts like amniotic membrane grafts to promote healing, and in some cases, employing tectonic reinforcement.

Marginal keratitis is due to type 3 hypersensitivity reaction (immune complex deposition). Characterized by peripheral stromal infiltrates, with a 1–2 mm clear cornea peripheral margin, associated with blepharitis. Usually no ulcer present, if ulceration with uptake, infectious causes need to be excluded by culture. If no clear margin present, consider Mooren's ulcer.

Terrien's marginal degeneration: a bilateral disease that is more in male around 20–40 years of age and characterized by peripheral corneal thinning with neovascularization, and lipid deposition along the leading edge, with intact epithelium (so painless). It starts superiorly and spreads circumferentially over time, but rarely reaches inferior cornea. It leads to against-rule-astigmatism.

Keep in mind that it lacks inflammation or epithelial defect, has neovascularization and lipids on the leading edge that slowly progressive from superior cornea.

The epithelium may be normal, thickened or thinned. Bowman's membrane is typically absent or degenerated.

Mooren's ulcer is severe and more likely bilateral in African, an evaluation for connective tissue disease is mandatory. Biopsy of the adjacent conjunctiva may show increased plasma cells. Mooren's ulcer causes peripheral circumferential ulcer with late central spread.

Table 15.5 Comparison between different types of peripheral ulcerative keratopathy

	Marginal keratitis	Dellen	Mooren	Terrien
Etiology	Hypersensitivity (type III mostly and to a lesser extent type IV) to Staph. Aureus	Poor lubrication in a localized area (e.g., surrounding pterygium or subconj hemorrhage)	Autoimmune, however, has a higher incidence after trauma, surgery (mostly ECCE), and infection with helminthic worms (cross antigenicity)	Idiopathic
Demographic			Elderly men at their 60–70 years. African populations are affected at younger age with worse prognosis (at their 20–30 years)	Male 20–40 years
Signs	Superficial stromal opacity with inferior punctate epithelial erosions. Infiltrates always have a clear margin of healthy cornea between them	Localized area of thinning	The condition is characterized by pain and is strictly peripheral, affecting only the superficial third of the cornea with a distinct leading edge. It is a stromal disease, meaning the epithelium, endothelium, and Descemet's membrane remain intact. The disease is progressive and presents more severely and bilaterally in younger patients, whereas it tend to be milder and unilateral in adults. It involves limbitis but does not progress to scleritis or associate with systemic disorder, which are more common in PUK linked to rheumatological causes	75% male 20–40 years. Asymptomatic, bilateral, against the rule astigmatism. Superior (very rare inferior) thinning and pannus with leading vascularization and lipid
Presence of clear corneal margin	Yes		No	
Treatment	Weak steroid, tetracycline for MGD	Lubrication	Strong topical steroids	Spectacles and contact lenses

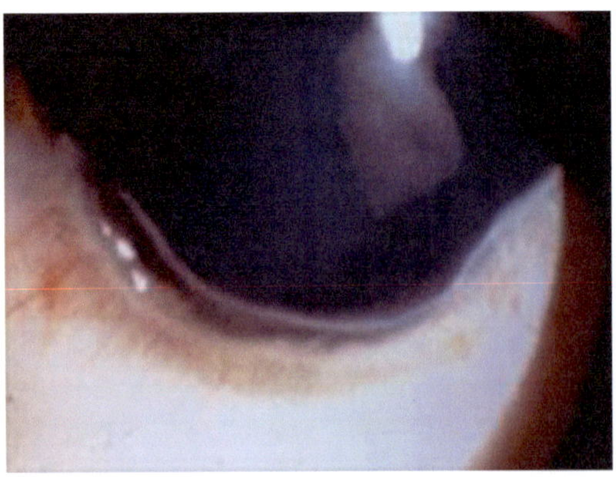

Fig. 15.3 Peripheral ulcerative keratitis from rheumatoid arthritis

*PUKs spread either circumferentially (e.g., Terrien) or centrally (e.g., Mooren).

In PUK, steroids should be avoided, which might lead to perforation. The systemic disease can be managed with immunosuppression.

Peripheral ulcerative keratitis is not associated with HIV infection or AID or Behcet (Fig. 15.3).

15.4 Metabolic Syndrome Affecting Cornea

Metabolic disorders can significantly impact the cornea, with the majority of these disorders being autosomal recessive (Table 15.6). Hunter

Table 15.6 Comparison between several metabolic syndromes affecting the cornea

	Cystinosis	Mucopolysaccharidoses (Hurler syndrome)	Fabry's disease	Tyrosinaemia type 2	Lecithin-cholesterol-acyltransferase deficiency (LCAT)	Immuno-protein deposition	Wilson disease
Inheritance	AR	AR (except type 2/Hunter, which is X-linked)	X-linked (All males affected develop disease)	AR	AR	Acquired	AR
Pathology	Lysosomal storage disorder resulting in deposition of cystine crystals	Lysosomal storage disorder of glycosaminoglycan caused by enzyme deficiency	Lysosomal storage disorder of alpha-galactosidase A	Enzyme deficiency leading to tyrosine accumulation	Lipoprotein metabolism	Systemic disease that involve Ig	Ceruloplasmin deficiency and accumulation of copper
Keratopathy	Crystal deposition	Diffuse stromal haze with punctate opacities	Vortex (swirl golden shaped) in 75%	Pseudodendritic keratitis with crystalline edges	Numerous minute grayish dots throughout the stroma, often concentrated peripherally	Band flake-like opacity at posterior stroma	Kayser–Fleischer (KF) rings, representing a brown copper deposition at Descemet of cornea, where it begins sup, then inf
Systemic	Nephropathy	Facial coarseness, skeletal, mental health, and heart abnormalities	Angiokeratoma. Burning pain in extremities and GI. Cardio and nephropathy	Painful hyperkeratosis forming calluses that develop at pressure points. CNS involvement	–	–	Liver, basal ganglia, and psychiatric disorders
Other ocular	–	Blue sclera, pigmentary retinopathy and optic neuropathy	Posterior cataract. Retinal and conjunctival vascular tortuosity	–	–	–	Anterior flower-shaped cataract
Notes	–	Keratopathy occurs in hurler, but does not occur in hunter and Sanfilippo	–	Managed by restriction of tyrosine and phenylalanine intake	–	–	The KF sign is pathognomonic and present in 95% of patients with neurological or psychiatric signs

syndrome and Fabry's disease serve as two notable exceptions, as they are X-linked recessive conditions.

Mucopolysaccharidoses affect the cornea and are often identified by corneal clouding, which is the most common ocular feature. Among these:

- Type 1 (Hurler syndrome) is most frequently associated with ocular manifestations, primarily corneal clouding and blue sclera.
- Type II (Hunter's syndrome), on the other hand, only occasionally exhibits corneal clouding, and this symptom is typically only observed in adults with a milder form of the disease.
- Type III (Sanfilippo syndrome) is almost never associated with corneal clouding.

All these disorders are autosomal recessive, apart from Hunter syndrome, which is X-linked. Moreover, retinal pigment epithelium (RPE) degenerations or pigmentary retinopathy have been detected in Hurler, Scheie, Hunter, and Sanfilippo's syndromes.

Fabry's disease, an X-linked disorder, affects male patients leading to renal failure, while female carriers generally remain unaffected.

Wilson's disease is characterized by copper deposition in Descemet's membrane, resulting in the formation of a Kayser–Fleischer ring. This ring is first detectable at the far periphery of the cornea superiorly and requires gonioscopy for early detection. Therefore, a slit lamp examination alone is insufficient for identifying early-stage copper deposition.

Gangliosidosis refers to a group of lipid storage disorders, often leading to a cloudy cornea, particularly prevalent in Type 1. These disorders follow an autosomal recessive pattern of inheritance.

Marfan syndrome, an autosomal dominant disorder linked to a defect in the fibrillin gene, is commonly associated with lens subluxation (without spherophakia), scleral thinning (resulting in blue sclera), and corneal flattening.

A variety of conditions can lead to blue sclera, such as Hurler syndrome, Marfan syndrome, osteogenesis imperfecta, Ehlers–Danlos syndrome, and Turner syndrome.

15.5 Keratoplasty

Keratoplasty, also known as corneal grafting, is performed for tectonic, therapeutic, or optical reasons. The most common indication for this procedure in adults is pseudophakic bullous keratopathy (PBK).

15.5.1 Types of Keratoplasty

- Penetrating Keratoplasty (PK): This was the first keratoplasty procedure, performed in 1905, and involves full-thickness corneal transplantation. PK can be performed for any indication but carries a higher risk of rejection. This procedure is primarily utilized for visually significant stromal scarring, opacities of uncertain endothelial status, or significant posterior corneal involvement. Selective removal of interrupted sutures can help reduce post-operative astigmatism. The ideal graft size is 7.5–8.0 mm, as larger grafts may predispose to glaucoma, while smaller grafts could lead to higher astigmatism. The maintenance of corneal sensation is crucial for successful post-operative re-epithelialization. Figure 15.4 showing corneal graft after PK.
- Anterior corneal keratoplasty: This procedure targets anterior corneal scarring and opacities, as well as corneal ectasia.
  - Deep Anterior Lamellar Keratoplasty (DALK): The first DALK surgery was performed in 1914. This technique is typically preferred for patients with keratoconus or scarring that doesn't involve Descemet's membrane or endothelium. Compared to PK, DALK offers lower rejection rates, faster recovery, and reduced astigmatism, although the final visual outcomes are roughly equivalent between the two procedures. However, recurrence of corneal dystrophy is higher with DALK than PK.

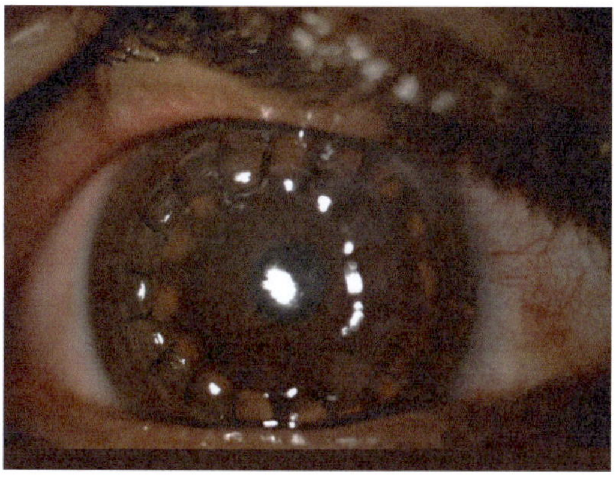

Fig. 15.4 A colored photograph showing corneal graft after penetrating keratoplasty

- Posterior cornea keratoplasty: This procedure is typically used to treat Fuchs' endothelial dystrophy and pseudophakic bullous keratopathy. While Posterior Lamellar Keratoplasty (PLK) and Deep Lamellar Endothelial Keratoplasty (DLEK) were introduced in 1990, these techniques are now rarely performed.
- Descemet Stripping Endothelial Keratoplasty (DSEK): In use since 2004, this technique involves manual dissection of both the donor and host corneas. Descemet's Stripping Automated Endothelial Keratoplasty (DSAEK) is a variation where the donor dissection is performed using a mechanical microkeratome. A common postoperative outcome is hyperopic shift. Descemet Membrane Endothelial Keratoplasty (DMEK): In use since 2006, this method transplants a pure Descemet's membrane and endothelium graft. DMEK allows faster visual recovery, superior postoperative visual acuity results, and lower rejection rates compared to DSAEK, largely because it eliminates the stroma-to-stroma graft-host interface. However, it is not widely practiced due to the complexity of donor preparation and the steep learning curve for surgeons. It can be done through a small incision, rather than 360, as in conventional keratoplasty (Fig. 15.5). DMEK adds a new Descemet's membrane and endothelium to the cornea, while DSEK also includes a layer of donor stroma. DMEK has proven to be superior to DSEK and other forms of keratoplasty regarding visual recovery.

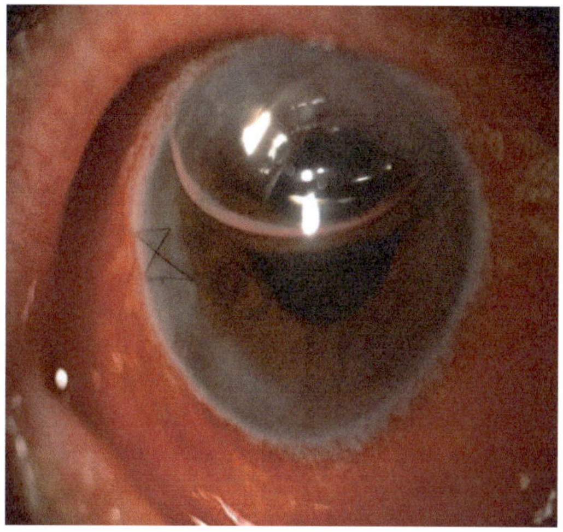

Fig. 15.5 Descemet membrane endothelial keratoplasty (DMEK) small incision and air bubble

15.5.2 Donor Cornea

Cornea with scleral rim must be claimed within 24H window from death and stored in soluble media (containing nutrients and antibiotic) for up to14 days.

Also can be stored for a short term (2–4 days) by extracting the whole eye.

Can be stored for up to a year in cryopreservation.

Corneal storage medium contains colorimetric pH indicators. Such a color change indicates a change in pH, which may be consistent with microbial contamination.

Contraindications for corneal donation:

- Prior corneal refractive surgery.
- Death from unknown cause.
- Certain systemic infections, including human immunodeficiency virus (HIV), viral hepatitis, syphilis, congenital rubella, tuberculosis, septicemia, and active malaria.

- History of high-risk behavior for HIV and hepatitis such as sexual activity with an HIV-positive individual, men who have sex with men, intravenous drug abuse, and prostitution.
- Infectious or potentially infectious diseases of the central nervous system, such as Creutzfeldt–Jakob disease.
- Receipt of a transplanted organ or human pituitary-derived growth hormone.
- Active lymphoma or leukemia.
- Presence of ocular disease, including inflammation or any condition likely to compromise graft success.

Intraocular malignancies (e.g., retinoblastoma, melanoma). Regarding age, no upper limit, but the lower limit is 2 years to prevent myopic shift.

Then the cornea assessed according to the following criteria (via slit lamp and specular microscopy):

- Epithelial defect
- Arcus senilis
- Stromal clarity
- Descemet folds
- Endothelial cell count (preferably >2000 cells/mm)
- Endothelial morphology

Corneas with good quality from donors through age 75 are suitable for transplantation.

15.5.3 Prognostic Factors for Graft Success

The indication for transplantation is the strongest predictor of graft survival. Transplants performed for conditions like keratoconus and stromal dystrophies generally have a better prognosis compared to those done for endothelial diseases, bullous keratopathy, and postinfective corneal scars.

Additional factors that can negatively impact graft success include the presence of corneal neovascularization, other ocular comorbidities such as herpetic eye diseases or glaucoma, aphakia, larger graft diameter, and the need for combined surgical procedures.

Grafts at high-risk of rejection usually defined as:

- when two or more quadrants have neovascularization or
- where previous rejection occurred

In those grafts, pre-op and post-on steroids, and continuing steroids for life should be considered.

15.5.4 Graft Failure and Rejection in Regards to PK

Graft failure is any irreversible change in the graft preventing recovery of useful vision.

Graft failure can be either primary or secondary. Common causes include immunologic allograft rejection, endothelial decompensation without documented immunologic reaction episodes, ocular surface disease, glaucoma, and astigmatism.

Primary graft failure is defined as persistent cornea edema from the immediate postoperative period, due to to inherent deficiencies in the donor graft, surgical trauma, or improperly stored tissue. Ideally, donor corneas should have at least 2000 cell/mm^2 and be stored for no more than 7 days.

Despite being an "immunologically privileged" site, the most common cause of graft failure is irreversible, immunologic allograft rejection. Diagnosis of rejection should only be made in grafts that have remained clear for at least 2 weeks following surgery. The diagnosis of immunologic graft failure is made if signs of rejection do not clear within 2 months of treatment. The risk of failure after rejection is 50%.

Risk of rejection is high up to 18 months.

Corneal neovascularization management may improve keratoplasty outcome, especially for deeper and large caliber vessels. Afferent vessels are generally thinner and deeper in the cornea with faster flow, while efferent vessels are larger and more superficial. Management modalities include:

- Corticosteroid in active inflammation, to prevent propagation of neovessels, ineffective for established vessels.
- Photocoagulation, where the afferent (arteriole) vessels should be treated first. This will induce less stasis of blood and allow better treatment of all vessels. All vessels should be treated till slight blanching is observed. Ineffective for extensive neovascularization.
- Cauterization (diathermy).
- Anti-VEGF (applied topically) are useful for small vessels, however, their use is not supported by large studies.

Several animal studies have demonstrated that blocking angiogenesis and/or lymphangiogenesis can improve graft survival.

Clinical signs of graft rejection (from most to least common regardless the layer) include:

- Corneal edema
- Keratic precipitates on the corneal graft but not on the peripheral recipient cornea
- Corneal vascularization
- Stromal infiltrates
- A Khodadoust line (separates immunologically damaged endothelium from unaffected endothelium)
- An epithelial rejection line
- Subepithelial infiltrates

Can be anatomically be classified into epithelial, stromal, or endothelial rejection (Table 15.7).

Epithelial rejection: Start as a peripheral line with uptake moving centrally. Minimal discomfort (unlike herpes).

Stromal rejection: mainly occurs in sensitized patients who have previously experienced rejection. It begins as stromal opacities at or below Bowman's layer, affecting only at the donor cornea while the recipient residual remains intact. This type of rejection rejection, characterized by significant haze and deep vascularization, can lead to corneal opacification and is more common after DALK compared to PK. In DALK, since the corneal endothelium is not transplanted; endothelial rejection cannot occur.

Endothelial rejection (most common): onset usually during the first 6 months up to 35 years. The risk of an endothelial graft rejection episode is 20%. Corneal graft rejection with endothelial rejection line (Khodadoust line) is a late sign of endothelium rejection, which starts in the periphery and moves centrally. Untreated the line will move across the cornea destroying the endothelium and cause irreversible damage. The line is made up of aggregates of lymphocytes.

Young age recipient is a risk factor for rejection, while the young age of the donor is a good candidate for donation.

Topical 1% prednisolone acetate is the primary treatment for acute graft rejection and is also used as postoperative prophylactic therapy for high-risk transplant recipients. For epithelial rejections, which have a higher rate of reversibility, topical corticosteroids can be applied six times per day, with a tapered dosing over 6–8 weeks. In contrast, severe endothelial rejection requires more intensive treatment, including hourly applications of topical corticosteroids (prednisolone acetate 1% q1h or difluprednate 0.05% q2h) in combination with systemic therapy. This often involves a single-pulse or three-pulse intravenous dose of 500 mg of methylprednisolone, with or without subconjunctival betamethasone 3 mg in 0.5 mL.

Table 15.7 Signs and management of different types of corneal rejections

	Epithelial	Stromal	Endothelium
Signs	Elevated line of abnormal epithelium	Deep haze and subepithelial infiltrates	Linear KPs, Khodadoust line
Steroid	Same pre-rejection dose	Higher dose	Topical + pulse intravenous

Due to high complications of high dose steroids, calcineurin inhibitors might be used: cyclosporine (CsA) and tacrolimus (FF-506). Although they are not superior to steroids, they can be used in low risk patients with good results, without raising IOP.

15.5.5 Keratoprosthesis (KPRO)

Keratoprosthesis (KPRO) is a surgical solution for severe corneal diseases, employed when traditional corneal transplantation has failed or carries a poor prognosis (Fig. 15.6). The most commonly used types initially included osteo-odonto-keratoprosthesis (OOKP) and AlphaCor artificial cornea. While OOKP uses a patient's tooth and alveolar bone as support for an optical cylinder, AlphaCor is a flexible device designed to integrate with natural tissues. However, both have largely been replaced by the Boston Type I Keratoprosthesis (Boston KPRO), which is now the most frequently used worldwide. The Boston KPRO uses a clear plastic plate, a titanium locking ring, and a back plate to house a donor cornea, providing improved visual rehabilitation, despite the need for long-term management and lifetime use of antibiotics and steroids to mitigate potential complications.

15.5.6 Surgical Hints in PK

- When performing Penetrating Keratoplasty (PK), it is essential to determine the optimal graft size. This decision involves balancing the optical benefits of a larger graft against the lower allograft rejection risks associated with smaller transplants. Generally, a recipient trephination of 7.5 mm and a donor graft of 7.75 mm are recommended, although larger sizes might be considered in cases of a re-do graft or corneal melting.
- Oversized grafts can lead to complications such as anterior bulging of the lens-iris diaphragm, peripheral synechiae formation, and glaucoma. It is worth noting that corneal transplants in children and young adults heal quickly, often requiring earlier suture removal.
- Suture pattern selection is also important. Continuous suturing usually results in a lower rejection rate, while interrupted suturing removes loose sutures and can help manage astigmatism. A combination of both techniques can also be applied.
- Postoperative care is crucial to ensure successful grafting. Premature suture removal may lead to graft dehiscence or unpredictable refractive error changes, while delayed removal tends to have a minimal impact on refractive error. Halting topical steroids too soon could leave the patient susceptible to graft rejection.
- Delayed epithelial healing can trigger a cycle of stromal melting, which may be challenging to manage. Therefore, any delay in epithelial healing beyond 2–3 weeks postoperatively should be proactively treated. Persisting epithelial defects after transplant surgery could indicate herpetic disease, in which case oral acyclovir might be beneficial. If patching is ineffective, a bandage lens trial or a temporary tarsorrhaphy might be worth considering.

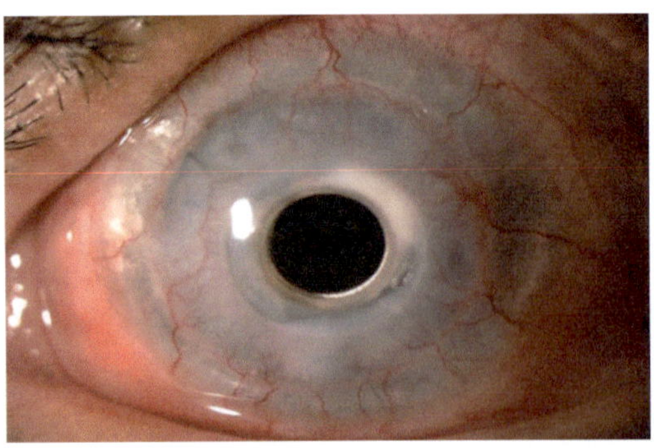

Fig. 15.6 Colored photograph showing keratoprosthesis with localized infiltrate at the supero-nasal edge

15.5.7 Conclusions from Major Cornea Clinical Trials

- Risk factors for penetrating keratoplasty graft failure include recipient age younger than 40, previous grafts, prior anterior segment surgery, prior glaucoma diagnosis, presence of anterior synechiae or stromal vessels, and primary diagnosis of chemical burns.

- Impact of donor age: 10-year analysis of the CDS data indicates higher success rates with donor corneas from individuals younger than 33 years and lower success rates with donor corneas from individuals older than 72 years, particularly in corneal endothelial disorders.

A non-inferiority study did not conclusively show that corneas preserved for 8–14 days had similar 3-year success rates to those preserved for 7 days or less. However, DSAEK success rates are higher with shorter donor tissue preservation times, and preservation times up to 11 days have minimal impact on outcomes.

15.6 Miscellaneous

15.6.1 Investigations

- **Confocal microscopy** has demonstrated efficacy in diagnosing patients with Acanthamoeba keratitis early. It allows rapid identification of Acanthamoeba cysts with a relatively high sensitivity and specificity, although it requires a skilled observer to interpret the images. Although confocal microscopy provides an in vivo highly magnified view of the corneal epithelium, stroma, and endothelium, it does not provide contour information.
- **Specular microscopy** allows imaging of the corneal endothelium.
- **Scheimpflug imaging system** can be best used to assess the posterior contour, a rotating scanning slit-beam device. This technology is particularly useful for evaluating subtle changes in the posterior corneal curvature and elevation that can indicate a higher risk for keratoconus or corneal ectasia in patients undergoing refractive corneal surgery.
- **Placido-disk imaging** employed in corneal topography only provides information about the anterior corneal surface.
- **Neurotrophic ulcer and its management**
- A keratopathy caused by corneal denervation (Fig. 15.7)
  - Initially with patching, increased lubrication, or placement of bandage contact lenses combined with careful monitoring.

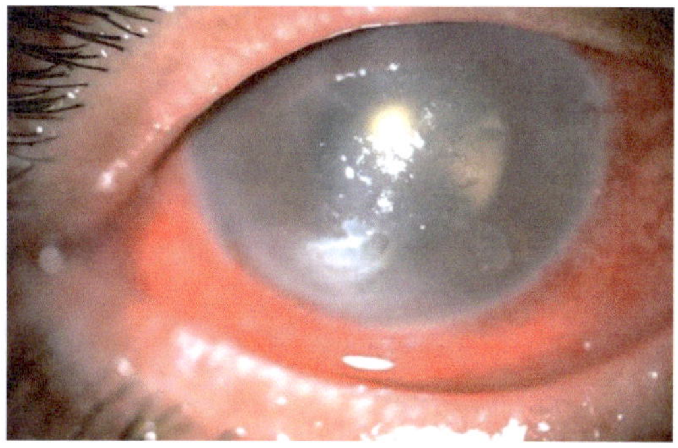

Fig. 15.7 Colored photograph showing neurotrophic ulcer

  - Then with Gundersen flap procedure and tarsorrhaphy.

  A Boston keratoprosthesis is indicated for end-stage corneal disease with significant corneal scarring. NSAIDs should be avoided in neurotrophic ulcer.

15.6.2 Corneal Perforation Management

Corneal perforations of 3 mm typically require emergent surgical closure with a corneal patch graft. Primary closure with nylon sutures is generally not feasible, particularly in eyes with acute infectious keratitis in which the surrounding tissue is also likely necrotic. Amniotic membrane grafts and cyanoacrylate glue are best suited for impending perforations or small perforations ($\leq$1 mm). They are unlikely to provide watertight closure of a large perforation.

15.6.3 Stem Cell Deficiency

Destruction of limbal stem cells is characterized by the loss of the limbal palisades of Vogt, abnormal corneal epithelium, and vascularization of the cornea. When limbal stem cells are damaged to the limbal stem cells, the conjunctival epithelium begins to cover the cornea.

Unilateral stem cell, often resulting from contact lens wear, is usually mild and can be managed effectively by discontinuing contact lens use and administering a short course of topical corticosteroids.

Limbal stem cell allograft transplantation is reserved for more severe cases of stem cell dysfunction, such as those associated with Stevens-Johnson syndrome or bilateral chemical injuries.

15.6.4 Chemical Burns

Chemical burns, particularly from alkali substances, cause significant damage to ocular tissues due to the saponification process, which affects the fatty acids and collagen fibers within the cornea. Alkali burns are particularly damaging because ocular tissues don't neutralize them effectively, unlike with acid burns where the denatured proteins can buffer the chemical reaction, leading to less overall damage.

Management of chemical burns can involve the use of topical steroids for short-term inflammation control, though prolonged use risks corneal melting. To protect corneal epithelial defects, therapeutic measures such as eyelid pressure patching or bandage contact lenses can be utilized. If needed, limbal stem cell transplantation may be conducted before a penetrating keratoplasty to enhance postoperative epithelial surface normalization.

The prognosis of chemical burns is largely influenced by the extent of perilimbal vessels blanching, which is a significant risk factor for poor outcomes. To reduce collagenase activity leading to stromal melting, topical collagenase inhibitors like L-cysteine, acetylcysteine, and disodium EDTA can be employed. Additionally, topical and systemic ascorbic acid and citrate can lower the likelihood of corneal ulceration and perforation. Ascorbic acid, particularly in high doses, is also believed to stimulate collagen synthesis. Oral tetracyclines can inhibit collagenolysis by chelating extracellular calcium, thereby impeding the activation of polymorphonuclear leukocytes (PMNs). Topical NSAIDs, however, have not shown significant effectiveness in managing chemical burns.

15.6.5 In Corneal Laceration Repair

To flatten the peripheral cornea, use widely spaced, longer sutures to close the laceration in the periphery. To steepen the central cornea, use closely spaced, shorter sutures to close the central portions of the laceration.

Cyanoacrylate glue is highly effective for closing small corneal perforations <3 mm in size. Larger perforations may be addressed with sutures or, in more difficult cases, may require tectonic corneal grafting.

Prominent corneal nerves are seen in ectodermal dysplasia, ichthyosis, acanthoamoeba keratitis, Refsum's disease, in addition to keratoconus.

Conflict of Interest None.

References

Austin A, Lietman T, Rose-Nussbaumer J (2017) Update on the management of infectious keratitis. Ophthalmology 124(11):1678–1689

Cabrera-Aguas M, Khoo P, Watson SL (2022) Infectious keratitis: a review. Clin Experiment Ophthalmol 50(5):543–562

Clinical Review of Uveitis: Part I

16

Ali Elobous, Saif Aldeen Alryalat,
Nakhleh E. Abu-Yaghi, and Ahmed A. Sallam

Abstract

This chapter offers high yield notes on uveitis, defined as inflammation of the uveal tract, which includes the iris, ciliary body, and choroid, as well as nearby structures such as the retina, vitreous, and optic nerve. It focuses on anterior and intermediate uveitis, with the following chapter covers posterior uveitis. The chapter also addresses various miscellaneous syndromes associated with uveitis, enhancing the understanding of its diverse presentations and potential complications. By providing detailed insights into the classification, clinical features, and implications of uveitis, the chapter aims to equip readers with the knowledge necessary for effective diagnosis and management in clinical practice.

Keywords

Uveitis · Anterior uveitis · Intermediate uveitis · Syndromes · Complications

16.1 Overview

Uveitis refers to the inflammation of the uveal tract, which includes the iris, ciliary body, and choroid, as well as nearby structures such as the retina, vitreous, and optic nerve. Depending on the area affected, uveitis can be anatomically categorized as:

- Anterior uveitis, which involves the anterior chamber, iris, and may extend to include some cells in the anterior vitreous.
- Intermediate uveitis, which involves the vitreous and peripheral retina, and is often characterized by "snowballs" in the vitreous or "snow banks" on the pars plana and ora serrata.
- Posterior uveitis, which involves the choroid, retina, retinal vessels, and the retinal pigment epithelium (RPE).
- Panuveitis, which denotes inflammation in all the aforementioned anterior, intermediate, and posterior regions.

A. Elobous (✉)
Department of Ophthalmology, Royal Medical Services, Amman, Jordan

Department of Ophthalmology, Indiana University School of Medicine, Indianapolis, IN, USA

S. A. Alryalat
Department of Ophthalmology, The University of Jordan, Amman, Jordan

The University of Colorado Anschutz Medical Campus, Aurora, CO, USA

N. E. Abu-Yaghi
Department of Ophthalmology, The University of Jordan, Amman, Jordan
e-mail: N.abuyaghi@ju.edu.jo

A. A. Sallam
Harvey and Bernice Jones Eye Institute, University of Arkansas for Medical Sciences (UAMS), Little Rock, AR, USA

S. A. Alryalat (ed.), *Ophthalmology Board and FRCS Part 2 Exams*,
https://doi.org/10.1007/978-981-96-1517-9_16

It is important to note that the term "panuveitis" should only be used when inflammation is present in all three anatomical regions. The emergence of posterior segment structural complications, such as macular edema, peripheral retinal vasculitis, optic disc edema, and retinal or choroidal neovascularization, does not influence the determination of a posterior uveitis diagnosis. For example, if a patient with HLA-B27–associated anterior uveitis develops macular edema, this does not imply the presence of concurrent posterior uveitis. Moreover, intermediate uveitis describes an inflammatory process primarily involving the vitreous base as the primary anatomical site. However, inflammation may also extend to the peripheral retina and its vasculature, manifesting as peripheral retinal vasculitis, and the pars plana, referred to as pars planitis.

In addition, uveitis can be classified depending on clinical behavior as:

- Acute: if a single attack with a duration ≤3 months or without recurrence within 3 months
- Chronic: when lasting >3 months or relapse occurring within 3 months off-treatment

A recurrence is defined if repeated episodes separated by ≥3 months period of inactivity without treatment occur (aka. Recurrent acute uveitis).

So, to diagnose a recurrence, we need attacks separated by a period (>3 months) without activity and without treatment.

Uveitis is considered to be resistant to treatment when there is no improvement after 3 months (Kanski 2019).

16.2 Anterior Uveitis

16.2.1 Overview

It is the most common type of uveitis. It may be isolated, part of panuveitis/intermediate uveitis, or part of a systemic disease. It can affect any age-group but generally becomes more common with age.

Clinical presentation:

1. Eye redness, pain, photophobia, and blurred vision
2. Ciliary injection, keratic precipitates (KPs) especially inferior one-third (Arlt's triangle), AC flare/cells/fibrin, hypopyon, posterior synechia, anterior vitreous cells (spillover), and possible CME/optic disc edema
3. Low intraocular pressure (IOP) (typical) due to ciliary body shutdown, but high IOP in:
   (a) Posner–Schlossman syndrome
   (b) Herpetic uveitis
   (c) Fuchs heterochromic iridocyclitis
   (d) Toxoplasmosis
   (e) Sarcoidosis
   (f) Secondary open angle glaucoma due to trabecular meshwork blockage by inflammatory cells or secondary angle closure glaucoma due to iris bombe and posterior synechiae
4. Often unilateral but can affect both eyes synchronously or sequentially
5. Can be recurrent or chronic as mentioned before

Anterior uveitis can be divided into granulomatous (mutton fat KPs) and non-granulomatous uveitis. All of the granulomatous causes can mimic non-granulomatous uveitis, but the non-granulomatous causes never look granulomatous.

Granulomatous causes include:

1. Sarcoidosis
2. Syphilis
3. Tuberculosis
4. Herpes Simplex
5. Lens-induced uveitis (phacoanaphylactic)
6. Intraocular foreign body
7. Sympathetic ophthalmia
8. Vogt–Koyanagi–Harada syndrome
9. Uveitis associated with multiple sclerosis
10. Other infectious agents: leptospirosis, brucellosis

The vast majority of anterior uveitis are as follows (Table 16.1):

Table 16.1 Comparison between HLA-B27 negative and positive uveitis

	HLA-B27 negative/ idiopathic	HLA-B27 positive
Age	Biphasic peaking at 30 and 60 years	Peaking at 30 years
Gender	M = F	M > F
Heredity	Not present	Positive family history
Course of inflammation	Acute but could be persistent	Acute episodic (explosive in nature)
Severity of inflammation	Less severe	More severe; more frequent AC fibrin, hypopyon, posterior synechiae (PS) and CME
Recurrences	Uncommon	Frequent

- Idiopathic (isolated, **HLA-B27 negative** with no underlying systemic disease).
- Or HLA-B27 related (**HLA-B27 positive**, may be associated with seronegative spondyloarthropathies like ankylosing spondylitis).

Other common causes should be kept in mind such as herpetic uveitis and Fuchs heterochromic iridocyclitis especially in the presence of atypical features.

16.2.2 HLA-B27 Associated Uveitis (Table 16.2)

- HLA-B27 is a class 1 molecule on chromosome 6.
- HLA-B27 is present in 8% of the general population but is seen in up to 40–50% of patients with non-granulomatous anterior uveitis.
- Lifetime risk of developing either uveitis or spondyloarthritis is 25%
- It is generally an acute anterior uveitis presenting unilaterally, recurrent, each episode is self-limited lasting 2–3 weeks, and can affect both eyes sequentially, i.e., alternating.
- The spondyloarthropathies are a group of inflammatory arthropathies featuring HLA-B27 positivity, inflammatory back pain, enthesitis, dactylitis, and asymmetric arthritis that affect lower limbs. In addition, these diseases have negative RF and ANA (hence the name seronegative spondyloarthropathies).
- They have male predominance (2X) (except psoriatic arthritis, where no gender predominance, and IBD, where females predominate)

16.2.3 Herpetic Uveitis

- HSV anterior uveitis is more likely to present in patients <50 years of age while VZV anterior uveitis in patients >50 years of age.
- Consider herpetic uveitis if associated with:
  - High IOP, common due to trabeculitis
  - Sectoral iris atrophy or transillumination defects near pupillary margin leading to semi-dilated/irregular pupil
  - Heavily pigmented KPs are common due to pigment shedding from herpes infection. Diffuse KPs may be noted
  - Reduced corneal sensation, esp. in VZV-related herpetic keratouveitis
  - Evidence of active or previous keratitis despite that iritis may occur either with or without corneal involvement
  - History of periocular herpetic disease is suggestive
- Viral PCR from an aqueous tap can confirm the diagnosis in suspected cases

16.2.4 Fuchs' Heterochromic Uveitis (FHU)

- Typically affects young to middle-aged adults. M = F
- Typically presents as unilateral low-grade inflammation; mild chronic anterior uveitis in a white eye. Bilateral in 10% of cases
- Rubella virus has been implicated as a causative factor
- Consider Fuchs' uveitis if associated with:
  - White gelatinous small stellate KPs, diffusely distributed over the corneal endothelium

Table 16.2 Comparison between disease entities causing HLA-B27 associated anterior uveitis

	Ankylosing spondylitis	Reactive arthritis (Reiter's syndrome)	Psoriatic arthritis	Inflammatory bowel disease
Manifestations	Young to middle-aged men with lower back pain and stiffness. Unilateral alternating acute anterior uveitis "flip-flop"	Young men with urethritis, conjunctivitis, and oligoarticular arthritis occurring after 1–4 weeks of UTI or GI infection caused by gram negative organisms such as Shigella, Klebsiella, Salmonella, Chlamydia, Ureaplasma, or Yersinia	Skin rash: raised scaly plaques (most common), or pustular type (more frequent in HLA-B27), finger nail (ungual) pitting and hyperkeratosis, "sausage digit" deformity. No gender predominance	More in women. They can develop episcleritis, scleritis, keratitis, iritis. May be associated with sacroilitis, pyoderma gangrenosum, erythema nodosum, and bloody stool
HLA-B27 +ve prevalence	90%	75%	~30% if without spondylitis, up to 70% if spondylitis exist	70% if spondylitis exist
Risk of anterior uveitis	25%	12% (Risk of conjunctivitis = 50%)	7%, tends to be bilateral, more insidious in onset and chronic in duration, with posterior involvement and worse prognosis	Anterior uveitis is present in 5–12% of ulcerative colitis and 2–3% of Crohn's patients. Uveitis is usually bilateral, posterior, insidious in onset, and/or chronic in duration
Notes	Rarely apical pulmonary fibrosis and aortitis with subsequent valvular insufficiency	Eye involvement is more common after GI (~75%) than urinary infection (~50%) Mucocutaneous- circinate balanitis (rash on penis), keratoderma blennorhagicum (scaling skin on the palms/ soles)	Uveitis typically occurs in patients with psoriatic arthritis, not just psoriasis which precedes the onset of arthritis by months or years	Crohn's disease has worse prognosis in relation to eye compared to UC. UC presents as partial thickness inflammation which always involves the rectum, while Crohn's presents as full thickness skip lesions with transmural inflammation at any part of GI tract

- Mild flare, few cells, and absence of PS or PAS
- Diffuse iris stromal atrophy; washed-out or moth-eaten appearance. Diffuse transillumination defects
- Iris atrophy can cause heterochromia. Usually the involved iris is lighter, however in patients with blue eyes, the affected iris may be darker
- Abnormal iris vessels
- Iris nodules and sometimes iris crystals
- Posterior subcapsular cataract—most common cause for blurred vision in affected patients
- Vitreous opacities—may cause floaters
- Gonioscopy: open angle, twig-like fine bridging blood vessels may be present in the angle, and these may bleed easily, especially during cataract surgery (Amsler sign)
- High IOP (secondary open angle glaucoma) in 10–30%

- Typically, patients with FHU does not have pigmented KPs, and posterior synechiae or significant CME are also uncommon. However, following cataract surgery, these signs can develop in FHU patients though.

16.2.5 Posner–Schlossman Syndrome (aka. Glaucomatocyclitic Crisis)

- Typically affects young to middle-aged adults. M > F
- Typically presents as unilateral recurrent mild anterior uveitis in a white eye associated with very high IOP (40–80 mmHg)
- CMV virus has been implicated as a causative factor
- Consider Posner–Schlossman syndrome if associated with:
  - Normal IOP and no uveitis signs between attacks
  - Painless episode of inflammatory glaucoma (high IOP) lasting from several hours to weeks; blurred vision and halos
  - Cornel edema and fine KPs
  - Mild flare, few cells, and absence of PS or PAS
  - Open angle on gonioscopy

Comparison between Fuchs Heterochromic Uveitis (FHU) and Posner–Schlossman syndrome (PSS) is provided in Table 16.3.

Table 16.3 Comparison between Fuchs Heterochromic Uveitis (FHU) and Posner–Schlossman syndrome (PSS)

	Fuchs Heterochromic uveitis (FHU)	Posner–Schlossman syndrome (PSS)
Inflammation	Mild recurrent unilateral inflammation with diffuse stellate KPs	Mild recurrent unilateral reaction
IOP	Usually normal primarily with 15% risk of glaucoma	High IOP with 25% risk of glaucoma
Iris	Iris heterochromia with prominent iris and angle vessels secondary to iris atrophy	Iris atrophy and heterochromia less than FHI, whereas posterior synechiae typically are not
Associations	Rubella, CMV	CMV
Notes	Cataract surgery might be complicated by hyphema (Amsler sign)	CMV anterior uveitis may mimic PSS

16.2.6 Schwartz–Matsuo Syndrome

- Typically presents with mild anterior uveitis and secondary open angle glaucoma in the presence of rhegmatogenous retinal detachment (RRD).
- Photoreceptor outer segments pass through the retinal break and enter the aqueous outflow pathways, leading to outflow obstruction and elevated IOP. Typically associated with detachments that are large in area (involving the macula); flat in height (shallow); and long in duration (chronic); where tears are located mostly around the ora serrata
- Following retinal detachment repair, IOP typically normalizes and prognosis is favorable
- Consider Schwartz–Matsuo syndrome if associated with:
  - AC cells without other signs of uveitis
  - High IOP with fluctuation
  - RRD
  - Open angle on gonioscopy

16.2.7 Tubulo-Interstitial Nephritis and Uveitis (TINU)

- Typically affects young females, median age 15 years (Mandeville et al. 2001).
- Typically presents as bilateral acute non-granulomatous anterior uveitis of sudden onset in a systemically-ill patient having acute renal failure (nephritis before uveitis)
- The uveitis is usually mild, and the nephritis is self-limited. However, recurrent or persistent uveitis may occur in over half of patients and chronic renal impairment in 11%

- Idiopathic condition, T-cell mediated disease (type 4 hypersensitivity), may be related to certain drugs or infections
- TINU is strongly associated with HLA-DQA1*01, HLA-DQB1*05, and HLA-DRB1*01
- Elevated levels of β2-microglobulin are usually present in the urine. So, increased β2-microglobulin level in a patient with uveitis should prompt the diagnosis of (TINU) syndrome

Diagnostic certainty for uveitis is classified into three categories:

- "Definite" is when typical uveitis is present alongside confirmed interstitial nephritis through renal biopsy or complete clinical criteria.
- "Probable" is assigned either when atypical uveitis accompanies a positive renal biopsy or when typical uveitis is present with incomplete interstitial nephritis criteria.
- "Possible" is when atypical uveitis exists with incomplete interstitial nephritis clinical criteria.

Interstitial nephritis, evaluated through clinical criteria, is considered "Complete" when all three criteria, including abnormal renal function, are met. If less than three criteria are met, it is termed "Incomplete."

16.2.8 Kawasaki Disease

- It is an acute febrile illness that typically affects children under 10 years old and is characterized by vasculitis of the medium-sized arteries.
- The disease is defined by a fever lasting five or more days accompanied by four of the following five criteria: conjunctival injection, skin rash, desquamation of extremities, cervical lymphadenopathy, and mucosal changes such as pharyngeal injection, red cracked lips, or strawberry tongue
- Eye manifestations include:
  - Bilateral bulbar conjunctival injection (>90%), which is nonexudative and typically sparing the limbus with absent follicles, papillae, and chemosis
  - Anterior uveitis (80%) which is typically bilateral and mild commonly in the first week of illness
- Cardiac abnormalities (coronary artery aneurysms) are serious complications of the disease
- Treatment: the drug of choice is aspirin

16.2.9 Lens-Induced Uveitis

- Lens proteins are immunogenic once they leave the confines of the capsular bag; for example, after traumatic release of lens material (**phacoantigenic uveitis/phacoanaphylactic uveitis**)
- The term, "phacoanaphylactic uveitis," is misleading because anaphylaxis involves immunoglobulin E (Ig E), mast cells, and basophils, none of which are involved in this condition
- Possible mechanisms for this uveitis include traumatic capsular rupture or post-operative retention of lens material. Typically presents as an acute severe anterior uveitis, days to weeks following the insult
- This insult may also cause immune sensitization of lens proteins. Consequently, lens protein exposure in the contralateral eye may be associated with an aggressive response occurring earlier (with 24 hrs of surgery)
- Histopathology shows zonal granulomatous inflammation surrounding a breach of lens capsule
- Clinically, it is associated with:
  - Exposed lens protein or retained lens fragment
  - Severe AC reaction (flare, cells, hypopyon)
  - Mutton-fat KPs
  - PS and PAS
  - IOP may be elevated but it is variable
- In contrast to infectious endophthalmitis, phacoanaphylactic uveitis is less painful and not involving the retina, choroid, or optic disc

- In contrast to phacoanaphylactic uveitis, phacolytic glaucoma occurs when soluble lens proteins pass through microscopic defects in the anterior capsule of hypermature cataract, leading to trabecular meshwork obstruction. These are HMW proteins from the liquefied cortex
  - The main concern is for high IOP, inflammation is milder
  - AC shows lens protein and foamy macrophages, may form pseudohypopyon
  - KPs are not typical

16.2.10 IOL-Induced Uveitis

- Intraocular chafing from intraocular lens (IOL) implants leading to a spectrum of disease ranging from mild iritis to Uveitis-Glaucoma-Hyphema (UGH) syndrome
- It was mostly due to iris-fixated and older style ACIOL lenses causing irritation of the iris by a lens haptic/optic. However, single piece IOLs placed in the sulcus can cause this as well. In addition, improper lens position; for example, dislocated or malpositioned IOL and misplaced haptics can lead to iris-lens contact and irritation. Rarely in patients with loose zonules, UGH can occur even with an IOL that is in the capsular bag and can be diagnosed by excessive IOL/bag movement with UBM.
- The incidence of IOL-induced uveitis has sharply declined as lens designs and materials improve.
- Clinically, it is associated with:
  - Variable AC reaction (cells, flare, hypopyon)
  - Microhyphema or hyphema
  - Iris transillumination defects, iris neovascularization
  - High IOP
  - Gonioscopy may show blood within the angle, increased pigmentation of the trabecular meshwork
  - CME

16.2.11 Juvenile Idiopathic Arthritis (JIA)-Associated Uveitis (Table 16.4)

- JIA is the most common rheumatic disease seen in children. It is a chronic, non-infectious arthritis that lasts for at least 6 weeks and begins before the age of 16 years (rarely develop before age 2).
  In children, up to 80% of all cases of anterior uveitis are associated with JIA, making JIA-associated uveitis being the most frequent extra-articular manifestation of the disease.
- There is typically little correlation between onset of uveitis and joint inflammation in JIA. Uveitis often begins shortly after the onset of arthritis, but it can also precede the arthritis. Approximately 90% of uveitis cases develop within 7 years of arthritis onset.
- The JIA subtypes particularly associated with uveitis include pauciarticular (oligoarthritis), polyarticular, psoriatic arthritis, and enthesitis-related arthritis. Uveitis almost never occurs in children with systemic arthritis and is very rare in those with RF +ve polyarticular subtype.
- Risk factors for the development of uveitis include:
  - Female gender
  - Early age of onset: <4 years
  - Oligoarthritis subtype
  - ANA positive
  - Others: involvement of lower extremity joints (Knees), and lack of involvement of the wrists.
- The major ocular manifestation of JIA is uveitis. It is typically a chronic non-granulomatous anterior uveitis that is usually bilateral (70%) but may present initially in one eye
- The eye is often externally white, and the patient is usually asymptomatic (hence the delayed diagnosis). Unfortunately, complications may have occurred at the time of presentation
- Clinically, it is associated with:
  - Small KPs

Table 16.4 Comparison between different subtypes of Juvenile idiopathic arthritis (JIA) that are associated with uveitis

Subtype	Clinical features
1. Systemic (Still's disease)	• Arthritis, fever, rash, splenomegaly, lymphadenopathy, serositis • Systemic features precedes arthritis • More in boys • RF and ANA are usually absent • Eye involvement is rare
2. Oligoarthritis	• The most common form, typically affecting young girls (F:M = 5:1) • Up to four joints affected during the first 6 months: – Persistent: affects no more than four joints throughout its course – Extended: affects five or more joints after the first 6 months • ANA present in up to 75% while RF usually absent • 80–90% of JIA related uveitis
3. Polyarthritis	• The second most common form (F:M = 3:1) • Five or more joints affected during the first 6 months: – RF positive, seen in adolescent girls. Similar to adult RA – RF negative, seen in young girls. ANA positive in 40% • 10% of JIA-related uveitis (esp. RF−ve)
4. Enthesitis-related arthritis	• Arthritis and enthesitis • More in older boys • May involve axial skeleton causing inflammatory back pain and sacroiliac joint tenderness • HLA-B27 more prevalent • Family history of HLA-B27-related disease
5. Psoriatic arthritis	• Arthritis and psoriasis • Bimodal: young girls and older (M = F) • Family history of psoriasis
6. Undifferentiated arthritis	Unknown cause of arthritis or not fitting any category

  - AC cells/flare
  - Posterior synechia (common)
  - Complications include: band keratopathy (60%), cataract (40%), glaucoma (10–25%), and CMO (10%)
  - Less commonly: vitritis, peripheral retinal vasculitis, and hypotony
- It is critical to screen children with systemic JIA for eye involvement. The initial screening exam should occur as soon as possible and no later than 6 weeks from referral. Further screening may occur at the following intervals:
  - For children <6 years age **and** disease duration &<4 years since arthritis began: Q3 months for ANA +ve and Q6 months in ANA −ve
  - For children >6 years age, **or** disease duration &>4 years: Q6 months for ANA +ve and Q12 months in ANA −ve
  - If both above: Q12 months regardless ANA
  - If Still disease: Q12 months
- Screening is generally more frequent in the first 4 years of diagnosis and in younger than 6 years of age. Screening may occur until 11–12 years old
- Treatment:
  - Steroids (topical, periocular, and systemic), NSAIDS, and steroid sparing agents may all play a role.
  - Given the severity of the disease and the high rate of complication, systemic immunosuppression is usually necessary to control both the systemic disease and uveitis in children with JIA. However, some children may only need topical steroids and a mydriatic to manage uveitis effectively. Long-term treatment is often necessary due to the chronicity of uveitis. However, when frequent topical steroid is needed to control the inflammation, steroid sparing agents such as methotrexate and anti-TNF agents may be considered.

16.3 Intermediate Uveitis

Intermediate uveitis is an anatomical description. It refers to inflammation primarily involving the vitreous and can also include the pars plana and the adjacent peripheral part of the retina. Primarily, it is characterized by vitritis and represents 10–15% of all uveitis cases, with up to a quarter of those occurring in children. This condition, most commonly appearing in young adults and again in middle-aged or elderly individuals, displays a bimodal distribution.

This form of uveitis, believed to be driven by T-cell mediated processes, is typically chronic, presenting subtly and recurring over time. It affects both sexes equally and is often bilateral, though it can manifest asymmetrically. Symptoms include floaters and reduced visual acuity due primarily to macular edema, though some patients may not exhibit any symptoms. The inflammation generally persists for a minimum of 3 years and tends to subside after 5–15 years.

Clinically it is associated with:

- Vitritis: Characterized by the presence of vitreal cells, snowballs, and snow banking (exudation at the ora serrata, most commonly, inferiorly but potentially occurring 360 degrees around)
  - Snowbank is composed of fibroglial and vascular elements
- Snowballs are composed of epithelioid cells and multinucleated giant cells. Peripheral periphlebitis is associated with increased risk for multiple sclerosis. Ischemia from peripheral vasculitis can cause neovascularization (10% of patients) as well as subsequent vitreous hemorrhage (≤5%)
- Some AC activity is common, but posterior synechiae is uncommon
- Macular edema is the commonest complication in 50% of intermediate uveitis. Other complications include papillitis, band keratopathy, cataract, glaucoma, ERM, tractional RD, and retinal tears. Hypotony may result from cyclitic membrane formation and traction (ciliary body detachment).

Intermediate uveitis can be caused by infectious and non-infectious causes.

The most common causes of intermediate uveitis are as follows:

- Pars planitis (the most common 85–90%, a diagnosis of exclusion)
- Multiple sclerosis (5–25%, second most common) (Fig. 16.1)
- Lyme disease (with intermediate uveitis being its most common eye manifestation)
- Sarcoidosis

Other less common causes include tuberculosis, syphilis, toxoplasmosis, and lymphoma. A useful mnemonic is **SIMPLE** (**S**arcoid/**S**yphilis, **I**nflammatory Bowel Disease, **M**ultiple sclerosis, **P**ars planitis, **L**ymphoma/**L**yme, and **E**tc (TB, Toxocariasis, Blau syndrome, VKH, and Whipple's disease).

Pars planitis, an idiopathic form of intermediate uveitis with no associated infection or systemic disease, predominantly affects young adults and children, exhibiting a bimodal age distribution: one peak in ages 5–15 and another in 25–35 years. This condition tends to affect younger females and older males more frequently. In children, it often manifests as strabismus, leukocoria, or most commonly, diminished visual acuity, often due to macular edema. Studies indicate a higher prevalence of asthma among young individuals with pars planitis than in the general population. As for its progression, pars planitis is persistent in 60% of cases, exhibits a remitting

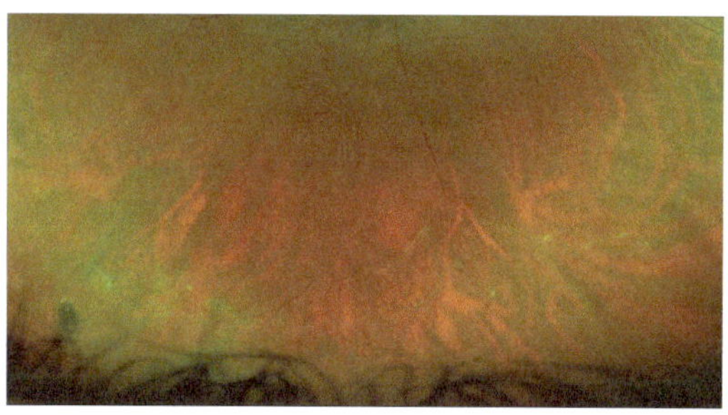

Fig. 16.1 The fundus image demonstrates a case of multiple sclerosis with stable inferior perivasculitis, characterized by "puff balls". Courtesy Retina Rocks®

and relapsing course in 30%, and is self-limited in 10%. In children, over 75% of pars planitis cases present as bilateral. If it is unilateral in a child, toxocariasis and diffuse unilateral subacute necrosis (DUSN) should be considered. Patients with pars planitis are typically young; therefore, if a patient in their 40s presents with intermediate uveitis, multiple sclerosis should be suspected, whereas for older patients, lymphoma should be ruled out, even though lymphoma often responds well to oral and topical corticosteroids.

Given the variety of potential differential diagnoses, a comprehensive evaluation plan is necessary for an accurate diagnosis. Typically, this includes complete blood count, urea and electrolytes, erythrocyte sedimentation rate, VDRL, TPHA, urinalysis, and chest X-ray for all patients, with additional investigations driven by specific clinical findings. Optical coherence tomography (OCT) or fundus fluorescein angiography (FFA) may be required to confirm cystoid macular edema.

Treatment:

- The treatment of noninfectious idiopathic intermediate uveitis typically involves managing inflammation, controlling symptoms, and preventing complications that could lead to long-term damage. Observation is reasonable if asymptomatic (VA > 6/12) and no CME or peripheral neovascularization
- If CME or visually disabling floaters, consider treatment as follows:
  - Topical steroids have minimal role, except for significant AC activity when topical steroids and mydriatics are used to control the inflammation.
  - Periocular (sub-tenon or orbital floor) and intraocular (intravitreal) steroids are preferred if disease is unilateral or very asymmetric (with dexamethasone implant working for 4–6 months and fluocinolone acetonide implant working for 3 years).
  - Systemic steroids (1–2 mg/kg/day) are indicated if disease is bilateral. Immunosuppressive agents also play a role especially when the disease is resistant with failure to get oral steroid dose to <7.5 mg/day and in case of intolerable steroid side effects. Because TNF inhibitors (e.g., infliximab and etanercept) can exacerbate MS, it is important to consider an extensive workup for MS before starting the treatment.
  - Laser or cryotherapy to the areas of nonperfusion/snow bank if steroids do not work or if they have neovascularization. It can be repeated, but cryotherapy carries the risk of epiretinal membrane formation and RRD
- Pars plana vitrectomy is mainly indicated for persistent vitreous opacities, VMT/ERM, and retinal detachment. It can be combined with cataract surgery as well. Whether PPV itself can decrease the inflammation and reduce the need for anti-inflammatory treatment is significantly debatable.

16.4 Miscellaneous

16.4.1 Endophthalmitis

Endophthalmitis is an inflammation of inner ocular layers, which can be clinically observed as inflammation in different layers of the eye, with inflammatory signs in the vitreous and aqueous (Fig. 16.2).

16.4.1.1 Specific Endophthalmitis Syndromes

A. Endogenous bacterial endophthalmitis: Patients are usually systemically unwell, and the mortality rate is relatively high, ranging from 5 to 10%. The prognosis for endogenous endophthalmitis is generally worse compared to postoperative endophthalmitis. This form of endophthalmitis typically results from hematogenous spread, with the infection often originating from a distant site. While Roth spots may develop in about 1% of cases of bacteraemia, most cases do not progress to full-blown ocular infection. Common pathogens associated with endogenous endophthalmitis include Klebsiella and other gram-negative bacilli.

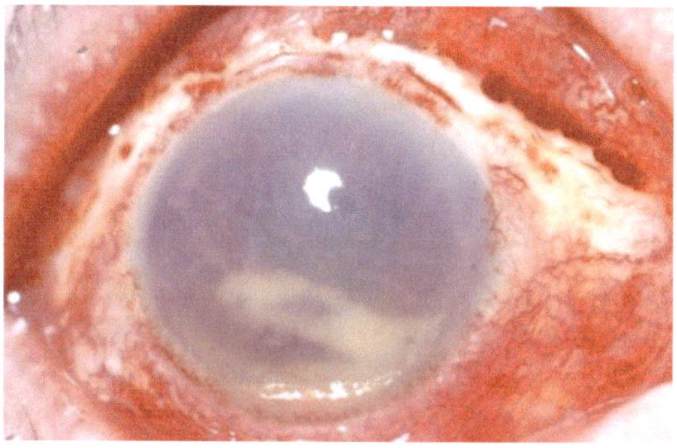

Fig. 16.2 Colored eye image showing signs of endophthalmitis involving the anterior segment. Courtesy Retina Rocks®

B. Posttraumatic endophthalmitis: Incidence after penetrating ocular trauma occurs in fewer than 10% of cases. The most common causative agents responsible are *Staphylococcus epidermidis* and Bacillus species, though many other organisms can be involved. The prognosis for visual recovery in this setting is generally poor, with final VA often being <20/200, especially when *Bacillus cereus* is implicated.

C. Endophthalmitis in IV drug abuse: The most common organisms are fungal and often occur without associated fungemia. Bacterial causes are primarily due to Staphylococcus species; with *B. cereus* being a less common pathogen. The incidence of endophthalmitis in this population is high due to the frequent introduction of contaminants through non-sterile needles.

D. Post-surgical endophthalmitis:

- Bleb-associated endophthalmitis, typically caused by Streptococcus species, particularly Streptococcus pneumoniae (gram-positive cocci in pairs or chains), and *Haemophilus influenzae* (gram-negative coccobacilli). Symptoms include sudden pain, vision loss, redness, and swelling of the eyelid and conjunctiva, along with signs of infection such as purulent discharge and hypopyon. Risk factors include bleb leakage, use of antimetabolites, and poor bleb healing.
- Cataract surgery-associated endophthalmitis, can occur as either early-onset or late-onset post-operative endophthalmitis. Early-onset infection commonly caused by *Staphylococcus aureus* (gram-positive cocci in clusters) and *S. epidermidis*, while late-onset infections are often associated with *Propionibacterium acnes (gram-positive, anaerobic bacterium)*. According to the Endophthalmitis Vitrectomy Study (EVS), patients with light perception (LP) vision who underwent immediate vitrectomy had a threefold increase in achieving a visual acuity of 20/40 or better (33% with PPV compared to 11% with TAP). They also had a twofold increase in achieving 20/100 or better (56% with PPV versus 30% with TAP), and a 50% reduction in the risk of severe visual loss, defined as vision worse than 5/200 (20% with PPV compared to 47% with TAP).

E. Candida endophthalmitis: It usually arises from candidemia, with the infection entering through the choroid. It typically presents with white, fluffy chorioretinal lesions, and overlying vitritis and is commonly treated with intravenous amphotericin. Candida is also the most frequent cause of fungal postoperative endophthalmitis.

16.4.2 Masquerade Syndromes

Masquerade syndromes are a group of ocular diseases that mimic the signs and symptoms of uveitis. They are named so because they "masquerade" or disguise themselves as uveitis, which can make them difficult to diagnose correctly. Here are some examples:

- Primary vitreoretinal lymphoma (PVRL)
- Other tumors, including choroidal melanoma and retinoblastoma
- Retinitis pigmentosa
- Ischemic syndromes
- RRD
- Pigment dispersion syndrome

16.4.2.1 Primary Vitreoretinal Lymphoma (PVRL)

- Primary vitreoretinal lymphoma (PVRL) is a rare but significant condition that often mimics uveitis, especially in elderly patients (around 70 years old). It is typically bilateral and considered a subset of primary central nervous system lymphoma (PCNSL). Approximately 60–75% of PVRL patients will develop CNS involvement within two years, even in the absence of neurological symptoms, necessitating a thorough CNS lymphoma evaluation.
- PVRL is predominantly of the B cell type, and rarely T cell variants.
- The main presenting symptoms of PVRL are decreased vision and floaters, and it can mimic many uveitis syndromes. Of note it does not typically cause macular edema, so visual acuity is usually preserved. It may respond to steroids, which can further complicate diagnosis, as steroid treatment might mask the underlying lymphoma.
- Diagnosis of PVRL should be suspected when patients do not respond to usual therapy. Typical signs include vitritis without CME, non-resolving retinitis or chorioretinitis, and the distinctive "leopard skin" pattern of yellowish lesions in the retinal pigment epithelium, along with subretinal infiltration of lymphomatous cells. A vitreous tap, often obtained via vitrectomy, should be performed for cytology and PCR analysis. In patients with lymphoma, interleukin-10 (IL-10) levels are elevated in the vitreous, whereas patients with inflammatory uveitis typically have high levels of IL-6. The ratio of IL-10 to IL-6 is often elevated in intraocular lymphoma. It is crucial to stop any corticosteroid treatments for a few weeks before a planned biopsy, as corticosteroids can reduce cell counts and interfere with diagnosis. Investigation should also include a lumbar puncture and brain imaging to assess for CNS involvement. Management of PVRL depends on CNS involvement. If CNS is involved, treatment typically includes a combination of intrathecal chemotherapy (such as methotrexate), IV cytotoxic agents, and both whole brain and ocular irradiation. In cases where the CNS is not involved, intravitreal chemotherapy, including methotrexate or rituximab, may be used to treat ocular lymphoma. Periocular and systemic steroids may also help reduce intraocular inflammation. The prognosis for PVRL patients is generally poor, with median survival dropping to about 6 months once CNS symptoms appear, highlighting that PVRL is considered a subset of primary CNS lymphoma.

16.4.3 Summary of HLA Associations

- HLA A11 is associated with sympathetic ophthalmia.
- HLA A28 is linked to intermediate uveitis.
- HLA A29 is strongly connected with birdshot retinochoroidopathy.
- HLA B5/B12 is associated with Behçet's disease.
- HLA B7 is linked to conditions such as presumed ocular histoplasmosis syndrome (POHS), serpiginous choroiditis, acute posterior multifocal placoid pigment epitheliopathy (APMPPE), and ankylosing spondylitis.
- HLA B8 has associations with conditions like Sjögren's syndrome, sarcoidosis, and intermediate uveitis.
- HLA B12 is related to ocular cicatricial pemphigoid (OCP).
- HLA B22 is associated with Vogt–Koyanagi–Harada syndrome.
- HLA B27 is linked to ankylosing spondylitis, Reiter's syndrome, inflammatory bowel disease (IBD), and psoriatic arthritis.
- HLA-B51 is associated with Behçet's disease.
- HLA Bw5 has associations with Posner–Schlossman syndrome.
- HLA DR2 is connected with conditions like intermediate uveitis or pars planitis, and APMPPE.
- HLA DR4 is linked to VKH Syndrome, OCP, and sympathetic ophthalmia.

- HLA DR15 and DQ6 are associated with multiple sclerosis (MS).
- HLA-DQA1*01, HLA-DQB1*05, and HLA-DRB1*01 are strongly associated with TINU

16.4.4 Immune-Related Uveitis

A. Immune recovery uveitis (IRU) is a condition observed in immune-deficient patients who have a history of cytomegalovirus (CMV) retinitis and experience an increase in intraocular inflammation following the initiation of HAART. This inflammation is presumed to be mediated by the recovery of immune responses targeting residual cytomegalovirus (CMV) antigens in the eye. Visual complications associated with IRU can include cataract, cystoid macular edema (CME), glaucoma, and epiretinal membrane formation. Risk factors for IRU include a low CD4 count at the start of HAART and larger areas of CMV retinitis.

B. Autoimmune retinopathy (AIR) can be broadly categorized into paraneoplastic retinopathy and nonparaneoplastic retinopathy. Paraneoplastic autoimmune retinopathy can be further subdivided into cancer-associated retinopathy (CAR), which is most commonly associated with small cell lung cancer, and melanoma-associated retinopathy (MAR), which is seen in patients with melanoma, particularly ocular melanoma. Nonparaneoplastic autoimmune retinopathy arises independently of cancer, and is a diagnosis of exclusion. It is associated with autoimmune disease, most commonly hypothyroidism.

Autoimmune retinopathy is characterized by progressive bilateral vision loss, visual field defects, and photoreceptor dysfunction. There have been a number of anti-retinal antibodies found to be associated with autoimmune retinopathy, mostly against recoverin, a photoreceptor-specific calcium-binding protein.

Investigations should focus on identifying an underlying malignancy through imaging (e.g., CT, MRI) and laboratory tests. The presence of anti-recoverin antibodies or other retinal antibodies (such as anti-ABCA4, anti-CRALBP) can be detected through blood tests and serve as diagnostic markers. Corticosteroids and nonbiologic immunosuppressive therapies (IMT) are generally first-line therapy, with the goal of reducing inflammation and immune-mediated damage to the retina. In cases of paraneoplastic retinopathy, it is crucial to address the underlying malignancy, as effective treatment of the cancer may help stabilize or improve visual function.

References

Kanski JJ (2019) Kanski's clinical ophthalmology e-book: a systematic approach, 6th and 9th edn. Elsevier Health Sciences

Mandeville JT, Levinson RD, Holland GN (2001) The tubulointerstitial nephritis and uveitis syndrome. Surv Ophthalmol 46(3):195–208. https://doi.org/10.1016/s0039-6257(01)00261-2

Clinical Review of Uveitis: Part II

17

Ali Elobous, Saif Aldeen Alryalat,
Nakhleh E. Abu-Yaghi, and Ahmed A. Sallam

Abstract

This chapter focuses on posterior uveitis, providing a detailed explanation of both noninfectious and infectious causes. Noninfectious uveitis is discussed in relation to conditions such as sarcoidosis, Behcet's disease, Vogt-Koyanagi-Harada syndrome, sympathetic ophthalmia, and various collagen vascular disorders, highlighting their pathophysiology and clinical implications. Infectious uveitis is also discussed, focusing on key pathogens including toxoplasmosis, tuberculosis, histoplasmosis, herpetic acute retinal necrosis (ARN), progressive outer retinal necrosis (PORN), cytomegalovirus (CMV), and cat scratch disease, alongside other less common etiologies. Additionally, the chapter covers inflammatory chorioretinopathy, particularly the white dot syndromes, elucidating their diagnostic features and management strategies.

Keywords

Posterior uveitis · Infectious · Noninfectious · White dot syndrome · Treatment

A. Elobous (✉)
Department of Ophthalmology, Royal Medical Services, Amman, Jordan

Department of Ophthalmology, Indiana University School of Medicine, Indianapolis, IN, USA

S. A. Alryalat
Department of Ophthalmology, The University of Jordan, Amman, Jordan

The University of Colorado Anschutz Medical Campus, Aurora, CO, USA

N. E. Abu-Yaghi
Department of Ophthalmology, The University of Jordan, Amman, Jordan
e-mail: N.abuyaghi@ju.edu.jo

A. A. Sallam
Harvey and Bernice Jones Eye Institute, University of Arkansas for Medical Sciences (UAMS), Little Rock, AR, USA

17.1 Posterior Uveitis

It includes retinitis, choroiditis, chorioretinitis, and neuroretinitis (Table 17.1) (Kanski 2019). It can be focal, multifocal, or diffuse. Similar to anterior uveitis, structural complications such as macular edema, retinal or choroidal neovascularization, and peripheral vasculitis are not regarded as essential components in the anatomical classification.

Posterior uveitis may also manifest as retinal vasculitis, the inflammation of retinal vasculature. It may be a primary ocular disease or can be associated with infection or systemic disease. Common possible causes include the following:

S. A. Alryalat (ed.), *Ophthalmology Board and FRCS Part 2 Exams*,
https://doi.org/10.1007/978-981-96-1517-9_17

Table 17.1 Comparison between posterior uveitis subtypes, including retinitis, choroiditis, chorioretinitis, and neuroretinitis

	Retinitis	Choroiditis	Chorioretinitis	Neuroretinitis
Features	White-yellow superficial retinal opacities (i.e., fluffy lesions) with relatively indistinct border due to retinal edema	White-yellow deep retinal or choroidal opacities, distinct border	Both features	Optic nerve edema with macular star formation
Causes	Infectious (i.e. viral retinitis, syphilis, toxoplasma retinitis), Behcet's disease	Sarcoidosis, white dot syndrome, VKH, sympathetic ophthalmia Infections particularly TB and fungal infection	Toxoplasmosis, TB, syphilis, Candida, Behcet, birdshot chorioretinopathy	Cat scratch disease, Lyme disease, syphilis, TB
Notes	May be associated with vasculitis. VZV most common, but HSV-2 is more common in pediatric age group	May be associated with exudative retinal detachment and BRVO. Can be focal (mostly infectious), multifocal (most common, usually noninfectious), or diffuse		

- Primarily retinal arteritis: ARN, systemic vasculitis (e.g., SLE, PAN), syphilis, IRVAN syndrome, Susac syndrome
- Primarily retinal phlebitis: MS, sarcoidosis, birdshot chorioretinopathy, HIV, Eales disease
- Involving both: Behcet's disease, toxoplasmosis, Wegener granulomatosis, Crohn's disease, TB

Diseases that commonly cause intermediate uveitis (pars planitis, MS, sarcoidosis) usually affect veins causing periphlebitis. It can be occlusive or nonocclusive, involving the posterior pole, periphery, or both.

Retinal vasculitis manifests clinically as perivascular sheathing of arteries, veins, or capillaries associated with retinal hemorrhages, vitritis, disc swelling, or CME. It may be complicated by B/CRVO, neovascularization, vitreous hemorrhage, and TRD.

Posterior uveitis can arise from a variety of causes, broadly categorized as infectious and noninfectious. In immunocompetent patients, ocular toxoplasmosis is the most common infective cause of posterior uveitis and is also the leading cause of this condition in adults overall. In pediatric patients, up to 50% of those with posterior uveitis are diagnosed with ocular toxoplasmosis as well. However, in immunocompromised patients, CMV retinitis is the most common infectious cause of posterior uveitis. In addition, unilateral uveitis should ring a bell for infectious etiology, so the first question to ask is whether the condition is unilateral or bilateral.

17.2 Noninfectious Entities

Most common etiologies include sarcoidosis, Behcet disease, Vogt-Koyanagi-Harada syndrome, sympathetic ophthalmia, and other collagen vascular disorders.

17.2.1 Sarcoidosis

- It is a systemic granulomatous disorder with predominant lung involvement in most cases. It is more common in African-Caribbeans, Irish, and Scandinavians, being 10 times higher in Blacks than Caucasians. It has a slight female predominance with peaks in the third and sixth decades of life.
- The presentation can be either acute or insidious. An acute presentation usually involves bilateral hilar lymphadenopathy and erythema nodosum, whereas an insidious presentation is more commonly associated with the gradual development of progressive pulmonary fibro-

sis. The characteristic histologic lesion in sarcoid biopsies is a noncaseating epithelioid cell granuloma, composed of Langhans-type multinucleated giant cells surrounded by a rim of lymphocytes. Granulomatous lesions can develop in various parts of the eye, ranging from KPs to peripheral choroidal lesions. Around 26–50% of patients with systemic sarcoidosis develop some form of uveitis. Ocular sarcoidosis is usually a chronic (60%), bilateral (70%) disease. Anterior uveitis occurs in >60%; posterior uveitis occurs in 30%. Lacrimal gland is involved in 25% of cases, classically as bilateral painless enlarged glands.

Clinically, it is associated with the following:

- Anterior uveitis: unilateral or bilateral granulomatous with mutton-fat KPs, AC cells/flare, posterior synechiae, iris granulomas, and nodules (Koeppe nodules are on the iris border; busacca nodules are on the mid-iris stroma; Berlin nodules are seen in the angle).
  - 2/3 persistent anterior uveitis; 1/3 acute anterior uveitis
- Intermediate uveitis: vitreous cells (vitritis is mild if present), snowballs, and snow banking.
- Posterior uveitis: CME, periphlebitis with perivenous exudates appearing as candle wax dripping, neovascularization developing peripherally, chorioretinal lesions (nodules, probably granulomata) which tend to be peripheral, mostly inferior. CNV may develop as a complication.
  - Peripheral multifocal choroiditis (appearing as punched-out lesions) is highly suggestive of sarcoidosis.
- In sarcoidosis, patients with posterior uveitis are thought to have a higher incidence of central nervous system involvement (35%) compared to those without posterior uveitis (5%). Optic disc swelling can occur from inflammatory papillitis, infiltrative granuloma, or papilledema secondary to CNS involvement.

In other words, typical presentation includes:

1. Granulomatous anterior uveitis
2. Vitritis/snowballs
3. Peripheral multifocal choroiditis and vasculitis
4. Optic disc inflammation and granulomas

Diagnosis:

- The diagnosis is essentially clinical but may be supported by some investigations. Tissue biopsy is the gold standard for definitive diagnosis (it may be taken from the lung or skin granulomata; look for conjunctival granulomas or lacrimal gland enlargement to biopsy although they are uncommon).
- Ocular sarcoidosis is established if tissue biopsy is positive with consistent uveitis that coexists. If biopsy is not taken, but systemic signs are suggestive of sarcoidosis with consistent uveitis, then "presumed" diagnosis is considered.
- Chest X-ray is abnormal in 90% of cases and often reveals bilateral hilar lymphadenopathy (BHL). Although CT thorax is more sensitive, it is generally not recommended unless there is a high clinical suspicion and the chest X-ray appears normal. Elevated serum levels of ACE, lysozyme, and calcium are seen.
- Increased helper/suppressor T cell ratio in bronchoalveolar lavage is almost suggestive of sarcoidosis.

Treatment:

- Steroids (topical, periocular, systemic) are the mainstay of treatment. Immunosuppressive agents such as methotrexate, azathioprine, cyclosporine, and anti-TNF agents are also useful. Treat the ocular inflammation and uveitic glaucoma aggressively.

Topical corticosteroids are usually effective in managing anterior uveitis caused by sarcoidosis; however, posterior uveitis often requires periocular or systemic corticosteroids. Retinal neovascularization due to inflammation generally responds well to systemic corticosteroids, while neovascularization resulting from retinal ischemia may benefit from scatter laser photocoagulation. CNV membrane in cases of sarcoidosis was found to respond well to oral steroids.

Specific sarcoidosis syndromes:

- *Löfgren syndrome* includes erythema nodosum, febrile arthropathy, bilateral hilar adenopathy, and acute iritis. This syndrome typically responds well to systemic corticosteroids and has a favorable long-term prognosis.
- *Heerfordt syndrome,* also known as uveoparotid fever, is characterized by uveitis, parotitis, fever, and facial nerve palsy.

Blau syndrome, a familial disorder that mimics sarcoidosis in children, is a challenging condition to treat. Blau syndrome, or familial juvenile systemic granulomatosis, is an AD disease caused by mutations in the *NOD2* (*CARD15*) gene. It presents with a triad of granulomatous arthritis, uveitis, and rash in childhood. Unlike sarcoidosis, Blau syndrome does not involve pulmonary disease or lymphadenopathy, and it often affects multiple family members. Chronic panuveitis with multifocal choroiditis is the most common ocular manifestation. The condition is difficult to treat and resistant to steroids.

17.2.2 Behcet's Disease

- It is a chronic multisystem disease that results in necrotizing vasculitis affecting small, medium, and large vessels.
- It is characterized by recurrent oral ulcers occurring more than three times in a 12-month period, along with at least two of the following major criteria: genital ulcers, uveitis, skin lesions (erythema nodosum, folliculitis, dermal vasculitis), and positive pathergy test. Positive pathergy test is defined by the formation of a sterile erythematous papule, 2 mm or larger in diameter, that appears 48 h after a skin prick with a sharp sterile needle.
- Other systemic manifestations which are not included as diagnostic criteria include arthritis (nonerosive/nondeforming), vascular thrombosis and aneurysms, bowel ulcers and GI bleeding, epididymitis, and CNS/psychiatric symptoms.
- It typically affects young adults (age of 25–35 years).
- It is more prevalent along the traditional Silk Route, affecting mostly patients of Japanese and Mediterranean (esp. Turkish) descent.
- The prevalence of Behcet's disease varies by gender depending on the region. In the Middle East, it is more common among males, whereas in Japan, it is slightly more prevalent in females. Males are also more likely to experience severe manifestations of the disease, such as eye inflammation.
- Behcet disease is a sporadic disease, but a familial aggregation is recognized, with HLA-B51 being the most strongly associated genetic factor. This association is particularly prevalent in Turkish, Middle Eastern, and Japanese population. Usually, patients have the systemic disease first before developing the eye findings.

Clinically, it is associated with:

- Ocular involvement in 70% of cases which is typically a bilateral non-granulomatous panuveitis with relapsing/remitting course, with each attack lasting 2–4 weeks. Rarely, Behcet disease may manifest solely as anterior uveitis, with mobile hypopyon being a characteristic sign:
  - Retinal vasculitis (occlusive vasculitis unlike sarcoidosis).
  - Severe vitritis is common.
  - Transient mobile hypopyon (cold hypopyon) is characteristic. It is present in 10–30% of cases.
  - Signs usually disappear after an initial attack, but devastating signs appear after recurrent attacks (probably due to occlusive disease).
  - It is typically a retinal disease, presenting with retinitis, and choroid is almost never involved.
  - Frequently associated with optic disc edema.

Table 17.2 Comparison between Behcet's disease and sarcoidosis

	Behcet	Sarcoidosis
Main presentation	Mostly posterior uveitis	Mostly anterior uveitis
Granulomatous inflammation	No	Yes, can also present as non-granulomatous
Type of vasculitis	Occlusive vasculitis	Nonocclusive, exudative vasculitis
Vitritis	Severe	Mild
Vascular involvement	Arteritis and phlebitis	Exclusive venous involvement
Retina and choroid involvement	Retinitis	Mainly choroiditis, retinitis rarely occurs

Behcet disease manifests as occlusive vasculitis (mostly veins), similar to Eales disease. However, it should be differentiated from sarcoidosis (Table 17.2).

Differential Diagnosis:

- Other causes of ischemic vasculitis include TB-delayed hypersensitivity uveitis (Eales), collagen vascular disease such as SLE, and antiphospholipid syndrome.
- Causes of infectious retinitis have to be ruled out, most importantly viral retinitis and syphilis, especially since these can present bilaterally.

Treatment:

- Systemic immunosuppression is required. Commonly used agents include systemic corticosteroids, azathioprine, chlorambucil, cyclophosphamide, colchicine, cyclosporine, and anti-TNF agents (e.g., infliximab).
- Without aggressive treatment, 50% of patients suffer from severe visual loss, and there is a high mortality rate if CNS involvement is present.

17.2.3 Vogt-Koyanagi-Harada Syndrome

- It is an idiopathic multisystem disorder that results in an autoimmune inflammation of melanocyte-containing tissues (e.g., eyes, ears, skin, hair, and meninges), so it is more common in darker-skinned patients.
- It typically manifests as bilateral granulomatous multifocal posterior uveitis with an associated anterior uveitis (i.e., panuveitis). The hallmark of VKH is the presence of multiple exudative retinal detachments with thickened choroid (pachychoroid).
- It is associated with HLA-DR1 and DR4.
- It is more common in women, with a peak in the fourth decade of life.
- Usually, it begins with a prodromal phase of fever, meningitis (+/− cranial nerve palsies), and auditory symptoms (tinnitus, deafness, and vertigo) for a few days before blurring of vision from uveitis develops. A convalescent phase then follows characterized by loss of pigments leading to areas of hypopigmentation including the retina (sunset glow fundus), limbus (Sugiura sign), and skin/hair (vitiligo, poliosis, and alopecia). In the chronic phase, recurrent or chronic anterior uveitis occurs (rarely posterior).
- Choriocapillaris is involved, unlike in sympathetic ophthalmia. However, Dalen-Fuchs nodules (choroidal granulomata) are seen like in sympathetic ophthalmia.
- FA typically reveals numerous punctate hyperfluorescent foci in the early stage of the study, followed by pooling of dye. Lumbar puncture might show lymphocytic pleocytosis (i.e., increased lymphocytes in CSF).

Diagnostic Criteria:

- No other causes
- No prior surgeries or trauma
- Bilateral uveitis
- Auditory or CNS signs
- Hypopigmentary changes after the beginning of inflammation.

VKH disease is termed "probable" when characteristic ocular inflammation is present without accompanying skin or neurologic symptoms. It is considered "incomplete" if either skin or neurologic symptoms are present, but not both. The disease is termed "complete" when both skin and neurologic symptoms are present along with the ocular inflammation.

Treatment:

- High-dose systemic steroids are the mainstay. A pulse methylprednisolone (0.5 mg) for 3 days, followed by oral (1–2 mg/kg/day). If anterior uveitis is present, then add topical management as stated in anterior uveitis. ERD often resolves with systemic steroids.
- Often, steroid-sparing agents such as cyclosporine, azathioprine, or anti-TNF agents are usually needed for 6–12 months.

17.2.4 Sympathetic Ophthalmia

- A bilateral granulomatous panuveitis (with multifocal choroidal lesions) (Fig. 17.1) occurs after trauma or intraocular surgery, mostly (in 65%) between 2 weeks and 3 months (90% occurring with 1 year of trauma).
- It is considered a type 4 (T-cell mediated) hypersensitivity reaction which bears remarkable parallels to VKH except for the cause being traumatic. The risk is higher after trauma (0.1%) compared to after surgery (0.01%).
- It is more common in two age groups: children under the age of 10 years (due to ocular injuries) and adults over the age of 60 years (due to surgical interventions).
- The exciting eye is the one that was injured. The fellow eye sympathizes with the exciting (injured) eye. The exciting eye exhibits more severe inflammation than the sympathetic eye. The exciting eye may be phthisical as well.
- Similar to VKH, ocular depigmentation may develop after inflammation subsides at the limbus ("Sugiura" sign), the trabecular meshwork ("Ohno" sign), or within the choroid ("sunset glow" sign).
- Systemic manifestations like vitiligo and poliosis can also occur similar to VKH, although they are less common.
- In histopathology, there is no difference between sympathetic uveitis and VKH syndrome.
- Imaging in both diseases may show choroidal thickening, hyperfluorescent spots, and exudative retinal detachment.

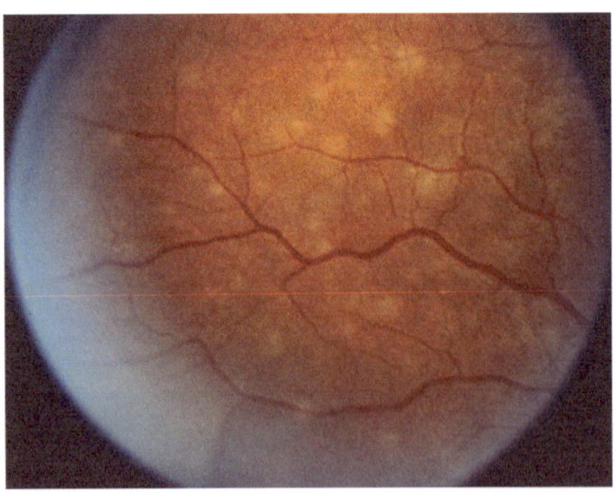

Fig. 17.1 Fundus image showing multifocal choroidal lesions in a patient with sympathetic ophthalmia. Courtesy Retina Rocks®

Dalen-Fuchs nodules are clusters of epithelioid histiocytes and lymphocytes situated between the RPE and Bruch's membrane, usually beneath the peripheral retina. These nodules are found in approximately one-third of patients with SO. However, they are not exclusive to SO and can also be observed in conditions like VKH syndrome, sarcoidosis, or tuberculosis.

Treatment:

- After penetrating ocular trauma, there is a brief window of up to 2 weeks during which enucleation of the injured eye can prevent the development of SO.
- Prevention strategies focus on the prompt closure of the traumatized eye and enucleation within this 2-week period for eyes that are blind and painful with no chance of regaining useful vision. Once SO has developed, enucleation of the injured eye offers no known benefit. After inflammation commences, treatment is limited to systemic immunosuppression. Steroids are

the mainstay of treatment. Steroid-sparing agents such as cyclosporine, mycophenolate, azathioprine, and anti-TNF agents are usually needed to be able to control the inflammation with a reduced dose of oral prednisone.
- With aggressive treatment, around 60% of patients may achieve >6/12 in the sympathizing eye.

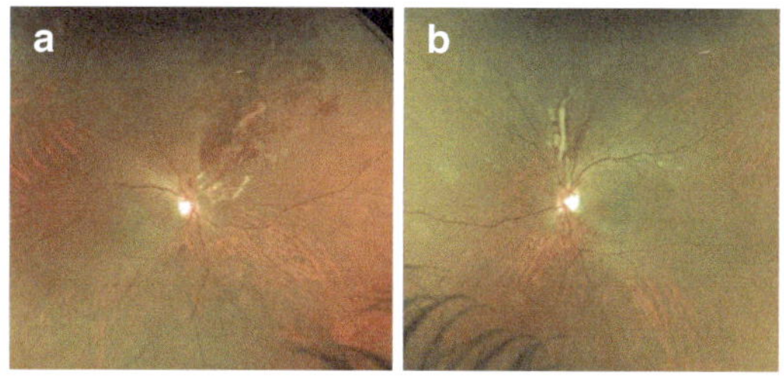

Fig. 17.2 Fundus images showing retinal vascular manifestations in a patient with systemic lupus erythematous (SLE); (**a**) right fundus (**b**) left fundus. Courtesy Retina Rocks®

17.2.5 Collagen Vascular Disorders

Vasculitis associated with collagen vascular disorders usually manifests as hypertensive retinopathy in young patients; posterior pole manifestations include hypertensive retinopathy, characterized by macular star formation, cotton-wool spots, intraretinal hemorrhages, retinal artery occlusions, and choroidal infarcts. Patients may have a retinal vasculitis or a vasculitis involving the posterior ciliary arteries and choroidal vessels, with resultant exudative retinal detachments.

The following are the common entities that cause hypertensive-like retinopathy picture:

- Systemic lupus erythematosus (SLE): affects primarily women of childbearing age, with higher incidence rates among African American and Hispanic persons. Ocular manifestations occur in 50% of patients with SLE with hypertensive-like retinopathy being the most common, including occlusive vasculitis, cotton wool spots, and hemorrhage (Fig. 17.2). Other manifestations include cutaneous lesions on the eyelids (discoid lupus erythematosus), secondary Sjögren syndrome, scleritis, cranial nerve palsies, optic neuropathy, retinal and choroidal vasculopathy, multiple pigment epithelial detachment like lesions, and, in rare cases, uveitis. Systemic manifestations include generalized fatigue, malar rash, oral ulcers, arthritis, kidney disease, and cerebritis. ANA and double-stranded ANA (dsANA) positivity can be observed.
- Polyarteritis nodosa (PAN): The disease presents in individuals between the ages of 40 and 60, with men being affected three times more often than women. The picture is also a hypertensive-like retinopathy. It is an uncommon systemic vasculitis marked by subacute or chronic, focal, necrotizing inflammation of medium-sized and small arteries. About 10% of patients with PAN test positive for hepatitis B surface antigen. Ocular involvement, occurring in up to 20% of PAN patients, results from the underlying vascular disease and can manifest as hypertensive retinopathy, retinal artery occlusions, or retinal vasculitis. PAN most commonly affects skin, nerves, kidneys, and gastrointestinal tract. Pulmonary arteries are typically spared in this condition.
- Granulomatosis with polyangiitis (GPA), aka Wegener's granulomatosis, is characterized by a classic triad of necrotizing granulomatous vasculitis of the upper and lower respiratory tract, focal segmental glomerulonephritis, and necrotizing vasculitis of small arteries and veins. A distinctive feature is involvement of the sinuses, often leading to a saddle nose deformity. Diagnosis is supported by the presence of ANCA antibodies, particularly c-ANCA, which has high diagnostic accuracy. Ocular manifestations of GPA can include necrotizing scleritis, peripheral ulcerative keratitis, orbital cellulitis, retinal vasculitis, or uveitis.
- Microscopic polyangiitis (MPA): Patients with MPA may have clinical features similar to those of GPA but lack granulomatous changes on biopsy.
- Susac syndrome: Mostly in young women. An inflammatory endotheliopathy, with a triad consisting of encephalopathy, hearing loss, and occlusive vasculitis (often manifesting as BRAO) (Fig. 17.3).

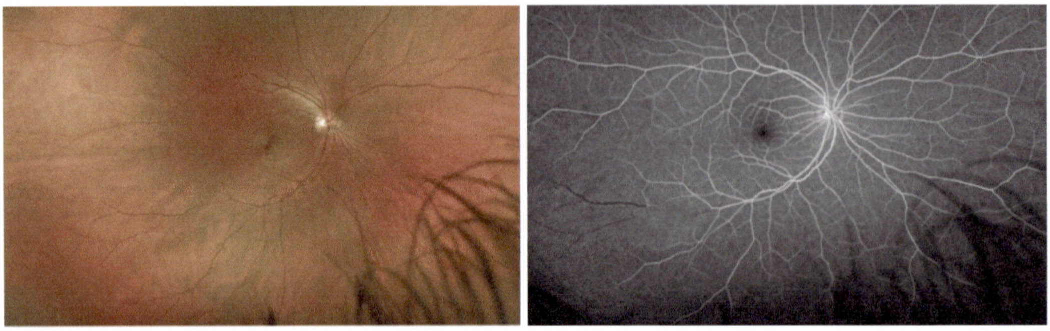

Fig. 17.3 Occlusive vasculitis in Susac syndrome manifesting as distal branch retinal artery occlusion (BRAO) along the inferotemporal arcade. Courtesy Retina Rocks®

Remember that Eales disease is a primary venous disease, compared to arterial disease for Susac. It is an idiopathic bilateral occlusive vasculitis involving the mid-peripheral retina characterized by neovascularization and recurrent vitreous hemorrhage in young men (20–45 years). It is a diagnosis of exclusion and does not have well-defined systemic abnormality. However, the vast majority of patients are PPD positive. It is currently being thought of as TB-delayed hypersensitivity vasculitis.

17.3 Infectious Entities

The most common causes of infectious uveitis are toxoplasmosis, tuberculosis, histoplasmosis, herpetic acute retinal necrosis (ARN), progressive outer retinal necrosis (PORN), CMV, and cat scratch disease. Less common etiologies are briefly mentioned according to pathogen.

17.3.1 Toxoplasmosis

- It is the most common cause of posterior uveitis in immunocompetent children and adults, comprising 20–60% of all posterior uveitis. It is unilateral in 75% of cases during active disease; however, inactive lesions are found bilaterally in 80% of cases.
- It is caused by *Toxoplasma gondii*, an obligate intracellular parasite. Cats are the definitive host, shedding oocysts in their feces, while humans and livestock serve as intermediate hosts. Human infection typically occurs through ingestion of the parasite from contact with contaminated soil, infected cat feces, drinking untreated water, or consuming undercooked meat. Transplacental transmission is also possible, with the transmission rate increasing from 15% in the first trimester to 60% in the third trimester, although the severity of the disease is greatest when the infection is acquired early in pregnancy. Bradyzoite form of *T. gondii* is inactive, while tachyzoite is the active form. The genetic makeup of toxoplasma affects its recurrence rate with some highly virulent genotypes resulting in a more severe ocular disease.
- Acquired cases of uveitis occur mostly due to reactivation of disease which is acquired congenitally or perinatally, with a mean age of 29 years. Postnatal infection represents 50% of toxoplasmosis cases.
- Clinical manifestations:
  - The characteristic lesion of toxoplasmosis is focal exudative necrotizing retinitis. Toxoplasma has a strong tendency to affect the posterior pole, especially the macular region, which is involved in over 50% of cases. Classically, the initial active lesion of toxoplasmosis begins in the superficial retina and progressively involves the full thickness of the retina, adjacent choroid, vitreous, and sometimes even the sclera. The lesion appears as a yellowish white or gray exudative spot with poorly defined borders due to surrounding retinal edema

(Fig. 17.4). The lesion can range in size from a fraction of the optic disc to about two quadrants of the retina. Associated features may include choroiditis, hemorrhage, and vasculitis. There can also be a significant overlying vitritis, leading to a "headlight in the fog" appearance.

- It can cause Kyrieleis plaques which indicate a segmental arteriolitis adjacent to active retinal lesion.
- Punctate outer retinitis, neuroretinitis, and optic neuritis are other manifestations of this disease.
- Anterior uveitis may occur, often with high IOP. Mutton-fat KPs may be dramatic in patients with toxoplasmosis.
- Inactive lesion manifests as healed scar which is usually well demarcated with pigmented border. Satellite lesions adjacent to old scars indicate reactivation. Peripheral retinochoroidal scars are the most common ocular finding, occurring in 82% of the patients.
- In congenital toxoplasmosis, the diagnostic feature is an asymptomatic punched-out macular cicatricial lesion. This lesion typically involves the retina, choroid, and vitreous, with a central necrotic zone. Other clinical features of congenital infection include microphthalmia, strabismus, coloboma, hydrocephalus, cerebral calcification, and hepatosplenomegaly. Secondary glaucoma is the most common complication.
- In patients with AIDS, increased activity of toxoplasmosis may indicate a worsening of AIDS and a drop in CD4 counts and may suggest CNS involvement. Ocular toxoplasmosis in AIDS is often associated with significantly more vitreous cells than in CMV retinitis. It also involves a larger area of necrosis. However, multiple and large active lesions are rare and should prompt HIV testing, too. It is of note that toxoplasma retinitis can also present with bilateral and multiple lesions in other causes of immunosuppression and in elderly patients.

Diagnosis

The diagnosis is mostly clinical, with positive serologic testing for anti-*T. gondii* IgG (starts after 2 weeks of infection and remains throughout life) or IgM (starts earlier and remains for 1 year) confirming exposure to the parasite. Negative antibody titer essentially rules out the diagnosis. PCR of aqueous/vitreous samples may be useful if the diagnosis is in doubt. However, it is important to note that PCR for toxoplasma antigen with intraocular fluid is specific but only 65% sensitive.

Treatment

- For acute toxoplasma retinochoroiditis in immunocompetent patients, routine antibiotic and steroid treatment is not strongly supported by evidence. Therefore, treatment is not mandatory and is only indicated in specific situations. The disease is generally self-limiting,

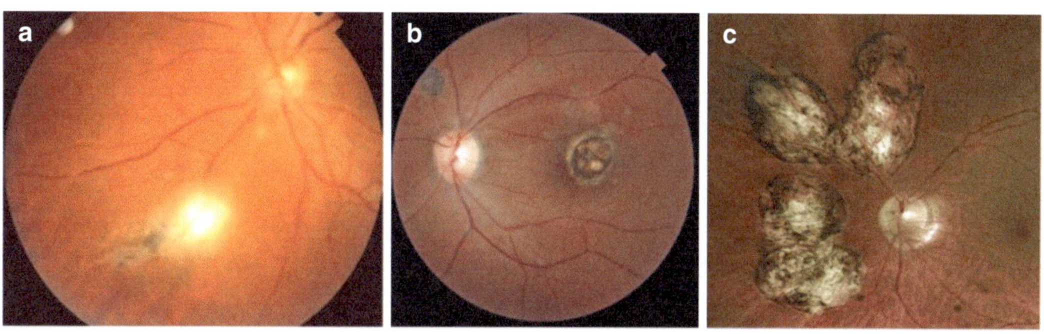

Fig. 17.4 Colored fundus images for an active toxoplasmosis lesion (**a**), congenital macular punched-out lesion (**b**), and completely inactive lesion (**c**). Courtesy Retina Rocks®

with spontaneous resolution typically occurring within 4–8 weeks. Treatment is necessary in the following cases:

- Lesion factors- involvement of the macula, papillomacular bundle, optic disc, or major vascular arcades; presentation with significant vitritis, decreased vision, multiple active lesions, or large ones (> disc diameter).
- Patient factors- immunocompromised state, pregnancy, or congenital infection.

Treatment usually lasts 4–6 weeks, and complete healing occurs over 4–6 months:

1. Systemic: Mostly in new infections (i.e., IgM positive). Consider adding oral steroids once the antibiotics have been started (after 2 days) as this may help clear up the vitritis. Regimens include:
   (a) Triple therapy: pyrimethamine + sulfadiazine + prednisolone
   (b) Quadruple therapy: pyrimethamine + sulfadiazine + clindamycin + prednisolone
   (c) Other antibiotic therapies: trimethoprim/sulfamethoxazole (Bactrim); azithromycin; atovaquone; spiramycin
      - Pyrimethamine can cause bone marrow suppression (aplastic anemia and thrombocytopenia), so these patients should be on leucovorin (folinic acid) to help reduce this risk.
      - Sulfa drugs can cause Stevens-Johnson syndrome, bone marrow suppression, and kidney stones.
      - Oral clindamycin can be useful, especially for patients with a sulfa allergy. It exhibits excellent ocular penetration. Rarely can it result in severe diarrhea due to *Clostridium difficile* superinfection.
      - Atovaquone can theoretically reduce recurrences as it is active against bradyzoites and tachyzoites (cysticidal).
      - The addition of azithromycin may reduce the number of recurrences, too.
      - Spiramycin can be used in pregnant women to reduce transplacental spread.
2. Intravitreal: It is an option in immunocompetent patients, esp. in pregnant women. It includes clindamycin (1 mg) and dexamethasone (400 μg) administered 3X 2 weeks apart.

Recurrence is common; reactivation of retinitis occurs on an average of 2X in each patient (80% have no more than three attacks). No eradication is reported; however, the aim is to reduce activity and resulting scar, with a decrease in the recurrence rate. Bactrim (Septrin) QOD may be used as prophylaxis to reduce the risk of recurrence in high-risk patients.

17.3.2 Syphilis

- It is caused by the spirochaete *Treponema pallidum*, which is usually transmitted by sexual contact (acquired syphilis) or transplacentally (congenital syphilis).
- It can be categorized into congenital and acquired infection, with each also subclassified as follows:
  – Congenital syphilis; see (Table 17.3)
  – Acquired syphilis; see (Table 17.4)
- Intraocular inflammation can be either granulomatous or non-granulomatous and may occur unilaterally or bilaterally (in about 50% of cases). It can affect either the anterior or the posterior segment of the eye. Ocular manifestations mostly occur in secondary syphilis. The most common ocular feature of both secondary and tertiary syphilis is anterior uveitis. It can be associated with roseola (vascular fronds on the iris), iris nodules, and high IOP.

Table 17.3 Congenital syphilis is subclassified into early and late infection

Early congenital (manifesting <2 years of life)	**Systemic**: mucocutaneous rash, lymphadenopathy, hepatosplenomegaly, osteochondritis **Ocular**: chorioretinitis and retinal vasculitis; salt-and-pepper fundus
Late congenital (manifesting >2 years of life)	**Systemic**: saddle nose, Hutchinson teeth, frontal bossing, sabre shins, deafness **Ocular**: interstitial keratitis

Table 17.4 Acquired syphilis is subclassified into primary, secondary, and tertiary infection

	Primary syphilis	Secondary syphilis	Tertiary syphilis
Timing	From 2 weeks after infection	From 2 months after infection	From 5 years after untreated infection
Systemic manifestations	Chancre with regional lymphadenopathy	Generalized lymphadenopathy and diffuse maculopapular rash	Categorized as benign, cardiovascular (aortitis), or neurosyphilis (**uveitis is considered a neurosyphilis**)
Ocular manifestations	Almost none	(10% uveitis) anterior or posterior	(5% uveitis) anterior or posterior Interstitial keratitis
Diagnosis	Direct visualization of spirochetes with dark-field microscopy	Serodiagnosis	Serodiagnosis
Treatment	Single-dose intramuscular penicillin (doxycycline is an alternative)	Single-dose intramuscular penicillin given weekly for 3 weeks (doxycycline is an alternative)	Same as secondary except for neurosyphilis, where IV penicillin given Q4H for 2 weeks

- Posterior uveitis is generally bilateral and nonprogressive. Typical active lesions are yellow plaque-like with overlying vitritis and retinal precipitates. Retinochoroiditis appears less opaque (diaphanous). Acute syphilitic posterior placoid chorioretinopathy (ASPPC) is marked by large, pale-yellowish subretinal lesions located in the posterior pole of the eye. It is a diagnostic feature of secondary syphilis. Nonulcerative stromal interstitial keratitis, frequently associated with anterior uveitis, is the most common inflammatory sign of untreated late congenital syphilis. It occurs in up to 50% of cases, with a higher prevalence in girls. Syphilis is called the great imitator as it can present as chorioretinitis, neuroretinitis, salt-pepper retinopathy, optic neuritis, papilledema, and optic perineuritis.

Diagnosis

Serologic tests fall into two categories based on the type of antibodies detected:

- Treponemal assays detect specific IgG and/or IgM antibodies directed against *T. pallidum*. These include fluorescent treponemal antibody absorption (FTA-ABS), *T. pallidum* particle agglutination (TP-PA), enzyme immunoassay (EIA), and multiplex flow immunoassay (MFI). They become positive during the secondary stage of syphilis and remain positive for life, as FTA-ABS does not normalize with treatment.
- Non-treponemal assays, such as rapid plasma reagin (RPR) and Venereal Disease Research Laboratory (VDRL) assays, detect antibodies reacting to cardiolipin-cholesterol-lecithin antigens. While these antigens are not specific to *T. pallidum*, they are present in most patients with syphilis. The titers typically correlate with disease activity, increasing during primary or secondary syphilis, and VDRL titer decreases with treatment. False-positive tests can occur in conditions such as SLE, leprosy, advanced age, and other spirochete infections.

The syphilis testing guideline includes treponemal (e.g., FTA) mostly and non-treponemal antibody (e.g., RPR) testing, and interpretation of syphilis testing can be as follows:

- If positive treponemal and positive non-treponemal → The patient has syphilis.
- If negative treponemal and negative non-treponemal → The patient does not have syphilis.
- If negative treponemal and positive non-treponemal → false-positive test, the patient has no syphilis.
- If positive treponemal and negative non-treponemal → need another treponemal test (mostly TP-PA). Accordingly:
  - Negative confirmatory TP-PA test → Negative for syphilis.

– Positive confirmatory TP-PA test → means either previously treated infection or latent syphilis. A thorough clinical assessment is warranted to adjudicate. With compatible clinical findings or suspicious new exposure, this should be treated with IV penicillin.

While a lumbar puncture with examination of cerebrospinal fluid (CSF) has been traditionally recommended for every case of syphilitic uveitis, many centers stopped performing lumbar puncture in these patients given that they will be receiving IV penicillin at a dosage that would treat any coexisting syphilitic CNS lesions.

Treatment

High-dose intravenous penicillin is the mainstay of treatment. Adjuvant systemic steroids might be considered to reduce inflammation.

Jarisch–Herxheimer reaction is a systemic response to treponemal antigens released on commencement of therapy and may include progression of ocular signs, managed by steroids.

17.3.3 Tuberculosis

- It is caused by *Mycobacterium tuberculosis*, a facultative intracellular bacterium. Only 1% of patients with systemic TB get ocular disease.
- *M. tuberculosis* has a preference for highly oxygenated tissues, which is why tuberculous lesions are frequently found in the apices of the lungs and in the choroid, an area with the highest blood flow rate in the body. The most common form of ocular involvement is hematogenous spread from pulmonary TB. Tuberculosis can affect the uveal tract either:
  – Primarily with direct ocular penetration from an exogenous source (infected lids or conjunctiva) or
  – Secondarily as a result of hematogenous spread of *M. tuberculosis* from a pulmonary focus or extrapulmonary site. Immune reaction to the released intraocular mycobacterium antigens plays an important role in the pathogenesis of the disease.
- Ocular TB can involve any part of the eye and can occur with or without evidence of pulmonary or extrapulmonary disease. It is commonly associated with normal CXR (50% of cases), so it may be difficult to diagnose.
- The most common ocular TB manifestation is granulomatous uveitis (caseating granulomatous inflammation with granuloma that can develop anywhere). Posterior uveitis with disseminated choroiditis is the most common manifestation of tuberculous uveitis that is usually bilateral (Fig. 17.5).
- Anterior uveitis, typically granulomatous with mutton-fat KPs and iris nodules, can also occur.
- Typically, these lesions, known as tubercles or choroidal granulomata, appear as white-yellow nodules primarily located in the posterior pole. They may be accompanied by disc edema, nerve fiber layer hemorrhages, exudative RD, and varying degrees of vitritis. The lesions may also liquefy into a subretinal abscess. Angiography confirms activity in choroiditis and reveals a classical ring-of-fire appearance around the subretinal abscess or choroidal granuloma. Other common patterns include a solitary tubercle or multifocal choroiditis
- Serpiginous-like choroidopathy is a pattern of choroiditis that is seen in patients with TB-delayed hypersensitivity rather than with acute infection (Table 17.5).
- Occlusive retinal periphlebitis can occur due to TB infection or due to delayed hypersensitivity reaction to TB (Eales disease).

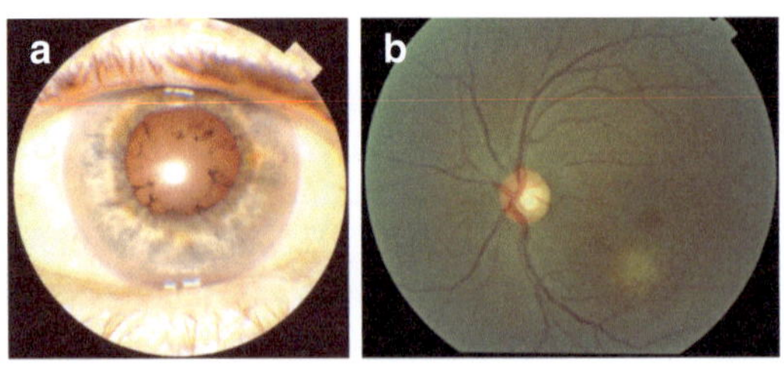

Fig. 17.5 Anterior segment (**a**) and fundus (**b**) involvement of *Mycobacterium tuberculosis*. Courtesy Retina Rocks®

Diagnosis

A definitive diagnosis of TB uveitis is only made when *M. tuberculosis*, or its DNA, is isolated from ocular fluids. Additionally, acid-fast bacilli can also be detected in sputum or early-morning urine sample.

However, ocular TB should be investigated by performing the following:

- CXR: it may show hilar lymph node enlargement, apical infiltrates or cavitation, consolidation, and pleural effusion.
- Tuberculin skin test (TST): it involves intradermal injection of 0.1 mL of 1:1000 tuberculin PPD and measuring the induration 72 h later. The interpretation can be variable depending on certain risk factors with several possible false-positive and false-negative results.
- Interferon-gamma release assay (IGRA): it includes tests such as QuantiFERON-TB Gold and T-SPOT which are more specific.

Table 17.5 Comparison between serpiginous-like choroidopathy and serpiginous choroiditis

Serpiginous-like choroidopathy	Serpiginous choroiditis
Usually does not extend to the disc	Spread centrifugally from the disc
Tends to spare the fovea even when the macula is involved	Macular involvement with the fovea
More multifocal and pigmented	Geographic with skip lesions
Significant vitritis	Mild vitritis

Treatment

It includes an initial induction phase with a daily regimen of isoniazid, rifampin, pyrazinamide, and ethambutol for 2 months. This is followed by a continuation phase lasting 4–7 months, during which isoniazid and rifampin are administered.

Adjuvant systemic steroids might be considered to reduce inflammation.

17.3.4 Histoplasmosis

An infection by inhaled *Histoplasma capsulatum* fungus. Ocular involvement represents an immune-mediated reaction to antigen, so-called presumed ocular histoplasmosis syndrome (POHS) (Fig. 17.6). Sixty percent of cases are bilateral and usually asymptomatic unless CNV develops (<5% of patients). Men and women are affected equally. Active retinitis is rarely caught, but the following signs are usually seen: multifocal atrophic white lesions (aka histo spots), with peripapillary pigment changes, and no vitritis. Treatment is directed to CNV. Risk of CNV is highest if spots are found in the macula. Active lesions show early hypofluorescence with late staining; such lesions may be treated with steroids (e.g., periocular), but the benefit is not clear. In contrast, areas of active CNV hyperfluoresce early and then hyperfluoresce in a leak.

The absence of vitritis and anterior segment inflammation is typical of OHS. Over 90% of patients with POHS have a positive histoplasmin skin reaction. Of note, antifungal agents have no benefit.

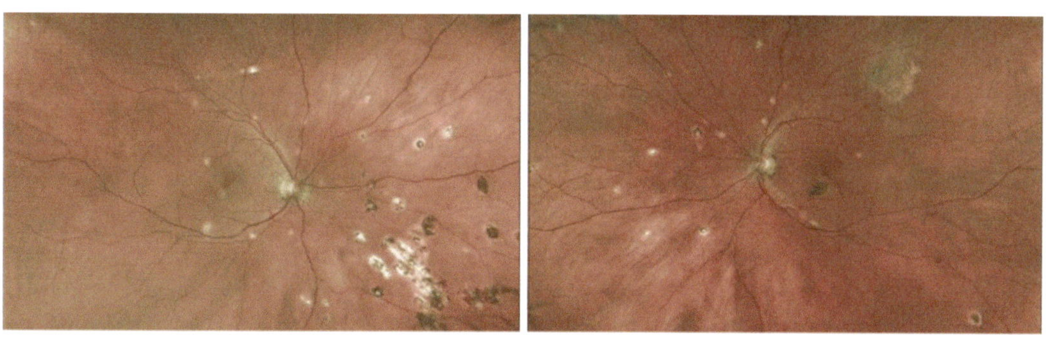

Fig. 17.6 Colored fundus photograph of both eyes showing signs of ocular histoplasmosis syndrome (OHS) involving the fovea. Courtesy Retina Rocks®

17.3.5 Herpetic Uveitis

17.3.5.1 Acute Retinal Necrosis (ARN)

Most forms of herpetic posterior uveitis are acute and fulminant, having poor visual acuity prognosis and often resulting in serious complications such as retinal detachment and optic atrophy. Herpetic retinitis can be:

- Necrotizing, e.g., ARN, PORN, and CMV retinitis
- Non-necrotizing, e.g., acute retinochoroiditis following acute VZV in children

The morphological appearance of herpetic retinitis depends largely on the immune status of the patient. Moreover, in HIV patients, different clinical presentations of the same disease may occur depending on CD4 count levels.

Acute retinal necrosis (ARN) is the classical presentation of herpetic viruses. It is caused by HSV-1, HSV-2, or VZV (most common cause). In younger patients, HSV-2 tends to be the causative organism, whereas in older patients (over 50), the cause tends to be VZV. Unlike CMV or PORN, patients with ARN are usually immunocompetent, but it also occurs in immunocompromised individuals. It usually presents in association with other forms of herpes infections, including encephalitis. There is a higher risk of encephalitis and meningitis among patients with ARN caused by HSV-1 infection than by VZV infection. In ARN, the majority of patients are 40–60 years old although it may occur at any age. The usual presentation is of unilateral eye involvement with blurred vision, floaters, and pain/discomfort, but fellow eye involvement occurs in around 30% (simultaneously to several years later). Second eye involvement usually occurs within 6 weeks, and around 80% of cases occur within 3 months.

Clinically, it is characterized by the following:

- Multifocal retinitis manifesting initially as one or more foci of small, patchy yellow-white areas of retinal necrosis with discrete borders located in the peripheral retina. Within few days to a week, the lesions grow and merge to form a confluent 360° creamy retinitis. This condition progresses in a posterior direction, leading to full-thickness retinal necrosis, arteriolitis, phlebitis, and occasional retinal hemorrhages. Because there is such a profound arteritis, there are relatively few intraretinal hemorrhages. Circumferential spread is a feature, with posterior pole being involved later (unlike PRN where central involvement occurs early).
- Occlusive vasculopathy is a feature, affecting arterioles.
- Because the inflammation is severe, there is moderate-to-severe vitritis and/or AC inflammation (cells may have large keratic precipitates) (Fig. 17.7).
- As the involved areas clear, it starts to take the appearance of Swiss cheese, and RPE stippling occurs. Other features include optic disc edema, optic neuropathy, retinal breaks, and retinal detachment (in up to 75%; rhegmatogenous or tractional). Retinal detachment may occur a few weeks to several months afterward but usually within 1–2 months.

Diagnosis: It is essentially a clinical diagnosis. Aqueous or vitreous tap with PCR is usually undertaken and confirms the diagnosis. However, viral DNA tests should include HSV, VZV, and CMV in addition to the test for toxoplasmosis and serological test for syphilis. The sensitivity of viral PCR in aqueous fluid and vitreous is very

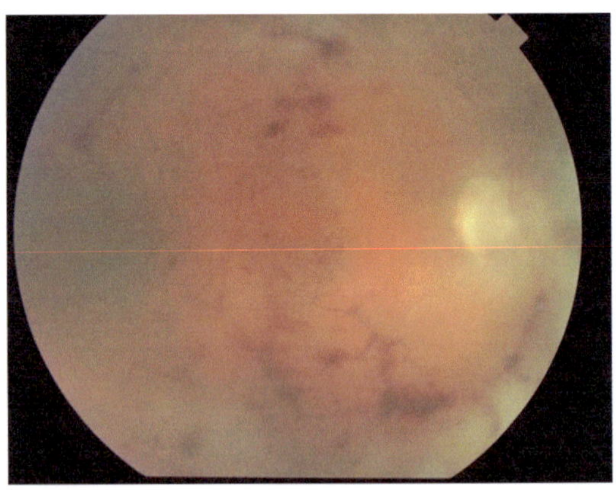

Fig. 17.7 Fundus image showing manifestations of acute retinal necrosis. Courtesy Retina Rocks®

high so that a negative sample makes the diagnosis very unlikely.

Treatment: Rapid progression is notable in the absence of antiviral therapy, so treatment should be commenced as soon as possible. Treatment entails IV acyclovir 10 mg/kg q8h for 2 weeks (or oral valacyclovir 2–3 g TID). Oral maintenance of 400–800 mg five times daily is then continued for 6–12 weeks (or oral valacyclovir 1 g TID).

Once antiviral therapy is initiated, systemic steroids may be added (prednisolone 0.5 mg/kg/day) and tapered over 3–6 weeks in immunocompetent individuals.

Without treatment, there will be second eye involvement in 20–70% of cases within 1 month. Systemic treatment reduces fellow eye ARN from 65% to 13% at 1 year.

17.3.5.2 Progressive Outer Retinal Necrosis (PORN)

It is a morphologic variant of acute necrotizing herpetic retinitis that typically occurs in individuals who are profoundly immunosuppressed, particularly in the context of advanced AIDS (CD4+ T lymphocytes ≤ 50 cells/μL). Although rare, PORN has also been reported in immunocompetent patients. The most common cause of PORN is VZV infection. Although ARN and PORN are considered distinct entities, they are essentially different manifestations of the same underlying disease, with variations in presentation due to differences in the host's immune status. PORN often presents bilaterally, affecting both eyes in around 70% of cases, and is characterized by rapid, painless loss of visual acuity with a generally poor visual prognosis. Similar to ARN, retina develops multifocal infiltrate that spreads rapidly leading to full-thickness necrosis and subsequent atrophy, holes, and detachment (also in 70% of patients). The typical "cracked mud appearance" is virtually diagnostic (Fig. 17.8).

Unlike ARN, it is characterized by:

- Early posterior pole and macular involvement
- Associated anterior uveitis and vitritis are rare
- Sparing of retinal vessels and perivascular retina
- Worse prognosis

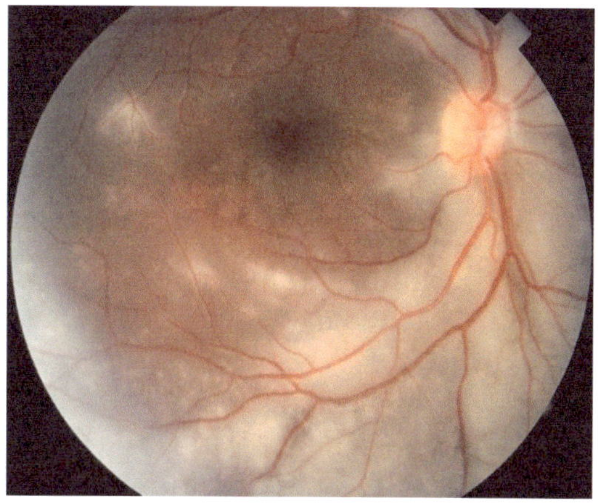

Fig. 17.8 Fundus image showing manifestations of progressive outer retinal necrosis (PORN). Courtesy Retina Rocks®

Diagnosis: It is essentially a clinical diagnosis with the aid of viral PCR from aqueous or vitreous. The immune status of the patient is the most important point to differentiate from other causes of retinitis.

Treatment: As for ARN, it consists of induction and maintenance regimens. However, PORN is often resistant to IV acyclovir alone and needs intravitreal combination. Some specialists initiate therapy with intraocular injection of ganciclovir 2 mg/0.1 mL or foscarnet 1.2–2.4 mg/0.1 mL, particularly when the macula or optic nerve is threatened, along with IV antiviral therapy (Table 17.6).

17.3.6 CMV Retinitis

Although CMV infection itself is common in general population, CMV retinitis only occurs in immunocompromised individuals such as AIDS patients (AIDS-defining illness) and those undergoing chronic immunosuppressive therapy. It is the most common infectious uveitis in AIDS, as it is highly correlated with CD4+ count (mostly when CD4+ T-cell counts are &<50/μL). Retinitis usually starts unilaterally and progresses to bilateral in 50% of patients without treatment. The retinitis begins peripherally in 90% of cases and appears as white lesions surrounded by hemorrhages (aka pizza appearance) (Fig. 17.9).

Table 17.6 Comparison between acute retinal necrosis (ARN) and progressive outer retinal necrosis (PORN)

	Acute retinal necrosis (ARN)	Progressive outer retinal necrosis (PORN)
Severity of inflammation	More severe; painful Prominent vitritis	Less severe; painless Minimal vitritis or none
Vasculitis and anterior uveitis	Yes (occlusive arteritis)	No
Clinical behavior	Starts in the periphery (usually adjacent/outside temporal arcades) and becomes confluent within a week, circumferential progression	No consistent direction, but early macular involvement and sparing of perivascular retina are features
Laterality	Unilateral (second eye involvement within 6 weeks occurs in 40%)	Bilateral (second eye involved in weeks in majority)
Response to treatment	Better	Less Extremely rapid progression
Immune status of patients	Immunocompetent or immunocompromised	Nearly exclusively immunocompromised

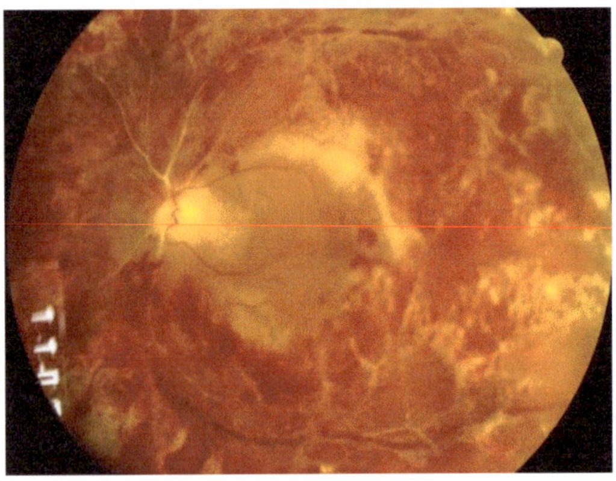

Fig. 17.9 Fundus image showing pizza appearance of an AIDS patient with CMV retinitis. Courtesy Retina Rocks®

Atrophy and holes after active infection subside, leading to RD in up to 50% of cases. It is treated by antiviral (e.g., ganciclovir, valacyclovir, or foscarnet) in combination with AIDS HAART therapy.

It is typically multifocal, with each lesion having the most activity in the borders. It has a characteristic granular or pizza pie appearance and a typical brushfire pattern of spread along the blood vessels.

The clinical appearance is similar regardless of clinical contexts, and it can be classified into three distinct variants:

- (1) A classic or fulminant retinitis with large areas of retinal hemorrhage set against a background of whitened, edematous, or necrotic retina. The retinitis usually manifests in the posterior pole, near the vascular arcades, and in the distribution of the nerve fiber layer, with involvement of blood vessels. (2) A granular or indolent variant is more commonly found in the retinal periphery and is characterized by minimal or no hemorrhage, edema, or vascular sheathing. Active retinitis may gradually progress from the borders of the lesion. (3) A perivascular form, often described as a variant of "frosted-branch" angiitis, is characterized by undifferentiated retinal perivasculitis. It was initially observed in immunocompetent children. Treatment consists of an induction phase followed by maintenance. Induction can be achieved using either IV ganciclovir or intravitreal antiviral therapy for CMV retinitis. Oral valganciclovir is equally effective as intravenous ganciclovir for induction therapy, which typically lasts for 14 days. After the retinitis is brought under control, maintenance therapy is continued until the CD4 count remains above 100–200 for 3–6 months. Ganciclovir slow-release implant had been used to treat unilateral CMV retinitis in HIV patients before the era of HAART. The implant is no longer manufactured.
- It is important to note that mortality rates are higher in patients with CMV retinitis who do not receive systemic anti-CMV therapy. Therefore, to improve outcomes and provide prophylaxis for the fellow eye, it is recom-

Table 17.7 Comparison between herpes simplex-caused acute retinal necrosis (ARN) and cytomegalovirus (CMV)-induced retinitis

	Acute retinal necrosis (ARN)	CMV retinitis
Affected patients	Immunocompetent mostly	Only immunocompromised
Manifestation	Occlusive arterial vasculitis	Periphlebitis (veins)
Vitritis	Severe	Mild to none
Retina	Periphery	Posterior pole
Treatment	Acyclovir or valacyclovir	Ganciclovir or valganciclovir

mended to place the patient on oral valganciclovir. Acyclovir is ineffective against CMV. In cases of ganciclovir-resistant CMV retinitis, intravenous foscarnet may be effective, though resistance can develop with long-term treatment. Congenital CMV infection is the most common congenital ocular infection, although it is mostly subclinical (unlike HSV). It is acquired during maternal viremia during pregnancy, rather than from the birth canal (which is the case for HSV) (Table 17.7).

Immune recovery uveitis (IRU) is the most common manifestation of immune reconstitution inflammatory syndrome in HIV-infected patients with cytomegalovirus retinitis who are undergoing HAART therapy. This condition is specifically associated with CMV infection.

17.3.7 Cat Scratch Disease (Bartonellosis)

It is caused by *Bartonella henselae* bacteria and affects the eyes in 5–10% of cases, typically presenting unilaterally. About 5% of patients develop Parinaud oculoglandular syndrome, characterized by unilateral granulomatous conjunctivitis and regional lymphadenopathy. The most common ocular manifestation is neuroretinitis, which typically involves the optic nerve head, retinitis, and a macular star. The disease primarily affects children under 10 years of age. The treatment of choice is doxycycline 100 mg. In this context, toxoplasma retinitis is an important differential diagnosis. Mild diseases are self-limiting, whereas severe diseases may require doxycycline treatment with or without steroid therapy.

17.3.8 Other Less Common Infectious Causes

Parasites

- **Toxocariasis**: It is caused by *Toxocara canis* parasite, with puppies (i.e., small dogs) being the primary host. It is a roundworm (i.e., not flat). It penetrates from soil through intestinal walls. It manifests mostly as visceral or ocular inflammation. Infections in humans, an end host, result in a focal granulomatous reaction in many organs, including the eye. Its most common presentation in the eye is retinal granuloma at the periphery (Fig. 17.10) with active uveitis, but it can also present as chronic endophthalmitis. The granuloma can be confused with retinoblastoma. It may appear as radial (rather than circular) retinal folds. Retinal granuloma is a fairly rare and specific finding and, in the context of panuveitis, is suggestive of toxocariasis. Treatment typically involves the use of local or systemic corticosteroids, while antihelminthic drugs (e.g., mebendazole) are used only in active infection (rather than inflammation). In most cases anthelmintic therapy has little or no therapeutic role.
- **Onchocerciasis**: It is the second most common cause of infectious blindness worldwide. The parasitic helminth *Onchocerca volvulus* is causative; the vector is the *Simulium* blackfly living around rivers (hence the name river blindness). It affects the skin (e.g., maculopapular rash), with the following ocular manifestations: keratitis, anterior uveitis, and posterior uveitis, with characteristic bilateral chorioretinitis that affects the macula only later in the disease. It is treated via ivermectin.

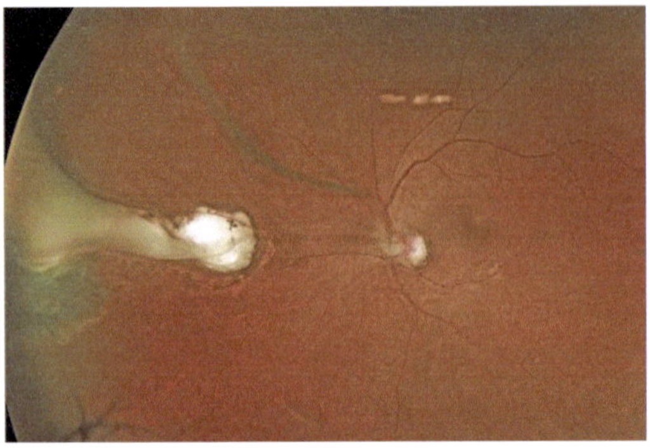

Fig. 17.10 Colored fundus image showing toxocariasis uveitis manifesting as a peripheral granuloma. Courtesy Retina Rocks®

- **Cysticercosis**: It is a parasitic infection by cysticercus cellulosae, the larval form of the pork tapeworm *Taenia solium*. The disease is characterized by cyst formation at lungs and brain with intense inflammation upon rupture. Ocular cyst can appear at eyelid, conjunctiva, AC, or even vitreous, where their rupture will induce intense inflammation. So, such cysts should be surgically removed, with steroid to ameliorate inflammation. Systemic albendazole should be used with caution.

Diffuse Unilateral Subacute Neuroretinitis (DUSN)

It is an inflammatory response triggered by the presence of a single motile subretinal nematode, often *Baylisascaris procyonis*. The nematode is visible in <50% of cases. Early signs include crops of gray–white outer retinal lesions with associated vitritis and vasculitis, reduced vision, vitreous cells, and optic disc edema. As the disease progresses, it can lead to optic atrophy, retinal vascular sclerosis, and diffuse pigmentary changes, ultimately resulting in unilateral wipe-out syndrome. Treatment involves photocoagulation of the worm if it is visible.

Viral Retinitis

Most common causes are herpes simplex, varicella zoster, and CMV.

Uveitis in HIV: It is linked to the depletion of CD4+ T cells. AIDS, which develops in about half of HIV-infected individuals within 10 years, is defined as an HIV infection with a CD4+ T-cell count below 200 cells/μL or the emergence of one or more AIDS-defining conditions. Cytomegalovirus (CMV) retinitis is one of the defining conditions. Retinal microangiopathy, the most frequent retinopathy in AIDS patients, occurs in up to 70% of cases and is characterized by hemorrhages and cotton wool spots that appear on the retina. This condition is associated with a declining CD4+ count and higher plasma HIV-RNA levels, serving as a marker for increased risk of cytomegalovirus (CMV) retinitis. Other manifestations include Kaposi sarcoma (affecting eyelid or conjunctiva) and various fungal or bacterial infections.

Rubella uveitis: The latent rubella virus can lead to chronic anterior uveitis that may not respond well to steroids and has been associated with Fuchs uveitis syndrome. The most frequent result of acquired Rubella infection is conjunctivitis. Rubella-related retinitis can cause diffuse pigment epithelial detachment, which may resolve on its own (Fig. 17.11). In congenital rubella syndrome (CRS), unilateral or bilateral pigmentary retinopathy is the most common ocular manifestation (25–50%), followed by cataracts (15%) and glaucoma (10%). The pigmentary changes are often described as a "salt-and-pepper" fundus. There is no specific antiviral treatment for congenital rubella, so management is supportive.

Epstein–Barr virus: Most common manifestation being conjunctivitis, but may cause a variety of posterior segment inflammations. No need for treatment.

Fungal Infections

Fungi are inhaled, leading to primary pulmonary disease, with associated systemic involvement, including ocular involvement. Fungal infections are usually suspected in the following cases: intravenous drug abuse, a septic focus associated with an indwelling catheter, chronic lung disease such as cystic fibrosis, general debilitation, and diabetes.

- *Candida albicans*: One-third of cases have ocular involvement, mostly bilateral. Significant vitritis with fluffy balls, overlaying

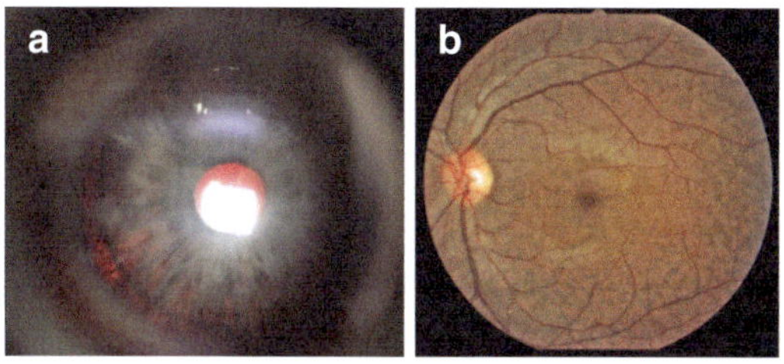

Fig. 17.11 Anterior segment (**a**) and fundus image (**b**) of a patient with congenital rubella syndrome. Courtesy Retina Rocks®

retinitis foci, can be seen. Amphotericin B is the treatment of choice.

- **Aspergillus**: It has worse prognosis than candida, with more macular involvement and occlusive vasculitis.
- ***Pneumocystis jirovecii*** and *Cryptococcus neoformans*: They lead to pneumocystis pneumonia and cryptococcosis, respectively. They also lead to progressive deep round yellow–orange lesions, usually without visual squeal. These pathogens are mostly found in AIDS patients.

Bacterial Infections

- **Lyme**: It is caused by the spirochaete *Borrelia burgdorferi*, transmitted by ticks (have eight legs to be distinguished from louse). Stage 1 represents erythema migrans at the site of lesion, followed by stage 2 representing mostly arthritis and other system involvement (including eye) occurring up to 4 months after the first stage, and stage 3 that includes chronicity. Ocular features mostly occur in stage 2, manifesting as uveitis, and most commonly as intermediate uveitis, but anterior and posterior uveitis (with signs similar to syphilis uveitis). Keratitis is the most common manifestation of stage 3. Serology is only positive after 1 month. Antibiotics are systematically used and include doxycycline, penicillin, and macrolides. Similar to syphilitic uveitis, intraocular inflammation associated with lyme disease should be considered a sign of CNS involvement, necessitating a thorough neurologic evaluation, including a lumbar puncture. The Jarisch–Herxheimer reaction has also been reported in Lyme disease cases. While Lyme disease is commonly associated with intermediate uveitis, in stage 3 Lyme disease, keratitis that responds to topical corticosteroids is the most frequent ocular manifestation.
- **Brucellosis**: Transmitted from animals to humans only, this disease is caused by gram-negative bacteria *Brucella melitensis* and *B. abortus*. Ocular involvement occurs in about 20% of cases and can include chronic anterior and posterior uveitis, papilledema, and retinal hemorrhages. Treatment typically involves doxycycline and streptomycin.
- **Leprosy**: A chronic granulomatous infection caused by *Mycobacterium leprae* and *M. lepromatosis*. It primarily affects the skin, peripheral nerves, upper respiratory tract, and eyes. If uveitis occurs, it is commonly in the form of chronic low-grade iridocyclitis, with iris pearls as pathognomonic features representing dead M. leprae. Posterior uveitis is rare.
- **Whipple disease** is a rare chronic infection caused by the bacterium *Tropheryma whipplei*. It primarily affects the small intestine but can involve multiple organs, including the eye, and result in various ocular manifestations. While anterior uveitis is more commonly seen in Whipple disease, posterior uveitis can also occur. The gold standard for diagnosing Whipple disease is a duodenal biopsy that reveals a periodic acid–Schiff (PAS)-positive bacillus within macrophages in the intestinal villi. Treatment typically includes long-term antibiotic therapy, with ceftriaxone or penicillin followed by trimethoprim-sulfamethoxazole for several months to years.

17.4 The Inflammatory Chorioretinopathies (White Dot Syndromes)

- Marked by numerous whitish-yellow inflammatory lesions found in the outer retina, retinal pigment epithelium, and choroid (Table 17.8) (Crawford and Igboeli 2013). Some of the white dot syndromes may be part

Table 17.8 Comparison between different white dot syndromes

	MEWDS	APMPPE	Serpiginous choroiditis	MCP	Punctate inner choroiditis	Birdshot	ARPE (Krill disease)	AZOOR	Subretinal fibrosis
Age-gender	Young <50 years-female	Young <50 years-equal gender	Older >50 years-male	Young <50 years-myopic female	Young <50 years-myopic female	Older >50 years-female	20–50 years	Young <50 years-myopic female	
Laterality	Unilateral	Bilateral	Bilateral	Bilateral	Bilateral	Always bilateral	Unilateral	Bilateral sequential	
Retina	Multiple small lesions sparing fovea. The fovea has a pathognomonic granular appearance	Multiple large placoid in appearance that arises at the fovea, which, as the name implies, causes acute onset of bilateral blurred vision	Multiple large placoid in appearance around disc (unlike APMPPE), and extends in a serpentine pattern around the disc	Initially choroidal yellowish lesions that become multiple small punched-out chorioretinal scars with pigmented borders in the posterior pole affecting fovea, along with vitritis in some cases	Multiple small lesions affecting fovea (unlike MEWDS), but not with vitritis (unlike MCP)	Multiple small cream-colored lesions sparing fovea, with vasculitis and vitritis in active disease. The lesions do not become pigmented over time (unlike others). Almost no anterior involvement (no PS, no KPs)	Fine pigment stippling in the macula surrounded by a hypopigmented halo. Observed as disrupted ellipsoid zone on OCT	Photoreceptor outer segment dysfunction. Can be observed as loss of ellipsoid zone on OCT	Significant anterior uveitis with vitritis, with later subretinal fibrosis
Recurrence	10%	50% (high)	Very common					1/3rd	
FAF	Hyperautofluorescence spots			Punctate hypoautofluorescence spots, but hyper if active		Hypoautofluorescent at RPE atrophy areas	Slight increased autofluorescence		
FA	Early hyperfluorescence of the dots in a 'wreath-like' cluster with late staining	Early dense hypofluorescence (aka early block) and late staining (characteristic!) for active lesions	Early dense hypofluorescence and late staining	Early hypofluorescence and late hyperfluorescence	Early hypofluorescence and late hyperfluorescence	Angiographically silent in early disease stages Extensive vascular leakage (disc leakage) in more advanced stages	Hyperfluorescence due to transmission defect with absent leakage	Normal	
Associations	may be preceded by a flu-like illness (also in APMPPE)	HLA-B7, HLA-DR2. Cerebral vasculitis and can cause stroke. Erythema nodosum. Mild vitritis	HLA-B7. Tuberculosis may cause similar lesions	Lesions are similar to histo lesions. Progressive subretinal fibrosis and uveitis syndrome can be thought of as a late complication	CNVs are more common, but macular edema, vitritis, or anterior uveitis is rare	HLA-A29 in 100% of patients	The characteristic OCT feature is a dome-shaped hyperreflective lesion at the photoreceptor outer segment layer disrupting the ellipsoid zone and interdigitation zone	Associated with autoimmune disease (e.g., subacute thyroiditis)	

CNV	Rare	Rare	35%	35% (as the patients are myopic, consider the possibility of myopic CNV)	70% (more than MCP), but less inflammatory components	Rare, good prognosis	Good prognosis		
Treatment	Recovery of vision within 2–10 weeks without treatment	When foveal involvement or CNS vasculitis (i.e., the patient will have severe headache) is present, systemic corticosteroid treatment is recommended. Otherwise, recovery of vision and lesions within 2–10 weeks without treatment	IMTs are first line, usually steroids are ineffective. Visual loss in 20%	Steroid with IMT	Mainly treatment of CNV when it happens. There is mixed evidence as to whether systemic corticosteroids and IMT may decrease disease activity and limit recurrence	Steroids with IMT are mandatory from the start and will lead to disease control	None	No treatment required, despite the need for 6 months to regain vision, with recurrent cases having worse outcome	Little benefit

of a shared spectrum, while others are etiologically distinct from each other. Includes the following:

- Multiple evanescent white dot syndrome MEWDS)
- Acute zonal occult outer retinopathy (AZOOR)
- Birdshot chorioretinopathy
- Acute posterior multifocal placoid pigment epitheliopathy (APMPPE)
- Serpiginous choroidopathy
- Multifocal choroiditis and panuveitis (MCP)
- Punctate inner choroidopathy (PIC)
- Acute retinal pigment epitheliitis (Krill disease)

General Rules:

- Bilateral involvement is the rule, except for MEWDS, and ARPE (Krill disease).
- Posterior pole involvement is the rule, mostly starting around the disc for placoid lesions.
- ICG usually shows more numerous lesions than appearing on FA, which also shows more lesions than FAF or clinically.
- Age: The majority of individuals are <50 years of age with the exception of birdshot chorioretinopathy and serpiginous choroiditis, which may affect older adults.
- Gender: MEWDS, birdshot chorioretinopathy, PIC and MCP are more commonly observed in women. Only serpiginous choroidopathy has slightly male predominance, and the other large lesion disease, APMPPE, has equal gender predominance.
- Laterality: The white dot syndromes may be unilateral (MEWDS, ARPE) or bilateral (others).
- Lesion shape: The white dot lesions may be small, discrete (MEWDS, PIC, MCP, birdshot chorioretinopathy), or more placoid (i.e., large) in appearance (APMPPE and serpiginous choroiditis).
- Vitritis severity: Vitritis is usually mild except in cases of birdshot chorioretinopathy and MCP.
- FFA: most of the white dot syndromes demonstrate early hypofluorescence and late hyperfluorescence, except for: MEWDS (early hyperfluorescence) and Birdshot chorioretinopathy (early normal or silent).

Associations:

- Birdshot: HLA-A29 (diagnostic)
- APMPPE: HLA-B7, HLA-DR2
- Serpiginous: HLA-B7

17.4.1 Specific Notes on White Dot Syndromes

- **Serpiginous**: Characterized by high recurrence rate, atrophic changes, and CNV (35%). Old, scarred lesions may be present in the newly diagnosed eye. Vasculitis and vitritis are rare (Fig. 17.12).
- **Tuberculosis (TB)-associated disease**: Known as multifocal serpiginoid choroiditis or serpiginous-like choroiditis. In this condition, lesions develop and advance in various areas instead of spreading outward. It is characterized by more pronounced vitritis and uveitis (Table 17.9).
- **Ocular histoplasmosis**: Has no vitritis and low risk of CNV, while punctate inner choroidopathy (PIC) has no vitritis with high risk

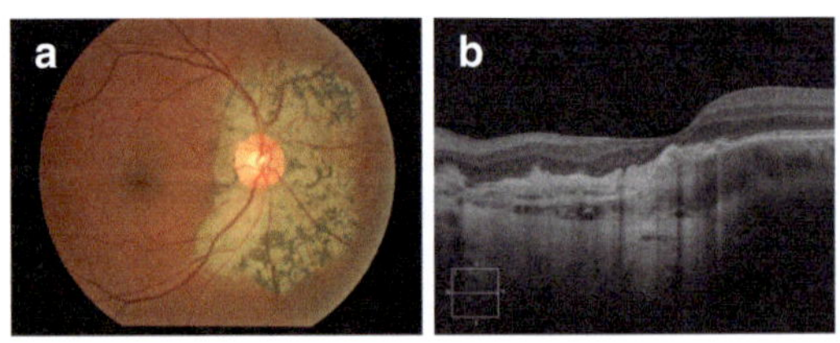

Fig. 17.12 Colored fundus photograph (**a**) and its corresponding OCT (**b**) of a serpiginous uveitis. Courtesy Retina Rocks®

Table 17.9 Comparison between tuberculous uveitis and serpiginous choroiditis

	Tuberculous uveitis	Serpiginous choroiditis
Laterality	Mostly unilateral	Mostly bilateral
Lesion color	Hyperpigmented	Hypopigmented
Fundus involvement	Diffuse	Mostly peripapillary

Table 17.10 Comparison between histoplasmosis uveitis and multifocal choroiditis and panuveitis (MCP)

	Histoplasmosis (POHS)	Multifocal choroiditis and panuveitis (MCP)[a]
Gender	Equal	Mostly female
Laterality	Mostly bilateral	Almost always bilateral
Inflammation	No vitritis	Presence of vitritis (100%) and AC inflammation (50%)
Treatment	No treatment required	Treated with steroid and IMT
Choroidal neovascularization (CNV) incidence	Lower incidence of CNV	Higher incidence of CNV

[a]Note that MCP initially appears as diffuse small yellow lesions, similar to birdshot and MEWDS

of CNV, and MCP has severe vitritis but lower risk of CNV (Table 17.10).

- **Relentless placoid chorioretinitis (RPC)**: It is a combination of serpiginous (around disc) + APMPPE (around the fovea). Placoid = large with scales.
- **Multiple evanescent white dot syndrome (MEWDS)**: Characterized by the presence of multiple small gray-white dots at the level of the deep retina/RPE in the posterior pole. Granular macular pigmentary change is usually present—a pathognomonic finding. This fovea pathognomonic granular appearance may persist even after the inflammation has subsided.
- **Birdshot retinochoroidopathy**: Always bilateral, no chorioretinal scar results from birdshot. Associated with macular edema and retinal vasculitis (periphlebitis).
- **Acute posterior multifocal placoid pigment epitheliopathy (APMPPE)**: An uncommon, usually bilateral inflammatory disorder characterized by acute-onset visual loss, usually followed weeks to months later by substantial or near-complete improvement. It is considered to be a type 4 hypersensitivity reaction.
- **Acute retinal pigment epitheliitis ARPE (Krill disease)**: A rare, idiopathic, self-limited condition affecting the RPE. It occurs unilaterally in 75% of cases and typically presents in young adults with mild disturbance in central vision. The lesions generally resolve on their own within 6–12 weeks, and vision usually returns to normal without the need for treatment.
- **Acute zonal occult outer retinopathy (AZOOR)** is characterized by acute-onset retinal dysfunction, associated with photopsia and visual field loss in young to middle-aged females (profound visual symptoms with minimal fundus signs). It is usually unilateral at presentation, but eventually the other eye becomes involved. It is identifiable by a loss of ellipsoid zone on OCT and central hypoautofluorescence on FA. ERG aids diagnosis, showing reduced amplitude and delayed flicker, indicating higher impact on cones than rods. Immunosuppression does not alter disease progression, and a 28% incidence of associated autoimmune diseases exists.

17.4.2 Other Relevant Observations

- Most entities described above are preceded by a prodrome of viral infection.
- Full-field ERG shows reduced amplitudes in both a-wave and early receptor potential (ERP), though these changes are reversible.
- When uveitis is unilateral, it is usually observed in the eye with higher myopia.
- The most common cause of decreased visual acuity in birdshot chorioretinopathy is cystoid macular edema.
- APMPPE usually affects young, healthy individuals and may be preceded by a viral prodrome. Unlike punctate inner choroiditis, APMPPE does not show a female predilection. APMPPE usually occurs after a viral illness, often involving both eyes rapidly once

symptoms start. In patients with APMPPE, fluorescein angiography reveals early blockage of lesions with late staining. In PIC, the angiography shows early hyperfluorescence and late staining of the lesions. For serpiginous choroiditis, fluorescein angiography demonstrates early choroidal flush blockage and staining of the active lesion edge in the later stages of the exam.

References

Crawford CM, Igboeli O (2013) A review of the inflammatory chorioretinopathies: the white dot syndromes. ISRN Inflamm 2013:783190. https://doi.org/10.1155/2013/783190

Kanski JJ (2019) Kanski's clinical ophthalmology e-book: a systematic approach, 6th and 9th edn. Elsevier Health Sciences

18 Clinical Review of Glaucoma: Part I

Khaled Ali Elubous and Hady Saheb

Abstract

This chapter on glaucoma provides a comprehensive overview of the disease, with a focus on high-yield notes for both clinical applications and ophthalmology exam boards. The chapter covers a wide range of topics, including primary and secondary glaucomas, tools and investigations for diagnosis and management, medical and surgical treatment options, and landmark trials in the field. The information presented is designed to be accessible and useful for both practicing clinicians and those preparing for board exams in ophthalmology. In addition, the chapter uses clear and concise language to explain complex concepts. Key points are highlighted throughout the text to help readers identify the most important information, and tables and figures are used to summarize and illustrate key concepts. Overall, the chapter on glaucoma is designed to be an effective study tool for those preparing for board exams in ophthalmology. By the end of the chapter, readers should have a solid understanding of the key concepts and best practices for managing patients with glaucoma.

Keywords

Glaucoma · Glaucoma risk factors Mechanism of glaucoma · Glaucoma management · Glaucoma surgery · Landmark trials · Open angle · Angle closure · Optical coherence tomography · Laser · Eye drops Glaucoma medication · High yield · Board exam · Ophthalmology

18.1 Overview

Glaucoma is defined as chronic progressive optic neuropathy which can be associated with characteristic visual field defects. The age-standardized prevalence of glaucoma is approximately 2–5% in the population aged 40 years and older worldwide, with primary open-angle glaucoma prevalence highest in Africa, whereas primary closed-angle glaucoma prevalence being highest in Asia (Tham et al. 2014). It carries a risk of blindness of up to 10% after 20 years (Kwon et al. 2001). It is the leading cause of irreversible blindness worldwide and ranked the fifth cause of global burden of disease (GBD) due to vision loss and blindness modeled in GBD 2019.

K. A. Elubous (✉)
Faculty of Medicine, The Hashemite University, Zarqa, Jordan

Department of Ophthalmology and Visual Sciences, McGill University, Montreal, QC, Canada
e-mail: khaled.elubous@hu.edu.jo

H. Saheb
Department of Ophthalmology and Visual Sciences, McGill University, Montreal, QC, Canada
e-mail: hady.saheb@mcgill.ca

S. A. Alryalat (ed.), *Ophthalmology Board and FRCS Part 2 Exams*,
https://doi.org/10.1007/978-981-96-1517-9_18

18.1.1 Optic Neuropathy with Corresponding Visual Field Defect

Glaucoma occurs due to damage to the nerve fiber layer that travels through the neuro-retinal rim at the optic disc, resulting in corresponding visual field defects. There are several theories present to explain the reason behind such damage, including a mechanical theory, where pressure inside the eye felt mostly by the posterior part, with more pressure on the fibers around the lamina cribrosa. Accordingly, longer fibers would be more susceptible to such damage. Figure 18.1 shows the nerve fiber layer (NFL) from different regions of the retina, as well as their insertion into the optic disc, and their corresponding visual field, where:

- Fibers from the fovea and the perifoveal region (red color) go straight to the temporal region of the optic nerve, and they are most resistant to damage and are last to be affected by glaucoma, and thus, central vision is usually preserved in glaucoma.
- Fibers from region temporal to the fovea (corresponding to nasal visual field) go around the fovea into the superior and inferior part of the optic nerve in an arcuate course (yellow and green color).
- Fibers nasal to the disc go into the nasal disc in addition to superior and inferior optic disc (blue color).

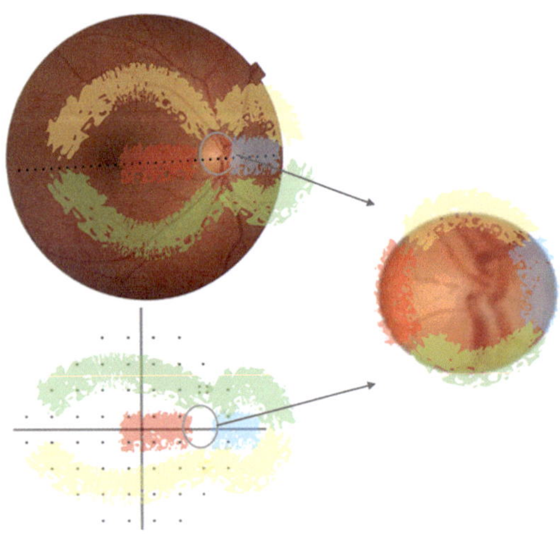

Fig. 18.1 Fundus image showing retinal nerve fiber layer from different retinal regions (upper image) and their corresponding insertion into the optic disc (right image) and visual field (lower image)

Typical optic neuropathy in glaucoma is characterized by enlarged optic disc cup in the superior and inferior region initially and then nasal and temporal quadrants (hence the ISNT rule), where green and yellow NFLs (in Fig. 18.1) are more susceptible to glaucomatous damage.

There are certain visual field defects that are characteristic for glaucoma that correspond to the damage in nerve fiber layer. These fields are shown in Fig. 18.2.

High-Yield Note
Visual field defects that respect horizontal midline mostly represent ocular pathologies, with glaucoma being the most common, while visual field defects respecting vertical midline represent neurological pathologies behind the optic chiasm (i.e., after optic nerve decussation).

18.1.2 Intraocular Pressure and Trabecular Meshwork

Glaucoma as a disease is associated with intraocular pressure (IOP) as it is the main modifiable risk factor, which exerts a pressure on the back of the eye leading to nerve fiber layer loss. IOP depends on aqueous humor dynamics, and understanding such dynamics will help better understand glaucoma treatments and interventions that will be mentioned in their respective sections below.

Aqueous humor is produced by ciliary body in the posterior chamber. The ciliary body is supplied by an anastomosis between two and three long posterior ciliary arteries (whereas the short posterior ciliary arteries supply the choroid) and anterior ciliary arteries (branches from arteries supplying the muscles), forming a major arterial arcade. The arcade has fenestrations to produce aqueous humor.

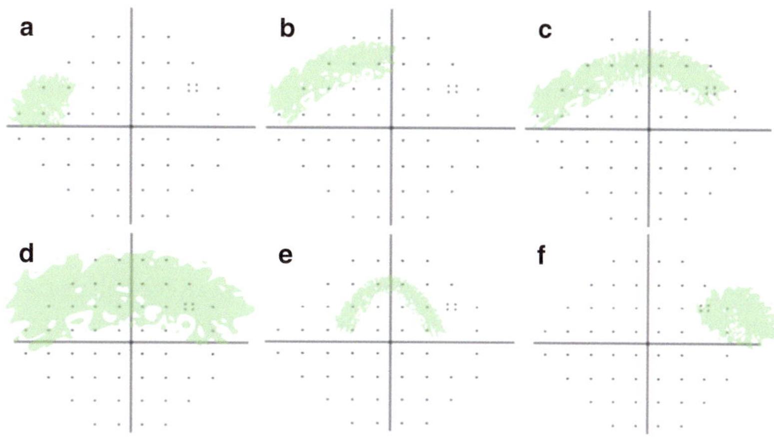

Fig. 18.2 Glaucomatous visual fields including nasal step (**a**); partial arcuate (**b**); arcuate (**c**); altitudinal (**d**); paracentral (**e**); and temporal wedge (**f**)

Aqueous then moves through the pupil to the anterior chamber and is then drained outside the eye mainly through the trabecular pathway (conventional) and the uveoscleral pathway (unconventional).

The trabecular retinaculum, or meshwork (TM), is formed by multiple layers or lamellae that extend between the scleral spur (anterior tip of internal scleral sulcus) and the Schwalbe's line. It can be defined into three regions:

- The uveal meshwork: The inner retinaculum contains about three layers of connective tissue beams that form irregular intertrabecular fenestrations. It represents the pigmented part of TM. These layers act as a primary filter of the aqueous humor through their fenestrations, and they hardly contribute to resistance.
- The corneoscleral meshwork: Beneath is the much denser corneoscleral meshwork composed of 8–15 layers of beams, and it represents the nonpigmented TM.
- The juxtacanalicular region (or cribriform region): Deep (posterior) to the corneoscleral, the fenestrations become narrower toward the scleral venous sinus (aka canal of Schlemm). The juxtacanalicular region is adjacent to the scleral venous sinus, attaching to its endothelium. It is thought to be the main contributor to the resistance of aqueous humor flow. Histologically, the JCT can be divided into three layers: trabecular endothelial layer, central connective tissue layer, and inner wall (IW) endothelium of SC.

Schlemm's canal (SC) or scleral venous sinus is a circular canal around the eye, behind the TM and embedded in the internal scleral sulcus (a shallow groove on the posterior surface of the corneoscleral junction). Aqueous humor is drained from the AC through the TM and into SC through SC endothelium, which then goes to the deep intrascleral plexus, draining to episcleral venous plexus, which drains into anterior ciliary veins and then into the superior ophthalmic vein. It is worth noting that the SC is not a continuous ring, as it has septations in it, so flow is not circumferential, as it goes from SC up into the intrascleral venous plexus (Francis et al. 2012). It is assumed that septation may occur in almost every 60', which is why it is recommended for some MIGS devices to be placed 2 clock hours apart to increase the chance of targeting different drainage segments of Schlemm's canal (Kaplowitz et al. 2014).

An increase in intraocular pressure will lead the TM to compress the SC, leading to further narrowing of SC (Kagemann et al. 2011). Trabecular retinacula endothelial cells have a phagocytic effect on the extracellular detritus. The progression of pathological glaucoma is promoted when the number of trabecular reticulum cells reduces significantly, resulting in dysfunction, increasing resistance through the narrowed fenestrations coupled with a decreased phagocytic effect of removing debris.

Unlike the trabecular pathway, the uveoscleral pathway is not a distinctive pathway with tubes and channels. Rather, it is a route whereby aqueous humor seeps through, around, and between tissues, including the supraciliary space, ciliary muscle, suprachoroidal space, choroidal vessels, emissarial canals, sclera, and lymphatic vessels, changed by pressure gradients through the uvea (Johnson et al. 2017). Uveoscleral outflow changes throughout life and in various syndromes associated with elevated IOP. It is reduced with aging and in exfoliation syndrome and ocular hypertension, but it increases in iridocyclitis and glaucomatocyclitic crisis. Uveoscleral outflow also slows every night, as reported in patients with ocular hypertension and in healthy adults of the same age.

18.2 Types of Glaucoma

18.2.1 Primary Open-Angle Glaucoma (POAG)

It is defined as optic neuropathy with anatomically open iridocorneal angle without secondary causes, typically with associated visual field defects. While it is the most common cause of optic neuropathy, it remains a diagnosis of exclusion.

Major risk factors for development or progression

- High IOP
- Age
- Thin CCT
- High C/D ratio
- Disc hemorrhage

Other risk factors

- Myopia
- Family history
- Race (black)
- Ethnicity (Latino, Asian)
- Perapapillary atrophy
- Anticardiolipin antibody
- Female sex
- Poor perfusion (low BP, low diastolic pressure, antihypertensive use, nocturnal dips)

Controversial risk factors

- Other cardiovascular diseases, sleep apnea, H. Pylori, hypothyroidism.

18.2.2 Target IOP

This is the IOP that is needed to be maintained to minimize progression of glaucomatous optic neuropathy. It is a range of IOP during management, aiming to control the glaucoma progression. Typically, low IOP target is usually required with advanced disease, fast progression, low baseline IOP, strong family history, and long life expectancy.

18.2.3 Normal-Tension Glaucoma (NTG)

Features

- Prevalence: East Asian > African > white European
- Risk factors: OSA, nocturnal hypotension
- Increased association with vasospastic disorders and ischemic vascular disease

Pathophysiology

- Mechanical theory:
  - Lamina cribrosa supply: high IOP negatively impacts the oxygen and nutrient supply to axons' intralamina cribrosa.
  - CCT: thinner CCT is associated with higher risk.
- Perfusion theory:
  - High IOP and systemic factors affect the perfusion of retinal ganglion cells.
  - Low systolic BP and nocturnal hypotension decreased perfusion.
- Vascular dysregulation:
  - Two main components: vascular endotheliopathy and autonomic dysfunction (decreased regulation of sympathetic and parasympathetic tone, measured by observing BP, heart rate variability).
  - Possible characteristics: vasospasm, elevated plasma endothelin-1 (ET-1), Flammer syndrome.

- Translaminar pressure difference theory:
  - Suggests an association between low CSF pressure and open-angle glaucoma.

Risk factors for progression:

- Disc hemorrhage, migraine, low ocular perfusion pressure, female.

  Differential diagnosis:

- Non-glaucomatous optic neuropathy, or resolved hypertensive glaucoma (steroid response, pigment dispersion, trauma, surgery).

  Common indications to commence treatment:

- Monocular, family history of blindness, advanced disease stage, documented structural or functional glaucoma progression, disc hemorrhage, pseudoexfoliation, female with migraine or Raynaud's.

Main Conclusion of (CNTGS)
- Reducing IOP by 30% significantly reduces the VF progression rate in NTG.
- At 5 years: 80% showed no VF progression in treated arm vs. 40% in untreated arm.

High-Yield Notes
In contrast to POAG:

- Paracentral scotoma early in course.
- Disc hemorrhage more common.
- Thinner neuroretinal rim.

18.2.4 Ocular Hypertension (OHTN)

- Definition: IOP >21 mmHg with no signs of glaucoma.
- High-risk group: high IOP, larger C/D ratio, lower CCT, older age, and high PSD.
- According to OHTS, the conversion risk over 5 years of treatment was reduced by 50%, from 9.5% to 4.4%.

High-Yield Notes
- High-risk factors.
- See the landmark trials chapter for more details on OHTS.

18.2.5 Angle Closure Glaucoma (ACG)

Angle closure glaucoma represents a spectrum of diseases that begin with primary angle closure suspect (PACS), followed by primary angle closure (PAC), followed by primary angle closure glaucoma (PACG) (Table 18.1). Within this spectrum, acute closure crises occur when the angle is closed in addition to angle closure symptoms (eye pain, redness, nausea and vomiting, corneal edema, and high IOP) (BMJ Publishing Group Ltd. BMA House 2021), with or without associated glaucomatous damage. PACG is more likely to be associated with blindness compared to POAG. Risk factors include short axial length, Asian ethnicity, older age, and female gender (F:M ratio of 3:1).

The definition of PACS (i.e., normal IOP, non-suspicious optic nerve examination findings [with OCT confirmation], no evidence of PAS on dynamic gonioscopy, and no history of an AAC episode). In such patients:

- In PACS, the cumulative risk of conversion to PAC appears to be relatively low in a community-based population with asymptomatic PACS (25% over 14 years, or 1–2% per year) (Yuan et al. 2024). The classical risk of progression to PAC is around 4%.
- ZAP trial: the hazard ratio for progression from PACS to PAC in LPI-treated eyes was 0.31 (95% CI, 0.21–0.46). PAC occurrence decreased approximately two-thirds following LPI (He et al. 2019).
- Higher IOP, shallower central and limbal anterior chamber depth (ACD), smaller trabecular iris space at 500 μm (TISA 500), and smaller light-room angle recess area at 750 μm (ARA

Table 18.1 The spectrum of primary angle closure suspect to primary angle closure glaucoma

	Primary angle closure suspect	Primary angle closure	Primary angle closure glaucoma
Definition	>180° Iridocorneal contact	+PAS or high IOP	+Optic nerve or field changes
Management	Risk-benefit discussion as below	If IOP <30, need LPI vs. lens extraction (especially >50 years). Otherwise, consider medical management, in addition to risk benefit discussion	Need LPI or lens extraction + glaucoma surgery based on severity
European glaucoma society	LPI in high-risk individuals, e.g., high hyperopia, patients requiring repeated pupil dilatation for fundus exam or with difficult access to healthcare facilities	LPI (age <50 years), LPI or CLE (age >50 years)	LPI (age <50 years), LPI or CLE (age >50 years)

750) at baseline were associated with an increased risk of progression from PACS to PAC over 14 years. Both AS-OCT measurements and ophthalmic examinations not using this technique allowed for the primary identification of PACS eyes at higher risk of PAC progression (Yuan et al. 2024).

Table 18.2 Differences between pupillary block and non-pupillary block angle closure

Relative pupillary block	Non-pupillary block
Posterior pushing	Anterior pulling
Relieved by iridotomy	Partially relieved
Shallow AC	Less shallow AC
Older	Younger
E.g., lens-related glaucoma	E.g., plateau iris, ICE syndrome, NVG

Mechanism

1. Pupil block (simultaneous activation of dilator and sphincter muscles → perpendicular force on lens → pupil block)
2. Plateau iris
3. Lens induced
4. Retrolenticular (vitreous hemorrhage, gas tamponade)
5. Iris volume (physiological component)

   Normally iris volume decreases with dilation, but in patients with PACG it increases.
6. Iris stiffness

Based on the mechanism, it can be classified into predominantly pupillary block vs. non-pupillary block (Table 18.2). The importance of differentiation can be appreciated for the use of parasympathomimetic (pilocarpine), which constricts the pupil (reduced iris thickness and iris root pull), but at the same time causes forward movement of the iris-lens diaphragm due to ciliary muscle contraction. While in pupillary block pilocarpine can relieve the block, it will have a paradoxical effect on spherophakia, and the highly convex lens is supported by long weak zonules that allow greater anterior movement of the iris-lens diaphragm. Other conditions include exfoliation syndrome (zonular weakness), phacomorphic glaucoma, and malignant glaucoma.

Precipitating Drugs

- Adrenergic agonists (phenylephrine, nebulizers).
- Anticholinergic effect (tropicamide, Botox, TCA, SSRI).
- Cholinergic effect (pilocarpine) → also forward iris-lens movement.
- Topiramate → ciliochoroidal effusion → forward iris-lens movement.

Both mydriatics and miotics may predispose to angle closure:

- Mydriatics are classically blamed for acute angle closure in predisposed patients, due to rolling of the iris toward the TM. Systemic drugs with adrenergic (sympathomimetic) or anticholinergic (parasympatholytic) activity have the potential to cause angle closure.

- Miotics, which were classically used to relieve angle closure, pull the peripheral iris away from the anterior chamber angle. However, strong miotics may also cause the zonular fibers of the lens to relax, allowing the lens-iris interface to move forward. Furthermore, their use results in greater iris-lens contact, thus potentially increasing pupillary block.

Management

Where iridotomy and cataract extraction remain the main modalities to prevent acute angle closure in patients with PACS based on ZAP and EAGLE studies, iridoplasty can be considered as second line, mainly to manage residual angle closure following peripheral iridotomy (Lim et al. 2019). An iridotomy with or without long-term use of ocular hypotensive medications controls the disease in most patients with PAC. However, the EAGLE study suggests that in PAC cases with IOP of ≥30 mm Hg, lensectomy may be the preferred treatment.

Management of acute primary angle closure (APAC) or intermittent APAC, which manifests as headache, rainbow halo, and blurred vision, with/out N/V: Begin by checking the patient's medications, as it is usually the precipitating factor. Gonioscopy is needed to diagnose and in some cases relieve the angle closure in appositional PAC. If the APAC is mild, it may be broken by cholinergic agents (pilocarpine 1–2%), which induce miosis that pulls the peripheral iris away from the trabecular meshwork. However, these agents may worsen some types of angle closure without pupillary block and exacerbate pupillary block in some eyes. Stronger miotics are ideally avoided, as they may increase the vascular congestion of the iris or rotate the lens-iris interface more anteriorly, increasing the pupillary block. Globe compression over the central cornea, dynamic gonioscopy, and careful paracentesis with a 30-gauge needle or sharp blade are all techniques to acutely lower the IOP in order to clear the corneal edema.

Plateau iris: IOP is a poor indicator for success, so serial gonioscopy should be carried out to confirm opening the angle. Plateau iris may be suspected if the central anterior chamber appears to be of normal depth, and the iris plane appears flat for an eye with angle closure. Plateau iris configuration is the term used to describe an eye with gonioscopic and/or imaging evidence of plateau iris in which a mydriatic provocative test does not induce IOP elevation. Conversely, in plateau iris syndrome, pharmacologic mydriasis induces IOP elevation of 6 mm Hg or more. In plateau iris syndrome, PAS formation has been reported to begin at the Schwalbe line (see Fig. 18.3) and then to extend in a posterior direction over the trabecular meshwork, scleral spur, and angle recess.

Peripheral Anterior Synechia (PAS)

These are tissue strands that extend from iris up to TM and beyond. It is differentiated from iris fibers by having a base in the iris and either an apex up (triangle shape) or wide apex (rectangle shape). PAS is one of the pathognomonic signs of angle closure.

Given that aqueous outflow occurs via the pigmented TM and the uveoscleral pathway, identifying "high" PAS (those obstructing PTM) and "low" PAS (adhesions forming posterior to PTM) is a key consideration when planning glaucoma management and assessing prognosis.

Ocular pathologies that may induce PAS formations include uveitis, iris neovascularization, and a previous history of trauma or intraocular surgery.

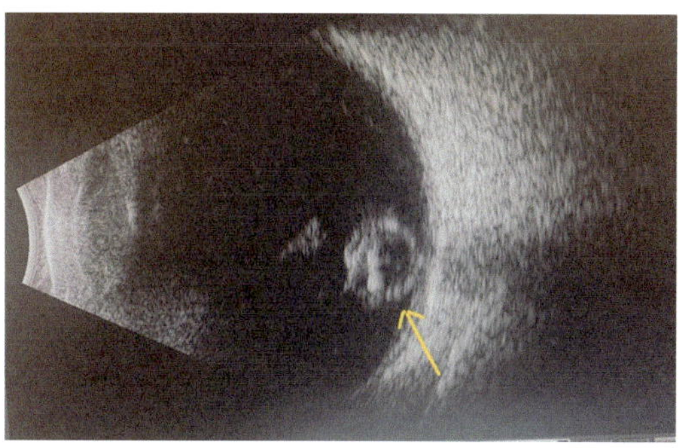

Fig. 18.3 This photo of a B-scan for a patient diagnosed with lens particle glaucoma, presented with acute rise in IOP, corneal edema, and aqueous flare. A dropped mature lens (yellow arrow) is shown in this scan

Table 18.3 Comparison between different types of glaucoma in regard to gender and ethnicity

Disease	Gender	Ethnicity
POAG	Equal	African-American
Normal tension glaucoma	Female	Japanese
Ocular hypertension	Male	
Congenital glaucoma	Male	
Angle closure glaucoma	Female	Asians
Pseudoexfoliation	Female	Caucasians/white
Pigment dispersion syndrome	Equal (but glaucoma is more common in male)	Caucasians/white
Iridocorneal dysgenesis	Female	
Anterior segment dysgenesis	Equal	

Table 18.4 Important pathogenic genes implicated in different glaucoma-related diseases

Gene	Disease	Note
TIGR/MYOC	Juvenile and adult POAG glaucoma	On GCL1A gene, AD inheritance
OPTN	Normal tension glaucoma	
CYP1B1	Isolated congenital glaucoma	Cytochrome p450 gene
LOXL1	Pseudoexfoliation	
LTBP2	Ectopia lentils with glaucoma	Megalocornea with zonular weakness. Glaucoma here is secondary, with lens removal being essential for treatment
RIEG1/PIXT2	Axenfeld-Rieger syndrome	Forkhead gene *FKHL7*
PAX6	Anterior segment dysgenesis; aniridia	

PAS in PAC mostly forms superiorly, compared to inferiorly in uveitis cases.

High-Yield Notes

Table 18.3 compares gender and ethnicity between different types of glaucoma. Table 18.4: Important pathogenic genes implicated in different glaucoma-related diseases.

18.3 Specific Glaucoma-Related Entities

18.3.1 Pseudoexfoliation Syndrome (PXF)

Features

- Elderly
- Scandinavians, Greeks, Middle Eastern
- Underlying systemic basement membrane disorder
- More resistant to medical treatment than POAG
- Possible risk factors: female, hyperhomocysteinemia, low-folate diet

Mechanism

- Deposition of fibrillogranular amyloid-like material obstructing TM

Clinical Features

- Gonioscopy: Patchy (uneven) deeply pigmented TM with Sampaolesi's line
- Moth-eaten pupillary iris
  - Increased risk of angle closure (forward lens displacement due to loose zonules)
- Increased risk of lens subluxation
- Good response to laser treatment

18.3.2 Pigment Dispersion Syndrome (PDS)

Features

- Myopia
- Male > female

- Young age (20–50 years)
- Predominantly in Caucasians

Symptoms
- Blurring of vision and halos especially after physical activity

Associations
- Peripheral retinal degenerations 20%
- RRD 5%
- Full-thickness retinal hole 10%

Mechanism
- Posterior insertion of iris, longer radial width of iris, and concave iris lead to:
- > Reverse pupillary block (contact between lens zonules and iris pigment epithelium)

Clinical Features
- Gonioscopy: iris bowing posteriorly, deeply pigmented TM with Sampaolesi's line
- Transillumination defect (TID) at midperiphery, spoke-like loss of iris pigment
- Krukenberg spindle on cornea
- Scheie's stripe: pigment on anterior lens capsule at zonule attachments
- Large IOP fluctuations
- Three phases: Active pigment dispersion (normal IOP), conversion to glaucoma/high IOP, and regression phase (normal IOP)

Treatment
- Laser peripheral iridotomy might be considered in early phase (flatten the iris).
- Drops that enhance outflow are more effective than aqueous suppressants.
- Pilocarpine is effective (by decreasing iris-zonules rubbing) but not well tolerated.
- ALT is equal or more effective than SLT.
- Need lower doses of laser (high risk of IOP spike).
- Angle based glaucoma surgery is effective.
- Myopic patient carries a risk of hypotony maculopathy after filtration surgery (Elubous 2024).

High-Yield Notes
- With lens rise, zonular-iris contact decreases and pigment dispersion may decrease.
- PDS is not associated with weak zonules as in PXF.
- PDS needs regular fundus exams.

18.3.3 Plateau Iris

Anatomical features: evident by UBM

- Anteriorly positioned ciliary processes.
- Narrow iridociliary sulcus angle [hallmark].
- Thicker peripheral iris.
- Anterior insertion of iris.

Table 18.5 provides a comparison between typical and atypical plateau iris syndrome.

Clinical Features
- Sharp angulation of the peripheral iris.
- Flat iris unless a concomitant lens rise.
- Plateau iris configuration: no angle closure evident after LPI.
- Plateau iris syndrome: persistent *appositional* angle closure and double-hump sign despite patent PI. Either (complete) closure with high IOP or (incomplete) closure with normal IOP.
- With time, PAS may develop and form a synechial closure.
- Double hump: created centrally by the lens and peripherally by anteriorly positioned ciliary process during indentation gonioscopy.

Table 18.5 Comparison between typical and atypical plateau iris syndromes

Typical plateau	Atypical plateau
Closed or narrow iridociliary sulcus angle +/- thick peripheral iris +/- anterior insertion of iris	Open iridociliary sulcus angle + thick peripheral iris + anterior insertion of iris

Treatment Options
- Laser iridoplasty
- Lens extraction
- Goniosynechialysis
- Filtration surgery

High-Yield Notes
Patients with plateau iris are more commonly female, at young age (30s–40s), and are less hyperopic than PACG.

18.3.4 Neovascular Glaucoma

- Etiology: retinal ischemia
- Stages
  - Rubeosis iridis (NVA and normal IOP).
  - Open-angle glaucoma (NVA and elevated IOP).
  - Angle closure glaucoma (NVA and elevated IOP and PAS).
- Predisposing factors
  - Ocular ischemic conditions
    CRVO (8.5% cumulative incidence of NVG, higher (40%) with severe ischemic CRVO, rare in nonischemic CRVO, 35% of nonischemic convert to ischemic in 3 years).
    PDR (20% risk of NVG).
    OIS (70% risk of NVG).
    CRAO (6–20% risk of NVG).
    BRVO
    BRAO (rare)
  - Inflammatory conditions
    Uveitis

18.3.5 Postsurgical Glaucoma

This includes malignant glaucoma, choroidal detachment (effusion vs. hemorrhage), and pupillary block. It is difficult to differentiate malignant glaucoma, choroidal effusion, suprachoroidal hemorrhage, or pupillary block, which can all occur post-surgery (Table 18.6).

18.3.6 Malignant Glaucoma

Uniform narrowing of the anterior chamber due to expansion of the choroid leading to anteriorization of the iris-lens diaphragm. The IOL and capsule appear to be pushed forward, especially on UBM and OCT.

Table 18.6 Comparison between etiologies to be suspected in postsurgical glaucoma with shallow anterior chamber

Aspect	Malignant glaucoma	Uveal or choroidal effusion	Suprachoroidal hemorrhage	Pupil block
Etiology	Forward movement of lens-iris diaphragm due to choroidal expansion	Accumulation of fluid in uvea or choroid and between uvea and sclera	Bleeding between choroid and sclera	Retropupillary push, closing the angle
Clinical picture	Uniformly shallow AC	Choroidal detachment	Pain with choroidal detachment	Pain, redness, nausea and vomiting
Management	• Cycloplegic agents with aqueous suppressants • YAG iridozonulohyaloidotomy (IZH)	Cycloplegics with steroid (topical and systemic). Discontinue pressure-lowering agents to avoid hypotony	Cycloplegics with steroid (topical and systemic). Discontinue pressure-lowering agents to avoid hypotony unless IOP elevated	Pilocarpine and iridotomy to break the pupil block along with pressure-lowering agents
	• Hyperosmotic agents			
	• Consider surgical options (e.g., iridozonulohyaloidovitrectomy (IZHV))			

Risk Factors

- Short axial length, plateau iris, history of contralateral malignant glaucoma, phakia, intraoperative anterior chamber decompression, female, angle closure, glaucoma surgery.

Clinical Presentation

- Typical presentation: high IOP, shallow AC despite patent PI after glaucoma surgery and absence of choroidal effusion or suprachoroidal hemorrhage on fundus exam and/or B-scan.
- AC swallowing centrally and peripherally.

Less Common Presentation

- Normal or low IOP (after a glaucoma surgery).
- Spontaneous onset
- Emmetropic or myopic eye
- Myopic shift
- Post-cataract surgery

Pathophysiology Theories

- Choroidal expansion
- Poor vitreous conductivity
- More common in hyperopic eye due to short axial length and relatively larger lens, which leads to faster expansion of vitreous and larger impact of AC shallowing.

Ultimately results in anterior rotation of ciliary body and forward displacement of lens-iris diaphragm.

Differential Diagnosis

- Pupillary block angle closure: shallow (periphery > centrally), nonpatent PI
- Suprachoroidal hemorrhage
- Choroidal effusion

Management

Malignant glaucoma medical management includes the triad of intensive cycloplegic therapy; aggressive aqueous suppression with b-adrenergic antagonists, a_2-adrenergic agonists, and carbonic anhydrase inhibitors; and dehydration of the vitreous with hyperosmotic agents. Miotics can make malignant glaucoma worse and should not be used. In aphakic and pseudophakic eyes, the anterior vitreous can be disrupted with the Nd:YAG laser. Laser photocoagulation of the ciliary processes reportedly has been helpful in treating this condition; this procedure may alter the adjacent vitreous face. In approximately half of the patients, malignant glaucoma can be controlled with laser and medical management; the other half require surgical intervention. The definitive surgical treatment is pars plana vitrectomy with iridozonulohyaloidovitrectomy (IZHV).

Chief Goal

- Establish a unicameral chamber
- Disruption of anterior hyaloid surface
- Vitreous body debulking

Stepwise Management

- Repeat LPI if nonpatent
- Medical therapy (atropine)
- Lens removal
- YAG or 30-gauge needle iridozonulohyaloidotomy (IZH)
- Iridozonulohyaloidovitrectomy (IZHV)

Recurrent Malignant Glaucoma

- Atropine drop → repeat YAG → repeat PPV + IZH (IZHV)

18.3.6.1 Malignant Glaucoma After Glaucoma Filtration Surgery

In this special setting, the IOP could be low, which may be misleading and therefore malignant glaucoma may be underdiagnosed.

The differential of shallow AC and hypotony after trabeculectomy:

- Hyperfiltration (high bleb)
- Wound leak
- Malignant glaucoma: failure to reform AC with OVD, absence of choroidal effusion

A choroidal detachment (CD) is defined by the abnormal presence of fluid or blood in the suprachoroidal space. It can be either serous (aka choroidal effusion or uveal effusion) or hemorrhagic (aka suprachoroidal hemorrhage). Serous detachment can also be classified into primary and secondary (e.g., post-surgery or trauma), while hemorrhagic cases are mostly secondary. Most commonly, this occurs due to post-op hypotony after glaucoma surgeries (>50% chance to happen in the other eye). Mostly, fundus exam is needed to see the choroidal detachment or B-scan if possible, but hemorrhagic cases are usually acute and painful compared to effusion. Pathophysiology of the primary syndrome includes thickened sclera that might result in a relative obstruction to venous outflow via the vortex veins, causing congestion of the choriocapillaris and subsequent uveal effusion (Elagouz et al. 2010).

Primary choroidal effusion or uveal effusion syndrome is related to a scleral abnormality, and congestion of the choroidal venous system caused by compression of the vortex veins by thick sclera was the cause of fluid accumulation in suprachoroidal and subretinal spaces. Uveal effusion syndrome is the idiopathic form of uveal effusion, and secondary causes must be excluded, including hypotony, intraocular inflammation, and intraocular tumor (Uyama et al. 2000). UES has been classified into:

- Type 1, nanophthalmic eyes (<21 mm axial length); the mean (SD) age 35.9 (12.2) years.
- Type 2, non-nanophthalmic eyes with clinically abnormal sclera (defined by abnormal scleral thickness or histology); the mean (SD) age 44.7 (8.2) years.
- Type 3, non-nanophthalmic eyes with clinically normal sclera.

The most striking features are choroidal elevation, subretinal fluid, and secondary RPE changes, often described as a leopard spot fundus. It characteristically begins in the periphery and may not be clinically apparent unless careful peripheral fundus examination is undertaken or if specifically looked for using ultrasonography. Shifting subretinal fluid is almost pathognomonic of a serous RD.

In uveal effusion patients with resolved serous RD, a diffuse, spotty pigmentation develops in and under the retina in those areas that were detached for an extended period of time. This pigmentation effect has been described as leopard skin spots, tessellation, and pseudoretinitis pigmentosa, or yellowish spots (Iida et al. 2002).

Primary cases can be surgically managed by sclerectomy with a small sclerostomy under the scleral flap (Uyama et al. 2000). However, for secondary cases, surgical management should be the last resort. B-scan can differentiate fluid type causing the choroidal detachment. In postsurgical cases, surgical drainage of choroidal effusion is indicated with failed medical therapy or with visual decline. However, for hemorrhagic cases, surgical drainage should be planned carefully and mostly delayed allowing for blood lysis and liquefaction and to avoid rebleeding (e.g., stopping blood thinner), owing to higher complication rate.

Other

After scleral buckle, angle closure can occur due to different mechanisms; each has unique management strategy in addition to the aqueous suppressants:

- Choroidal effusion, which can be managed conservatively (e.g., cycloplegics).
- Compression on vortex veins, which needs readjustment of the buckle.

Drug-induced secondary angle closure patients experience sudden bilateral vision loss with acute myopia, bilateral ocular pain, and headache, usually within 1 month of starting topiramate or other sulfa medications (including acetazolamide), which is an idiosyncratic reaction. In addition to discontinuing the agent, aqueous suppressants and cycloplegics aid in treatment. Peripheral iridotomy is not indicated (i.e., non-pupillary block mechanism). The secondary angle closure usually resolves within 24–48 h with medical treatment, and the myopia resolves within 1–2 weeks of discontinuing topiramate.

18.3.7 Inflammatory Glaucoma

- Most commonly open angle (e.g., herpetic, Posner, FHI, JIA, granulomatous).
- Angle closure (e.g., idiopathic, HLA B27, JIA, granulomatous).
- Ciliary body anterior rotation angle closure (e.g., VKH, sympathetic ophthalmic).

Mechanisms

- Open angle (decrease TM outflow facility, steroid response, or trabeculitis).
- Pupillary block angle closure (with seclusio or occlusio pupillae and iris bombe).
- Non-pupillary block angle closure (broad PAS or ciliary body swelling).
- Neovascular glaucoma may rarely develop in chronic cases.

Special Types

- **Posner-Schlossman Syndrome**

Features:

- Acute, unilateral, recurrent short attacks of elevated intraocular pressure (IOP)
- Mild anterior chamber inflammation and no or mild pain
- Normal between attacks
- No synechiae develop

- **Fuchs Heterochromic Iridocyclitis (FHI)**

A triad of heterochromia, glaucoma, and recurrent anterior uveitis:

- Iris texture changes
- Glaucoma (15%) is usually an open angle
- Mild anterior uveitis
- Diffuse stellate KPs
- Neovascularization and Amsler sign (not pathognomonic): bleeding of the vessel upon AC penetration
- Associated with posterior subcapsular cataract

Table 18.7 compares between Fuchs heterochromic iridocyclitis (FHI) and Posner-Schlossman syndrome.

- Peripheral anterior synechiae start inferiorly in patients who have uveitic glaucoma.
- Peripheral anterior synechiae start superiorly in patients with angle closure glaucoma.
- Reversible granulomatous or non-granulomatous anterior uveitis has been reported with alpha-agonists.

Management

- Mitotics should be avoided (associated with breakdown of blood aqueous barrier).
- First-line medical therapy includes beta-blocker and carbonic anhydrase inhibitor.
- Prostaglandin analogues could be used in a quiet eye (anterior uveitis, CME, reactivation of herpes have been reported).
- SLT (but not ALT) can be considered (lower success rate than other glaucomas).
- Surgical iridectomy for angle closure with iris bombe (high rate of failure with LPI).
- Surgery poses a higher risk of failure than POAG:
  - Trabeculectomy +MMC.
  - Tube valved or non-valved (complications include tube/plate exposure, hypotony, poor encapsulation of plate, and flare of uveitis).
  - Other options (deep sclerectomy, canaloplasty, and goniotomy in JIA).
- Need good control of uveitis pre- as well as post-surgery.
- Cyclodestructive procedures pose higher risk of hypotony and flare.

Table 18.7 Comparison between Fuchs heterochromic iridocyclitis (FHI) and Posner-Schlossman syndrome

	Fuchs heterochromic iridocyclitis (FHI)	Posner-Schlossman syndrome
Inflammation	Mild recurrent unilateral inflammation with diffuse stellate KPs	Mild recurrent unilateral reaction
IOP	15–60% risk of glaucoma	High IOP with 25% risk of glaucoma
Gender	No difference between male and female	More in men
Iris	Iris heterochromia with prominent iris and angle vessels secondary to iris atrophy	Iris atrophy and heterochromia less than FHI
Associations	Rubella, CMV	CMV, HSV

18.3.8 Lens-Induced Glaucoma

Could be open (e.g., phacolytic, phacoanaphylactic, and lens-particle glaucoma) or closed angle (e.g., phacomorphic glaucoma) (see Fig. 18.3).

18.3.8.1 Phacolytic Glaucoma

- Develops from leakage of lens proteins in an eye with a mature cataract through an intact capsule.
- These proteins as well as protein-laden macrophages compromise the trabecular meshwork outflow.

Signs
- Acute rise in IOP
- Conjunctival injection
- Pain
- Diffuse corneal edema
- Aqueous flare
- Mature cataract

Management
- Antiglaucoma medication
- Steroid eye drops
- Urgent cataract surgery

18.3.8.2 Phacoanaphylactic Glaucoma

Features
- Granulomatous uveitis
- Traumatic or surgical lens disruption
- Immune complex formation not IgE mediated (misnomer)

Presentation
- Onset (days–years)
- Uveitis
- Retained lens material
- IOP (normal or high)

Mechanism

Open or closed angle mechanisms:
- Trabecular outflow may become compromised by inflammatory cells and high-molecular-weight proteins
- Or synechiae may develop leading to chronic angle closure or pupil block.

Management
- **B-scan**: to exclude endophthalmitis, intraocular foreign body, dropped lens nucleus, retinal detachment.
- **Surgical removal**
- **Histopathology** of specimen: zonal granulomatous infiltrate

18.3.8.3 Lens-Particle Glaucoma

Features
- Liberated lens material (after cataract sx, YAG capsulotomy, or trauma)
- White fluffy debris
- AC reaction
- IOP elevation (TM clogged by lens particles or from synechia formation)

Management
- Antiglaucoma medication
- Steroid eye drops
- Surgical removal (if there is substantial retained cortical material)

18.3.9 Steroid Response Glaucoma

Risk Factors
- Children and elderly
- Glaucoma suspect and POAG
- Family history of POAG
- Route and potency (intraocular > peribulbar > eye drop > systemic > inhaler > intranasal)
- Ocular risk factors (PDG, high myopia)
- Systemic risk factors (DM1, connective tissue diseases)

Features
- Onset
  - Usually 1–4 weeks with topical steroids
  - Weeks to years with systemic steroids
  - Rarely, rapid onset may occur
- Resolution
  - Reversible
  - Mirrors the onset
  - May last up to 2 months after discontinuation of steroid drops.

Pathophysiology
- Increased deposition of extracellular matrix proteins
- Inhibition of metalloproteinases and upregulation of their inhibitors
- Reorganization of the cytoskeletal cellular network and production of cross-linked actin networks (CLANs)
- Significant increase in TM cell size leads to thickened trabecular beams
- Decreased intertrabecular spaces

Management
- Discontinuation if possible
- Regular follow-up examinations
- Medical therapy (e.g., PGAs, Rho kinase inhibitors)
- SLT (high success rate)

18.3.10 Angle Abnormalities

18.3.10.1 Cyclodialysis
- Separation of the longitudinal ciliary muscle fibers from the scleral spur (Fig. 18.4)
- Causes: mostly blunt trauma or iatrogenic
- Features: hypotony, IOP spike after cleft closure

Management
- Cycloplegics
- Miotics are contraindicated (it may predispose to prolonged opening of the cleft)
- In cases of persistent hypotony >2 months, possible treatment options include:
  - Argon laser application to small cleft + atropine drops
  - Cyclodiode laser
  - For larger cleft direct suture cyclopexy or vitrectomy with gas tamponade or sulcus IOL/CTR

18.3.10.2 Angle Recession

Features
- Glaucoma affects about 8% of patients with angle recession.
- Contralateral involvement more than 50%.

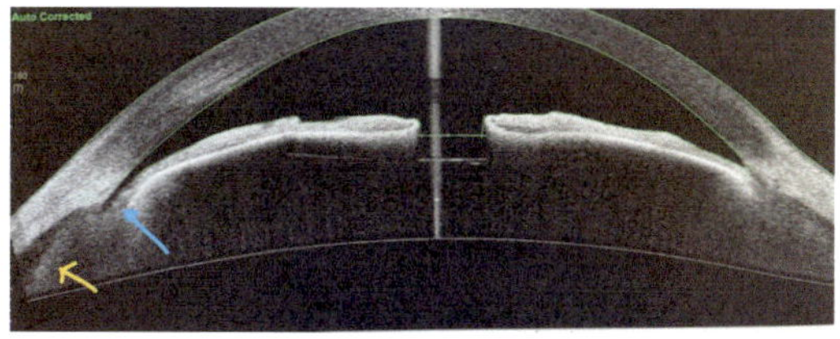

Fig. 18.4 This photo of anterior segment OCT shows a cyclodialysis cleft (blue arrow), with associated hypotony (with shallow AC), and ciliochoroidal effusion (yellow arrow) following Kahook dual-blade trabeculotomy

- Glaucoma results from degenerative changes of TM.

Risk Factors
- Blunt trauma
- >180 degrees of angle recession
- Hyphema

Signs
- Abnormally white scleral spur
- Broad ciliary body band
- Torn iris processes
- Localized depression

Management Options
- Medical therapy (avoid miotics)
- SLT (high failure rate >55%)
- Trabeculectomy or tube (failure rate at 5 years is 34–50%)
- Ab externo canaloplasty

18.3.11 Iridocorneal Endothelial (ICE) Syndromes

It can be divided into three distinct entities (Table 18.8).

Features
- Unilateral
- Women, 20–50 years of age
- Endothelial overgrowth at cornea, iris, and trabecular meshwork, leading to three syndromes
- Progression to glaucoma in 50% (open and closed mechanism)
- Definitive treatment is glaucoma drainage device

Table 18.8 Comparison between the three entities in iridocorneal endothelial (ICE) syndrome, including Chandler syndrome, iris nevus (Cogan-Reese) syndrome, and essential progressive iris atrophy

	Chandler syndrome	Iris nevus (Cogan-Reese) syndrome	Essential progressive iris atrophy
Signs	Unilateral abnormal corneal endothelium with silver hammer appearance	Large nevus ± multiple nodules	Severe atrophy with associated corectopia, pseudopolycoria
Frequency	Most common, milder glaucoma	Less	Least common
Prevalence of iris atrophy	40%	50%	100%

- Hypertonic saline for corneal edema
- Peripheral anterior synechiae (PAS) **extending beyond the Schwalbe's line**
- PCR suggesting a possible herpes simplex viral origin to the disease process
- Pseudopolycoria is an additional opening in the iris that does not react to light, unlike polycoria.

18.3.12 Pediatric Glaucoma

18.3.12.1 Primary Congenital Glaucoma

Features

- Bilateral (70%)
- Usually sporadic
- Most familial cases are autosomal recessive
- Classified into neonatal, infantile, late onset, and spontaneously arrested
- Male preponderance
- Most frequent identified gene is CYP1B1
- Abnormal angle appearance
- Symptoms of photophobia, epiphora, and blepharospasm
- Buphthalmos, Haab striae, optic disc cupping, large cornea, and high IOP
- Risk of PCG in the second child is <3%, and up to 25% in the third child
- Primary treatment is surgery

18.3.12.2 Juvenile Open-Angle Glaucoma

Features

- Usually bilateral
- Autosomal dominant inheritance
- Age of onset (4–40) years
- Male preponderance
- Associated with MYOC gene mutation
- Angle phenotypes (normal, high iris insertion, prominent iris process, or featureless angle) ± prominent iris crypts
- Very high IOP (40s–50s)
- Associated with myopia
- Difficult to control with medical therapy

18.3.13 Syndromic Congenital Glaucoma

It represents constellation of signs and symptoms that present in patients with congenital glaucoma (Table 18.9).

- Surgical management of secondary congenital glaucoma (with nonacquired ocular or systemic associations) requires a glaucoma drainage device or cyclodestructive procedure as a definite control of high IOP if medical therapy fails.
- Sturge–Weber syndrome poses a high risk of suprachoroidal hemorrhage with filtration surgery due to elevated EVP mechanism.

18.3.14 Aniridia

Classifications

- Autosomal dominant
  - PAX6 gene (on chromosome 11)
  - No systemic involvement
  - Most common type
- Sporadic
  - PAX6 and WF1 gene
  - Systemic association (WAGR syndrome)

Table 18.9 Characteristics of different syndromes of congenital glaucoma

	Characteristic feature	Laterality	Systemic association	Glaucoma prevalence	Genes	Inheritance (most commonly)
Axenfeld-Rieger syndrome (spectrum of disease)	Axenfeld: Iridocorneal adhesions Rieger: Iris anomaly Syndrome: Systemic association	Bilateral	Anomalies: Dental Deafness Cardiac Craniofacial	50%	PITX2 FOXC1 REIG2	Autosomal dominant (AD)
Peters anomaly — Type 1	Central corneal leukoma — No lens touch	Unilateral	Unlikely	50%	PAX6, PITX2	Sporadic
Peters anomaly — Type 2	Central corneal leukoma — Lens touch	Bilateral	Possible	50%	PAX6, PITX2	Sporadic
Sturge–Weber syndrome	Port-wine stain Iris heterochromia Elevated EVP Episcleral hemangioma	Unilateral	– Facial hemihypertrophy – CNS anomaly	Rare (8%) 50% with port-wine stain	GNAQ	Sporadic
Neurofibromatosis type 1	Eyelid neurofibroma (a feature associated with glaucoma) Iris hamartomas (Lisch nodules)		Criteria ≥2: – CAL spot *6 – Axillary/groin freckling – Family history (first degree) – 1 plexiform neurofibroma/2 any type – Two Lisch nodules – Optic glioma – Bone lesion	Rare (1–2%) 50% with plexiform neurofibroma	NF1 (ch 17)	Autosomal dominant (AD)

- Autosomal recessive
  - Systemic association (Gillespie syndrome: cerebellar ataxia and intellectual disability)
  - Very rare

Features
- Limbal stem cell deficiency, foveal hypoplasia, cataract, and nystagmus

Mechanisms
- **Synechiae closure of the angle by tissue extends from iris processes to the angle, with rotation of pupillary iris stump**
- Synechiae closure by avascular tissue with flat iris processes
- Absence of Schlemm's canal
- Abnormality of TM

Treatment
- Prophylactic goniotomy
- Therapeutic trabeculotomy
- Trabeculectomy with MMC (high risk of failure)
- GDD (beyond early childhood)
- CPC

High-Yield Notes
- Synechial closure and rotation of the iris stump are the major mechanisms of glaucoma.
- Sporadic cases are associated with Wilms tumor and need regular investigations.

18.3.15 Nanophthalmos and Microspherophakia

Nanophthalmos

- Normal structure but short axial length <20 mm.
- Bilateral involvement.
- Thick sclera impedes the vortex vein drainage.
- Risk of choroidal effusion, macular edema, and malignant glaucoma after ocular surgery.
- Predispose to angle closure glaucoma (need of LPI or iridoplasty).
- Considerations during cataract surgery include vitreous dehydration with mannitol, prophylactic sclerotomies, or iridozonulohyaloidovitrectomy.

Microspherophakia

- Congenital spherical lens and weak zonules lead to lens subluxation/dislocation.
- Bilateral involvement.
- Characterized by a triad of lenticular myopia, shallow AC, and angle closure glaucoma.
- Most commonly isolated, uncommon associations include Weill–Marchesani syndrome and homocystinuria.
- Management:
  - Significant lens subluxation might need lens aspiration.
  - Lensectomy requires special considerations due to weak zonules including CTR, CTS, and SFIOL.
  - May combine with trabeculectomy/tube surgery if glaucoma was progressive or with extensive PAS.

18.3.16 Raised Episcleral Venous Pressure (EVP)

Causes

- Venous congestion
- Thyroid eye disease, superior vena cava syndrome, cavernous sinus thrombosis, retrobulbar mass, carotid-cavernous fistula, orbital varices, Sturge–Weber syndrome
- Idiopathic

EVP Measurement

- Venomanometer
- Hemoglobin video imaging
- Erythrocyte-mediated angiography

Features

- IOP elevation
- Dilated tortuous episcleral vessels
- Proptosis
- Vascular bruit (in case of high-flow AV fistula)

Mechanism

- Direct effect on IOP
- Reduced outflow facility (TM degeneration with chronic IOP elevation)
- Angle closure (venous stasis in the vortex vein may cause choroidal detachment and anterior displacement of the lens–iris diaphragm)
- Neovascular glaucoma (ocular ischemia, treatment complication)

Treatment

- Treatment of the underlying cause if possible
- Medical therapy (aqueous suppressant is most effective)
- Cyclophotocoagulation (CPC)
- Glaucoma surgery (intraocular surgery should be performed with caution given high risk of suprachoroidal hemorrhage)

High-Yield Notes

- Glaucoma surgery poses a high risk of suprachoroidal hemorrhage in high EVP cases.
- Lasers and drugs that facilitate outflow are not as effective in acute cases.
- Gonioscopy feature: blood in Schlemm's canal; see Fig. 18.5.

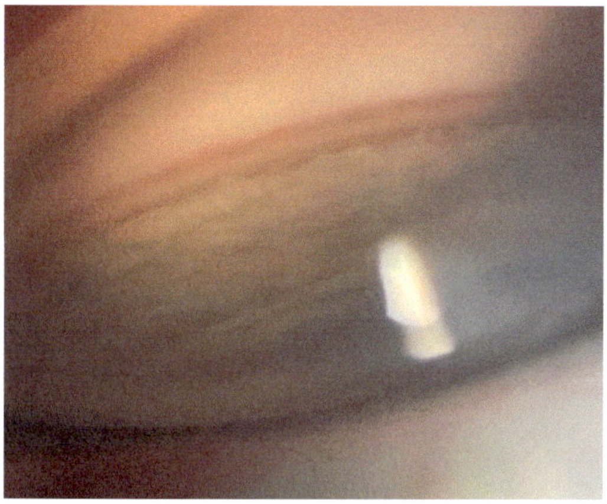

Fig. 18.5 Blood in Schlemm's canal in a patient with elevated episcleral venous pressure

18.4 Tools and Investigations

18.4.1 Optic Nerve Imaging

Optical Coherence Tomography (OCT)

- Uses low-coherence interferometry to generate cross-sectional images (Table 18.10).
- RNFL thickness measurement differs between different devices, a point to consider while monitoring glaucoma progression from different machines.
- Green disease: reduction in RNFL but still labeled statistically normal (green).
- Red disease: statistically abnormal RNFL (red) due to anatomic variant or non-glaucomatous issues like pathological myopia improperly diagnosed as glaucoma.
- Floor effect: The more advanced the disease state, the closer the RNFL will be to its minimum level. A well-measured RNFL thickness does not reach zero even in absolute glaucoma because Muller cells, astroglia, and blood vessels do not degenerate completely.
- Floor RNFL: around 50 (Spectralis), 57 (Cirrus).
- Once the RNFL approaches the floor, RNFL thickness measurement becomes less useful for disease monitoring.
- Other available options after reaching RNFL floor effect (advanced glaucoma) are using visual field (24-2, 10-2) or ganglion/macular OCT.
- Progression monitoring:
  - Event-based analysis: detect progression when a measurement exceeds an established threshold for change from baseline at an individual location within visual field.
  - Trend-based analysis: evaluating the change of a parameter over time (slope).
- Typically, structural loss occurs before functional loss.
- Broken-stick model indicates nonlinear structural function relationship.
- In advanced glaucoma (RNFL <55, md >10), VF monitoring may be more useful than structural testing.
- Common artifacts:
  - Segmentation error: abnormal determination of anterior and posterior boundaries of NFL (as in ERM, optic nerve swelling, myelinated NFL, cataract, corneal haze, vitreous detachment, or debris).
  - Decentration error: not centered on optic disc (most commonly in peripapillary atrophy, myopia).
  - Motion artifacts (less with faster scanning speeds with SD-OCT).
  - Poor signal strength.

Other Modalities

- Heidelberg retina tomograph® (HRT)
- Scanning laser polarimetry (GDx)

18.4.2 Tonometers

Contact Tonometry

- **Applanation**
  - Gold standard
  - Principle: Imbert-Fick
  - Contact (e.g., Goldmann)
  - Noncontact (e.g., pneumatic)
  - False high readings (excessive amount of fluorescein, corneal scar)
  - False low readings (corneal edema, thin cornea)
- **Indentation**
  - E.g., Tonopen®
  - Principle: transducer measures force required for corneal indentation

Table 18.10 Comparison between different types of optical coherence tomography (OCT)

	Time domain (TD)	Fourier domain	
		Spectral domain (SD)	Swept source (SS)
Examples	Stratus OCT	Cirrus® (Zeiss®) Spectralis® (Heidelberg®) RTVue-100® (Optovue®)	DRI (Topcon®)
Note	• Movable reference mirror	• Reduced acquisition time • Increased signal-to-noise ratio • Improved image quality • Less motion artifacts • Highest resolution • Fixed reference mirror	• Faster scanning speed • Deeper penetration (longer wavelength) • Wider field • Uniform sensitivity over different depths (no drop-off sensitivity like in SD) • Sweeping light
Laser type	Near-IR diode	Near-IR diode	Tunable laser
A-scan/sec (commercial devices)	400	Cirrus® (27,000) Spectralis® (40,000) Optovue® (26,000)	>100,000
Axial resolution	10 μm	Cirrus® (5 μm) Heidelberg® (7 μm) Optovue® (5 μm)	
Light bandwidth	Broadband (20 nm)	Broadband (150 nm)	Narrowband
Center wavelength	Shorter (810)	Shorter (840 nm)	Longer (1050 nm)
Deep penetration (choroid-sclera)	No	No	Yes
Lamina cribrosa visualization	No	Only with enhanced depth imaging (EDI-SD)	Yes
Image dimension's ability	2D	3D	3D
Reflected light detection		Spectrometer (CCD camera for diffraction)	Photodetector
Glaucoma diagnosis ability	Same		
Glaucoma progression (sensitivity)		Better	

  - Better for corneal edema, post-LASIK, or scarring
  - Tear film thickness is not a source of error measurement
- **Rebound**
  - (e.g., Icare®)
  - Principle: use a magnetized probe that is propelled toward the cornea. The device measures the deceleration of the probe when it contacts the cornea to provide an IOP measurement.

Noncontact Tonometry

- **Ocular response analyzers** (ORA)
  - Measure corneal hysteresis.
  - Use air impulses to assess IOP and corneal biomechanics based on corneal deformation.
  - The ORA measures the force at initial flattening and as the cornea returns to its original shape.
  - It produces two IOP summary measures, a Goldmann-correlated IOP and a corneal compensated IOP.

18.4.3 Gonioscopy

- Indirect non-indentation
- Indirect indentation (dynamic, compression)
- Direct (image not inverted)

To see the angle better:

- Ask the patient to look toward the mirror.
- Tilt the gonio-lens opposite to mirror and toward the angle quadrant of interest.

Angle Grading Systems

- The **Spaeth** system: describes visible static and dynamic angle structure, iris contour, angle grade, and degree of pigmentation.
- **Scheie** system: uses Roman numbers to describe the angle, with higher numbers indicating narrower angle (unlike other gradings).
- **Shaffer** system: grades the angle from 0 to 4 with wider angle with increasing number (unlike Scheie).

Conflict of Interest No conflict of interest to disclose.

References

BMJ Publishing Group Ltd., BMA House, Tavistock Square (2021) European glaucoma society terminology and guidelines for glaucoma, 5th edition. Br J Ophthalmol 105(Suppl 1):1–169. https://doi.org/10.1136/bjophthalmol-2021-egsguidelines

Elagouz M, Stanescu-Segall D, Jackson TL (2010) Uveal effusion syndrome. Surv Ophthalmol 55(2):134–145. https://doi.org/10.1016/j.survophthal.2009.05.003

Elubous KA (2024) Navigating hypotony challenges with XEN gel implantation. Expert Rev Med Devices 21(4):277–284. https://doi.org/10.1080/17434440.2024.2327529

Francis AW et al (2012) Morphometric analysis of aqueous humor outflow structures with spectral-domain optical coherence tomography. Invest Ophthalmol Vis Sci 53(9):5198–5207. https://doi.org/10.1167/iovs.11-9229

He M et al (2019) Laser peripheral iridotomy for the prevention of angle closure: a single-centre, randomised controlled trial. Lancet 393(10181):1609–1618. https://doi.org/10.1016/S0140-6736(18)32607-2

Iida T et al (2002) Leopard-spot pattern of yellowish subretinal deposits in central serous chorioretinopathy. Arch Ophthalmol 120(1):37–42. https://doi.org/10.1001/archopht.120.1.37

Johnson M, McLaren JW, Overby DR (2017) Unconventional aqueous humor outflow: a review. Exp Eye Res 158:94–111. https://doi.org/10.1016/j.exer.2016.01.017

Kagemann L et al (2011) 3D visualization of aqueous humor outflow structures in-situ in humans. Exp Eye Res 93(3):308–315. https://doi.org/10.1016/j.exer.2011.03.019

Kaplowitz K, Schuman JS, Loewen NA (2014) Techniques and outcomes of minimally invasive trabecular ablation and bypass surgery. Br J Ophthalmol 98(5):579–585. https://doi.org/10.1136/bjophthalmol-2013-304256

Kwon YH et al (2001) Rate of visual field loss and long-term visual outcome in primary open-angle glaucoma. Am J Ophthalmol 132(1):47–56. https://doi.org/10.1016/s0002-9394(01)00912-6

Lim DK et al (2019) Quantitative assessment of changes in anterior segment morphology after argon laser peripheral iridoplasty: findings from thc EARL study group. Clin Experiment Ophthalmol 47(1):33–40. https://doi.org/10.1111/ceo.13374

Tham Y-C et al (2014) Global prevalence of glaucoma and projections of glaucoma burden through 2040: a systematic review and meta-analysis. Ophthalmology 121(11):2081–2090. https://doi.org/10.1016/j.ophtha.2014.05.013

Uyama M et al (2000) Uveal effusion syndrome: clinical features, surgical treatment, histologic examination of the sclera, and pathophysiology. Ophthalmology 107(3):441–449. https://doi.org/10.1016/S0161-6420(99)00141-4

Yuan Y et al (2024) Long-term risk and prediction of progression in primary angle closure suspect. JAMA Ophthalmol 142(3):216–223. https://doi.org/10.1001/jamaophthalmol.2023.5286

Further Readings

Ah-Kee EY, Egong E, Shafi A, Lim LT, Yim JL (2015) A review of drug-induced acute angle closure glaucoma for non-ophthalmologists. Qatar Med J 2015(1):6. https://doi.org/10.5339/qmj.2015.6

AlObaida I, Aljasim LA (2020) Selective laser trabeculoplasty in patients with angle recession glaucoma: a small case series. Am J Ophthalmol Case Rep 19:100835. https://doi.org/10.1016/j.ajoc.2020.100835

Amini H, Razeghinejad MR (2005) Transscleral diode laser therapy for cyclodialysis cleft induced hypotony. Clin Experiment Ophthalmol 33(4):348–350. https://doi.org/10.1111/j.1442-9071.2005.01008.x

Anderson DR, Normal Tension Glaucoma Study (2003) Collaborative normal tension glaucoma study. Curr Opin Ophthalmol 14(2):86–90. https://doi.org/10.1097/00055735-200304000-00006

Andole S, Senthil S (2023) Ocular surface disease and anti-glaucoma medications: various features, diagnosis, and management guidelines. Semin Ophthalmol 38(2):158–166. https://doi.org/10.1080/08820538.2022.2094714

Asanad S, Park A, Pottenburgh J, Siddiqui A, Mayo L, Saeedi OJ (2021) Erythrocyte-mediated angiography: quantifying absolute episcleral blood flow in humans. Ophthalmology 128(5):799–801. https://doi.org/10.1016/j.ophtha.2020.09.010

Baez KA et al (1994) Long-term results of ab externo neodymium: YAG cyclophotocoagulation. Ger J Ophthalmol 3(6):395–399

Billant J et al (2022) Use of selective laser trabeculoplasty as an alternative in patients who developed ocular hypertension after intravitreal dexamethasone implants: a series of 35 eyes. Graefes Arch Clin Exp Ophthalmol 260(11):3665–3673. https://doi.org/10.1007/s00417-022-05725-3

Bodh SA, Kumar V, Raina UK, Ghosh B, Thakar M (2011) Inflammatory glaucoma. Oman J Ophthalmol 4(1):3–9. https://doi.org/10.4103/0974-620X.77655

Broadway DC et al (1994) Adverse effects of topical antiglaucoma medication. II. The outcome of filtration surgery. Arch Ophthalmol 112:1446–1454

Chauhan BC et al (2008) Canadian Glaucoma Study: 2. risk factors for the progression of open-angle glaucoma. Arch Ophthalmol 126(8):1030–1036. https://doi.org/10.1001/archopht.126.8.1030

Cheng H et al (2023) Clinical outcomes of penetrating canaloplasty in patients with traumatic angle recession glaucoma: a prospective interventional case series. Br J Ophthalmol 107(8):1092–1097. https://doi.org/10.1136/bjophthalmol-2021-320659

Choy BNK, Lai JSM, Yeung JCC, Chan JCH (2018) Randomized comparative trial of diode laser transscleral cyclophotocoagulation versus Ahmed glaucoma valve for neovascular glaucoma in Chinese - a pilot study. Clin Ophthalmol 12:2545–2552. https://doi.org/10.2147/OPTH.S188999

Christakis PG et al (2016) The Ahmed versus Baerveldt study: five-year treatment outcomes. Ophthalmology 123(10):2093–2102. https://doi.org/10.1016/j.ophtha.2016.06.035

Conlon R, Saheb H, Ahmed II (2017) Glaucoma treatment trends: a review. Can J Ophthalmol 52(1):114–124. https://doi.org/10.1016/j.jcjo.2016.07.013

Dhingra D, Grover S, Kapatia G, Pandav SS, Kaushik S (2020) Phacolytic glaucoma: a nearly forgotten entity. Eur J Ophthalmol 30(5):NP32–NP35. https://doi.org/10.1177/1120672119841972

Feldman RM, Bell NP (2013) Complications of glaucoma surgery. Oxford Academic, New York

Flammer J et al (2013) The primary vascular dysregulation syndrome: implications for eye diseases. EPMA J 4(1):14. https://doi.org/10.1186/1878-5085-4-14

Fukushima M, Yunoki T, Otsuka M, Hayashi A (2020) Association of deepening of the upper eyelid sulcus with the incidence of blepharoptosis after glaucoma filtration surgery. Semin Ophthalmol 35(7–8):348–351. https://doi.org/10.1080/08820538.2020.1863435

Garway-Heath DF et al (2015) Latanoprost for open-angle glaucoma (UKGTS): a randomised, multicentre, placebo-controlled trial. Lancet 385(9975):1295–1304. https://doi.org/10.1016/S0140-6736(14)62111-5

Gazzard G et al (2023) Laser in glaucoma and ocular hypertension (LiGHT) trial: six-year results of primary selective laser trabeculoplasty versus eye drops for the treatment of glaucoma and ocular hypertension. Ophthalmology 130(2):139–151. https://doi.org/10.1016/j.ophtha.2022.09.009

Gedde SJ, Vinod K, Prum BE Jr, Primary Tube Versus Trabeculectomy Study Group (2023) Results from the primary tube versus trabeculectomy study and translation to clinical practice. Curr Opin Ophthalmol 34(2):129–137. https://doi.org/10.1097/ICU.0000000000000928

Gedde SJ et al (2012) Treatment outcomes in the tube versus trabeculectomy (TVT) study after five years of follow-up. Am J Ophthalmol 153(5):789–803.e2. https://doi.org/10.1016/j.ajo.2011.10.026

Gedde SJ et al (2022) Treatment outcomes in the primary tube versus trabeculectomy study after 5 years of follow-up. Ophthalmology 129(12):1344–1356. https://doi.org/10.1016/j.ophtha.2022.07.003

Ghosh S et al (2014) Efficacy of transscleral diode laser cyclophotocoagulation in patients with good visual acuity. Eur J Ophthalmol 24(3):375–381. https://doi.org/10.5301/ejo.5000389

González-Martín-Moro J et al (2017) Cyclodialysis: an update. Int Ophthalmol 37:441–457. https://doi.org/10.1007/s10792-016-0282-8

Gordon MO, Kass MA (2018) What we have learned from the ocular hypertension treatment study. Am J Ophthalmol 189:xxiv–xxvii. https://doi.org/10.1016/j.ajo.2018.02.016

Hayashi K, Yoshida M, Sato T, Manabe SI (2019) Effect of topical hypotensive medications for preventing intraocular pressure increase after cataract surgery in eyes with glaucoma. Am J Ophthalmol 205:91–98. https://doi.org/10.1016/j.ajo.2019.03.012

Hayreh SS, Rojas P, Podhajsky P, Montague P, Woolson RF (1983) Ocular neovascularization with retinal vascular occlusion-III. Incidence of ocular neovascularization with retinal vein occlusion. Ophthalmology 90(5):488–506. https://doi.org/10.1016/s0161-6420(83)34542-5

Heijl A et al (2002) Reduction of intraocular pressure and glaucoma progression: results from the Early Manifest Glaucoma Trial. Arch Ophthalmol 120(10):1268–1279. https://doi.org/10.1001/archopht.120.10.1268

Hong EH et al (2019) Comparison of repeatability of swept-source and spectral-domain optical coherence tomography for measuring inner retinal thickness in retinal disease. PLoS One 14(1):e0210729. https://doi.org/10.1371/journal.pone.0210729

Horsley MB, Chen TC (2011) The use of prostaglandin analogs in the uveitic patient. Semin Ophthalmol

26(4–5):285–289. https://doi.org/10.3109/08820538.2011.588650
Jansook P, Loftsson T (2022) Aqueous prostaglandin eye drop formulations. Pharmaceutics 14(10):2142. https://doi.org/10.3390/pharmaceutics14102142
Jat NS, Tripathy K (2023) Peters anomaly. In: StatPearls. StatPearls Publishing
Jung YH et al (2016) Incidence and clinical features of neovascularization of the iris following acute central retinal artery occlusion. Korean J Ophthalmol 30(5):352–359. https://doi.org/10.3341/kjo.2016.30.5.352
Junttila TL, Alberto N, Winkels M, Greenwood MD (2020) Successful reduction of intraocular pressure in a patient with glaucoma secondary to Sturge–Weber syndrome using a suprachoroidal shunt. J Curr Glaucoma Pract 14(1):43–46. https://doi.org/10.5005/jp-journals-10078-1266
Kalogeropoulos D, Sung VC (2018) Pathogenesis of Uveitic glaucoma. J Curr Glaucoma Pract 12(3):125–138. https://doi.org/10.5005/jp-journals-10028-1257
Kaplowitz K et al (2015) Current concepts in the treatment of vitreous block, also known as aqueous misdirection. Surv Ophthalmol 60(3):229–241. https://doi.org/10.1016/j.survophthal.2014.12.004
Karaconji T, Zagora S, Grigg JR (2022) Approach to childhood glaucoma: a review. Clin Experiment Ophthalmol 50(2):232–246. https://doi.org/10.1111/ceo.14039
Kass MA et al (2002) The ocular hypertension treatment study: a randomized trial determines that topical ocular hypotensive medication delays or prevents the onset of primary open-angle glaucoma. Arch Ophthalmol 120(6):701–830. https://doi.org/10.1001/archopht.120.6.701
Kass MA et al (2021) Assessment of cumulative incidence and severity of primary open-angle glaucoma among participants in the ocular hypertension treatment study after 20 years of follow-up. JAMA Ophthalmol 139(5):558–566. https://doi.org/10.1001/jamaophthalmol.2021.0341
Kaushik J et al (2022) Evaluation of primary Ahmed Glaucoma valve implantation in post-traumatic angle recession glaucoma in Indian eyes. Int Ophthalmol 42(3):817–827. https://doi.org/10.1007/s10792-021-02047-x
Kesav N et al (2020) Current management of uveitis-associated ocular hypertension and glaucoma. Surv Ophthalmol 65(4):397–407. https://doi.org/10.1016/j.survophthal.2019.12.003
Kim YH, Sung MS, Park SW (2017) Clinical features of ocular ischemic syndrome and risk factors for neovascular glaucoma. Korean J Ophthalmol 31(4):343–350. https://doi.org/10.3341/kjo.2016.0067
Knier CG et al (2020) Three-decade evaluation of cerebrospinal fluid pressure in open-angle glaucoma at a tertiary care center. J Ophthalmol 2020:7487329. https://doi.org/10.1155/2020/7487329
Krag S, Larsen D, Albertsen BK, Glerup M (2021) Risk of ocular hypertension in children treated with systemic glucocorticoid. Acta Ophthalmol 99(8):e1430–e1434. https://doi.org/10.1111/aos.14820
Landsend ECS et al (2021) Congenital aniridia - a comprehensive review of clinical features and therapeutic approaches. Surv Ophthalmol 66(6):1031–1050. https://doi.org/10.1016/j.survophthal.2021.02.011
Lee BL et al (2003) Ocular hypertension treatment study (OHTS) commentary. Curr Opin Ophthalmol 14(2):74–77. https://doi.org/10.1097/00055735-200304000-00003
Lee SS, Robinson MR, Weinreb RN (2019) Episcleral venous pressure and the ocular hypotensive effects of topical and intracameral prostaglandin analogs. J Glaucoma 28(9):846–857. https://doi.org/10.1097/IJG.0000000000001307
Leske MC, Heijl A, Hyman L, Bengtsson B (1999) Early manifest glaucoma trial: design and baseline data. Ophthalmology 106(11):2144–2153. https://doi.org/10.1016/s0161-6420(99)90497-9
Macovei ML, Canache M, Neagoe BM (2021) Phacolytic glaucoma - case report. Rom J Ophthalmol 65(2):191–195. https://doi.org/10.22336/rjo.2021.38
Massaoutis P et al (2007) Bilateral symptomatic angle closure associated with a regular dose of citalopram, an SSRI antidepressant. Br J Ophthalmol 91(8):1086–1087. https://doi.org/10.1136/bjo.2006.107185
Meier-Gibbons F, Töteberg-Harms M (2023) Follow-up studies of the classical landmark studies in Glaucoma. Curr Opin Ophthalmol 34(2):116–122. https://doi.org/10.1097/ICU.0000000000000926
Muñoz-Negrete FJ et al (2015) Current approach in the diagnosis and management of uveitic glaucoma. Biomed Res Int 2015:742792. https://doi.org/10.1155/2015/742792
Musch DC, Gillespie BW, Lichter PR, Niziol LM, Janz NK, CIGTS Study Investigators (2009) Visual field progression in the collaborative initial glaucoma treatment study the impact of treatment and other baseline factors. Ophthalmology 116(2):200–207. https://doi.org/10.1016/j.ophtha.2008.08.051
Na K-S et al (2010) Autonomic dysfunction in normal tension glaucoma: the short-term heart rate variability analysis. J Glaucoma 19(6):377–381. https://doi.org/10.1097/IJG.0b013e3181c4ae58
Ng DS, Ching RH, Chan CW (2015) Angle-recession glaucoma: long-term clinical outcomes over a 10-year period in traumatic microhyphema. Int Ophthalmol 35(1):107–113. https://doi.org/10.1007/s10792-014-0027-5
Ondrejka S, Körber N, Dhamdhere K (2022) Long-term effect of canaloplasty on intraocular pressure and use of intraocular pressure-lowering medications in patients with open-angle glaucoma. J Cataract Refract Surg 48(12):1388–1393. https://doi.org/10.1097/j.jcrs.0000000000001000
Peng M et al (2022) Cross-linked actin networks (CLANs) affect stiffness and/or actin dynamics in

transgenic transformed and primary human trabecular meshwork cells. Exp Eye Res 220:109097. https://doi.org/10.1016/j.exer.2022.109097

Podoleanu AG (2012) Optical coherence tomography. J Microsc 247(3):209–219. https://doi.org/10.1111/j.1365-2818.2012.03619.x

Pujari A, Selvan H, Behera AK, Gagrani M, Kapoor S, Dada T (2020) The probable mechanism of traumatic angle recession and cyclodialysis. J Glaucoma 29(1):67–70. https://doi.org/10.1097/IJG.0000000000001358

Razeghinejad MR, Nowroozzadeh MH (2010) Anti-glaucoma medication exposure in pregnancy: an observational study and literature review. Clin Exp Optom 93(6):458–465. https://doi.org/10.1111/j.1444-0938.2010.00526.x

Razeghinejad R, Lin MM, Lee D, Katz LJ, Myers JS (2020) Pathophysiology and management of glaucoma and ocular hypertension related to trauma. Surv Ophthalmol 65(5):530–547. https://doi.org/10.1016/j.survophthal.2020.02.003

Ritch R et al (2003) Angle closure in younger patients. Ophthalmology 110(10):1880–1889. https://doi.org/10.1016/S0161-6420(03)00563-3

Rudkin AK et al (2010) Bilateral simultaneous acute angle closure glaucoma precipitated by non-prescription cold and flu medication. Emerg Med Australas 22(5):477–479. https://doi.org/10.1111/j.1742-6723.2010.01338.x

Sadeghi R et al (2023) Management of malignant glaucoma. J Curr Ophthalmol 34(4):389–397. https://doi.org/10.4103/joco.joco_147_22

Selvan H, Gupta S, Wiggs JL, Gupta V (2022) Juvenile-onset open-angle glaucoma - a clinical and genetic update. Surv Ophthalmol 67(4):1099–1117. https://doi.org/10.1016/j.survophthal.2021.09.001

Senthil S, Dangeti D, Battula M, Rao HL, Garudadri C (2022) Trabeculectomy with mitomycin-C in post-traumatic angle recession glaucoma in phakic eyes with no prior intraocular intervention. Semin Ophthalmol 37(2):171–176. https://doi.org/10.1080/08820538.2021.1945116

Senthilkumar VA, Ramesh S (2022) Lens particle glaucoma after penetrating injury. Ophthalmol Glaucoma 5(2):218. https://doi.org/10.1016/j.ogla.2021.12.004

Shaarawy T, Sherwood MB, Hitchings RA, Crowston JG (2014) Glaucoma e-book. Elsevier Health Sciences

Shue A, Wong MO, Freedman SF (2022) Primary congenital glaucoma. In: Albert DM, Miller JW, Azar DT, Young LH (eds) Albert and Jakobiec's principles and practice of ophthalmology. Springer, Cham. https://doi.org/10.1007/978-3-030-42634-7_168

Stefan C, Iliescu DA, Batras M, Timaru CM, De Simone A (2015) Plateau iris--diagnosis and treatment. Rom J Ophthalmol 59(1):14–18

Varma DK et al (2014) Malignant glaucoma after cataract surgery. J Cataract Refract Surg 40(11):1843–1849. https://doi.org/10.1016/j.jcrs.2014.02.045

Venkataraman P et al (2022) A systematic approach to the management of microspherophakia. Indian J Ophthalmol 70(7):2262–2271. https://doi.org/10.4103/ijo.IJO_2888_21

Wang RX, Li N, Chen XY (2022) Ultrasound cyclo-plasty for moderate glaucoma: eighteen-month results from a prospective study. Front Med (Lausanne) 9:1009273. https://doi.org/10.3389/fmed.2022.1009273

Yuen NSY et al (2006) New method of surgical repair for 360-degree cyclodialysis. J Cataract Refract Surg 32(1):13–17. https://doi.org/10.1016/j.jcrs.2005.05.035

Zuo C et al (2021) Associations between the choroidal vascularity index and malignant glaucoma after trabeculectomy for primary angle closure glaucoma. Front Med (Lausanne) 8:747720. https://doi.org/10.3389/fmed.2021.747720

19 Clinical Review of Glaucoma: Part II

Khaled Ali Elubous and Hady Saheb

Abstract

This chapter on glaucoma provides a comprehensive overview of the disease, with a focus on high-yield notes for both clinical applications and ophthalmology exam boards. The chapter covers a wide range of topics, including primary and secondary glaucomas, tools and investigations for diagnosis and management, medical and surgical treatment options, and landmark trials in the field. The information presented is designed to be accessible and useful for both practicing clinicians and those preparing for board exams in ophthalmology. In addition, the chapter uses clear and concise language to explain complex concepts. Key points are highlighted throughout the text to help readers identify the most important information, and tables and figures are used to summarize and illustrate key concepts. Overall, the chapter on glaucoma is designed to be an effective study tool for those preparing for board exams in ophthalmology. By the end of the chapter, readers should have a solid understanding of the key concepts and best practices for managing patients with glaucoma.

Keywords

Glaucoma · Glaucoma risk factors Mechanism of glaucoma · Glaucoma management · Glaucoma surgery · Landmark trials · Open angle · Angle closure · Optical coherence tomography · Laser · Eye drops Glaucoma medication · High yield · Board exam · Ophthalmology

19.1 Glaucoma Management

19.1.1 Medications

Different classes of medications can be used in glaucoma management medically, including classical classes (Table 19.1) and newly approved classes (Table 19.2) that target different structures in the eye (Fig. 19.1). Table 19.3 also lists anti-glaucoma medications with their preservatives, while Table 19.4 provides anti-glaucoma agents that can be used as combination therapy.

K. A. Elubous (✉)
Faculty of Medicine, The Hashemite University, Zarqa, Jordan

Department of Ophthalmology and Visual Sciences, McGill University, Montreal, QC, Canada
e-mail: khaled.elubous@hu.edu.jo

H. Saheb
Department of Ophthalmology and Visual Sciences, McGill University, Montreal, QC, Canada
e-mail: hady.saheb@mcgill.ca

S. A. Alryalat (ed.), *Ophthalmology Board and FRCS Part 2 Exams*,
https://doi.org/10.1007/978-981-96-1517-9_19

Table 19.1 Classes of glaucoma medications classically used for medical management of glaucoma

	Examples	Effect	Side effect	Contraindications and cautions	Notes
Cholinergic	Pilocarpine	– Miosis – Opening of TM – Decreases uveoscleral outflow	– Miosis—Headache – Increased risk of retinal detachment – Bradycardia – myopia	Neovascular glaucoma, uveitis, and malignant glaucoma	More effect on blue eyes
Anticholinergics	Atropine	– Mydriasis – Loss of accommodation – Shifts the lens-iris diaphragm posteriorly – Deepens the anterior chamber	– Narrows the iridocorneal angle – Anticholinergic (salivation, lacrimation, tachycardia)	Angle closure glaucoma	– Atropine effect can last for up to 2 weeks – Used to treat malignant glaucoma – Used to treat hypotony
Alpha-2 agonist	– Apraclonidine – Brimonidine	– Decreases aqueous production – Increases the uveoscleral flow	– Dry nose and mouth, conjunctival blanching (early and transient) – ↓ BP (concentration dependent) – Allergic conjunctivitis 20% (early or late) – Anterior uveitis (early or late)	Relative contraindication in the pediatric population (crosses blood-brain barrier and causes apnea) Caution in severe cerebrovascular diseases and peripheral vascular insufficiency	– Tachyphylaxis (apraclonidine > brimonidine) – Brimonidine has a neuroprotective effect – Apraclonidine is used prophylactically to decrease IOP before laser – Allergic reaction is lower with Purite preservative than BAK – Less allergy with BB combination – Three times better than twice-daily regimen
Beta-blocker (B1 present in cardiac muscles, B2 in bronchioles)	– Betaxolol (Betoptic®) (selective B1) – Apimol – Timolol (Timoptic®) (B1, B2)	– Decrease the aqueous production—Mildly decrease the outflow	– Ocular surface disease due to BAK – Exacerbation of myasthenia gravis – Reduce HDL—Blockage of the systemic response to hypoglycemia in diabetic patients	– Asthma, COPD (non elective) – Heart block or bradycardia (both selective and nonselective)	– Long washout period ≥24 h – Less effective during night – Nonselective BBs are more effective than selective ones in lowering IOP – Contraindicated in bundle branch block but not contraindicated in heart failure

	Examples	Effect	Side effect	Contraindications and cautions	Notes
Prostaglandin analogues	– Bimatoprost (Lumigan) – Travoprost (Travatan) – Latanoprost (Xalatan)	– Latanoprost and travoprost enhance uveoscleral outflow—Bimatoprost enhances both uveoscleral and trabecular outflow	– Pigmentation (MC) and eyelash growth – Cystoid macular edema—Keratitis and uveitis, meiosis—Vasodilation with increased permeability – Periorbital fat atrophy – Iritis and iris cyst	Active uveitis, keratitis	Twice-daily dosing is less effective than a single dose and may increase IOP – Latanoprostene bunod (Vyzulta) has nitric oxide-dilating effect, and it enhances trabecular meshwork and uveoscleral outflow
Carbonic anhydrase inhibitors	Acetazolamide (Dimox), dorzolamide (Trusopt), and brinzolamide (Azopt) →Renal excretion Methazolamide → hepatic excretion	Decrease aqueous production	– Hypersensitivity reactions – Bitter taste With topical (dorzolamide more than brinzolamide): – Corneal edema – Irritation With systemic: Blood dyscrasia – Hypokalemia – Paresthesia – Loss of libido – Acidosis – Nephrocalcinosis – Transient myopia—Shallowness in the anterior chamber	– Severe renal failure (CrCl <30 mL/min) – Sulfa allergy—Pregnancy and lactating – Newborns	– Chemically related to sulfonamide antibiotics – Can be used for macular edema. Neuroprotective-Systemic agents may cause choroidal effusion angle closure. Combining topical and systemic CAI does not usually give an additive effect – Effective in IOP reduction post-phacoemulsification (preferred) – Chronic systemic use needs hematologic workup
Osmotic agents	Mannitol (1.5–2 g/kg IV infused over 30–60 min) 1–1.5 h before surgery	Creating an osmotic gradient so that water is “drawn out” from the vitreous into the blood	– Electrolyte imbalance (hypo/hyper K, Na, Ca) worsens cardiac function – Hypernatremia (encephalopathy) – Hypervolemia (exacerbates congestive heart failure) – Hypovolemia – CNS toxicity	– Anuria – Pulmonary congestion – Active intracranial bleeding – Severe hypovolemia – Caution with renal impairment with concomitant nephrotoxic drugs	

Table 19.2 New anti-glaucoma medications, including Rho kinase inhibitors and latanoprostene bunod (LBN)

Drug	Mechanism of action	Effect	Side effect	Notes	Available agents
Rho kinase inhibitors	Inhibition of Rho kinase (ROCK) (a protein kinase) decreases contractility of the trabecular meshwork (TM) endothelial cells and the cells of Schlemm's canal (SC). This is done by inhibiting myosin light chain (MLC) phosphorylation, thus reducing the resistance of trabecular cells, leading to relaxation of the TM and expansion of the juxtacanalicular network	Enhancing the trabecular meshwork drainage. They also stimulate corneal endothelial cell regeneration and have neuroprotection properties presumed to be due to vascular endothelial effect (decrease optic nerve vasoconstriction)	Conjunctival hyperemia, corneal verticillata, and conjunctival hemorrhage		Rhopressa® (netarsudil ophthalmic solution) 0.02% applied once a day. Ripasudil is approved in Japan
Latanoprostene bunod (LBN) 0.024%	Is metabolized into latanoprost acid (F2α analog) and a nitric oxide (NO)-donating moiety, thus increasing the outflow of aqueous humor through the uveoscleral and trabecular routes	Latanoprost acid reduces IOP by increasing uveoscleral outflow, whereas NO facilitates trabecular outflow through relaxation of the trabecular meshwork and Schlemm's canal			

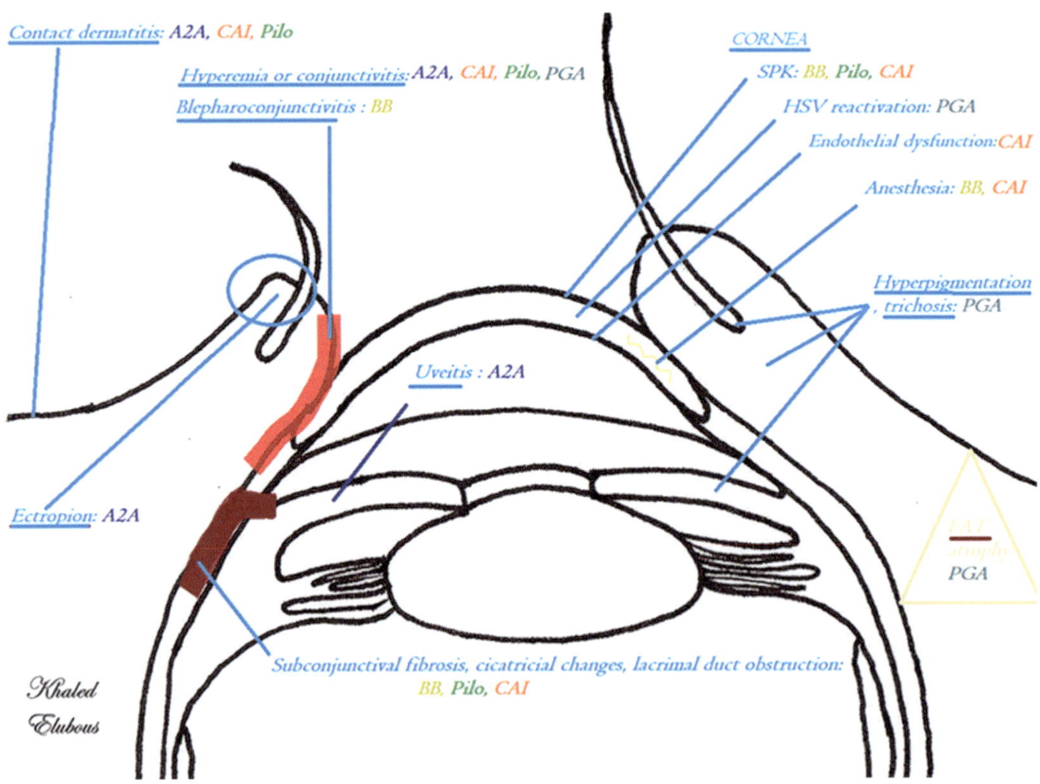

Fig. 19.1 Diagrammatic representation of some medication side effects

Table 19.3 Anti-glaucoma with their preservatives (have antimicrobial effect)

Anti-glaucoma	Preservative used	Components, notes
Azopt, Lumigan, Timolol, Xalatan	Benzalkonium chloride BAK	Quaternary ammonium compound, penetrate epithelium
Alphagan P	Purite	Stabilized oxychloro complex (SOC) (H_2O, Na, Cl, O_2), less toxic
Travatan Z	SofZia	Borate, propylene glycol, sorbitol, and zinc chloride Less toxic than BAK
Lubricants (Tears Naturale II) Travoprost, Travatan	*Polyquad*	Polyquaternium-1
Genteal	*GenAqua*	Sodium perborate

Table 19.4 Anti-glaucoma used as combination therapy

Combinations drops	Brand name	Preservatives	Non-preservatives' brand name
Travoprost/Timolol	DuoTrav	Polyquad	
Latanoprost/Timolol	Xalacom	BAK	
Bimatoprost/Timolol	Ganfort	BAK	Ganfort UD
Tafluprost/Timolol			Taptiqom
Brimonidine/Timolol	Combigan	BAK	
Dorzolamide/Timolol	Cosopt	BAK	Cosopt preservative free
Brinzolamide/Timolol	Azarga	BAK	
Brimonidine/Brinzolamide	Simbrinza	BAK	

- Uveoscleral outflow is increased by cycloplegia.
- Rho kinase inhibitors (netarsudil, ripasudil) increase trabecular outflow and reduce episcleral pressure.
- Alpha agonist (brimonidine) is the safest in pregnancy (Class B), while most other drugs are class C.
- In the **first** trimester:
  - **Brimonidine** and **prostaglandin** analogues can be used.
  - Avoid beta-blockers and carbonic anhydrase inhibitors.
- In the **second and third** trimesters (*except last month*):
  - **Brimonidine** can be used.
  - Other eye drops need special caution: topical carbonic anhydrase inhibitors (K level monitoring), beta-blockers (fetal heart and growth monitoring), and prostaglandin analogues (attention to premature labor).
- In the **late third trimester and during lactation:**
  - **Topical carbonic anhydrase inhibitors** can be used.
  - Avoid brimonidine.
  - Caution with prostaglandin analogues (attention to premature labor) and beta-blockers.
- Preservatives can cause ocular surface changes.
- In healthy corneal surface, no significant changes were found between BAK and preservative-free drops.
- Using preservative-free drops is justified in eyes with preexisting ocular surface disease or that need multiple bottles of medications.
- Minimizing medication pre-filtration surgery might be helpful (4 weeks pre-op if needed).

19.1.2 Laser

Laser trabeculoplasty enhances aqueous outflow, probably by shrinking the meshwork and releasing mediators (Table 19.5).

- Optimal ALT settings: spot size: 50 µm, duration: 0.1 s, energy: 700 mW.

Table 19.5 Comparison between different glaucoma lasers

	Argon laser (ALT)	Selective laser (SLT)	Micropulse laser
Laser type	Argon (488–514 nm)	YAG (532 nm)	Thermal 810 nm
Features	Use high energy, variable spot size starting with 50 μm	Lower energy and number of shots, same spot size 400 μm	Laser (multiple pulses) so lowest energy
Mechanism	Tissue reaction	Tissue reaction	No tissue reaction
Repeatable with benefit	No	Yes	–
Coagulation	Higher	Lower	Lower
Side effects	Inflammation with IOP elevation acutely, PAS formation	Inflammation with IOP elevation acutely (less than argon)	Minimal SE

- Although initial success rates are high after laser trabeculoplasty, the success rate declines over time to approximately 50% after 3–5 years and 30% after 10 years.
- Other complications of lasers include iritis, hyphema, postoperative IOP spike (most common), and anterior synechiae formation (with ALT).
- Laser trabeculoplasty may result in reactivation of uveitis in inflammatory glaucoma as well as IOP spike.
- Pigmentary glaucoma has a very good response although there is a high risk of IOP spike which could be unmanageable medically; therefore, it is advisable to consider proceeding with sequential partial treatments, at lower laser energy level.
- Argon laser produces a characteristic white burn when applied to the epithelial membrane on the iris surface. Such a coagulation reaction would confirm the diagnosis of epithelial downgrowth.
- Give steroid drops after SLT in case of pain during laser, or a history of pain after previous SLT laser.

Laser iridoplasty is a procedure in which argon laser burns are applied to the peripheral iris to cause contraction and flattening. This technique has been shown to be useful in opening an angle that remains narrow after an iridotomy, as with plateau iris syndrome and nanophthalmos.

Cyclophotocoagulation

- **Continuous-wave Transscleral cyclophotocoagulation (TS-CPC)**
  - Is the most commonly used technique
  - Using a semiconductor diode laser of 810 nm
- **Endoscopic cyclophotocoagulation**
  - Commonly performed in combination with cataract surgery
  - Allows direct visualization of ciliary process
  - Reduces thermal damage to surrounding tissues
- **The micropulse technique**
  - Delivers repetitive bursts of laser energy in on/off phases
  - The "off phase" allows time for surrounding tissues to cool
- **Ultrasound cycloplasty**
  - Use high-intensity focused ultrasound for selective CB destruction.
- Pops mean excessive coagulation leads to boiling of intracellular water (vaporization).
- Better approach is with low (but not too low) energy and a long exposure time ("slow burn" technique).
- Highly pigmented eyes need less energy.
- The main significant parameter that correlates with IOP reduction post-CPC laser is the ciliary body process **width**.
- Complications include transient corneal edema, inflammation, pain, acute or late hypotony, decrease in visual acuity, phthisis bulbi, sympathetic ophthalmia, and malignant glaucoma.
- Lower success rate in uveitic or secondary glaucomas.
- TS-CPC approach as suggested by Douglas Gaasterland:

  - Brown iris: 1.25 W, 4.0–4.5 sc
  - Non-brown: 1.5 W, 3.5–4.0 sc
  - Adjusted by 0.25-W up or down according to pop

19.2 Surgeries

19.2.1 Penetrating Glaucoma Surgery

19.2.1.1 Trabeculectomy

Definitions

- Goniotomy: incision at the trabecular meshwork, typically performed ab interno.
- Trabeculotomy: incision at the trabecular meshwork, typically performed ab externo.
- Trabeculectomy: The term refers to removal of part or all the trabecular meshwork; the actual procedure is a keratectomy, which is removing part of the peripheral cornea. It can be done as limbal based (conjunctival incision away from limbus) or fornix-based (conjunctival incision at limbus) flaps.

Advantages

- Possible to achieve low pressure in single digits.
- Patient is less dependent on drops postoperatively (desired in case of noncompliance or intolerance).
- Effective with low baseline IOP or normotensive glaucoma.

Risk Factors for Failure

- African race
- Prior surgery involving conjunctiva
- Secondary glaucoma (except pseudoexfoliation glaucoma)
- Young age
- Diabetes
- Pseudophakia and combined phaco-trabeculectomy:
  - Old patients, whites, phakic, with PXF or pigmentary dispersion, all good prognostic factors

Antimetabolites

- Complications: scleral melting, hypotony, wound leak, and increased risk of infection.
- Mitomycin is 100 times more potent than 5-FU and has a more permanent antiproliferative effect, and it is safer for the corneal epithelium, unlike 5-FU.

Iridectomy Indications

- Iris prolapses during the surgery.
- Secondary glaucoma with high risk of broad PAS (NVG, ICE).
- Side effects of iridectomy include increased risk of vitreous prolapse and the risk of inflammation postoperatively; therefore, it can increase the risk of failure.

Bleb Morphology

The most desirable blebs are:

- Shallow
- Widespread
- Relatively avascular
- Covered by the lid
- Show epithelial microcysts

*Indiana Bleb Grading scale assesses HEVS: the height (H), elevation (E), vascularity (V), and Seidel (S).

19.2.1.2 Postoperative Management and Interventions

High IOP and Deep AC

- Tight sutures → treated by suture lysis (preferably not on POD 1 due to higher risk of hypotony).
- Blockage by debris (patent ostomy) → observe or gentle digital pressure on sclera or do suture lysis to increase the flow.
- Blockage by iris or vitreous → treated by YAG laser or iridectomy.
- Vascularized bleb → 5-FU injections, suture lysis, increase steroid drops.
- Tenon's cyst → Medical therapy or needling.

*Anti-glaucoma drops could be added in the management.

Low IOP (Fig. 19.2) could be due to:

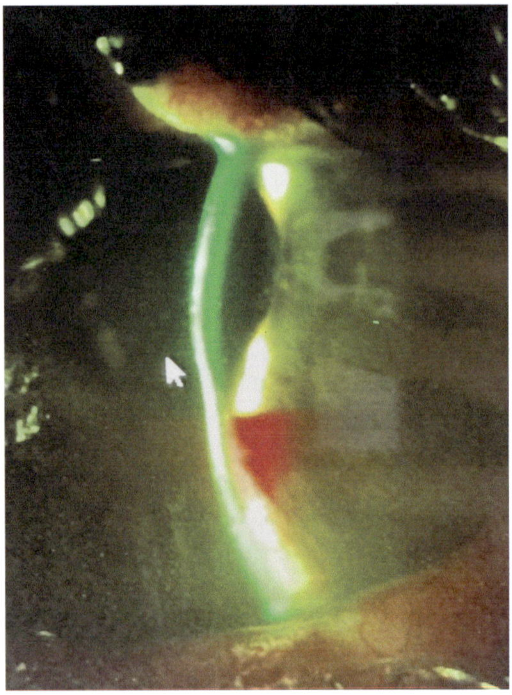

Fig. 19.2 This photo of a slit-lamp biomicroscopy for a patient status post-trabeculectomy had hypotony with shallow anterior chamber, with iridocorneal contact. Patient improved without surgical intervention

- Wound leak → large bandage contact lens (BCL) +/− aqueous suppressant +/− reduce steroid drops, autologous blood injection, resuturing.
- CB shutdown (immobile cells in AC, low bleb, formed AC) → increase steroid drops (reduce inflammation).
- Overfiltration (high bleb, deep or shallow AC) → reduce steroid drops (to enhance episcleral fibrosis). If overfiltration leads to persistent complications of hypotony → resuturing.

*Also add atropine drop to deepen the AC.

*Observe choroidal effusions, unless kissing choroidal effusions, cornea-lens touch, and hypotony maculopathy, which can be treated initially by dispersive OVD injection.

High-Yield Notes
Shallow Chamber DDX

Low IOP
- Wound leak
- Hyperfiltration
- Malignant glaucoma

High IOP
- Malignant glaucoma *(discussed elsewhere)*
- Suprachoroidal hemorrhage *(discussed elsewhere)*

Other complications

- Blebitis (most common organisms are *Streptococcus* and *Haemophilus influenzae*)
- Reduced axial length (mean reduction is 0.4 mm)
- Refractive changes
- Cataract (usually posterior subcapsular)
- Reduced visual acuity (common in the first 3 months postoperatively)
- Suprachoroidal hemorrhage (usually within first 2 weeks postoperative)
- Hypotony maculopathy (more common in young myopic patients)
- Blepharoptosis

19.2.1.3 Glaucoma Drainage Device (GDD)

- Valved anti-glaucoma devices: Ahmed (AGV) and Krupin.
- Non-valved devices: Molteno, Baerveldt (BGD), Ahmed, Clearpath, Paul.
- Each has a different plate surface area and material that may affect the device efficacy.

Indications High risk of trabeculectomy failure

- Previous ocular surgery (unless no conjunctival scarring).
- High risk of conjunctival scarring.
- Uveitic or neovascular glaucoma.

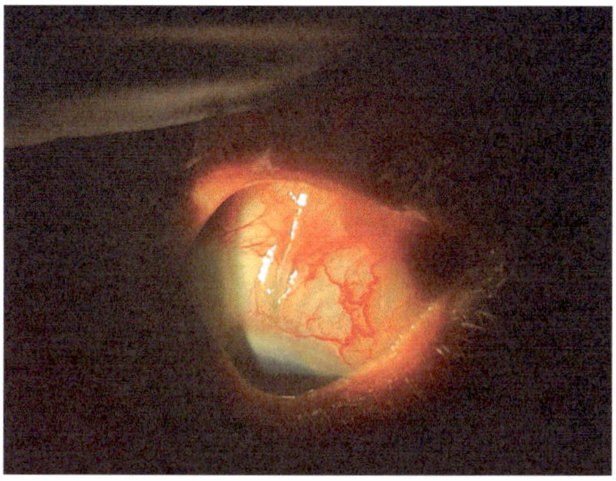

Fig. 19.3 This slit lamp photo shows an exposed drainage tube after prolonged use of steroidal and nonsteroidal eye drops postoperatively. The patient required tube revision surgery

Complications and Post-surgery Issues

- Tube erosion (Fig. 19.3) (risk factors: thin conjunctiva, multiple surgeries, eye rubbing, long-term anti-glaucoma medications, patch graft melting, uveitic glaucoma).
- Tube malposition (retraction or migration).
- Corneal decompensation (less with sulcus implantation).
- Hypotony (Fig. 19.4) (DDX: excessive drainage, ciliary body shutdown, wound leak).
- Hypertensive phase (capsular fibrosis, 1–3 months after valved devices).
- Strabismus

Factors Affecting the Choice of Device

- Severity of glaucoma (better result with BGD 350).
- Compliance with medical therapy (less need for drops with BGD comparing to AGV).
- Ocular factors like pediatric group, small orbit (AGV FP8 or BGD 250 is a good choice).
- Risk of suprachoroidal hemorrhage (previous cyclodestructive laser, previous pars plana vitrectomy); use a ripcord with BGD or AGV.
- Risk of hypotony due to chronic uveitis (like in juvenile rheumatoid arthritis).
- Available space for device placement (conjunctival scarring, scleral thinning, previous tube, buckle).

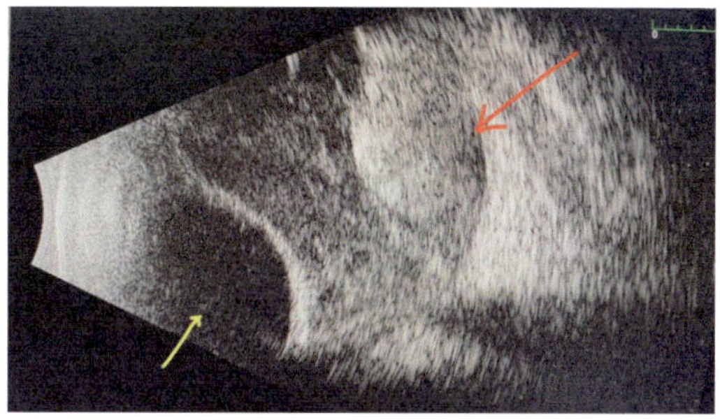

Fig. 19.4 This photo of a B-scan for a patient with inflammatory glaucoma underwent Baerveldt tube implant. Postoperatively, the patient developed hypotony with choroidal effusions (yellow arrow), with hemorrhagic component (red arrow)

IOP Elevation Post-glaucoma Surgery

Tube

- Steroid response (2 weeks and more after surgery)
- Hypertensive phase (due to hyperencapsulation) 2–8 weeks after *valved* GDD, or after tube opening in non-valved GDD
- Tube retraction

Trabeculectomy

- Failure of filtration (bleb encapsulation or scleral fibrosis, blockage of osteotomy by heme, iris or vitreous, tight sutures)

19.2.1.4 Cataract and Glaucoma

- Previous bleb with high or borderline IOP has a risk of failure after cataract surgery.
- Combination of bleb needling and cataract surgery as well as medical therapy control preoperatively may reduce the risk of bleb failure.
- Cataract or clear lens extraction with or without trabeculectomy is an effective treatment for primary angle closure glaucoma.
- Solo cataract removal may reduce IOP.

19.2.1.5 Minimally Invasive Glaucoma Surgeries (MIGSs)

Classification

- Trabecular outflow enhancement.
  Ab interno (e.g. iStent, Hydrus, Kahook Blade, trabeculotomy).

Ab externo (e.g. canalostomy, canaloplasty).

- Suprachoroidal outflow enhancement.
  - Ab interno (e.g., Cypass, Miniject).
  - Ab externo (e.g., gold shunt, STARflo).
- Subconjunctival drainage.
  - Ab interno (Xen gel).
  - Ab externo (Xen gel, Preserflo).

19.3 Major Glaucoma Trials

Tables 19.6 and 19.7 provide a summary of landmark glaucoma trials.

Table 19.6 A summary of the main landmark trials in glaucoma

Study	F/up results at _ years	Disease	Specifications	#Eyes	Intervention	IOP	Medication (MD ± SD)	Success or failure rate note	Conclusion
PTVT	5	POAG (90%)	– No history of incisional Sx – IOP (18–40) on TMT	242	BGD 350	13.4 ± 3.5	2.2 ± 1.3	Comparable failure rate	Similar IOP, but fewer med after trabeculectomy
					Trab/MMc 0.4 mg/mL/2 min	13.0 ± 5.2	1.3 ± 1.4		
AVB	5	– OAG (50%) – NVG (20%) – Uveitic (10)%	– Uncontrolled IOP on MTMT – Included cases with previous trab (37%)	238	AGV-FP7	16.6 ± 5.9	1.8 ± 1.5	– BGD had a lower failure rate and a lower IOP on fewer medications – Corneal edema (~10%), graft need (4–7%)	– Risk of hypotony in BGD – NVG and no history of trabeculectomy are risks for failure
					BGD 350	13.6 ± 5.0	1.2 ± 1.3		
TVT	5	POAG (85%)	– History of incisional Sx (cataract or glaucoma) – IOP >18 on MTMT	212	BGD 350	14.4 ± 6.9	1.4 ± 1.3	Tube had a higher success rate	– Similar IOP and medication in both groups – Reoperation more in trabeculectomy group
					Trab/MMc 0.4 mg/mL/2 min	12.6 ± 5.9	1.2 ± 1.5		

Table 19.7 A summary of the main landmark trials in glaucoma

Study	F/up results at _ years	Disease	Specifications	#Eyes	Intervention	IOP mmHg	Visual field progression	Conclusion
CIGTS	5 and 8	POAG (95%) PG (5%)	Newly diagnosed POAG	607	Medical therapy	14.4 ± 3.8	25%	– Favor initial surgery for mod-advanced – More cataract in surgery arm – Diabetic patient had more VF loss with initial surgery regimen
					Trab ±(5-FU) *In both arms, next step was ALT	17.7 ± 2.6 *At 5 years	21% *At 8 years	
CNTGS	5	NTG	IOP ≤24	140	Observation	16	35%	– Most patients do not progress without treatment – Other risk factors for progression were female, migraine, Drance hemorrhage
					30% IOP reduction by (Med, ALT, or Sx)	10	12%	
LiGHT	6	POAG OHTN		718	Eye drops	15.4 ± 3.9	27	– Less disease progression – Less need for trabeculectomy and cataract surgery with SLT – No significant difference in QoL – 70% ≤ target IOP with SLT
					SLT	16.3 ± 4.0	20	
EMGT	6	OAG	Excluded advanced and any mean IOP >30	255	Betaxolol and ALT	Reduction of 25%	45%	– Treatment significantly delayed progression – Every 1 mmHg IOP reduction decreases progression by 10% – NNT is 6
					Observation	Reduction of 0%	62%	
UKGTS	2	OAG (mild or moderate)	Excluded advanced, IOP >30, PDG	516	Latanoprost	3.8 mmHg reduction	15% reached deterioration endpoint at 24 months	– First masked, placebo-controlled RCT showed preservation of VF by anti-glaucoma medication – Time to first deterioration was significantly longer in the latanoprost – NNT is 10
					Placebo	0.9 mmHg reduction	25.6%	

Abbreviations: *OHTS* ocular hypertension treatment study, *EMGT* early manifest glaucoma trial, *CIGTS* collaborative initial glaucoma treatment study, *CNTGS* collaborative normal tension glaucoma study, *TVT* trabeculectomy vs. tube, *PTVT* primary tube versus trabeculectomy, *AVBS* Ahmed versus Baerveldt study, *LiGHT* laser in glaucoma and ocular hypertension study, *UKGTS* The United Kingdom glaucoma treatment study, *AGV* Ahmed glaucoma valve, *BGD* Baerveldt glaucoma valve, *NNT* number need to treat, to prevent 1 from progression, *PDG* pigment dispersion glaucoma

Acknowledgments I am deeply grateful to my esteemed colleague, Dr. Saif Al-Ryalat, for his invaluable contributions throughout the development of this chapter.

Conflict of Interest No conflict of interest to disclose.

Further Readings

Ah-Kee EY, Egong E, Shafi A, Lim LT, Yim JL (2015) A review of drug-induced acute angle closure glaucoma for non-ophthalmologists. Qatar Med J 2015(1):6. https://doi.org/10.5339/qmj.2015.6

AlObaida I, Aljasim LA (2020) Selective laser trabeculoplasty in patients with angle recession glaucoma: a small case series. Am J Ophthalmol Case Rep 19:100835. https://doi.org/10.1016/j.ajoc.2020.100835

Amini H, Razeghinejad MR (2005) Transscleral diode laser therapy for cyclodialysis cleft induced hypotony. Clin Experiment Ophthalmol 33(4):348–350. https://doi.org/10.1111/j.1442-9071.2005.01008.x

Anderson DR, Normal Tension Glaucoma Study (2003) Collaborative normal tension glaucoma study. Curr Opin Ophthalmol 14(2):86–90. https://doi.org/10.1097/00055735-200304000-00006

Andole S, Senthil S (2023) Ocular surface disease and anti-glaucoma medications: various features, diagnosis, and management guidelines. Semin Ophthalmol 38(2):158–166. https://doi.org/10.1080/08820538.2022.2094714

Asanad S, Park A, Pottenburgh J, Siddiqui A, Mayo L, Saeedi OJ (2021) Erythrocyte-mediated angiography: quantifying absolute episcleral blood flow in humans. Ophthalmology 128(5):799–801. https://doi.org/10.1016/j.ophtha.2020.09.010

Baez KA et al (1994) Long-term results of ab externo neodymium: YAG cyclophotocoagulation. Ger J Ophthalmol 3(6):395–399

Billant J et al (2022) Use of selective laser trabeculoplasty as an alternative in patients who developed ocular hypertension after intravitreal dexamethasone implants: a series of 35 eyes. Graefes Arch Clin Exp Ophthalmol 260(11):3665–3673. https://doi.org/10.1007/s00417-022-05725-3

BMJ Publishing Group Ltd., BMA House, Tavistock Square (2021) European glaucoma society terminology and guidelines for glaucoma, 5th edition. Br J Ophthalmol 105(Suppl 1):1–169. https://doi.org/10.1136/bjophthalmol-2021-egsguidelines

Bodh SA, Kumar V, Raina UK, Ghosh B, Thakar M (2011) Inflammatory glaucoma. Oman J Ophthalmol 4(1):3–9. https://doi.org/10.4103/0974-620X.77655

Broadway DC et al (1994) Adverse effects of topical antiglaucoma medication. II. The outcome of filtration surgery. Arch Ophthalmol 112:1446–1454

Chauhan BC et al (2008) Canadian Glaucoma Study: 2. risk factors for the progression of open-angle glaucoma. Arch Ophthalmol 126(8):1030–1036. https://doi.org/10.1001/archopht.126.8.1030

Cheng H et al (2023) Clinical outcomes of penetrating canaloplasty in patients with traumatic angle recession glaucoma: a prospective interventional case series. Br J Ophthalmol 107(8):1092–1097. https://doi.org/10.1136/bjophthalmol-2021-320659

Choy BNK, Lai JSM, Yeung JCC, Chan JCH (2018) Randomized comparative trial of diode laser transscleral cyclophotocoagulation versus Ahmed glaucoma valve for neovascular glaucoma in Chinese - a pilot study. Clin Ophthalmol 12:2545–2552. https://doi.org/10.2147/OPTH.S188999

Christakis PG et al (2016) The Ahmed versus Baerveldt study: five-year treatment outcomes. Ophthalmology 123(10):2093–2102. https://doi.org/10.1016/j.ophtha.2016.06.035

Conlon R, Saheb H, Ahmed II (2017) Glaucoma treatment trends: a review. Can J Ophthalmol 52(1):114–124. https://doi.org/10.1016/j.jcjo.2016.07.013

Dhingra D, Grover S, Kapatia G, Pandav SS, Kaushik S (2020) Phacolytic glaucoma: a nearly forgotten entity. Eur J Ophthalmol 30(5):NP32–NP35. https://doi.org/10.1177/1120672119841972

Feldman RM, Bell NP (2013) Complications of glaucoma surgery. Oxford Academic, New York

Flammer J et al (2013) The primary vascular dysregulation syndrome: implications for eye diseases. EPMA J 4(1):14. https://doi.org/10.1186/1878-5085-4-14

Fukushima M, Yunoki T, Otsuka M, Hayashi A (2020) Association of deepening of the upper eyelid sulcus with the incidence of blepharoptosis after glaucoma filtration surgery. Semin Ophthalmol 35(7–8):348–351. https://doi.org/10.1080/08820538.2020.1863435

Garway-Heath DF et al (2015) Latanoprost for open-angle glaucoma (UKGTS): a randomised, multicentre, placebo-controlled trial. Lancet 385(9975):1295–1304. https://doi.org/10.1016/S0140-6736(14)62111-5

Gazzard G et al (2023) Laser in glaucoma and ocular hypertension (LiGHT) trial: six-year results of primary selective laser trabeculoplasty versus eye drops for the treatment of glaucoma and ocular hypertension. Ophthalmology 130(2):139–151. https://doi.org/10.1016/j.ophtha.2022.09.009

Gedde SJ, Vinod K, Prum BE Jr, Primary Tube Versus Trabeculectomy Study Group (2023) Results from the primary tube versus trabeculectomy study and translation to clinical practice. Curr Opin Ophthalmol 34(2):129–137. https://doi.org/10.1097/ICU.0000000000000928

Gedde SJ et al (2012) Treatment outcomes in the tube versus trabeculectomy (TVT) study after five years of follow-up. Am J Ophthalmol 153(5):789–803.e2. https://doi.org/10.1016/j.ajo.2011.10.026

Gedde SJ et al (2022) Treatment outcomes in the primary tube versus trabeculectomy study after 5 years of follow-up. Ophthalmology 129(12):1344–1356. https://doi.org/10.1016/j.ophtha.2022.07.003

Ghosh S et al (2014) Efficacy of transscleral diode laser cyclophotocoagulation in patients with good visual acuity. Eur J Ophthalmol 24(3):375–381. https://doi.org/10.5301/ejo.5000389

González-Martín-Moro J et al (2017) Cyclodialysis: an update. Int Ophthalmol 37:441–457. https://doi.org/10.1007/s10792-016-0282-8

Gordon MO, Kass MA (2018) What we have learned from the ocular hypertension treatment study. Am J Ophthalmol 189:xxiv–xxvii. https://doi.org/10.1016/j.ajo.2018.02.016

Hayashi K, Yoshida M, Sato T, Manabe SI (2019) Effect of topical hypotensive medications for preventing intraocular pressure increase after cataract surgery in eyes with glaucoma. Am J Ophthalmol 205:91–98. https://doi.org/10.1016/j.ajo.2019.03.012

Hayreh SS, Rojas P, Podhajsky P, Montague P, Woolson RF (1983) Ocular neovascularization with retinal vascular occlusion-III. Incidence of ocular neovascularization with retinal vein occlusion. Ophthalmology 90(5):488–506. https://doi.org/10.1016/s0161-6420(83)34542-5

Heijl A et al (2002) Reduction of intraocular pressure and glaucoma progression: results from the Early Manifest Glaucoma Trial. Arch Ophthalmol 120(10):1268–1279. https://doi.org/10.1001/archopht.120.10.1268

Hong EH et al (2019) Comparison of repeatability of swept-source and spectral-domain optical coherence tomography for measuring inner retinal thickness in retinal disease. PLoS One 14(1):e0210729. https://doi.org/10.1371/journal.pone.0210729

Horsley MB, Chen TC (2011) The use of prostaglandin analogs in the uveitic patient. Semin Ophthalmol 26(4–5):285–289. https://doi.org/10.3109/08820538.2011.588650

Jansook P, Loftsson T (2022) Aqueous prostaglandin eye drop formulations. Pharmaceutics 14(10):2142. https://doi.org/10.3390/pharmaceutics14102142

Jat NS, Tripathy K (2023) Peters anomaly. In: StatPearls. StatPearls Publishing

Jung YH et al (2016) Incidence and clinical features of neovascularization of the iris following acute central retinal artery occlusion. Korean J Ophthalmol 30(5):352–359. https://doi.org/10.3341/kjo.2016.30.5.352

Junttila TL, Alberto N, Winkels M, Greenwood MD (2020) Successful reduction of intraocular pressure in a patient with glaucoma secondary to Sturge-Weber syndrome using a suprachoroidal shunt. J Curr Glaucoma Pract 14(1):43–46. https://doi.org/10.5005/jp-journals-10078-1266

Kalogeropoulos D, Sung VC (2018) Pathogenesis of uveitic glaucoma. J Curr Glaucoma Pract 12(3):125–138. https://doi.org/10.5005/jp-journals-10028-1257

Kaplowitz K et al (2015) Current concepts in the treatment of vitreous block, also known as aqueous misdirection. Surv Ophthalmol 60(3):229–241. https://doi.org/10.1016/j.survophthal.2014.12.004

Karaconji T, Zagora S, Grigg JR (2022) Approach to childhood glaucoma: a review. Clin Experiment Ophthalmol 50(2):232–246. https://doi.org/10.1111/ceo.14039

Kass MA et al (2002) The Ocular Hypertension Treatment Study: a randomized trial determines that topical ocular hypotensive medication delays or prevents the onset of primary open-angle glaucoma. Arch Ophthalmol 120(6):701–830. https://doi.org/10.1001/archopht.120.6.701

Kass MA et al (2021) Assessment of cumulative incidence and severity of primary open-angle glaucoma among participants in the ocular hypertension treatment study after 20 years of follow-up. JAMA Ophthalmol 139(5):558–566. https://doi.org/10.1001/jamaophthalmol.2021.0341

Kaushik J et al (2022) Evaluation of primary Ahmed Glaucoma valve implantation in post-traumatic angle recession glaucoma in Indian eyes. Int Ophthalmol 42(3):817–827. https://doi.org/10.1007/s10792-021-02047-x

Kesav N et al (2020) Current management of uveitis-associated ocular hypertension and glaucoma. Surv Ophthalmol 65(4):397–407. https://doi.org/10.1016/j.survophthal.2019.12.003

Kim YH, Sung MS, Park SW (2017) Clinical features of ocular ischemic syndrome and risk factors for neovascular glaucoma. Korean J Ophthalmol 31(4):343–350. https://doi.org/10.3341/kjo.2016.0067

Knier CG et al (2020) Three-decade evaluation of cerebrospinal fluid pressure in open-angle glaucoma at a tertiary care center. J Ophthalmol 2020:7487329. https://doi.org/10.1155/2020/7487329

Krag S, Larsen D, Albertsen BK, Glerup M (2021) Risk of ocular hypertension in children treated with systemic glucocorticoid. Acta Ophthalmol 99(8):e1430–e1434. https://doi.org/10.1111/aos.14820

Landsend ECS et al (2021) Congenital aniridia - a comprehensive review of clinical features and therapeutic approaches. Surv Ophthalmol 66(6):1031–1050. https://doi.org/10.1016/j.survophthal.2021.02.011

Lee BL et al (2003) Ocular hypertension treatment study (OHTS) commentary. Curr Opin Ophthalmol 14(2):74–77. https://doi.org/10.1097/00055735-200304000-00003

Lee SS, Robinson MR, Weinreb RN (2019) Episcleral venous pressure and the ocular hypotensive effects of topical and intracameral prostaglandin analogs. J Glaucoma 28(9):846–857. https://doi.org/10.1097/IJG.0000000000001307

Leske MC, Heijl A, Hyman L, Bengtsson B (1999) Early Manifest Glaucoma Trial: design and baseline data. Ophthalmology 106(11):2144–2153. https://doi.org/10.1016/s0161-6420(99)90497-9

Macovei ML, Canache M, Neagoe BM (2021) Phacolytic glaucoma - case report. Rom J Ophthalmol 65(2):191–195. https://doi.org/10.22336/rjo.2021.38

Massaoutis P et al (2007) Bilateral symptomatic angle closure associated with a regular dose of citalopram, an SSRI antidepressant. Br J Ophthalmol

91(8):1086–1087. https://doi.org/10.1136/bjo.2006.107185
Meier-Gibbons F, Töteberg-Harms M (2023) Follow-up studies of the classical landmark studies in Glaucoma. Curr Opin Ophthalmol 34(2):116–122. https://doi.org/10.1097/ICU.0000000000000926
Muñoz-Negrete FJ et al (2015) Current approach in the diagnosis and management of uveitic glaucoma. Biomed Res Int 2015:742792. https://doi.org/10.1155/2015/742792
Musch DC, Gillespie BW, Lichter PR, Niziol LM, Janz NK, CIGTS Study Investigators (2009) Visual field progression in the collaborative initial glaucoma treatment study the impact of treatment and other baseline factors. Ophthalmology 116(2):200–207. https://doi.org/10.1016/j.ophtha.2008.08.051
Na K-S et al (2010) Autonomic dysfunction in normal tension glaucoma: the short-term heart rate variability analysis. J Glaucoma 19(6):377–381. https://doi.org/10.1097/IJG.0b013e3181c4ae58
Ng DS, Ching RH, Chan CW (2015) Angle-recession glaucoma: long-term clinical outcomes over a 10-year period in traumatic microhyphema. Int Ophthalmol 35(1):107–113. https://doi.org/10.1007/s10792-014-0027-5
Ondrejka S, Körber N, Dhamdhere K (2022) Long-term effect of canaloplasty on intraocular pressure and use of intraocular pressure-lowering medications in patients with open-angle glaucoma. J Cataract Refract Surg 48(12):1388–1393. https://doi.org/10.1097/j.jcrs.0000000000001000
Peng M et al (2022) Cross-linked actin networks (CLANs) affect stiffness and/or actin dynamics in transgenic transformed and primary human trabecular meshwork cells. Exp Eye Res 220:109097. https://doi.org/10.1016/j.exer.2022.109097
Podoleanu AG (2012) Optical coherence tomography. J Microsc 247(3):209–219. https://doi.org/10.1111/j.1365-2818.2012.03619.x
Pujari A, Selvan H, Behera AK, Gagrani M, Kapoor S, Dada T (2020) The probable mechanism of traumatic angle recession and cyclodialysis. J Glaucoma 29(1):67–70. https://doi.org/10.1097/IJG.0000000000001358
Razeghinejad MR, Nowroozzadeh MH (2010) Anti-glaucoma medication exposure in pregnancy: an observational study and literature review. Clin Exp Optom 93(6):458–465. https://doi.org/10.1111/j.1444-0938.2010.00526.x
Razeghinejad R, Lin MM, Lee D, Katz LJ, Myers JS (2020) Pathophysiology and management of glaucoma and ocular hypertension related to trauma. Surv Ophthalmol 65(5):530–547. https://doi.org/10.1016/j.survophthal.2020.02.003
Ritch R et al (2003) Angle closure in younger patients. Ophthalmology 110(10):1880–1889. https://doi.org/10.1016/S0161-6420(03)00563-3
Rudkin AK et al (2010) Bilateral simultaneous acute angle closure glaucoma precipitated by non-prescription cold and flu medication. Emerg Med Australas 22(5):477–479. https://doi.org/10.1111/j.1742-6723.2010.01338.x
Sadeghi R, Momeni A, Fakhraie G et al (2023) Management of malignant glaucoma. J Curr Ophthalmol 34(4):389–397. https://doi.org/10.4103/joco.joco_147_22
Selvan H, Gupta S, Wiggs JL, Gupta V (2022) Juvenile-onset open-angle glaucoma - a clinical and genetic update. Surv Ophthalmol 67(4):1099–1117. https://doi.org/10.1016/j.survophthal.2021.09.001
Senthil S, Dangeti D, Battula M, Rao HL, Garudadri C (2022) Trabeculectomy with mitomycin-C in post-traumatic angle recession glaucoma in phakic eyes with no prior intraocular intervention. Semin Ophthalmol 37(2):171–176. https://doi.org/10.1080/08820538.2021.1945116
Senthilkumar VA, Ramesh S (2022) Lens particle glaucoma after penetrating injury. Ophthalmol Glaucoma 5(2):218. https://doi.org/10.1016/j.ogla.2021.12.004
Shaarawy T, Sherwood MB, Hitchings RA, Crowston JG (2014) Glaucoma e-book. Elsevier Health Sciences
Shue A, Wong MO, Freedman SF (2022) Primary congenital glaucoma. In: Albert DM, Miller JW, Azar DT, Young LH (eds) Albert and Jakobiec's principles and practice of ophthalmology. Springer, Cham. https://doi.org/10.1007/978-3-030-42634-7_168
Stefan C, Iliescu DA, Batras M, Timaru CM, De Simone A (2015) Plateau iris--diagnosis and treatment. Rom J Ophthalmol 59(1):14–18
Varma DK et al (2014) Malignant glaucoma after cataract surgery. J Cataract Refract Surg 40(11):1843–1849. https://doi.org/10.1016/j.jcrs.2014.02.045
Venkataraman P et al (2022) A systematic approach to the management of microspherophakia. Indian J Ophthalmol 70(7):2262–2271. https://doi.org/10.4103/ijo.IJO_2888_21
Wang RX, Li N, Chen XY (2022) Ultrasound cyclo-plasty for moderate glaucoma: eighteen-month results from a prospective study. Front Med (Lausanne) 9:1009273. https://doi.org/10.3389/fmed.2022.1009273
Yuen NSY et al (2006) New method of surgical repair for 360-degree cyclodialysis. J Cataract Refract Surg 32(1):13–17. https://doi.org/10.1016/j.jcrs.2005.05.035
Zuo C et al (2021) Associations between the choroidal vascularity index and malignant glaucoma after trabeculectomy for primary angle closure glaucoma. Front Med (Lausanne) 8:747720. https://doi.org/10.3389/fmed.2021.747720

20 Clinical Review of Cataract and Power Calculation: Part I

Saif Aldeen Alryalat, Mutasem Elfalah, Mohammad Elfalah, and Kenneth Hoffer

Abstract

This chapter provides a comprehensive exploration of cataract surgery, beginning with an overview of cataract risk factors that contribute to the development of this common ocular condition. It delves into phacoemulsification, outlining key concepts, including innovative photodynamic fluidic techniques and various chopping methods that enhance surgical efficiency. Detailed surgical technique tips are offered, addressing special situations such as preoperative preparations, intraoperative considerations, and postoperative care, along with patient-specific cautions to optimize outcomes. The chapter also discusses the role of anesthesia in cataract surgery and emphasizes the importance of antimicrobial measures to prevent infection. Additionally, ophthalmic viscosurgical devices are examined for their critical role in maintaining surgical conditions during the procedure. The chapter focuses on a discussion of potential complications associated with cataract, to ensure safe and effective surgical practices.

Keywords

Cataract surgery · Phacoemulsification Anesthesia · Antimicrobial · Ophthalmic viscosurgical devices

20.1 Overview

Cataract is a clouding or opacification of the eye's natural lens that might lead to a decrease in vision. It typically occurs due to aging but can also result from trauma, radiation exposure, diseases such as diabetes, and certain medications like corticosteroids or can be congenital. The lens, located behind the iris and the pupil, focuses the light entering the eye onto the retina to produce a clear, sharp image. As the opacity increases, the light passing through the lens is scattered, causing visual disturbances. The overall incidence of cataract is greater in women than in men. References for this chapter include the American Academy of Ophthalmology resources in addition to several specific ones (Liu and

S. A. Alryalat (✉)
Department of Ophthalmology, The University of Jordan, Amman, Jordan

The University of Colorado Anschutz Medical Campus, Aurora, CO, USA

M. Elfalah
Department of Ophthalmology, The University of Jordan, Amman, Jordan
e-mail: M.Alrabie@ju.edu.jo

M. Elfalah
School of Medicine, The University of Jordan, Amman, Jordan

K. Hoffer
The University of California, Los Angeles, CA, USA
e-mail: khoffermd@startmail.com

S. A. Alryalat (ed.), *Ophthalmology Board and FRCS Part 2 Exams*,
https://doi.org/10.1007/978-981-96-1517-9_20

Bardan 2021; Infant Aphakia Treatment Study Group 2010; Lee et al. 2018; Bowen et al. 2018).

Aging is associated with different changes in the lens and its surrounding structures. The following changes occur with aging:

- Increase in the lens curvature, which results in more refractive power.
- Increase in water-insoluble proteins, decreasing the index of refraction and decreasing lens power, offsetting the increased power by the increase in curvature.
- Equatorial zonules are lost with increasing age, so the anterior and posterior zonules predominate.
- As we age, the lens of the eye can lose elasticity and become less flexible, a condition called presbyopia, leading to difficulties focusing on close objects.

Cataracts can be classified into different types based on their location within the lens (nuclear, cortical, posterior subcapsular, or a combination) and the cause (age-related, traumatic, secondary, and congenital). They can also be characterized by their severity and the impact they have on the individual's vision.

20.1.1 Types of Cataract

The three classical and most common types are the following:

- Anterior and posterior subcapsular cataracts: These cataracts involve fibrous metaplasia of the anterior lens epithelium, leading to the posterior migration of lens epithelial cells. These cells then swell along the posterior capsule, forming what are known as Wedl or bladder cells.
- Nuclear sclerotic cataract is characterized by homogenous loss of cellular laminations, along with deposition of urochrome pigment appearing as a yellowish hue. It is best assessed with an oblique slit lamp beam. African-Americans have lower rates of nuclear opacity incidence.
- Cortical cataracts associated with hydropic swelling of the lens fibers with eosinophilic globules in between called morgagnian globules. It typically starts inferonasally.

20.1.1.1 High-Yield Note

Cataract histopathology: Posterior subcapsular cataracts: posterior migration of the lens epithelial cells from the lens equator. Nuclear sclerotic: increased number of lamellar membrane whorls. Cortical: local swelling and disruption of lens fiber cells.

A rarer type of cataract is the polar cataract, which includes both anterior and posterior polar cataracts. These can be inherited in an autosomal dominant manner or occur sporadically:

- Anterior polar cataracts are usually small and nonprogressive and usually do not significantly affect vision. They may be associated with conditions such as microphthalmos, persistent pupillary membrane, and anterior lenticonus.

Posterior polar cataracts are larger and tend to cause more visual impairment compared to anterior polar cataracts. They may be associated with posterior lenticonus or a remnant of tunica vasculosa lentis.

Congenital cataract is also classified into different types. Lamellar cataracts are the most common type of congenital and infantile cataracts. Congenital cataracts are usually AD or sporadic (unlike congenital glaucoma, which is AR).

20.1.2 Important Definitions

Glaukomflecken: represents focal infarcts of the lens epithelium and is pathognomonic of a previous acute congestive angle closure.

Soemmering's ring: is a deposition of retained equatorial lens epithelial cells that continue to proliferate and form new cortical fibers between anterior and posterior capsules within the bag.

Elschnig ring: Accumulation of clusters of proliferated epithelial cells outside the bag, mostly post-cataract surgery. These cells lack any basement membrane unlike the Soemmering's ring.

Morgagnian cataract: is a hypermature cataract in which the liquefaction of the lens cortex has caused the denser nucleus to sink to the bottom of the lens. **Vossius ring** is a circular deposit of pigment on the anterior lens capsule, usually resulting from blunt trauma. It forms a complete or incomplete ring. **Lens coloboma** is a wedge-shaped defect or indentation at the lens periphery. It occurs as an isolated anomaly or is secondary to the absence of ciliary body or zonular development, often resulting in a missing part of the lens with an associated zonular defect. Cortical lens opacification or thickening of the lens capsule may be present adjacent to the defect. Lens colobomas are typically found inferiorly and may be associated with colobomas of the uvea.

20.2 Cataract Risk Factors

While cataract is mainly associated with aging, other risk factors and causes can also contribute to its development. Chronic anterior uveitis is the most common cause of secondary cataract. Table 20.1 summarizes conditions and the associated cataract type with each of them.

Patients over the age of 50 are particularly susceptible to cataracts. Following vitrectomy, almost 90% of phakic eyes may develop a significant nuclear sclerotic cataract within 2 years. Procedures like trabeculectomy and keratoplasties could also enhance cataract risk.

Despite not increasing the chance of cataracts, psoralen plus ultraviolet A (PUVA) treatment can escalate the risk of squamous cell carcinoma. Various drugs, including amiodarone, phenothiazine, all types of steroids, and echothiophate, are associated with cataract formation.

Conditions like Alport syndrome, Waardenburg syndrome, and spina bifida are linked with anterior lenticonus. Cataract formation can be accelerated due to retained iron foreign bodies, leading to siderosis bulbi, often visible as darker iris color and pigments beneath the lens capsule. The preferred pre-surgical investigation is a CT scan to identify any retained iron.

It is important to remember that neither hypoglycemia nor hypercalcemia contributes to the development of cataracts. Cataract-related changes in the lens can be triggered by allopurinol, which manifests as modifications in the anterior and posterior lens capsules and the formation of anterior subcapsular vacuoles.

Rubella syndrome, often resulting from infection during the first trimester of pregnancy, is associated with various complications, including cataracts. Additional findings may include microphthalmos, a shallow anterior chamber, a "salt-and-pepper" appearance of the fundus, hearing loss, and abnormalities of the heart, valves, and genitourinary system. Rubella-related cataracts are characterized by the retention of fetal cell nuclei within the cataractous lens nucleus, with the virus potentially persisting in the lens for up to 3 years after birth.

Traumatic cataracts develop swiftly due to a breach of the lens capsule and consequent hydration of the lens, with the lens itself being susceptible to various reactive oxygen species (ROS).

Chalcosis, a copper deposition, can occur in Descemet's membrane, lens capsule, and other intraocular basement membranes. This condition could lead to a "sunflower" cataract, which is usually not visually significant.

Various factors related to metabolic syndrome can lead to cataracts, including diabetes, hypocalcemia, and myotonic dystrophy. Electrical injury and alkali ocular burns can also induce cataracts. With burns, however, only alkali burns are implicated in cataract formation, not acid burns.

The risk of cataract development may be decreased by foods rich in vitamin C, specifically the nuclear cataract.

The lens is the most radiosensitive structure of the eye.

Table 20.1 Conditions and the associated cataract type with each of them

Condition	Associated cataract	Notes
Atopic dermatitis	Anterior subcapsular (shield-like) cataract	Usually bilateral, and develops in 10–25% of severe cases by fourth decade
Acute hyperglycemic attack (classic diabetic cataract)	Snowflake cortical cataract	May resolve or progress to persistent cortical cataract. The main enzyme responsible is aldose reductase
Blunt trauma	Stellate or rosette-shaped cataract at the posterior capsule axially	Posterior lens capsule might be disrupted
Penetrating trauma (with capsule disruption)	Cortical changes that may remain focal if small or may progress rapidly to total cortical opacification	
Myotonic dystrophy	Christmas tree cataract	90% of patients will develop Christmas tree nuclear cataract by the third decade. Polychromatic iridescent crystals (red and green in color) in the lens cortex, non-visually significant
Galactosemia	Oil droplet	Appears within the first few weeks of life, reversed with milk elimination from diet
Neurofibromatosis type 2	Posterior subcapsular cataract	60% of patients
Hereditary fundus dystrophies	Posterior subcapsular cataract	
Chalcosis	Sunflower subcortical cataract	Copper deposition beneath the capsule, non-visually significant
Steroids	Posterior subcapsular cataract	
High myopia	Posterior subcapsular cataract	
Hypocalcemia	Anterior and posterior subcortical cataract	Bilateral, hypocalcemic (tetanic) cataracts are punctate iridescent opacities in the anterior and posterior cortex
Phenothiazines and amiodarone	Stellate anterior subcapsular cataract	Non-visually significant stellate-like deposition on anterior lens capsule Amiodarone may also cause PSCC
Cholinergics (e.g., pilocarpine or echothiophate)	Vacuoles at posterior capsule	
Statin and tamoxifen	Cataract	Higher risk with prolonged use
Rubella congenital infection	Nuclear	Bilateral nuclear. Retained nuclei within cells. Induces excessive inflammation if part of the cataract is left. Occurs when mother is infected during the first trimester

20.3 Phacoemulsification

20.3.1 Phacoemulsification Concepts

The core component of the phacoemulsification handpiece is a transducer that converts electrical energy into mechanical movement of the phacoemulsification tip. Electrical input causes crystals with piezoelectric properties to oscillate, converting electricity energy into vibrating motion and vice versa.

This oscillation is transmitted to the phacoemulsification tip through an ultrasonic horn, which also functions as an amplifier, resulting in the longitudinal (backward and forward) movement of the phacoemulsification needle, known as the stroke. In traditional longitudinal phacoemulsification, the needle moves back and forth, mechanically cutting the lens material during the forward movement, a process often referred to as the *jackhammer effect*. Additionally, this rapid movement generates microcavitation bubbles, though the impact of these bubbles is still a topic of debate.

Cavitation: It is the formation of gas bubbles arising from the aqueous humor due to pressure changes at the tip of the phacoemulsification needle. These bubbles expand and contract, and their implosion generates localized intense heat and pressure, leading to the emulsification of lens material. If the ultrasonic power is set too high relative to the density of the cataract, achieving tip occlusion becomes challenging because excessive cavitation occurs. The energy released by cavitation emulsifies too much nuclear material at the phaco tip, reducing the likelihood of achieving proper tip occlusion. **Chatter** occurs when the ultrasonic stroke surpasses the vacuum or "holding power," causing the nuclear fragments to be pushed away from the ultrasonic tip. As more power is applied, the chatter effect intensifies, leading to greater repulsion of the pieces and reducing their followability.

(*Ultrasonic* refers to frequencies above the range of human audibility or greater than 20,000 Hz.)

Stroke: This is the linear distance the tip moves to impact lens material. In phacoemulsification, stroke length varies by device and typically ranges from 0.05 mm to 0.10 mm.

Power: This represents a percentage of the maximum stroke length. Increasing power has the benefits of producing cavitation, shock waves, shear forces, and heat at the tip; however, the downside is an increase in chatter.

The phacoemulsification handpiece generates ultrasound power through converting electrical energy into mechanical vibration through piezoelectric crystals. Piezoelectric crystals are used in handpieces, when an electric charge is applied to opposite faces of these crystals; a strain appears in the structure, which results in deformation. This is how ultrasonic movement and energy are created in phaco handpieces. The movement of crystals will dictate how the power is delivered:

- Longitudinal: Traditionally, the probe delivers power in a linear, back-and-forth motion, with the phaco needle moving forward and backward.
- Lateral *torsional*: In this method, the phaco tip oscillates rotationally along its primary axis, working best with an angled phaco needle. This torsional oscillation creates a side-to-side movement at the tip's end. The cataract is cut through shearing rather than the jackhammer effect, minimizing lens bulk repulsion and enhancing followability. The repulsion of the lens bulk is minimized, improving followability.

Lateral *transversal* is where the phaco tip moves in an elliptical path, and this method works equally well with either a straight or angled needle. The advantage of lateral movement is the reduction of piece repulsion from the handpiece, as occurs with vertical movement.

Lower phacoemulsification power setting is used when using burst mode as compared to pulse or continuous modes.

Absolute phacoemulsification time (APT) = Power given (in %) * duration.

Depressing the foot pedal in position three adjusts the power, which affects the stroke length—the distance the tip moves from rest to its maximum forward displacement in a single cycle—without changing the frequency. The stroke frequency is preset by the manufacturer and cannot be modified by the surgeon. The machine displays power as a percentage of the maximum stroke length, typically representing the electrical power supplied to the crystals, which then oscillate, creating vibrational movement at the titanium tip.

Pedal position:

- Single linear, where position 1 is irrigation, position 2 is aspiration, and position 3 is phaco ultrasound power
- Dual linear, where phaco ultrasound power is achieved by moving the pedal sideways, and positions 2 and 3 for aspiration

Phacoemulsification power can be delivered in three main modes:

- Continuous mode: Where ultrasound power is delivered continuously as long as the pedal is on position 3, with its amount of power dependent on pedal push.
- Pulse mode: Where the interval between ultrasound power is constant, but the delivered power increases with pedal push on position 3. Reduction in the energy delivered is accomplished by decreasing the time that the power is on by altering the ratio of the on:off pulses, not by changing the number of pulses per second. Lower pulse rate is better for emulsification, while higher pulse rate is better for sculpting. Duty cycle is the ratio of on to off, with the default being 50% to 50%, while variable duty cycle may vary.

Burst mode: each burst of energy is delivered at the same power level, but the interval between bursts decreases as the foot pedal is further depressed, meaning bursts are delivered more rapidly. The more the foot pedal is pressed, the shorter the "off" period becomes between each burst. At a maximum foot pedal depression, the bursts of energy merge into a continuous delivery of energy (the ratio of the "on" to "off" pulses is called the duty time). The advantages of pulse and burst modes are the allowance of a pause period to aspirate pieces and to allow the tip to cool.

Irrigation from probe side ports maintains AC pressure during aspiration, and there are some fluids at the phacoemulsification tip to cool the probe from the ultrasound power.

The term *followability* describes a relatively feathery and continuous aspiration of the lens fragments into the phacoemulsification tip; it is opposite to chatter.

Phacoemulsification tips differ in the angle of the tip and the size of the lumen. The end configurations can be round, ellipsoid, bent, or flattened. A tip with a steeper bevel has an oval port with a larger surface area, which can generate more holding force and increase cutting efficiency. However, the drawback of steeper bevels is that the larger opening can be more challenging to occlude, making it harder to achieve full vacuum.

20.3.2 Photodynamic Fluidic Concepts

Aspiration (flow rate, mL/min): An active fluid withdrawal from AC to the tubing system, which can be represented by the flow rate measured in milliliters per minute (mL/min).

Vacuum (mmHg): Upon phaco tip occlusion, a negative pressure builds up in the tubing system known as vacuum (measured in (mm Hg)), which aims to hold material into the tip. So, vacuum is the magnitude of negative pressure created in the tubing.

Rise time: The rate at which vacuum builds after the aspiration port is occluded, which depends on the aspiration flow rate.

Followability: The ability of a fluidic system to attract and hold nuclear or cortical material onto the tip of an ultrasonic or irrigation/aspiration (I/A) handpiece until vacuum forces evacuate the material.

Inflow: The introduction of fluid into the AC.

Surge: A phenomenon that occurs when a vacuum has built up due to an occlusion, and the occlusion is suddenly broken, causing the fluid in the higher-pressure (positive) anterior chamber to rush into the lower-pressure (negative) phaco tip.

**** Adjusting the flow rate can enhance the ability to attract nuclear or cortical material to the distal end of the handpiece, while adjusting the vacuum level determines how firmly the occluded material is held by the phaco tip.*

- There are three main types of aspiration pumps used in phaco machines: peristaltic pumps, diaphragm pumps, and Venturi pumps. **Peristaltic (flow) pumps:** Vacuum is generated only when the tip becomes occluded. Once occlusion occurs, the pump slows and stops when a set maximum vacuum is achieved. It pulls fluid and lens material into the phaco tip by compressing tubing over variable speed rollers. The speed of these rollers allows for linear control of aspiration, which indirectly controls the vacuum.

Diaphragm pumps: This type of pump system produces a slower rise in vacuum compared to peristaltic pumps. With continued occlusion of the aspiration port, the vacuum increases exponentially. Diaphragm pumps have the slowest vacuum buildup among the three types.

Venturi (vacuum) pumps: The vacuum buildup depends on the machine, rather than the occlusion. These pumps create a negative pressure (Vacuum) in a vessel by passing compressed gas across its entrance, which indirectly drives aspiration. There is generally no independent control over the AFR, as it is regulated by the vacuum. Depressing the foot pedal increases vacuum toward a preset maximum, independent of occlusion, ensuring that the tip vacuum is always available. Venturi pump provides the most rapid rise in vacuum. Although a vacuum limit is set on the machine, the peristaltic pump does not directly produce the level of vacuum. Rather, it controls the aspiration flow rate (AFR), which indirectly produces vacuum. In contrast, a Venturi (or vacuum) pump directly creates the vacuum based on the Venturi effect. Direct control of vacuum level in the pump cassette then indirectly produces flow (while the aspiration port is not occluded) by "pulling" on the fluid in the aspiration tubing. In the absence of significant occlusion, higher vacuum levels produce a faster AFR.

20.3.3 Surgical Technique Tips

Here are some crucial tips and tricks for cataract surgical techniques.

When deciding on the incision's location, there are several considerations to take into account. Superior incisions have the advantages of not interfering with a pterygium site and being associated with lower instances of endophthalmitis. Temporal incisions, on the other hand, can correct with-the-rule astigmatism, are easier to perform in sunken eyes, and can avoid a prior trabeculotomy site. However, keep in mind that clear corneal incisions generally have a higher risk of endophthalmitis.

In cases of zonular dialysis of less than 180 degrees, if the intraocular lens (IOL) is in the bag, place the haptic parallel to the dialysis site. If the IOL is in the sulcus, the haptics should be placed perpendicular to the dialysis site. This is crucial to prevent or minimize decentration by resisting the contraction of the capsule.

To mitigate the effects of floppy iris syndrome intraoperatively, consider reducing the aspiration flow rate and vacuum, using mechanical iris expansion devices, applying intracameral epinephrine, employing highly retentive viscoelastic, and avoiding an incision that is overly large or posterior (to reduce the risk of iris prolapse).

The primary wound should ideally be 2.4–3.2 mm wide, depending on the phaco machine handpiece. This width is necessary to fit the wound and prevent any leakage. Clear corneal cataract incisions can function similarly to arcuate incisions used to correct astigmatism. They can flatten the cornea in the meridian of the incision and, by virtue of "coupling," steepen the cornea 90 degrees away.

In the event of a capsulorhexis radializing, consider implementing Little's technique. This involves injecting OVD and attempting a pull toward the center at 90 degrees. If unsuccessful, you can switch to the "can-opener" technique. The continuous curvilinear capsulorhexis (CCC) should be large enough for cataract removal and small enough to overlap the anterior optic edge of the intraocular lens (IOL). In terms of hydrodissection, be cautious as the fluid that passes behind the lens can cause the lens to move more anteriorly, shallowing the chamber leading to capsular block syndrome.

In terms of chopping techniques, there are several methods:

- "Divide and conquer" involves sculpting a tunnel vertically and horizontally to fracture the nucleus into four pieces.
- "Stop and chop" is after a single sculpt and dividing the nucleus into two pieces, chopping into smaller pieces without sculpts.
- Horizontal chop: where the phaco tip is buried into the nucleus via high aspiration; then a chopper is used to fracture the nucleus into two pieces by moving both hands horizontally toward the center.
- Vertical chop: same as horizontal, but the movement of phaco tip is upward and chopper downward.

In intraocular lens (IOL) insertion, it is essential to place the leading haptic in the bag. The trailing haptic can be either placed directly or dialed. Avoid using a single-piece acrylic IOL for the ciliary sulcus due to the possible development of uveitis-glaucoma-hyphema (UGH) syndrome.

In case of vitreous prolapse and lens material drops, never proceed with phacoemulsification as this can lead to retinal tractions. However, the course of action will depend on when this occurs. If it happens at the beginning (for instance, during sculpting), then either close the wound and refer or insert an anterior chamber intraocular lens (ACIOL) and refer. If it occurs at the end of the surgery with cortical material dropped, insert a sulcus IOL and refer to a vitreoretinal surgeon.

IOL exchange can be considered for cataract surgeries performed within the past 3 months, particularly if there was a refractive surprise. The management of a large Descemet's detachment involves filling half the chamber with SF6 gas and positioning the head to aid sealing. If striae appear in the cornea incision after introducing the phaco probe, consider enlarging the internal and external lips to allow more room for the phacoemulsification needle. This should relax the tight fit and make the striae disappear.

20.3.4 Special Situations

20.3.4.1 Preoperative Preparations

Several precautions are necessary when dealing with patients who have specific medical histories. For instance, patients with a history of herpes keratitis should be prescribed prophylactic oral acyclovir (400 mg*2). Those who have undergone keratoplasty and are scheduled for cataract surgery should have all sutures removed prior to the procedure. Furthermore, patients with preexisting diabetic macular edema should receive treatment for the condition before undergoing cataract surgery. For those with high-risk proliferative diabetic retinopathy (PDR), laser photocoagulation should be performed 1–2 months prior to cataract surgery to ensure its effectiveness. Uveitic patients should also be inflammation-free for a period of 3 months prior to the operation, with oral and topical steroids prescribed preoperatively for 3 days.

Clear cornea standard cataract surgery achieves a visual acuity of 20/40 or better in over 90% of patients.

During cataract surgery, a piece of the cataract falls posteriorly through a posterior capsular tear. Postoperatively, the lens remnant is noted in the inferior vitreous compartment in a "quiet" eye. The best immediate course of action is continuation of routine corticosteroid eye drop therapy and close observation.

The intraocular pressure on the first postoperative day is 38 mm Hg. The best course of action is "burp" the wound so that a small amount of aqueous is removed. It can be repeated one time.

20.3.4.2 Intraoperative Surgical Considerations

Zonular dialysis: In the management of zonular dialysis to prevent the dislocation of the intraocular lens (IOL), if the IOL is placed in the bag, the haptics should be aligned parallel to the dialysis site. If the IOL is placed in the sulcus, the haptics should be positioned perpendicular to the dialysis site.

Management of vitreous prolapse with posterior capsular rupture (PCR): If the break is enlarging, it is advisable to stop the procedure and convert to an extracapsular approach. Avoid using cotton tips to check for vitreous in the wound, as this can induce vitreous traction and increase the risk of retinal tears. Remove cortical material by pulling it toward the break, rather than away from it, to prevent the opening from extending. Remember that phacoemulsification does not cut vitreous, and vitreous will clog the probe. The strong vacuum can increase the risk of retinal tractions.

Dealing with dropped nuclear parts: In cases of dropped nuclear parts, factors that support the removal of retained lens fragments rather than watchful waiting include large fragment size, significant nuclear density, associated retinal tears or detachment, risk of endophthalmitis, and prolonged elevated intraocular pressure or inflammation unresponsive to medical therapy.

IOL considerations in patients with PCR: The ideal IOL for patients with PCR is sulcus three-piece IOLs or scleral sutured three-piece IOLs. When single-piece acrylic IOLs are the only option, iris fixation using McCannel sutures should be performed. Single-piece IOLs are not ideal for sulcus placement or scleral suturing in complicated cataract surgeries.

Zonular dialysis: For a patient with 90° of zonular dialysis, management may include continued phacoemulsification capsular tension ring (CTR) placement, or a three-piece IOL in the bag with haptic parallel to dialysis. When zonular dialysis ranges from 90° to 180°, the capsular bag can be stabilized by suturing it to the ciliary sulcus.

Misdirection syndrome: During cataract surgery, the phenomenon of misdirection syndrome can occur, characterized by a persistent, forward shift of the posterior capsule during irrigation/aspiration. This occurs when infusion fluid flows through intact zonules or zonular dehiscence, leading to fluid accumulation between the anterior hyaloid and posterior capsule, resulting in forward displacement of the capsule and shallowing of the anterior chamber.

20.3.4.3 Specific Patient Conditions and Related Precautions

Posterior polar cataract: In the case of patients with a posterior polar cataract, the risk of posterior capsular disruption should be anticipated. The incidence of posterior capsule rupture (PCR) in normal cataracts is approximately 1.1%, whereas for posterior polar cataracts, the reported incidence ranges between 6% and 36%. To mitigate these risks, several measures should be taken during surgery:

- The continuous curvilinear capsulorhexis (CCC) should be enlarged to prepare for out-of-the-bag phacoemulsification.
- Hydrodissection should be avoided in favor of hydrodelineation.
- Nucleus removal techniques that involve sculpting should be replaced with chopping techniques.
- To clean the epinucleus from the posterior capsule, ophthalmic viscosurgical devices (OVDs) should be used instead of direct irrigation/aspiration.

Understanding and managing intraoperative floppy iris syndrome (IFIS): Intraoperative floppy iris syndrome (IFIS) is an intraoperative phenomenon characterized by three features: an iris that billows and exhibits floppiness, iris prolapse into the surgical incisions, and progressive pupillary miosis. This condition is often caused by alpha-antagonists, particularly tamsulosin, which is commonly used for prostate symptoms. Tamsulosin has been observed to cause IFIS more frequently than other alpha-antagonists due to its effect of competitively inhibiting the receptors. It is important to note that the severity of IFIS is not linked to the duration of tamsulosin intake. Discontinuing alpha-antagonists even 1 week prior to operation does not significantly reduce the risk of developing IFIS. Other possible causes of IFIS include pseudoexfoliation (PXF) syndrome and the use of anti-glaucoma medications, among others.

Pseudoexfoliation syndrome: Manifestations of PXF to be considered in cataract surgery:

- Poor dilatation
- Iridodonesis, phacodonesis, and zonulopathy
- Defective corneal endothelium
- Weak capsule, leading to complications in capsulotomy

Patients with prior keratoplasty: When treating patients who have previously undergone keratoplasty and are now scheduled for cataract surgery, it is vital to ensure that all sutures from the keratoplasty have been removed before proceeding with the cataract surgery. This helps mitigate potential complications and ensures a safer surgical process.

Patients with preexisting diabetic macular edema and proliferative diabetic retinopathy (PDR): For those with preexisting diabetic macular edema, the condition should be managed and treated before proceeding with cataract surgery. In cases of high-risk PDR, preoperative laser photocoagulation, performed 1–2 months before the cataract surgery, is recommended to give ample time for the treatment effect to occur.

Patients with Parkinson's disease: Given that individuals with Parkinson's disease often have reduced blink frequency, leading to severe keratopathy and impaired epithelial wound healing due to increased exposure, it is recommended to create a cataract incision under the lid and covered by conjunctiva, such as a superior scleral tunnel incision.

Patients with hyperopia (AL <22 mm): These patients are expected to have a shallow anterior chamber (AC) due to vitreous push. IV mannitol administration pre-op may decrease the vitreous push. Choroidal hemorrhage and effusion are more common in such patients.

Patients with myopia (AL >26): These patients should have an IOL placed even if plano is recommended to act as a barrier against vitreous prolapse. Silicon IOLs should be avoided due to the risk of future vitrectomy with silicon oil implant.

20.3.4.4 Postoperative Considerations

Management of residual error after multifocal IOL implantation: Following the implantation of multifocal intraocular lenses (IOLs), some degree of residual refractive error may be observed. This can be managed by the following:

- Mild residual refractive errors: Can typically be managed with glasses or contact lenses. These corrective methods can help to fine-tune vision by addressing minor discrepancies in refractive error.
- Significant residual refractive errors: These are best managed more definitively with procedures like photorefractive keratectomy (PRK), laser-assisted in situ keratomileusis (LASIK), IOL exchange, or implantation of piggyback IOLs. It is important to note that refractive stability should be achieved prior to these interventions, which typically occurs about 3–6 months postoperatively.

Use of steroids and anti-glaucoma medications: Uncomplicated phacoemulsification surgery lowers IOP between 10% and 34%, on average, in some eyes. It can therefore be considered as a stand-alone procedure in eyes with early to moderate glaucoma.

Some patients may experience intraoperative floppy iris syndrome (IFIS) due to certain medications such as alpha-antagonists, especially tamsulosin, and anti-glaucoma medications, or in cases of pseudoexfoliation syndrome (PXF). However, cessation of these medications even a week pre-op may not help reduce the IFIS. Also, the severity of the condition is not associated with the duration of tamsulosin intake.

IOL exchange considerations: If a patient is not satisfied with the operative power outcome, consider IOL exchange if surgery was performed within a 3-month window. This decision should be made after thorough consideration of the potential risks and benefits. Note that postoperative hyperopia is the complicated refractive outcome that is more common in patients who have undergone previous refractive surgery.

Postoperative vision suboptimality: In cases where vision is not optimal after an uncomplicated cataract surgery and normal postoperative exam, consider corneal topography when looking for irregular astigmatism as a potential cause.

20.3.4.5 Patient-Specific Cautions

Patients with a history of herpes keratitis: Such patients should be prescribed prophylactic acyclovir orally (400 mg*2) as a preventative measure from 1 day before to 1 week after the surgery.

Patients with uveitis: Patients with chronic uveitis should be treated, and the uveitis should be under control for at least 3 months before the surgery. A perioperative injection of intravitreal triamcinolone (4 mg/0.1 mL) may be considered to decrease post-op inflammation.

Patients with a history of scleritis and episcleritis: Similar to patients with uveitis, these patients must be under control for at least 3 months before the surgery. Also, such patients should be given topical and systemic NSAIDs 1 day before to 1 month after the surgery.

Patients with a history of rhegmatogenous retinal detachment: Patients with a history of rhegmatogenous retinal detachment (RRD) should get a thorough retinal examination before the surgery. They should also get prophylactic retinal laser treatment if predisposing factors like lattice degeneration and retinal tears are present.

Patients with Fuchs' dystrophy: Care should be taken in patients with Fuchs' dystrophy, as it is important to keep the corneal endothelium as healthy as possible during cataract surgery. To help manage the condition, a slow, careful phacoemulsification is performed. Postoperatively, the use of topical steroids should be minimized as it can exacerbate the disease.

Pediatric cataract surgery: Pediatric cataract surgery requires different planning and has distinct considerations compared to adult cataract surgery. Children have a significantly stronger healing response, which can lead to postoperative inflammation and potential complications such as aggressive posterior capsular opacification. Therefore, a thorough follow-up is necessary.

Nanophthalmos cataract surgery: Nanophthalmos cataract surgery involves special considerations due to the unique anatomy of nanophthalmic eyes, which have an axial length of less than 20 mm. These eyes typically have shallow anterior chambers, narrow angles, and thickened sclera, leaving limited room for the surgical maneuvers. A notable risk during and after surgery is the possibility of intraoperative or postoperative uveal effusion.

20.3.5 Anesthesia

Anesthesia plays a crucial role in the successful outcome of cataract surgery, ensuring both patient comfort and optimal surgical conditions. There are several options available, each with its own advantages, disadvantages, and specific precautions:

1. **Retrobulbar block:** This type of anesthesia is administered via a 25-gauge needle through the skin or conjunctiva. The injection is given behind the muscle cone, providing a superior level of anesthesia compared to peribulbar methods. However, this technique carries a higher risk of optic nerve damage. The last muscle to be rendered akinetic with a retrobulbar anesthetic block is the superior oblique. A serious complication of retrobulbar anesthesia is retrobulbar hemorrhage, which can be managed with canthotomy and cantholysis to relieve pressure around the optic nerve.
2. **Peribulbar block:** Given through the skin or conjunctiva with a 27-gauge needle, the injection is administered within the muscle cone. This method generally provides less effective anesthesia and akinesia than a retrobulbar block, but it carries a reduced risk for optic nerve and dura penetration (Table 20.2).
3. **Topical anesthesia:** This method involves the use of drops or gel (proxymetacaine 0.5%, tetracaine 1% drops, lidocaine 2% gel). Topical anesthesia can be augmented with intracameral preservative-free lidocaine (0.2–1%), which is often infused during hydrodissection.
4. **Sub-tenon anesthesia:** For this type of anesthesia, a conjunctival incision is made posteriorly, and lidocaine is injected via a blunt cannula (aka air cannula) into the sub-tenon space.
5. **Facial nerve block:** This type of block is particularly useful for patients with blepharospasm.

Keep in mind that patients on anticoagulation medication are at a higher risk of retrobulbar

Table 20.2 Comparison between retrobulbar block and peribulbar block

	Retrobulbar block	Peribulbar block
Injection site	Through the skin	Either through skin or conjunctiva
Anesthesia efficiency	Better	Less, with fourth nerve (i.e., superior oblique) not anesthetized
Specific risks	Optic nerve and dura penetration	Less risk to almost none
Needle gauge	27 (larger)	25 (smaller) and shorter
IOP impact	Less increase	Higher increase
Chemosis	Less frequent	More frequent

hemorrhage or periocular ecchymosis with retrobulbar and peribulbar anesthesia.

The last muscle to be rendered akinetic with a retrobulbar anesthetic block is the superior oblique.

One of the most serious complications of retrobulbar anesthesia is retrobulbar hemorrhage, characterized by lid ecchymosis, subconjunctival hemorrhage, and proptosis that appear immediately after injection. It should be managed by canthotomy and cantholysis to relieve the pressure around the optic nerve.

When a patient develops allergy to one anesthetic type, always avoid others from the same group, and consider anesthetics from a different group:

- Ester-linked local anesthetics: tetracaine, benzocaine, and butacaine
- Amide-linked local anesthetics: lidocaine, bupivacaine, and mepivacaine

The most commonly used agents in periocular anesthesia are a combination of lidocaine and bupivacaine. Lidocaine, a short-acting anesthetic, offers immediate pain relief, while bupivacaine provides a longer duration of anesthesia. However, it is important to be cautious with bupivacaine, as it can induce respiratory arrest if accidentally administrated into an artery.

Axial high myopia is a risk factor for ocular perforation with a retrobulbar injection. It is a relative, not an absolute, contraindication.

20.3.6 Antimicrobial Measures

100,000 AC bacteria are needed to cause endophthalmitis, while only 5 in vitreous are needed. So, if posterior capsular rupture occurs, the use of intracameral antibiotics is most needed.

20.3.6.1 Proven Measures

- Treat patients with blepharitis preoperatively, in addition to good draping intraoperatively.
- A 5% (which is half the concentration of the usual) povidone-iodine solution (not scrub or soap) placed in the conjunctival fornix prior to surgery has been associated with a reduction in endophthalmitis.
- Intracameral antibiotics (i.e., moxifloxacin or cefuroxime) administered at the end of cataract surgery significantly reduced the rate of endophthalmitis.
- Sutureless corneal wound hydration prevents pathogen influx into AC, decreasing the risk of endophthalmitis.

Molecular studies have confirmed that most intraocular infections are caused by organisms from the patient's own eyelids. Therefore, patients with significant blepharitis or meibomianitis should be treated aggressively before surgery, as meibomian glands can be colonized by bacteria. Similarly, patients with acne rosacea or seborrheic dermatitis should receive systemic doxycycline preoperatively to reduce the risk of bacterial contamination in the operative field.

20.3.6.2 Not Proven Measures

The use of antibiotics pre-op or post-op has not been proven to reduce the risk of endophthalmitis, in addition to its use within the irrigation bottle.

The European Premed study showed that the NSAID Bromfenac is most useful to reduce macular edema after cataract surgery compared to the steroid dexamethasone, while the combination is most useful.

Reference: European multicenter trial of the prevention of cystoid macular edema after cataract surgery in nondiabetics: ESCRS PREMED study report 1

20.3.7 Ophthalmic Viscosurgical Devices (OVDs)

What most viscoelastic agents have in common is that they are solutions of long-chain biopolymers. OVDs contain one or more of the following substances in varying concentrations:

- Sodium hyaluronate: half-life of approximately 1 day in aqueous and 3 days in vitreous
- Chondroitin sulfate
- Hydroxypropyl methylcellulose

Table 20.3 Comparison between cohesive, adaptive, dispersive ophthalmic viscosurgical devices

	Cohesive	Adaptive (both functions)	Dispersive
Composition	Long chain, high molecular weight	Medium molecular weight	Short chain, low molecular weight
Composition	Sodium hyaluronate		Chondroitin sulfate + hydroxypropyl methyl cellulose
Examples	Healon, Amvisc, Provisc	Discovisc	Viscot, OcuCoat
Viscosity	Higher viscosity	Moderate viscosity	Lower viscosity
Function	Create space and induce and sustain pressure	–	Prolonged retention with high coatability (so protects endothelium) and partition spaces
Coating ability (surface tension)	Low		High
Removability	Easily aspirated		Difficult, so might be retained in the eye
Uses	Pupil dilatation, maintain AC		Protect cornea, coat a PCR to prevent vitreous prolapse

Important properties for OVDs (Table 20.3):

Viscosity refers to fluid resistance to flow, essentially describing its "thickness" or "thinness." Viscosity is primarily determined by the fluid's molecular weight and concentration.

Elasticity is the ability of a material to maintain space and its shape and return to its original shape after being stressed.

Pseudoplasticity: In clinical terms, this describes how an OVD behaves under different conditions. At zero shear force, an OVD acts as a lubricant and coats tissues well. However, when forced through a small-gauge cannula, it behaves like a liquid. This property allows the OVD to transform from a gel to a liquid under pressure. **Surface tension** (coatability) describes how a fluid's surface tends to adhere to another surface. This property is inversely related to surface tension; thus, an OVD with low surface tension coats tissues better but is harder to remove from the eye.

Incomplete removal of the viscoelastic agent can, in some cases, lead to problems with elevated intraocular pressures, but not corneal endothelial cell loss.

OVDs produce significant pressure elevations at 4 ± 1 h postoperatively.

3% Sodium hyaluronate (HA) and 4% sodium chondroitin sulfate (CS) are used as dispersive ophthalmic viscosurgical devices.

Most viscoelastic agents have in common the fact that they are solutions of long-chain biopolymers.

20.4 Cataract Surgery Complications

20.4.1 Intraoperative

Posterior capsular rupture: Marked by a sudden deepening and momentary pupillary dilatation. Vitreous in AC can be stained via triamcinolone.

20.4.1.1 Loss of Lens Fragments or IOL

Suprachoroidal hemorrhage (aka expulsive hemorrhage) (0.04%)**:** Bleeding into the suprachoroidal space from a ruptured posterior ciliary artery (not vein). It is marked by partial loss of red reflux and associated with severe pain and agitation and a rise in IOP. The most important part of immediate management is quick closure of the wound ASAP. Clinically, suprachoroidal effusion may be difficult to differentiate from suprachoroidal hemorrhage. It is mostly seen in large wound open surgeries that lead to hypotony, with the presence of associated hypertension.

Phaco corneal wound burn: This occurs due to failure of phaco tip cooling, which can be by a plug on the irrigation port. Higher frequency with bimanual technique as the ultrasound tip has no overlaying cooling.

AC flattening: This could be due to leakage from the wound, extensive pressure from behind the lens (e.g., anxiety), fluid misdirection to vitreous from ruptured PC, or suprachoroidal hemorrhage (checked by red reflux loss):

- A shallow or flat anterior chamber in the immediate postoperative period may be associated with a low or high intraocular pressure (IOP).
- A low IOP with shallow AC: wound leak, retinal detachment, or cyclodialysis cleft.
- High IOP with shallow AC:
  - If shallow AC centrally and peripherally → Aqueous misdirection.
  - If shallow AC only peripherally → Pupillary block.

20.4.2 Postoperative

Corneal edema: It can be either epithelial or stromal epithelial edema and typically resolves within 4–6 weeks after surgery, particularly if the corneal periphery remains clear. In contrast, stromal edema, which results from endothelial loss, often does not resolve and can lead to bullous keratopathy. Persistent corneal edema beyond 3 months is unlikely to clear. Treatment options include hyperosmotic agents and steroids, with surgical intervention like keratectomy, cross-linking, and finally endothelial keratoplasty or full-thickness keratoplasty considered if medical therapy is insufficient.

Endothelial loss: Studies on endothelial cell loss following cataract surgery have shown average losses of 20% with anterior chamber phacoemulsification, 14% with posterior chamber phacoemulsification, 7% with extracapsular cataract extraction (ECCE), and 4% with intracapsular cataract extraction. Superior clear-corneal incisions tend to result in more endothelial cell loss (average 15%) compared to temporal incisions (average 7%). This difference is attributed to the fact that superior incisions are closer to the central endothelium, while temporal incisions are more peripheral and posterior.

Phaco done below the anterior capsule is presumed to have minimal impact on endothelial loss.

High IOP: It is mostly due to retained OVD, which peaks 4–6 h post-op; if more than 40, a gentle pressure on the paracentesis wound (never from the main wound!) to release it from the eye might be successful. If lower than 40, go for topical hypotensive medications.

Endophthalmitis (0.1%): Acute endophthalmitis, occurring within the first 6 weeks after surgery, is most commonly caused by staph epidermis and aureus. Chronic endophthalmitis, which develops several months post-surgery, is often caused by *P. acnes*, *S. epidermidis*, and *Candida*, though other organisms like *P. granulosum*, *Achromobacter*, and *Corynebacterium*, have also been reported.

Diagnosing endophthalmitis can be challenging. If inflammation signs are mild, a trial of topical steroid therapy with an early follow-up (6–24 h) is appropriate. If there is no significant improvement, endophthalmitis management should be considered. This includes a vitreous tap for culture followed by intravitreal antibiotic (ceftazidime and vancomycin). If VA is above LP, this procedure can be performed in the clinic; however, immediate PPV is reserved for vision of LP or worse. Delayed-onset endophthalmitis, developing after 4 weeks, often involves low virulence organisms like *P. acnes*, which can become trapped within the capsular bag, leading to mild-to-moderate inflammation. In such cases, a trial of topical antibiotic may be beneficial before more aggressive treatments such as IOL and bag removal, secondary IOL implantation, and intravitreal antibiotics. The main ddx is TASS. Endogenous endophthalmitis is bilateral in 25% of cases. For fluid samples from suspected endophthalmitis cases, at least 0.2 mL of liquid vitreous should be collected. Preventive measures include using 5% (half concentration) iodine-povidone on the conjunctiva before surgery and administering intracameral cephalosporins at the end of surgery.

Note: Temporal incision has been associated with a higher risk of endophthalmitis. Most isolates are Gram-positive (about 90%), and 10% Gram-negative, with *Staphylococcus epidermidis* being the most common, typically originating from eyelid and conjunctival flora.

Studies indicate a higher incidence of endophthalmitis with clear corneal incisions, although the exact mechanism remains unclear.

Posterior capsular opacity (PCO): PCO is the most common late complication of cataract surgery, affecting about 25% of patients. The incidence of PCO is reduced when the capsulorhexis opening is in complete contact with the anterior surface of the IOL. PCO is treated via YAG capsulotomy, with proposed maximum energy of 80 mJ. It is not related to post-op steroids or other medications. The type of IOL can influence the rate of PCO development, with hydrogel IOLs having the highest incidence, followed by PMMA, silicone, and hydrophobic acrylic materials leading to the lowest rate. IOL shape also plays a significant role; truncated-edge designs are associated with lower rates of PCO in both silicone and acrylic IOLs, although these lenses may increase the incidence of unwanted optical reflections and positive dysphotopsias.

Capsular phimosis: It is the circumferential fibrosis of anterior capsule, leading to glare mostly at night, and may displace IOL. It can be managed by YAG.

CME (aka Irvine-Gass syndrome) occurs usually 6–10 weeks post-op and is managed by topical NSAIDs and steroids four times daily, which may take 3 months usually. Sub-tenon steroid might be considered in chronic cases. Topical use of NSAIDs post-op alone or combined with steroid reduces its incidence better than steroid alone. So, corticosteroids and NSAIDs are the mainstay of treatment for routine postoperative CME. Discontinuing prostaglandin analogue might also be helpful. In resistant cases, consider oral acetazolamide and anti-VEGF. Clinical CME is present in 5% of patients, and FFA evidence of CME is present <40% of the time.

Toxic anterior segment syndrome (TASS): It is an acute sterile postoperative inflammation. TASS presents within hours of surgery, whereas acute infectious endophthalmitis typically develops 2–7 days postoperatively. TASS is limited to AC and treated with extensive steroids. If endophthalmitis cannot be ruled out, it is treated as endophthalmitis.

Retained vitreous in AC: Which might lead to raised IOP, corneal edema, iris distortion, or a band might stick to the wound acting as a wick that leads to pathogens entering the eye.

Rhegmatogenous retinal detachment: Occurs most frequently up to 1 year post-op.

IOL sublimation or dislocation: most commonly on top of PXF.

Uveitis-glaucoma-hyphema (UGH) syndrome or Ellingson syndrome is a mechanical irritation of AC from intraocular lens (IOL), mostly with ACIOL and less commonly with sulcus and other lenses. It occurs mostly within the first 6 months of surgery. Common manifestations include mild-moderate uveitis, pigmentary dispersion to micro-hyphemas and hyphemas, and elevated intraocular pressure (IOP). It can also be characterized by chronic inflammation, cystoid macular edema (CME), secondary iris neovascularization, recurrent hyphemas, and glaucomatous optic neuropathy. Surgical IOL exchange is often required as definitive treatment. Upside-down placement of IOLs might also lead to severe ocular inflammation. Single-piece IOL should not be placed in the sulcus, as it might be unstable and lead to UGH syndrome.

Cataract surgery, using routine phacoemulsification and in-the-bag IOL on an urgent basis, is the best course of therapy.

Epithelial ingrowth: It is the epithelial proliferation over the corneal endothelium or any surface. Elevated IOP can be a sign, and whitening on argon laser may confirm the Dx.

Corneal decompensation may result from long-term shallow AC.

Postoperative capsular block syndrome is caused by a trapped viscoelastic or aqueous fluid behind an IOL in an intact capsular bag, leading to a large space between the IOL and the posterior capsule. The posterior capsular distention pushes the IOL forward, uniformly shallows the anterior chamber, and causes a myopic refractive shift. The anterior chamber narrowing can lead to a rise in IOP. Aqueous misdirection also leads to a uniformly shallow anterior chamber with an anteriorly displaced IOL. This condition can also cause elevated IOP. Neither aqueous misdirection nor capsular block syndrome is associated with peripheral choroidal detachment.

Ptosis: 10% of cataract surgeries are complicated by ptosis, which is acutely related to edematous changes. However, the chronic persistent form is the one that needs management. Causes of persistent or chronic ptosis usually involve damage (either chemical by anesthesia or mechanical) to the levator aponeurosis or scarring to the levator complex.

It is managed by mullerectomy for mild 1–2 mm cases. If more severe ptosis, the etiology is usually dehiscence of levator, manifesting as increased lid crease height and a superior sulcus defect secondary to retraction of the preaponeurotic fat pad. This should be managed by levator resection (aka advancement).

Dysphotopsia can be classified as follows:

- Positive dysphotopsia (PD) is characterized by bright light artifacts, such as arcs, streaks, starbursts, rings, or halos that appear centrally or mid-peripherally in the visual field. It is commonly associated with decentered PCIOLs of all types.

Negative dysphotopsia (ND) refers to the absence of light on a portion of the retina, presenting as a dark, temporal arcing shadow. This phenomenon occurs when light rays entering the eye from the temporal periphery interact with the nasal edge of a well-centered IOL in the capsular bag, casting a shadow (penumbra) on the nasal retina. Negative dysphotopsia is observed with all types of IOLs placed in the capsular bag but is most frequently seen with smaller, square-edge optic designs. Negative dysphotopsia does not occur with ACIOLs.

20.4.2.1 Endothelial Cell Loss

The site of phacoemulsification significantly influences endothelial cell loss, with losses increasing as the proximity to the endothelium decreases. The average cell loss is 20% for anterior chamber procedures, 14% for posterior chamber procedures, 7% for in situ phacoemulsification, and 4% for intracapsular extraction. Extracapsular extraction has been associated with an average cell loss of about 7%, similar to that seen with in situ phacoemulsification.

Furthermore, superior clear-corneal incisions have shown greater cell loss, averaging 15% compared to temporal incisions, which average 7%.

Eyes with very high axial lengths are at risk for **lens–iris diaphragm retropulsion syndrome (LIDRS)**, in which a reverse pupillary block occurs, and the anterior chamber becomes very deep, causing pain. Eyes with lax zonular fibers are more prone to this issue. Lifting the iris off the capsule with a second instrument and lowering the infusion bottle might help correct this problem.

Toxic anterior segment syndrome (TASS) usually manifests within hours of surgery, while infectious endophthalmitis typically develops 2–7 days after the procedure.

Risk factors for **expulsive choroidal hemorrhage** include myopia, glaucoma, atherosclerotic vascular disease, hypertension, and previous expulsive hemorrhage in the opposite eye.

Statistically significant risk factors for suprachoroidal expulsive hemorrhage, according to an age-adjusted analysis, include glaucoma, increased axial length, elevated intraocular pressure, generalized atherosclerosis, and elevated intraoperative pulse.

In classical teaching, IOL implantation is contraindicated in **pediatric patients with uveitis** (active or inactive), especially patients with juvenile rheumatoid arthritis-associated iridocyclitis. For further details:

- If IOL is inserted during active inflammation, patients will have poor visual recovery, severe inflammatory sequelae, and sight-threatening complications if an IOL is inserted.
- If patients have stable uveitis without activities for >3 months, insufficient evidence with or against IOL implantation.

The long-term **sequela of a postoperative shallow or flat anterior chamber** is corneal decompensation.

In patients with a **prior history of pars plana vitrectomy**, excessive mobility of the posterior capsule is expected during cataract surgery, increasing complication rates.

YAG capsulotomy: It is better if delayed to allow fusion in the peripheral capsule and prevent vitreous prolapse and to decrease the risk of CMO and RD (preferably 6 months).

The association between Nd:YAG capsulotomy and development of RD includes several risk factors: longer axial length, myopia, a history of RD or lattice degeneration, younger age, and ocular trauma following cataract surgery. Gender does not appear to be a risk factor.

A large, prospective cohort study found no increased risk of hemorrhagic complications in **patients** undergoing cataract surgery while **on anticoagulant or antiplatelet therapy**.

Sunrise syndrome, also known as superior subluxation of an intraocular lens, occurs when one haptic of the lens is positioned in the capsular bag and the other in the ciliary sulcus.

Posterior iris chafing by the loop or the optic portion of sulcus-fixated posterior chamber lens implants can lead to various issues, including iris-pigment epithelial defects, pigment dispersions with or without intraocular pressure elevation, intermittent micro-hyphemas with transient visual obscurations, and uveitis-glaucoma-hyphema (UGH) syndrome.

The primary cause of **phaco burn** is occlusion of the phaco tip, which impedes or halts fluid evacuation through the phaco handpiece. This leads to an accumulation of heat within the handpiece and subsequently transfers thermal energy to the incision. To prevent phaco burn, measures include using lower ultrasound power, aspirating of OVD, employing more easily aspirated cohesive OVDs, increasing aspiration flow rates and vacuum levels, and ensuring a loose fit between the phaco handpiece and the incision. These strategies enhance fluid flow through the handpiece and/or the incision, reducing thermal energy transfer.

Posterior infusion syndrome is a rare complication occurring during cataract surgery, characterized by shallowing of the anterior chamber not in the postoperative period. It typically happens during hydrodissection when fluid is misdirected into the vitreous cavity, causing forward displacement of the lens.

PCO has two forms:

- Fibrous: involves abnormal proliferation of lens epithelial cells (LECs) and is characterized by wrinkles and folds on the posterior capsule where the anterior and posterior capsules fuse. Histological examination typically reveals extracellular matrix (ECM) accumulation and elongated fibroblast cells.

Pearl (also referred to as proliferative): It is made up of normally differentiated LECs lining the equatorial lens region. It presents as clusters of swollen, opacified, and differentiated LECs, known as bladder or Wedl cells. This form is responsible for the majority of visual loss associated with PCO. In piggyback IOL, **interlenticular membranes** have been reported to occur between two acrylic IOLs, especially when both lenses are implanted in the capsular bag. The preferred treatment is to remove the IOLs.

Acknowledgments None.

Conflict of Interest None.

References

Bowen RC, Zhou AX, Bondalapati S, Lawyer TW, Snow KB, Evans PR, Bardsley T, McFarland M, Kliethermes M, Shi D, Mamalis CA, Greene T, Rudnisky CJ, Ambati BK (2018) Comparative analysis of the safety and efficacy of intracameral cefuroxime, moxifloxacin and vancomycin at the end of cataract surgery: a meta-analysis. Br J Ophthalmol 102(9):1268–1276. https://doi.org/10.1136/bjophthalmol-2017-311051. Epub 2018 Jan 11. PMID: 29326317; PMCID: PMC6041193

Infant Aphakia Treatment Study Group, Lambert SR, Buckley EG, Drews-Botsch C, DuBois L, Hartmann E, Lynn MJ, Plager DA, Wilson ME (2010) The infant aphakia treatment study: design and clinical measures at enrollment. Arch Ophthalmol 128(1):21–27. https://

doi.org/10.1001/archophthalmol.2009.350. PMID: 20065212; PMCID: PMC2983098

Lee JY, Lee EK, Lee HJ, Jeong J, Lee SY, Kim JY (2018) Postoperative hemorrhagic occlusive retinal vasculitis with intracameral vancomycin. Korean J Ophthalmol 32(5):430–431. https://doi.org/10.3341/kjo.2018.0043. PMID: 30311469; PMCID: PMC6182214

Liu C, Bardan AS (eds) (2021) Cataract surgery: pearls and techniques. Springer Nature

21 Clinical Review of Cataract and Power Calculation: Part II

Mutasem Elfalah, Saif Aldeen Alryalat, Mohammad Elfalah, and Kenneth Hoffer

Abstract

This chapter delves into the critical aspects of intraocular lenses (IOLs) used in cataract surgery. It begins with a detailed classification of IOLs, addressing their focality and the specific sites for lens placement, which are essential for achieving optimal visual outcomes. The chapter further explores the intricacies of IOL power calculation, an important step in ensuring proper lens selection tailored to individual patient needs. Additionally, it discusses lens dislocation and subluxation, highlighting their causes, implications, and management strategies. The chapter also examines congenital cataracts, providing insights into their etiology and treatment options. Lastly, miscellaneous topics such as ectopic lentis, IOL tenting, decentration, and axial movement are addressed, enhancing the understanding of various complications and considerations in IOL management. This comprehensive overview prepares readers with vital knowledge for successful cataract surgery and IOL implantation.

Keywords

Intraocular lens · Power calculation
Congenital cataract · Miscellaneous · Lens dislocation

M. Elfalah
Department of Ophthalmology, The University of Jordan, Amman, Jordan
e-mail: M.Alrabie@ju.edu.jo

S. A. Alryalat (✉)
Department of Ophthalmology, The University of Jordan, Amman, Jordan

The University of Colorado Anschutz Medical Campus, Aurora, CO, USA

M. Elfalah
School of Medicine, The University of Jordan, Amman, Jordan

K. Hoffer
The University of California, Los Angeles, CA, USA
e-mail: khoffermd@startmail.com

21.1 Intraocular Lenses

References for this chapter include the American Academy of Ophthalmology resources in addition to several specific ones (Liu and Bardan 2021; Infant Aphakia Treatment Study Group 2010; Lee et al. 2018; Bowen et al. 2018).

21.1.1 Intraocular Lens Classifications

Intraocular lenses (IOLs) can be classified based on multiple parameters including material, design, haptic flexibility, and additional features. This classification helps us understand the varying characteristics and applications of these lenses.

S. A. Alryalat (ed.), *Ophthalmology Board and FRCS Part 2 Exams*,
https://doi.org/10.1007/978-981-96-1517-9_21

21.1.1.1 Classification Based on Design

- Single-piece design: IOLs of this type are made from a single material. They offer ease of insertion and are widely used.
- Multipiece design: Typically referred to as three-piece lenses, these are constructed with separate optic and haptic components. The haptics, or the support structure, is made from a different material than the optic, or the lens, itself.

21.1.1.2 Classification Based on Haptic Flexibility

- Flexible: These lenses have haptics that can fold, facilitating insertion via injectors. They are available in multiple materials.
- Rigid: These IOLs require a larger incision for insertion, typically 5 or 6 mm. Rigid lenses are only available in polymethylmethacrylate (PMMA) material.

21.1.1.3 Classification Based on Hydrophilic vs. Hydrophobic

These terms are determined by the angle a water drop forms on the lens surface. Hydrophobic materials result in a more obtuse angle, while hydrophilic materials create a more acute contact angle.

- Hydrophilic IOLs are deemed more biocompatible due to their lower risk of uveitis, though they are generally thicker and carry a higher risk of posterior capsule opacification (PCO).
- Hydrophobic IOLs (water content <1%), while thinner and less susceptible to PCO, might carry a higher risk of uveitis due to their reduced biocompatibility. They have a greater refractive index than hydrophilic lenses and are consequently thinner, though this can result in dysphotopsia.

The hydrophilic or hydrophobic nature of an IOL has implications for individuals with a history of ocular inflammation, such as uveitis. Since the lens is surrounded by aqueous humor, hydrophilic materials, which attract water, may be more compatible than hydrophobic materials in eyes with uveitis.

To summarize, IOL can be:

Hydrophilic: More biocompatible, so lower risk of uveitis, but generally thicker. More risk of PCO
Hydrophobic: Less biocompatible, so higher risk of uveitis, but generally thinner. Lower risk of PCO

21.1.1.4 Classification Based on Material (Table 21.1)

- Polymethylmethacrylate (PMMA) IOL (hydrophobic): PMMA was the first material introduced for IOLs. It is economical and reliable, although it is associated with higher posterior capsule opacification (PCO) rates and an increased incidence of uveitis. Heparin-coated PMMA IOLs are hydrophilic, exhibiting lower immunogenicity.

Table 21.1 Comparison of different characteristics between available intraocular lens (IOL) materials

	PMMA	Silicon	Hydrophobic acrylic	Hydrophilic acrylic
Refractive index	1.49	1.41–1.46	Up to 1.53	1.43
Thickness[a]	Moderate	Thickest	Thinnest	Thick
Optic diameter	5–7 mm	5.5–6.5 mm	5.5–7 mm	5.5–7 mm
Foldable	No	Yes	Yes	Yes
PCO	Highest	Moderate	Lowest	Low
Contrast sensitivity	Highest	Moderate	Lowest	Lowest
Dysphotopsia		Low	High (higher)	High (lesser)
Notes[b]		Higher risk of postoperative infections and silicon oil adhesion	Less biocompatible	More biocompatible

[a]A higher refractive index means the lens can be made thinner for an equivalent power
[b]All above absorb UV light

- Acrylic IOL (hydrophilic or hydrophobic): Acrylic IOLs are more biocompatible, but have a higher PCO incidence. Hydrophobic acrylic IOLs (with water content <1%) have a higher refractive index than hydrophilic lenses, making them thinner. However, this could cause dysphotopsia and trigger a stronger reaction in eyes with uveitis.
- Silicone IOL (hydrophobic): These are available in loop haptic (one- or three-piece) and plate haptic (one-piece) designs. Silicone IOLs exhibit greater biocompatibility than hydrophobic acrylic IOLs, but can cause problems in silicone oil-filled eyes. They are not recommended for patients with uveitis nor in patients planned for pars plana vitrectomy with silicon implantation.
- Collamer IOL: These collagen-based IOLs are principally marketed based on their high biocompatibility.

21.1.1.5 Classification Based on Additional Features

- Sharp (square) edge optic (based on the original Hoffer ridge principle): This design lowers the incidence of PCO but might lead to a higher rate of dysphotopsia.
- Blue light filters: These additional filters minimize retinal damage caused by light.
- Aspheric optic: This feature decreases corneal spherical aberrations.
- Heparin coating: This coating decreases the immunogenicity of IOLs.

Dysphotopsia represents an annoying visual phenomenon. Round-edged IOLs and silicone material IOLs may be less liable to result in dysphotopsia than acrylic IOLs and square edges. A square optic edge appears to inhibit PCO, though it may have a higher rate of dysphotopsia.

The higher the refractive error, the lower the thickness, with acrylic having the highest refractive index:

Refractive index:

Silicon < PMMA < acrylic

Thickness:

Acrylic < PMMA < silicon

Example: A 6-mm-diameter optic with a biconvex shape and 21 diopters of power has different thickness depending on the material: 0.75 mm with an acrylic, 0.93 mm with PMMA, 1.27 mm with hydroxyethylmethacrylate (HEMA), and 1.82 mm with first-generation silicone.

21.1.2 Focality of IOL

Intraocular lenses (IOLs), integral components in cataract surgery and vision correction procedures, come in various designs intended to address a range of visual needs and conditions. The focality of an IOL, or its focusing capability, is one of the key factors that determine its functionality and the quality of vision it provides.

21.1.2.1 Monofocal Lenses

Monofocal intraocular lenses are the traditional form of IOLs that have been used in cataract surgery for decades. These lenses have a single focal point, generally set for clear distance vision. While they provide excellent clarity for distance tasks such as driving or watching television, they usually require the patient to wear reading glasses for near-vision tasks, as they do not adjust or "accommodate" to different distances. Monofocal lenses are widely regarded for their visual quality and minimal visual disturbances, such as glare and halos.

21.1.2.2 Accommodative Lenses

Accommodative IOLs are a relatively new class of lenses designed to mimic the eye's natural ability to change focus, or "accommodate," from distant to near objects. They do this by changing shape or position within the eye, in response to the focusing muscles in the eye. This means that these lenses can potentially provide a range of vision—distance, intermediate, and near—without the need for glasses. However, the effectiveness of accommodative IOLs can vary depending on individual factors such as the health of the eye's focusing muscle. Additionally, their accommodative performance tends to decrease over time, so some patients may still require glasses for certain tasks.

21.1.2.3 Toric Lenses

Toric IOLs are specifically designed to correct regular astigmatism, a condition where the cornea is more oval than round, leading to blurry vision at all distances. The positioning of the toric IOL is critical as it needs to align with the patient's astigmatism for optimal correction. More than 90% of toric IOLs generally remain within 30 degrees off the intended axis. If the IOL rotates between 30 and 40 degrees, it essentially functions like a spherical IOL, while rotation of more than 40 degrees can induce astigmatism in another axis.

21.1.2.4 Multifocal Lenses

Multifocal IOLs (MIOLs) aim to provide a broader range of vision—near, intermediate, and far—by incorporating multiple focus points within the lens. They come in two primary forms: refractive and diffractive. Refractive MIOLs typically offer superior distance vision, whereas diffractive MIOLs excel in providing near vision and reading ability, along with equivalent intermediate vision. They also reduce unwanted photic phenomena and tend to offer a higher degree of spectacle independence. However, one drawback is that all multifocal lenses can potentially cause visual disturbances like halos. Although most patients experience a decrease in such symptoms over several months due to neuroadaptation, persistent and disruptive halos may necessitate an IOL exchange to a monofocal lens.

21.1.3 Site of IOL Placement

The placement of the intraocular lens (IOL) during surgery is a vital aspect that determines the success of the procedure and the visual outcomes. Depending on the clinical scenario and specific patient conditions, an IOL can be placed in different locations within the eye. These include the posterior chamber in-bag placement, posterior chamber scleral suture, sulcus placement, anterior chamber, and anterior chamber iris fixated.

21.1.3.1 Posterior Chamber In-Bag Placement

Posterior chamber in-bag placement is a common technique for intraocular lens (IOL) implantation. It involves positioning the IOL in the capsular bag, which is the natural lens envelope remaining after cataract extraction. This method mimics the natural positioning of the human lens and is usually preferred for its stability and low complication rate. In addition, this method reduces the risk of posterior capsule opacification, as the lens is entirely surrounded by the capsule, thus limiting cell migration. However, the successful in-bag placement demands the integrity of the capsular bag during surgery, which may be compromised in cases of posterior capsule rupture or zonular weakness.

21.1.3.2 Sulcus Placement

The sulcus is the area between the iris base and ciliary body, and it has 12 mm in diameter, requiring 14 mm length lenses to be stable there. This means that placing the usual PCIOL lenses in sulcus will result in unstable lenses (i.e., will be easily rotated and moved), which also means that you cannot put a toric lens in sulcus. Sulcus placement of an intraocular lens (IOL) is usually not a preferred option for surgeons, but certain intraoperative circumstances may necessitate it. This placement is typically considered when there is zonular dehiscence, severe pseudoexfoliation, an unstable capsular bag, or subluxation. The main methods for sulcus placement are optic capture and suturing. The optic capture method is often chosen when the posterior capsule cannot support the IOL but the anterior capsule remains intact. This method ensures long-term stability only when the anterior capsule allows the optic to be captured into the bag. If optic capture is not feasible, the IOL may eventually decenter. Suturing is an alternative when there is insufficient support in the sulcus, such as in cases of zonular loss or absence of an anterior capsular rim. In these situations, the haptics can be sutured to the iris or sclera to provide additional support and stability. The choice of lens is also crucial, with three-piece lenses being preferred over single-piece lenses for sulcus placement due to their thinner haptics, posterior vaulting, and rigidity. Finally, power adjustment of the IOL is necessary when moving the lens forward inside the eye, where the sulcus is 0.5 mm anterior to posterior bag, so requiring around 0.5–1D reduction for PCIOL with PCIOL powers 17–27D (see IOL power calculation).

A scleral-sutured IOL is preferred for its low complication rates, significantly reducing the risk of corneal endothelial loss and CME from iris irritation. An acrylic posterior-chamber IOL with Prolene haptics is the ideal choice for ciliary sulcus placement. In contrast, plate silicone lenses and one-piece acrylic posterior-chamber IOLs are specifically designed for in-the-bag placement. The ciliary sulcus is located approximately 0.85 mm posterior to the limbus in the horizontal meridian and 0.45 mm posterior to the vertical meridian. The needle should be inserted about 0.75 mm posterior to the limbus. To minimize the risk of damaging the long ciliary arteries and nerves, which typically run in the vertical meridian, an oblique needle insertion at the 2 o'clock and 8 o'clock or 10 o'clock and 4 o'clock positions is recommended.

21.1.3.3 Anterior Chamber Placement

Anterior chamber placement involves inserting the IOL in the anterior part of the eye, in front of the iris, and just behind the cornea. This method is typically used when posterior placement is not possible due to reasons like insufficient posterior capsular or zonular support. Anterior chamber IOLs are specially designed to avoid contact with the cornea and the angle structures, thereby reducing potential complications. However, despite these precautions, anterior chamber placement can have potential risks, such as corneal endothelial cell loss, glaucoma, and inflammation, due to the proximity of the lens to the cornea and iris. It is essential to carefully evaluate the risk-benefit ratio when considering anterior chamber IOL placement. Regular patient monitoring post-operation is necessary to manage any potential complications.

In iris fixation, the haptic claws can be clamped to anterior iris, which is easier but carries a higher endothelial cell loss, or posterior iris. The haptics of iris fixation lenses are designed as pincers or claws that grasp the immobile part of the peripheral iris. This design helps to avoid the difficulties in pupil dilation commonly encountered with iris clip lenses and allows for excellent fundus visualization. One particular concern with all types of anterior chamber lens is a reduction in corneal endothelial cell density. Another concern is angle closure, so ACIOL patients should undergo regular gonioscopy to confirm the position of haptics, in addition to pachymetry and specular microscopy.

Notes

Following complicated cataract surgery, predominantly after posterior capsule rupture, the following options are available: Sulcus placement if capsular support is available. If no capsular support, consider trans-scleral fixation (via either sutured scleral fixation or Yamane ISHF), anterior chamber, or iris fixation (e.g., via iris claws).

21.1.4 IOL Power Calculation

Intraocular lens (IOL) power calculation is critical to preoperative cataract surgery planning. Estimating IOL power requires optimizing three key elements: biometric measurements, devices used, and choice of the IOL power calculation formula (or method).

Biometric measurements: Three core parameters are pivotal to optimal IOL power estimation: axial length (AL), keratometry (K), and IOL lens constant.

- Axial length: The main parameter for IOL calculation is the AL, which can be measured via ultrasound (immersion only; do not use contact) or optical methods. Optical methods are generally more accurate and repeatable. It is important to be sure that the instrument gives an approval of the reading. The difference between both eyes should not exceed 0.3, unless explanation exists (e.g., prior surgery or anisometropia).

- Keratometry: The second most important parameter is keratometry (aka corneal power), including the power at the flattest and steepest meridians (K1 and K2). Conventional methods include manual keratometers and old corneal topography that assumes the cornea to be part of a perfect sphere, obtains several points on the curvature, and estimates both anterior and posterior corneal powers. This estimation in patients who underwent laser refractive surgeries is not accurate, as the corneal curvatures are asymmetrical now, and the estimation becomes inaccurate, leading to hyperopic refractive surprise. Newer tomographers are better suited due to their ability to directly measure, rather than estimate, corneal powers.

IOL lens constant: This is somewhat misleading, as it is actually subject to considerable variability. It depends on several factors including the type, material, and position of the IOL; the surgeon's technique and placement of the incision; adjustments in keratometry (K) and axial length (AL) measurements; and the method used for biometry. The most accurate results are achieved when the constant is optimized for a specific IOL and surgical technique.

Additional measurements like anterior chamber depth (ACD, measured from corneal epithelium to lens), lens thickness (LT), horizontal corneal diameter (CD), and central corneal thickness (CCT) can further enhance the accuracy of IOL calculations, particularly in certain cases.

Keratometry in patients with prior refractive surgeries such as radial keratotomy (RK) or corneal laser refractive procedures poses unique challenges in determining IOL power. Traditional methods like manual keratometry often lead to a hyperopic outcome. To better estimate IOL power for these patients, the use of computerized videokeratography (CVK) values at the 1 and 2 mm zones is recommended. It is noteworthy to mention that these patients do not exhibit a higher likelihood of irregular astigmatism or myopia post-cataract extraction compared to those without previous refractive surgeries. Further, no change in AL calculation is required post-RK for IOL power estimation.

21.1.4.1 Devices

IOL calculation can be performed using optical or ultrasound methods, which can further be done by direct contact or immersion.

- Optical methods: These utilize various laser technologies, with the most recent advancement being Swept Source OCT (SS-OCT). There are over 13 different companies producing optical biometers, offering the benefits of noncontact procedures along and greater accuracy. However, these methods may be less accurate or difficult to use in cases of very dense cataracts.
- Ultrasound methods: This approach can be performed through direct contact or immersion techniques. Contact ultrasound measurements are more prone to subjective errors due to potential corneal compression. The immersion method, on the other hand, avoids corneal compression, measuring axial length (AL) based on the speed at which sound travels through the different intraocular media.
- Adjustments must be made to AL calculations for eyes filled with silicone oil to avoid large errors in AL measurement. It is best to use optical methods in these eyes.

21.1.4.2 Formula

IOL calculation formulas can be broadly categorized into three generations, each employing more complex mathematics and incorporating a greater number of biometric variables to improve the precision of IOL power prediction.

First-Generation Formulas

First-generation formulas, such as the Fyodorov ('67), Colenbrander ('73), Hoffer ('74), and Binkhorst ('75), used basic thin lens optics and a single lens constant (ACD) for all IOLs and all eyes. The SRK I introduced the use of regression formulas.

Second-Generation Formulas

Second-generation formulas were introduced by Hoffer with his Hoffer ACD/AL formula followed by Binkhorst 2 and SRK II which varied the ACD lens constant based on the AL.

Third-Generation Formulas

Third-generation formulas were introduced by Holladay using both K and AL to predict the "ACD" (or estimated lens position (ELP)) in his Holladay 1 formula. This was followed by the SRK/T and the Hoffer Q (using the tangent of K for ELP prediction):

1. All three formulas performed well in normal AL eyes (22–24.5 mm).
2. Hoffer Q was shown more accurate for short eyes (<22 mm axial length).
3. Holladay 1 provides excellent results in medium long eyes (24.5–26 mm).

SRK/T showed better results in very long AL eyes (>26 mm)

Fourth-Generation Formulas

These formulas represent the addition of multiple factors to predict ELP. They were initiated by Olsen and followed by Holladay with his Holladay 2 formula incorporating multiple variables to predict ELP. They consider additional factors like lens thickness, corneal diameter, and even preoperative lens position.

1. Holladay 2: Requires more parameters but provides excellent results, particularly for short ALs but not better than Holladay 1 in all other ALs.
2. Olsen 4 factor: This formula incorporates four factors, including lens thickness, and performs well across a range of ALs.
3. Barrett Universal II: A robust formula that performs well across all ALs.

Despite their complexity, the third-generation formulas have been incorporated into most biometers, making them accessible for everyday use.

21.1.4.3 Artificial Intelligence Formulas

The future of IOL calculation may lie in artificial intelligence (AI) and machine learning. These technologies can learn from large datasets of patient outcomes, potentially creating formulas with even greater accuracy than currently possible.

Hoffer and Savini showed that gender and race play a significant part in human biometry.

1. Kane: incorporated gender in his formula.
2. EVO formula.
3. Radial basis function (RBF).
4. Pearl-DGS.
5. Hoffer QST gender was incorporated in this update of the Hoffer Q using AI.

It is essential to remember that IOL power calculations are just predictions, and individual patient outcomes may still vary. Careful preoperative measurements, meticulous surgery, appropriate formula selection based on the patient's unique ocular characteristics, and postoperative refraction checks to fine-tune future calculations are all crucial components of achieving the best possible refractive outcomes.

Remember that formulas commonly differ by 0.5–1 diopters, and the least accurate and the most accurate formulas in regular patients do not differ much.

Notes

In patients planned for simultaneous IOL and silicone oil implantation, certain considerations are essential:

- Choice of formula: Regression formulas in eyes filled with silicone oil yield an average of 4.0 D of hyperopic shift due to the oil acting as a minus lens in the eye.
- Choice of IOL type: Consider using a convex-plano IOL, as this lens configuration eliminates some of the reduction in power of the posterior surface that occurs with biconvex or plano-convex IOLs. A meniscus lens eliminates this factor but is no longer produced. This IOL type also minimizes the change in refraction if silicone is later removed.
- AL measurement: Silicone oil in the vitreous cavity can lead to falsely long AL measurement by A-scan biometry due to slower ultrasound velocity in silicone oil. Therefore, an adjustment must be made for this slower speed.

Preoperative power calculation usually aims for in-bag IOL placement, and adjustment is needed if placement in the anterior chamber or sulcus. This first includes lens constant adjustment if the IOL will be substituted with another one. Then, adjustment related to IOL position change should be considered as follows:

Anterior chamber placement: an anterior chamber intraocular lens (ACIOL) will typically require a power approximately 1–3 diopters (D) lower than a planned in-the-bag posterior chamber IOL (PCIOL), depending on AL and K.

Sulcus placement: The adjustment here is less than that of ACIOL, due to the proximity to the bag, with adjustment ranging from 0 to 1 D less than the original in-bag placement. The "rule of nines" system to calculate the necessary reduction in lens power can be used. In a nutshell, if the lens power is between 0 and 9 D, you do not need to change the power when you move it forward. If it is between 9.5 and 18 D, you subtract 0.5 D from the power. If it is between 18.5 and 27 D, you subtract 1 D. If it is above 27 D, subtract 1.5 D. And so forth.

21.2 Lens Dislocation and Subluxation

The most common cause of sublimated lens is a mutation in the FBN1 (fibrillin-1) gene with AD inheritance. Although it may present with just eye findings, it is important to consider Marfan syndrome and to do an echocardiogram to rule out aortic dilatation. The other consideration is homocystinuria and appropriate blood and urine testing. The (lens) zonules are usually broken (in homocystinuria) rather than stretched (as with Marfan syndrome) (Table 21.2).

- Isolated ectopia lentis (AD): An autosomal dominant condition, typically presenting with the lens being displaced superiorly and temporally. The condition is usually bilateral and symmetric. While it is most inherited as an AD trait, the onset can vary occurring either at birth or later in life. Late-onset cases often involve the developments of glaucoma. Additionally, some patients with heterozygous mutations in *FBN1* gene (which is associated with Marfan syndrome) may present with isolated ectopia lentis without other systemic involvement, ectopia lentis et pupillae (AR) bilateral displacement of the pupil, usually inferotemporally, and dislocation of the lens (which is usually microspherophakia) in the opposite direction.
- Marfan syndrome (AD): Lens dislocation superior-temporal (up and out). AD caused by mutations in *FBN1*, which provides instructions for making the protein fibrillin-1. Patients are tall with lax joints, with cardiac abnormalities as a potential cause of death. No intellectual abnormalities are seen. Ocular abnormality is present in 80% of patients with lens subluxation being the most common. They have high axial length (i.e., myopia, thin sclera and retina, so higher RD risk, glaucoma) and poorly dilating pupils with iris transillumination. Decreased corneal curvature (unlike KC) is seen. So, many ocular associations are there, but KC not among them!
- Homocystinuria (AR): An autosomal recessive disorder, typically presenting with bilateral lens dislocation around the age of 3 years, with 30% of cases occurring in infancy and 80% by the age of 15. The condition arises from mutations in the gene encoding cystathionine β-synthase, leading to the accumulation of

Table 21.2 Comparison between Marfan syndrome and homocystinuria

	Marfan	Homocystinuria
Direction of subluxation	Upwards (superior-temporal)	Downwards (inferonasal)
Inheritance	AD	AR
Zonular integrity and accommodation	Intact (hyper-stretched)	Absent
Intellectual dysfunction	Absent	Present

homocysteine and methionine in the plasma and their excretion in the urine, while cysteine levels are low. This results in abnormal, brittle zonules, which are distinct from the stretched zonules seen in Marfan syndrome. A urine homocysteine test is diagnostic for the condition. Urine homocysteine test is diagnostic. Dietary management involves dietary restriction, such as a low-methionine diet with supplemental cysteine, and supplementation with pyridoxine (vitamin B6), which helps alleviate systemic problems in about 50% of cases. Patients with homocystinuria often exhibit skeletal features similar to Marfan syndrome, including tall stature and light-colored hair, but they are normal at birth. Over time, they may develop seizures, mental retardation, scoliosis, and osteoporosis. Central nervous system abnormalities occur in approximately 50% of patients, and intellectual disability and seizures are the most common. A significant concern in homocystinuria is the high risk of arterial thrombotic disease, such as myocardial infarction, necessitating ongoing monitoring for cardiovascular events. Interestingly, there is not an increased risk for venous events like deep vein thrombosis (DVT).

- Weill-Marchesani syndrome, which can be inherited in either an autosomal recessive or a dominant pattern, presents as the clinical opposites of Marfan syndrome. Patients are typically short in stature, with brachydactyly (short fingers) and short limbs. Mutations in the *ADAMTS10* gene are often implicated in this condition. A hallmark of the syndrome is the presence of microspherophakic lenses, which are abnormally small and spherical. This lens shape predisposes patients to angle-closure glaucoma, particularly aggravated by meiosis, while cycloplegia may reduce the risk. Over time, the lenses may dislocate into the anterior chamber, leading to pupillary block glaucoma. For this reason, prophylactic laser peripheral iridectomy or lensectomy may be necessary to prevent these complications.

Sulfite oxidase deficiency (molybdenum cofactor deficiency), a very rare hereditary disorder related to sulfur metabolism, is associated with severe neurologic disorders and ectopia lentis. The deficiency in the enzyme interferes with the conversion of sulfite to sulfate, leading to increased sulfite excretion in the urine. Diagnosis can be confirmed by detecting the absence of sulfite oxidase activity in skin fibroblasts. Neurologic abnormalities include infantile hemiplegia, choreoathetosis, and seizures, with irreversible brain damage and death typically occurring by the age of 5.

More commonly, lens displacement is associated with systemic syndromes, such as Marfan syndrome, homocystinuria, and Weill-Marchesani syndrome. It can also be associated with other ocular disorders such as aniridia, pseudoexfoliation syndrome, and congenital glaucoma. Other less common conditions associated with ectopia lentis include Ehlers-Danlos syndrome, sulfite oxidase deficiency, hyperlysinemia, congenital syphilis, Apert's (not Alport) disease, ectopia lentis et pupillae, spherophakia, iris coloboma, retinitis pigmentosa, and Rieger syndrome.

***Note that the syndromes causing congenital cataract are not associated with ectopia lentis.

Microspherophakia: It is characterized by a round lens with small diameter, resulting in high converging power and causing myopia. This condition increases the risk of pupillary block, which can be worsened by miotic agents. On the other hand, mydriatic agents can alleviate the block by tightening the zonules, which pulls the lens backward and reduces the risk of pupillary block.

Astigmatism induced by lens displacement is expected to cause lenticular cylinder in a direction parallel to the axis of the lens displacement. In plus cylinder format, this is in the same direction of the displacement. In minus cylinder format, this would be 90 degrees different from the direction of displacement.

A superior-temporal lens subluxation would induce $-7.00 + 6.00 \times 135$

Hyperlysinemia is associated with lens subluxation but not cataract

Hypocalcemia but not hypercalcemia is associated with cataract

Hypoglycemia in utero is associated with cataract

Table 21.3 Different lens subluxation syndromes and their mode of inheritance

Disease	Inheritance
Galactosemia	AR
Lowe's (oculocerebrorenal)	X-linked
Alport	X-linked
Nance-Horan syndrome	X-linked
Marfan	AD
Fibrillin gene	AD
Ectopia lentis et pupillae	AR
Homocystinuria	AR
Weill-Marchesani syndrome	AR

Ectopia lentis is associated with (Table 21.3):

- Familial ectopia lentis
- Marfan syndrome
- Weill-Marchesani
- Homocystinuria
- Familial microspherophakia
- Hyperlysinemia
- Sulfite oxidase deficiency
- Stickler syndrome
- Sturge-Weber syndrome
- Crouzon syndrome
- Ehlers-Danlos syndrome
- Aniridia

21.3 Congenital Cataract

Pediatric cataracts can be classified by the age of occurrence into the following:

- Congenital cataracts: present at birth or within the first 2 months of life, although they may not be identified until later.
- Infantile cataracts are present during the first year of life.
- Juvenile cataract is present afterward during the pediatric age.

Crystalline gene mutation is present in almost 50% of congenital cataracts and is inherited as AD.

Two-thirds of congenital cataract cases are bilateral (similar to congenital glaucoma), mostly AD (unlike congenital glaucoma), while unilateral cataract is mostly sporadic.

Posterior polar or posterior lenticonus are generally unilateral, even in syndromic cases (Lowe's syndrome). On the other hand, anterior lenticonus are generally bilateral (e.g., Alport).

Assessed by visibility of red reflux, where:

- Dense cataract impedes visualization of red reflux.
- Less dense, where red reflux can be seen via indirect method only.
- Visually insignificant, where red reflux can be seen both with direct and indirect methods.

Unilateral cataracts in the pediatric population are most commonly caused by trauma, posterior lenticonus, and persistent hyperplastic primary vitreous. Less common but significant causes include intraocular inflammation, such as toxocariasis, and intraocular tumor like retinoblastoma. For patients with visually significant cataracts measuring 3 mm or greater, daily pharmacologic dilation is not an appropriate treatment.

21.3.1 Congenital Cataract Depending on the Cataract Appearance

- Anterior polar cataract: Clinically insignificant with <3 mm on anterior capsule, generally not amblyogenic. If unilateral, anisometropia should be suspected to be a cause of amblyopia.
- Posterior polar cataract: May be associated with posterior lenticonus or fetal vascular remnants including a Mittendorf dot.
- Persistent fetal vasculature (PFV), previously known as *persistent hyperplastic primary vitreous*, is the most common cause of a unilateral cataract in children. PFV typically presents as an isolated, sporadic ocular malformation, though bilateral cases can be associated with systemic or neurologic abnormalities. Affected eyes are often smaller than normal, and surgical intervention carries a higher risk of complications. Posterior sutural cataracts: female carriers of X-linked Nance-Horan syndrome.

- Congenital nuclear cataract: Mostly bilateral, with around 3 mm opacity at the center of lens. Unilateral causes may result in smaller involved eyes.
- Lamellar/zonular cataract: Mostly bilateral. It occupies the zone of the fetal nucleus and occurs in one of the cortical layers with >5 mm diameter. It can be congenital or it can be acquired during the first years of life due to tetany or rickets.
- Posterior lenticonus: Cone-shaped deformation of the posterior lens surface caused by progressive thinning of the central capsule. When the deformation is global, lentiglobus occurs. It appears as oil droplet red reflux. Posterior capsular tear may develop and results in total lens opacity. The opacities are almost always *unilateral*, and the affected eye is normal in size. It develops in female carriers of Lowe (oculocerebrorenal) syndrome by puberty.
- Sectoral cataract: Usually a result of trauma or underlying focal pathology (e.g., tumor).
- Peripheral vacuolar cataract: Incidental finding, which is visually insignificant and resolves spontaneously.

Posterior polar or posterior lenticonus is generally unilateral, even in syndromic cases (Lowe's syndrome). On the other hand, anterior lenticonus is generally bilateral (e.g., Alport).

21.3.2 Syndromes Causing Cataract

- **Galactosemia** is an autosomal recessive (AR) disorder caused by a deficiency in the enzyme galactose-1-phosphate uridyl transferase, leading to elevated levels of galactose in the urine. Approximately 70% of affected individuals develop anterior and posterior subcapsular cataracts before fully maturing. Early dietary intervention can sometimes reverse cataract formation. A milder form, known as "forme fruste" galactosemia, occurs in young adults (35–55 years of age), due to a partial deficiency of galactose-1-phosphate uridyl transferase, resulting in early-onset posterior subcapsular cataract. Classic galactosemia presents within the first few weeks of life with symptoms such as malnutrition, hepatomegaly, jaundice, and intellectual disability. The cataracts in this condition typically exhibit an "oil droplet" appearance on retro illumination due to increasing opacification of the nucleus and deep cortex. There are three known types of galactosemia: type 1 (classic) galactosemia is autosomal recessive and is caused by deficiency of galactose-1-phosphate uridyl transferase. Children are generally unwell, including failure to thrive, hepatosplenomegaly, CNS disease, and renal disease, and the cataract is typically a central oil droplet.
- Type 2 and type 3 galactosemia are also autosomal recessive, but they are less common than type 1 and children are less systemically unwell. Cataract is classically lamellar rather than oil droplet. Type 2 is caused by deficiency of galactokinase, while type 3 is caused by deficiency of UDP galactose epimerase.

Lowe syndrome (oculocerebrorenal syndrome) is an X-linked (i.e., mostly in men) inborn error of amino acid metabolism with a mutation in the OCRL gene, leading to the loss of an enzyme called PIP2–5-phosphatase. Majority have visually significant cataracts since birth in both eyes.

Ocular: posterior subcapsular progression to nuclear at late stages, with posterior lenticonus. Glaucoma at 1–2 years of age.

Cerebral: hypotonia, intellectual disability.

Renal: proximal tubular acidosis, aminoaciduria, low-molecular-weight proteinuria, Fanconi's syndrome.

Can be assessed via proteinuria.

Females who carry the X-linked gene for Lowe's syndrome (oculocerebrorenal syndrome) have been reported to have an increased likelihood of posterior polar and cortical lens opacities after the age of 10 years.

Alport syndrome is an X-linked disease affecting type 4 collagen (aka basement membrane collagen), leading to renal, ocular, and ear manifestations (Table 21.4). The following are the manifestations:

Table 21.4 Comparison between Lowe's syndrome and Alport syndrome

	Lowe	Alport
Inheritance	X-linked	X-linked
Mutation target	Amino acid metabolism (a phosphatase enzyme)	Basement membrane collagen
Cataract	Posterior subcapsular with posterior lenticonus (*unilateral*)	Anterior polar with anterior lenticonus (*bilateral*)
Other ocular	Glaucoma	Posterior polymorphous corneal dystrophy, fleck retinopathy
Renal	Proteinuria	Hematuria
Other systems	Hypotony with intellectual disability	Deafness

- Ocular: anterior lenticonus and anterior polar cataracts. Other ocular associations include posterior polymorphous corneal dystrophy and dot-fleck retinopathy.
- Renal failure, with hematuria always present.
- Deafness due to cochlear involvement.

Note that 75% of anterior polar cataracts are non-syndromic.

Retinitis pigmentosa leads to PSCC.

Usher's syndrome accounts for half of all cases of combined deafness and blindness in childhood with pigmentary retinopathy developing before puberty.

Cataract-dental syndrome, also known as Nance-Horan syndrome, is an X-linked genetic disorder that often presents at birth with congenital cataracts. This condition is primarily characterized by dental abnormalities and lens opacities, leading to poor vision. While the syndrome typically affects males, female carriers may exhibit posterior sutural cataract.

Congenital infections:

- Rubella
- Toxoplasmosis
- CMV
- Varicella

Most neonatal HSV is contracted at the time of delivery caused by passage through an infected birth canal. By contrast, most neonatal CMV is caused by maternal viremia during, or shortly before, pregnancy and passage of the virus from the mother to the fetus across the placenta. Unlike congenital CMV, which is mostly asymptomatic, congenital HSV infection is usually symptomatic with vesicular dermatitis, keratoconjunctivitis, pneumonitis, or meningoencephalitis.

Remember

Down syndrome is associated with bilateral cataract in 75% in early childhood.

Hallermann–Streiff syndrome features cataracts in 90%.

Nance-Horan syndrome is X-linked, where females have Y suture cataract.

21.3.3 Management of Pediatric Cataract

Results from Infant Aphakia Treatment Study (IATS) and its follow-up trials:

- There was no significant difference in visual acuity at 1 year or 10 years between infants who had an intraocular lens (IOL) implanted before 6 months of age and those who were left aphakic and treated with contact lens.
- Infants who received an IOL before 6 months of age had a five-times increase in the rate of intraoperative complications and required more additional intraocular procedures within the first year. This raises concerns about early IOL implantation for infantile cataracts.
- Follow-up studies indicate that IOL implantation after 6 months of age is associated with lower overall complication rates while maintaining similar visual outcomes.

In bilateral visually significant cataract, perform surgery on one eye with immediate aphakic correction; perform surgery on the other eye before 3 months of age.

Sometimes, these children can be treated with glasses or contact lenses alone. What is the best-corrected vision? Also measure by refracting around the lens (aphakic visual axis) with the pupil dilated. This is another way to get the best vision. If refraction is not helpful, surgery may be indicated understanding that there is likely some irreversible amblyopia. Lensectomy with or without IOL (suture or iris-fixated) is indicated when inadequate visual acuity is obtained from these refraction efforts.

Investigations: When there is no family history and a unilateral complete cataract is present, screening labs are not warranted. However, urine protein and reducing substance analysis should be conducted to screen for conditions like Lowe's syndrome or galactosemia, particularly in cases of bilateral cataracts. Bilateral cataracts are also associated with chromosomal abnormalities, including trisomy 13 and Turner syndrome. If the fundus cannot be visualized, a B-scan ultrasonography is necessary to rule out secondary causes, such as intraocular tumors, that may lead to unilateral cataracts.

21.3.4 Timing

Surgery optimally should be delayed to >4 weeks of age to reduce the risk of glaucoma.

A visually significant unilateral cataract should be removed before age 6 weeks.

Visually significant bilateral cataracts should be removed before age 10 weeks (3 months).

For visually nonsignificant cataract, close follow-up is needed.

Surgery for older children is usually indicated when the VA drops to <20/40.

When to implant an IOL is a subject of debate; if babies are more than 1 year of age, implantation is generally safe; for younger children, rate of complications with early implantation is high, so it is advisable to delay implantation to after 1 year of age. If possible, for infants who undergo cataract surgery within the first 7 months of life, it is often preferable to leave them aphakic and use a contact lens, planning to implant an intraocular lens [IOL] a few years later. However, in cases where families have developmentally delayed child, live far from the doctor, or may struggle with contact lens care, early IOL implantation might be a better option.

In Infant Aphakic Treatment study, the authors found no significant visual outcome in early vs. delayed IOL implantation.

21.3.5 IOL Choice

IOL implantation for infants <1 year of age is associated with higher rate of complications and larger shifts in refractive error, so aphakic glasses and patching are indicated for such children, followed by secondary IOL after 1–2 years of age.

- Studies have indicated that in aphakic pediatric eyes, there is a variable myopic shift in refractive error, averaging approximately 7.00–8.00 D between the ages of 1 year and 10 years, with considerable variability. This suggests that if a child is made emmetropic with an IOL at 1 year of age, their refractive error at 10 years could be −8.00 D or higher. The refractive changes in children younger than 1 year are even less predictable. This projection assumes that an IOL does not affect the normal growth pattern of the aphakic eye, which may not hold true based on findings from animal and early human studies. So we have two options:

  Either aim for hyperopia and correct it with glasses post-op, to allow the progression of myopia correcting it with age, thus aiming for adulthood emmetropia, or

  Aim for childhood emmetropia to enhance amblyopia management, and do secondary surgery in adulthood to correct the resulting myopia.

Patching in unilateral cases and some bilateral cases is necessary after surgery.

21.3.6 Special Technique for Pediatric Cataract Surgery

In young children who experience rapid posterior capsule opacification, a controlled posterior capsulotomy and anterior vitrectomy should be performed during cataract surgery if the patient is under 5 years of age. For older children, YAG capsulotomy is a viable option. Whenever possible, adequate peripheral lens should be preserved to allow for future implantation of a secondary posterior chamber IOL. This procedure can be approached through a limbal incision or a pars plana approach.

21.3.7 Complications of Pediatric Cataract Surgery

- PCO: Occurs 18–24 months after cataract extraction, which is why posterior capsulotomy should routinely be done.
- Glaucoma: The earlier the surgery, the higher the risk; most risk for <4 weeks. Usually develops several years after surgery.
- Refractive errors with difficult-to-predict power.
- Strabismus: decompensation of eso or exo.
- Secondary membrane: When post-op uveitis is severe without aggressive treatment.
- Proliferation of lens epithelium, forming a Soemmering's ring.
- Others are rare, including corneal decompensation, RD, and endophthalmitis.

21.4 Miscellaneous

21.4.1 Ectopia Lentis

- Isolated AD, where displacement occurs superotemporal.
- Ectopia lentis et pupillae: AR, ectopia lentis with pupil in opposite direction.
- Aniridia.
- Marfan: superotemporal bilateral dislocation in 80%, with intact zones.
- Weill-Marchesani syndrome: AR, the opposite of Marfan, with short stature and inferior ectopia lentil in 50%. Microspherophakia, predisposing to angle closure.
- Homocystinuria: Degenerated zonules in untreated patients. Ectopia lentis, typically inferonasal, is almost universal by the age of 25 years in untreated cases.
- Stickler and Ehlers-Danlos syndromes.

***Microspherophakia is most often and characteristically seen in patients with Weill-Marchesani syndrome.

21.4.2 Abnormal Lens Shape

- Anterior lenticonus: bilateral axial projection of the anterior surface of the lens into the AC. The "oil droplet" sign can be seen on retroillumination. Almost all patients have Alport syndrome.
- Posterior lenticonus: mostly due to deficient posterior capsule. Most cases are *unilateral*, sporadic, and not associated with systemic disease.
- Microspherophakia: small spherical lens. Mostly isolated AD, or associated with Marfan and Weill-Marchesani syndromes, hyperlysinemia, and congenital rubella.

*** Lens coloboma is simply zonular deficiency, rather than true absence of lens tissue.

Proliferations of the lens epithelium are common (e.g., posterior and anterior subcapsular cataracts), but neoplasms, such as phacomas, do not occur since birth.

The cataract in galactosemia (autosomal recessive) usually is an anterior and posterior subcapsular opacity. The cataract can become nuclear before it matures. A form-fruste type of galactosemia can occur in young adults.

The difference in magnification between an intraocular lens and the original crystalline lens is approximately 1.5%.

The most accurate calculations occur with a normal-size eye with moderate astigmatism.

Corneal edema is the most common complication of iris-supported intraocular lenses.

When performing separate procedures for phacoemulsification and PKP, there is an increased risk of graft failure compared to performing a combined procedure.

Placing an IOL in the sulcus of an aphakic eye is generally not advisable due to the lack of posterior support, which increases the likelihood of the IOL migrating into the vitreous cavity.

Intraoperative iris prolapse can occur for several reasons, including entering the anterior chamber too posteriorly near the iris root, use of systemic tamsulosin by the patient for urinary issues, and rarely impending choroidal effusion or expulsive hemorrhage. Additionally, injecting a viscoelastic agent posterior to the iris can exacerbate the problem.

21.4.3 IOL Tilting, Decentration, and Axial Movement

Tilting and decentration occur most commonly in scleral fixation IOL, with incidence reaching 5–10%. They mostly occur spontaneously.

Lens tilt is defined as the angle between the IOL optical axis and the baseline axis.

Decentration refers to the vertical distance between the center of the IOL and the baseline.

Tilting a plus lens around its axis increases its spherical power of the lens and adds approximately three times as much cylinder in the direction of the tilt. In this example, tilting a +10 D lens around the vertical axis will result in increased plus power and plus cylinder, with the cylinder axis aligned at 90°.

Conversely, tilting a plus lens introduces plus cylinder power with the axis aligned with the tilt direction, while tilting a minus lens induces minus cylinder power in the direction of the tilt. Axial movement of IOL (a positive lens) would result in myopic shift in anterior movement and hyperopic shift in posterior movement.

Monovision: The goal is to achieve emmetropia for distance vision in the eye and aim for refractive outcome of approximately −1.25 D sphere in the second eye following cataract surgery. Patients who achieve 6/9 or better UCVA in the first eye are given the option to target either emmetropia or modest myopia (−1.25 D) in the second eye. Monocular blur is known to negatively impact and contrast sensitivity. The reduction in stereopsis, a key drawback of monovision, affects depth perception, making it one of the significant challenges in using this method to correct presbyopia.

Most patients with a first-day elevation of pressure will respond nicely to "burping" the wound and draining aqueous fluid.

Hyperventilating a patient will decrease vitreous pressure.

Acknowledgments None.

Conflict of Interest None.

References

Bowen RC, Zhou AX, Bondalapati S, Lawyer TW, Snow KB, Evans PR, Bardsley T, McFarland M, Kliethermes M, Shi D, Mamalis CA, Greene T, Rudnisky CJ, Ambati BK (2018) Comparative analysis of the safety and efficacy of intracameral cefuroxime, moxifloxacin and vancomycin at the end of cataract surgery: a meta-analysis. Br J Ophthalmol 102(9):1268–1276. https://doi.org/10.1136/bjophthalmol-2017-311051. Epub 2018 Jan 11. PMID: 29326317; PMCID: PMC6041193

Infant Aphakia Treatment Study Group, Lambert SR, Buckley EG, Drews-Botsch C, DuBois L, Hartmann E, Lynn MJ, Plager DA, Wilson ME (2010) The infant aphakia treatment study: design and clinical measures at enrollment. Arch Ophthalmol 128(1):21–27. https://doi.org/10.1001/archophthalmol.2009.350. PMID: 20065212; PMCID: PMC2983098

Lee JY, Lee EK, Lee HJ, Jeong J, Lee SY, Kim JY (2018) Postoperative hemorrhagic occlusive retinal Vasculitis with Intracameral vancomycin. Korean J Ophthalmol 32(5):430–431. https://doi.org/10.3341/kjo.2018.0043. PMID: 30311469; PMCID: PMC6182214

Liu C, Bardan AS (eds) (2021) Cataract surgery: pearls and techniques. Springer Nature

Clinical Review of Retina and Vitreous Diseases: Part I

22

Mo'ath AlShawabkeh, Saif Aldeen Alryalat, Mohammed Abu-Ameerh, and Ahmed A. Sallam

Abstract

This chapter provides a comprehensive overview of various retinal diseases, beginning with age-related macular degeneration, a leading cause of vision loss in older adults. It then discusses diabetic retinopathy, highlighting its stages, risk factors, and management strategies. The chapter also covers hypertensive retinopathy, detailing the effects of systemic hypertension on the retina. It explores retinal vascular occlusions, both central and peripheral, discussing their etiology, clinical presentation, and treatment options. In addition to these common conditions, the chapter addresses other vascular diseases, including sickle cell retinopathy, idiopathic juxtafoveal telangiectasia, retinal artery macroaneurysm (RAMA), Coats disease, Eales disease, Susac syndrome, and trauma-associated retinopathy. Finally, pathological myopia is examined, emphasizing its implications on the retina. By providing a thorough understanding of these diverse retinal disorders, the chapter equips readers with essential knowledge for effective diagnosis and management in clinical practice.

Keywords

Retina · Age-related macular degeneration
Retinopathy · Vascular occlusion · Myopia

M. AlShawabkeh (✉)
Department of Ophthalmology, The Hashemite University, Zarqa, Jordan

S. A. Alryalat
Department of Ophthalmology, The University of Jordan, Amman, Jordan

The University of Colorado Anschutz Medical Campus, Aurora, CO, USA

M. Abu-Ameerh
The University of Jordan, Amman, Jordan

A. A. Sallam
Harvey and Bernice Jones Eye Institute, University of Arkansas for Medical Sciences (UAMS), Little Rock, AR, USA

22.1 Overview

Disorders of the retina are vitreous humor; despite being widely variable, they are generally quite common worldwide and potentially blinding if left untreated or when diagnosis is delayed.

While many vitreoretinal disorders may remain asymptomatic until late stages, visual symptoms associated with these diseases can include sudden or gradual vision loss, visual field defects, visual distortion (metamorphopsia), night blindness, floaters and flashing lights, and many more.

The diagnosis of such conditions relies primarily on clinical examination with slit lamp and indirect ophthalmoscope; however, imaging

S. A. Alryalat (ed.), *Ophthalmology Board and FRCS Part 2 Exams*,
https://doi.org/10.1007/978-981-96-1517-9_22

modalities such as optical coherence tomography (OCT) and fluorescence angiography (FFA) are extremely helpful tools to support diagnosis and monitor treatment.

This chapter discusses various vitreoretinal diseases including age-related macular degeneration, diabetic and hypertensive retinopathies, retinal vascular disorders, pathological myopia, hereditary retinal dystrophies, retinopathy associated with systemic diseases and some drugs, retinal detachment, and vitreous and vitreomacular surface disorders.

Other less common conditions including choroidal disorders, retinopathies, and endophthalmitis are summarized in the miscellaneous section. Discussion for each entity includes a brief overview of the pathology, signs and symptoms, diagnostic modalities, and treatment options. High-yield designs in concordance with the standards of eye yield series were maintained in the discussion of each disease entity; these include comparison tables summarizing differentiating points between any potentially conflicting entities, high-yield notes to highlight information that has high potential or has appeared in prior ophthalmology exams, as well as an overall up-to-the-point style of writing useful for exam revisions.

The chapter also reviews various forms of imaging modalities used in vitreoretinal disorders including optical coherence tomography, OCT-angiography, fundus autofluorescence, fundus fluorescein angiography, and indocyanine green angiography. Since these technologies provide valuable information in many retinal conditions, ophthalmologists should master interpretation of all these modalities, so here the chapter provides a simple guide for this purpose.

As with other branches of medicine, treatment of retinal disease should be guided by evidence-based practice. This chapter also provides summary tables for the results of the most important and recent clinical trials in the treatment of retinal vein occlusion, age-related macular degeneration, diabetic retinopathy and diabetic macular edema, and endophthalmitis.

Finally, as different types of lasers are commonly used in the treatment of various retinal conditions, the chapter briefly summarizes the high-yield notes about photocoagulation lasers used in clinical practice.

For readers interested in further more comprehensive and detailed information, the following references are useful (Kim 2021; Kanski and Bowling 2015; Kertes and Conway 1998; Karampelas et al. 2020; Scott et al. 2020; Heeren et al. 2020; Reed 2001; Doft et al. 1995).

22.2 Age-Related Macular Degeneration

22.2.1 Introduction

Age-related macular degeneration (AMD) is a progressive disorder that affects the macula, the part of the retina responsible for sharp, central vision. Predominantly seen in individuals over 65, AMD is a leading cause of blindness in the developed world. This condition is generally bilateral, characterized by various clinical findings such as drusen (tiny yellow or white deposits under the retina), pigmentary disturbances, geographic atrophy (GA), macular neovascular membrane (MNV), and pigment epithelial detachment (PED), among others.

22.2.2 Risk Factors

- Age is the most significant risk factor, with AMD being more common in individuals over the age of 65.
- Demographic factors: AMD is more prevalent in females, Caucasians, and those with blue irises.
- Environmental factors: Smoking doubles the risk of AMD. Other risk factors include obesity and excessive sunlight exposure.
- Genetic factors: A family history of AMD, along with variations in certain genes such as complement factor H and ARMS2, can increase susceptibility to the disease.
- Miscellaneous: Cardiovascular disease, prior cataract surgery, hyperopia, and frequent aspirin use have also been associated with an increased risk of AMD.

Table 22.1 Comparison between age-related macular degeneration (AMD) types

Dry AMD	Wet AMD
Non-neovascular/nonexudative	Neovascular/exudative
More common	Less common
Slow vision loss	Rapid vision loss
Includes Drusen, pigmentary changes, and geographic atrophy	Includes macular neovascular membrane (MNV), pigment epithelial detachment (PED), retinal angiomatous proliferation (RAP) lesions, polypoidal choroidal vasculopathy (PCV), and disciform scar

22.2.3 Normal Age-Related Maculopathy

Normal aging involves a range of changes in the retina, retinal pigment epithelium (RPE), and Bruch's membrane. These include the following:

- A reduction in the density of photoreceptors, which are light-sensitive cells in the retina.
- A decrease in melanin, the pigment that protects the eye from harmful ultraviolet light, and an increase in lipofuscin granules in the RPE. Lipofuscin granules are a byproduct of cellular waste and can accumulate over time.
- Progressive age-related changes in the choriocapillaris, the fine network of capillaries that supply the outer retina.
- The formation of basal laminar and basal linear deposits, which are accumulations of waste material between the RPE and Bruch's membrane.

22.2.3.1 AMD Types

AMD is broadly classified into two main types: dry AMD and wet AMD. Table 22.1 demonstrates the major differences between these types.

22.2.3.2 Dry AMD

Drusen are extracellular small round yellow deposits along the basal surface of RPE.

Classification of drusen:

1. **Small drusen (droplets):** ≤63 μm (1/2 width of retinal vein at optic disc margin)
2. **Intermediate drusen:** 64–125 μm
3. **Large drusen:** >125 μm

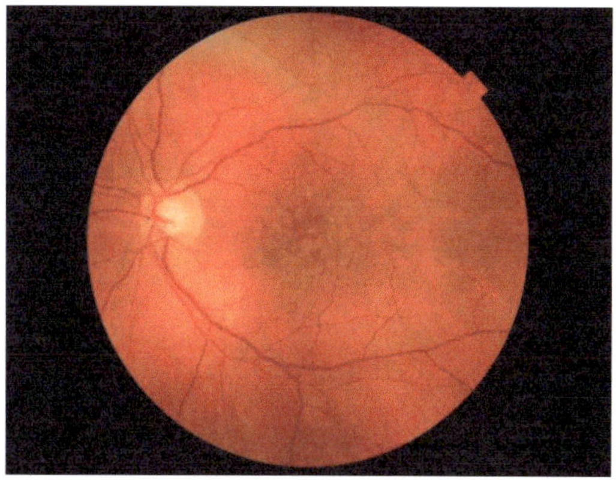

Fig. 22.1 Soft drusen in dry AMD (Courtesy of Retina Rocks®)

22.2.3.3 Other Classification

1. **Soft drusen**: Amorphous and poorly demarcated and usually large (Fig. 22.1). Associated with higher risk of AMD.

   On FFA, show early hypo- and late hyperfluorescence due to pooling.
2. **Hard drusen**: Discrete and well demarcated and usually small (Fig. 22.2).

   Lower AMD risk.

   On FFA, show early hyperfluorescence with window defect due to RPE atrophy or loss.
3. **Confluent drusen**: contiguous drusen without clear boundaries (Fig. 22.3).

22.2.3.4 Risk Factors for Progression of Dry AMD into Wet Type

1. The presence of pigmentary disturbances
2. Size of drusen

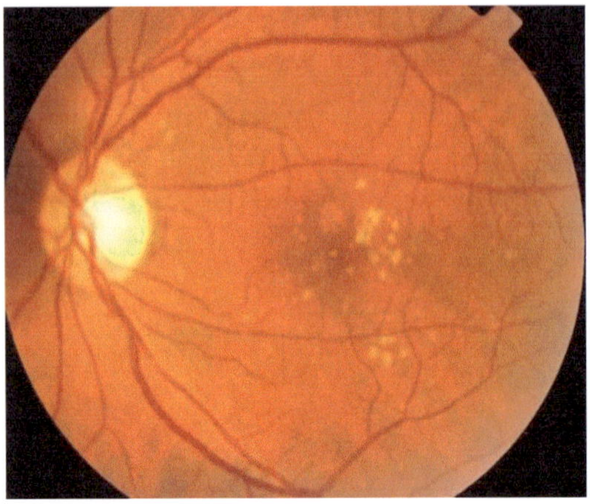

Fig. 22.2 Hard drusen with pigmentary disturbances (Courtesy of Retina Rocks®)

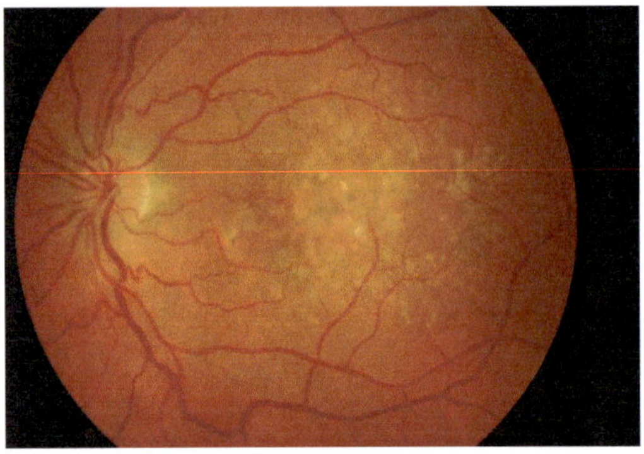

Fig. 22.3 Confluent drusen (Courtesy of Retina Rocks®)

22.2.3.5 OCT Changes of Dry AMD

1. Drusen which appear as a hyper-reflective nodular sub-RPE elevations
2. RPE atrophy
3. Photoreceptor loss
4. Outer retinal tubulations
5. Outer retinal corrugations

22.2.3.6 Management of Dry AMD

1. Patient education and follow-up
2. Amsler grid self-testing
3. Lifestyle modifications, especially smoking cessation
4. Dietary changes: Age-Related Eye Disease Study (AREDS) formula (see Table 22.2)
5. Low vision aids

Table 22.2 Comparison between Age-Related Eye Disease Study 1 (AREDS 1) and AREDS 2 formula

AREDS 1	AREDS 2
Vitamin E 400 IU	Same
Vitamin C 500 mg	Same
Beta-carotene 15 mg	Lutein 10 mg + zeaxanthin 2 mg
Zinc 80 mg	Zinc 25 mg
Copper 2 mg	–

22.2.3.7 Indications for AREDS Formula

1. Extensive medium-sized drusen
2. Large-sized drusen
3. Unilateral or bilateral non-subfoveal geographic atrophy
4. Unilateral advanced AMD (MNV or subfoveal GA)
5. Intravitreal treatment to slow the progression of GA. Pegcetacoplan injection (SYFOVRE) binds to C3 and its activation fragment C3b, regulating the cleavage of C3 and the generation of downstream effectors of complement activation. Results show a reduction in GA extension of approximately 20% after 24 months.

22.2.3.8 Wet (Neovascular) AMD

This form of AMD is characterized by the development of a macular neovascular membrane (MNV), formerly known as a choroidal neovascular membrane (CNV). The balance of angiogenesis and neovascularization from the choriocapillaris is maintained by an intact Bruch's membrane and retinal pigment epithelium (RPE), complemented by substances like the pigment epithelial derived factor (PEDF) and complement factor H.

However, degenerative changes in the RPE and Bruch's membrane (as seen in AMD and pathological myopia), or disruptions to their normal function (due to trauma, neoplasia, or uveitis), can upset this balance and create a proangiogenic environment. This stimulates the choriocapillaris to form new blood vessels. The neovascular complex that forms can extend through the damaged Bruch's membrane into one of the three possible areas:

1. Sub-RPE space (type 1 MNV): If these vessels bleed or leak, it can result in a fibrovascular pigment epithelial detachment (PED).
2. Subretinal space (type 2 MNV): If these vessels bleed or leak, it can cause subretinal hemorrhage.
3. Intraretinal deep capillary plexus (type 3 MNV): In some cases, neovessels originating from this area can grow towards the RPE, a condition also known as retinal angiomatous proliferations (RAP).

The bleeding and leakage from the fibrovascular complex can disrupt the usual interactions between the RPE and photoreceptors. This disruption can cause acute or subacute vision loss and metamorphopsia (visual distortion) and, if left untreated, can culminate in a disciform scar.

22.2.3.9 Macular Neovascular Membrane (MNV) Classifications

Fundus Fluorescein Angiography (FFA)-Based Classification

1. Classic MNV: This anatomically corresponds to type 2 MNV, characterized by an early well-defined lacy hyperfluorescence with progressive late leakage.
2. Occult MNV: This represents anatomically type 1 MNV, featuring ill-defined, irregular, granular-pattern leakage.
3. Predominantly classic MNV: A mix of the two types where over 50% of the lesion is classic.
4. Minimally classic MNV: A mix of the two types where less than 50% of the lesion is classic.
5. Retinal angiomatous proliferation: This represents anatomically type 3 MNV, showing focal intraretinal hyperfluorescence along with occult-type features.

Anatomical Classification of MNV

1. Subfoveal MNV: The lesion is within 200 um from the center of the foveal avascular zone (FAZ).
2. Extrafoveal MNV: The lesion is more than 200 um from the center of FAZ.

22.2.3.10 Key Presentations of Neovascular Age-Related Macular Degeneration (nAMD)

- RPE detachment (PED): This refers to a separation of the RPE from Bruch's membrane's inner collagenous layer due to disrupted hydraulic adhesions and conductivity. PED can be serous, hemorrhagic, fibrovascular, or drusenoid.
- RPE tears/rips: These are crescent-shaped discontinuities of the RPE, usually accompanied by a folded flap at the junction between attached and detached RPE. They can occur spontaneously or after treatment.
- Polypoidal choroidal vasculopathy (PCV): This condition involves a network of branching choroidal vessels with terminal aneurysmal dilations, typically affecting African and East Asian females in their late middle ages.

22.2.3.11 Imaging in nAMD

Subretinal or choroidal neovascularization typically requires prompt FFA for diagnosis, but indocyanine green angiography (ICGA) can be used for higher sensitivity MNV detection in some situations. OCT imaging is widely used for diagnosing and monitoring MNV and guiding treatment regimens.

High-yield notes: PCV should be considered in cases of recurrent serosanguineous PED without drusen, particularly in relatively young, black or Asian race, females. ICGA is the gold standard for diagnosing PCV, and prognosis is generally better than MNV associated with nAMD. Combined photodynamic therapy (PDT) and anti-VEGF treatment is preferred according to the EVEREST study.

22.2.3.12 Management of nAMD

Anti-VEGF Intravitreal Injections

This is now considered the mainstay of treatment.

Four main types of anti-VEGF are currently used in practice (see Table 22.3).

All MNV subtypes respond to anti-VEGF, but only those with "active lesions" will benefit

Table 22.3 Types of anti-VEGF agents used in clinical practice

	Bevacizumab (Avastin®)	Ranibizumab (Lucentis®)	Aflibercept (Eylea®)	Brolucizumab (Beovu®)	Faricimab (Vabysmo®)
Composition	Full anti-VEGF A	Fab fragment	Recombinant fusion protein: Fab portion of VEGF fused to Fc portion of IgG1	Humanized monoclonal single-chain variable fragment (scFv)	Bispecific antibody
MW (KDa)	149	48	115	26	146
Binding target	VEGF-A	VEGF-A	VEGF-A, VEGF-B, PIGF	VEGF-A	VEGF-A and angiopoietin-2 (Ang-2)
Dose for macular edema	1.25 mg in 0.05 mL (25 mg/mL)	0.5 mg in 0.05 mL (10 mg/mL)	2 mg in 0.05 mL (40 mg/mL)	0.6 mg in 0.05 mL	6 mg in 0.05 mL
Half-life in normal eyes	5–7 days	7–9 days	10 days (longest)	3 days	3 days
Systemic half-life	21 days	2 h	11 days	4–5 days	7.5 days
Supporting studies for AMD	CATT study	ANCHOR, MARINA, SEVEN-UP	VIEW1, VIEW2	HAWK and HARRIER	TENAYA and LUCERNE

visually especially so if their outset visual acuity is good.

Remember: Active lesion is evident by the presence of subretinal fluid, hemorrhage, leakage on FFA, enlarging MNV membrane, or deteriorating visual acuity.

Treatment Protocols

A: Regular monthly injections.

B: As-needed regimen (PRN): treatment is administered regularly until the macula appears dry both clinically and on OCT. Afterward, treatment is only resumed if there are signs of recurrent exudation. As described in the PRONOTO study, patients should still be seen every month. However, in clinical practice, follow-up is usually extended, and this may result in worse outcomes due to the delay in administering treatment.

C: Treat-and-extend regimen: regular monthly treatment is administrated until the macula is dry; after that, treatment continues with progressively increasing intervals as long as the macula remains dry, and intervals are decreased if fluid reappears. This cautiously treats inactive MNV by extending the time between injections to prevent sudden recurrence of exudation, in contrast to the as-needed approach, which only treats active disease.

Notes

While brolucizumab was generally well tolerated in the HAWK trial compared to aflibercept, there was a higher incidence of intraocular inflammation. Specifically, uveitis and iritis occurred in 2.2% of patients treated with brolucizumab, compared to 0.3% (uveitis) in those treated with aflibercept. Additionally, recent reports have highlighted the risk of retinal vasculitis with intravitreal brolucizumab injections.

The ranibizumab portal delivery system (RPDS) (Susvimo™) is an implantable, refillable reservoir that requires surgical implantation. This reservoir can be refilled as needed in a clinical setting, providing a long-term solution to maintain visual outcomes.

Photodynamic Therapy (PDT)

Light-activated drug (verteporfin) is given intravenously and is taken up by dividing cells including neovessels; when activated by diode laser, it induces thrombosis and regression of MNV.

PDT is now infrequently used for managing exudative AMD, except in cases involving PCV. The most serious adverse effects associated with PDT are photosensitivity reactions caused by the photosensitizer, which can range from mild skin irritation to second-degree burns on sun-exposed areas.

Laser Photocoagulation

Thermal argon or diode laser ablation of MNV is seldom used due to collateral retinal damage risk and loss of vision.

22.2.3.13 High-Yield Notes

Vitreoretinal interface status may significantly modify the response to therapy with anti-VEGF agents:

Hyaloidal separation seems to enhance drug penetration, potentially reducing the frequency of injections needed, although it does not impact visual acuity. Eyes with an epiretinal membrane may require more frequent injections due to anatomic disturbance, reduced drug penetration, or associated inflammation. A serous PED is typically seen as an area of hypofluorescence on ICGA. In contrast, a vascularized PED will have a hyperfluorescent notch or plaque associated with the MNV. Drusenoid may appear hypo- or iso-fluorescent.

AMD can be staged as

Stage one (normal aging): few small drusen

Stage two (early AMD) (risk of progression to stage 4 is 1.3%): many small drusen or few intermediate drusen

Stage three (intermediate AMD) (risk of progression to stage 4 is 18%): the presence of at least 1 large drusen (≥125 μm), extensive intermediate drusen (63–124 μm diameter), or non-subfoveal GA

Stage four (advanced AMD): vision loss due to neovascular AMD or subfoveal GA in only one eye

22.3 Diabetic Retinopathy

Diabetic retinopathy is the leading cause of permanent blindness in working-age adults, aged 20–64 years.

22.3.1 Diabetic Eye Disease

Diabetes affects various structures in the anterior and posterior segments of the eye. These manifestations are collectively called diabetic eye disease, which is demonstrated in Table 22.4.

22.3.1.1 Pathogenesis

All manifestations of diabetic retinopathy and maculopathy arise from two major pathological processes; the first is microvascular leakage in which the loss of pericytes leads to development of microaneurysms and to break of blood-retinal barriers, which result in hard exudates and various types of hemorrhage and edema. The second pathological process is microvascular occlusion in which hyperglycemia-induced glycosylation of cellular elements and generation of free radicals involving the capillary walls cause thickening of the basement membranes, endothelial cell damage, deformation of RBCs and platelets, and activation of coagulation cascade with resultant

Table 22.4 Various manifestations of diabetic eye disease

	Manifestations
Refraction	Unstable refraction; hyperglycemia causes a myopic shift, and hypoglycemia causes a hyperopic shift
Eyelid	Tear film instability, dry eye, blepharitis, recurrent styes
Cornea	Decreased corneal sensation, marginal keratitis, unstable epithelium causing recurrent erosions
Iris	Minor transillumination defects, poor pupillary dilatation, rubeosis iridis
Lens	Acceleration of senile cataract, true diabetic (snowflake) cataract, decreased amplitude of accommodation
Retina	Diabetic retinopathy, diabetic maculopathy
Neuro-ophthalmology	Diabetic papillitis, non-arteritic anterior ischemic optic neuropathy (NAAION), light-near dissociation, ocular motor nerve palsies including III, IV, and VI
Others	Wolfram syndrome, orbital mucormycosis

ischemia that is responsible for soft exudates, vascular shunts, and development of neovascularization. It is important to note that certain conditions including hypertension, hypercholesterolemia, renal disease, and pregnancy can increase the severity and progression of diabetic retinopathy.

22.3.1.2 High-Yield Notes

- The best predictor of diabetic retinopathy is the duration of the disease. Disease control is also important.
- Pathologically, apoptosis of retinal capillary pericytes is the earliest finding in diabetic retinopathy.
- Clinically, microaneurysms are the first ophthalmoscopically detectable change in diabetic retinopathy.
- Proliferative vessels usually arise from retinal veins.
- The greatest protection against the development of proliferative diabetic retinopathy is provided by a complete posterior vitreous detachment (PVD).

22.3.2 Classification of Diabetic Retinopathy

As shown in Table 22.5, diabetic retinopathy is broadly classified into non-proliferative diabetic retinopathy (NPDR) (see Fig. 22.4) and proliferative diabetic retinopathy (PDR) (Fig. 22.5) with further subclassifications for each type.

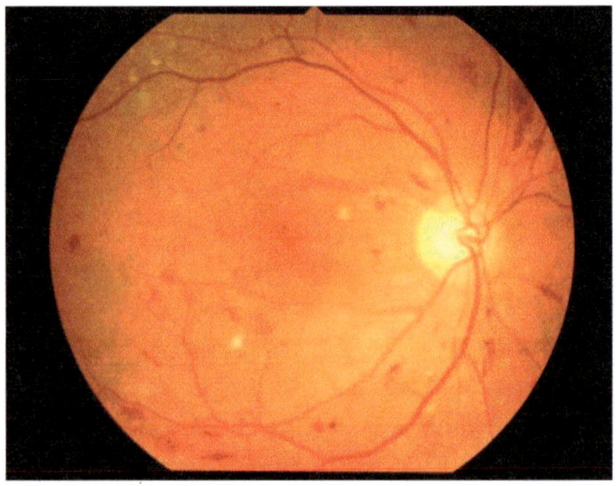

Fig. 22.4 Features of severe NPDR (Courtesy of Retina Rocks®)

Table 22.5 Classification of diabetic retinopathy

Non-proliferative diabetic retinopathy (NPDR)	Mild NPDR	Microaneurysms only
	Moderate NPDR	– Retinal hemorrhages in 1–3 quadrants – Venous beading in one quadrant – Cotton wool spots
	Severe NPDR	*One* of the following 4:2:1 rule – Microaneurysms or blot hemorrhages in 4 quadrants – Venous beading in 2 quadrants – Intraretinal microvascular abnormality (IRMA) in 1 quadrant
	Very severe NPDR	*More than one* of 4:2:1 rule
Proliferative diabetic retinopathy (PDR)	Neovascularization of the disc (NVD) Neovascularization elsewhere (NVE) Neovascularization of the iris (NVI) Neovascularization of the angle (NVA)	High-risk PDR: – Any NVD with VH or preretinal hemorrhage – NVD $\geq$ ¼ disc area – NVE $\geq$ 1/2 disc area with VH or preretinal hemorrhage
Advanced diabetic retinopathy	Vitreous hemorrhage, tractional retinal detachment or rubeosis iridis	

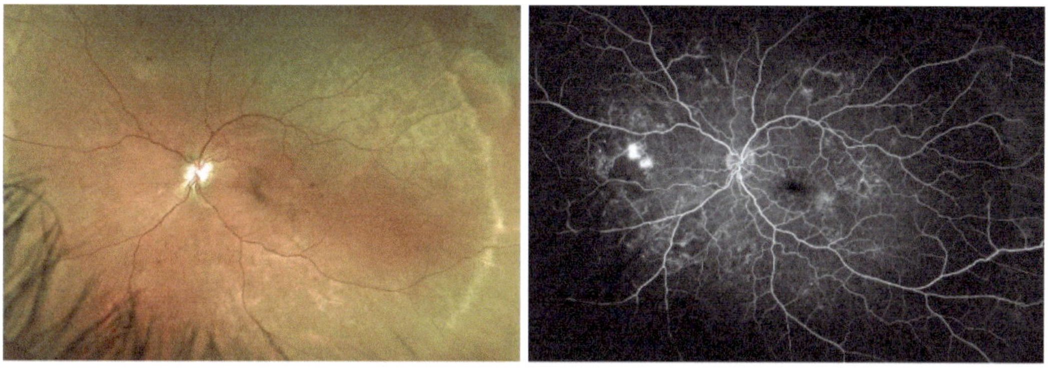

Fig. 22.5 Features of PDR (Courtesy of Retina Rocks®)

Table 22.6 Common retinal signs and their associated pathology

Sign	Pathology
Cotton wool spots (aka soft exudates)	Ischemic infarcts of nerve fiber layer (NFL)
Hard exudates	Damage of deep capillaries at the outer plexiform layer (OPL) with subsequent lipid deposition
Microaneurysm	Localized saccular retinal capillary dilatation due to loss of pericytes
Dot and blot hemorrhages	Damage to inner blood-retinal barriers (BRBs) and hemorrhage in the inner nuclear and plexiform layers
Flame-shaped hemorrhage	Hemorrhage in the NFL
Boat-shaped hemorrhage	Subhyaloid hemorrhage
Intraretinal microvascular abnormalities (IRMAs)	Dilated intraretinal telangiectatic arteriolar-venular shunts
Cherry red spot	An orange reflex from the intact choroid at the foveola, contrasts with the surrounding pale retina
Cystoid macular edema	Transudation across the inner BRB (i.e., retinal vessels) into the OPL, particularly in Henle's loop
Retinal neovascularization	Retinal ischemia leads to the formation of secondary fragile vessels that originate from existing retinal vessels. These new vessels penetrate the internal limiting membrane (ILM) and extend into the vitreous

Table 22.6 shows the pathological levels for each of the diabetic retinopathy features.

22.3.3 Management of Diabetic Retinopathy

In cases of non-proliferative diabetic retinopathy (NPDR), the primary approach is typically to control diabetes and other risk factors. Regular scheduled checkups are also crucial, with the frequency of these visits being determined by the severity of the condition. While aspirin intake might reduce cardiovascular issues, it does not seem to affect outcomes for retinopathy or macular edema.

For patients with severe NPDR, it is worth noting that approximately 50% will progress to proliferative diabetic retinopathy (PDR) within a year. Treatment can be considered at any stage of PDR but is typically mandatory if the condition is high risk.

Laser photocoagulation is the standard treatment for PDR, with anti-VEGF therapies often used as adjunctive treatments in specific circumstances, including:

- Initial treatment of rubeosis iridis
- Addressing persistent vitreous hemorrhage
- Prior to surgery for advanced PDR to minimize bleeding during the operation

Signs of successful laser treatment include:

- The tips of the vessels appearing blunt and a decrease in vein caliber
- Shrinking and disappearance of new blood vessels
- Retinal hemorrhages being reabsorbed
- Regression of intraretinal microvascular abnormalities (IRMAs)

Note: Previously, a pale optic disc was considered a sign of successful panretinal photocoagulation (PRP) treatment. However, it is now thought of as a sign of overtreatment and is not required.

Side effects of laser photocoagulation can include peripheral vision loss and defects in night and color vision. However, most patients do not report symptoms. Other possible side effects include the development or worsening of cystoid macular edema (CME), risk to central vision, and choroidal effusion, which could lead to angle-closure glaucoma.

The laser treatment should be applied starting from 2 disc diameters away from the fovea, 2000 micron nasal to the disc, extending to the periphery.

There is no long-term vision benefit in administering multiple- versus single-session laser treatments, and there is no significant difference in macular thickness. Therefore, the decision on the number of treatment sessions should be determined on an individual basis.

Vitrectomy is recommended in diabetic retinopathy when:

- Persistent non-clearing vitreous hemorrhage
- Persistent dense pre-macular hemorrhage
- Tractional retinal detachment (Fig. 22.6)
- Combined tractional and rhegmatogenous retinal detachment
- Refractory neovascular or ghost cell glaucoma
- Progressive severe proliferative retinopathy despite complete laser treatment

22.3.4 Diabetic Maculopathy

Diabetic macular edema (DME) can be present in any severity level of diabetic retinopathy (DR). However, the more severe the DR, the more likely the DME.

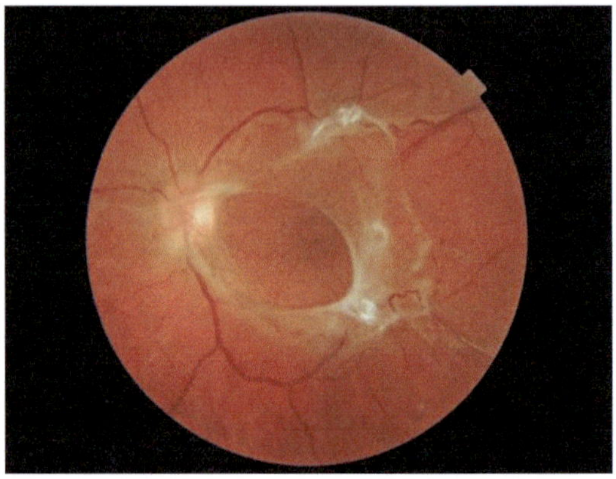

Fig. 22.6 Advanced PDR with TRD involving macula (Courtesy of Retina Rocks®)

Fluid accumulation primarily occurs in the outer plexiform layer. It can be categorized as center-involving (CI) DME or non-center (NCI) DME, depending on whether there is retinal thickening within the central 1 mm of the macula. Non-center-involved DME is generally unlikely to impact vision unless it progresses to involve the center. The term clinically significant macular edema (CSME) is a clinical diagnosis that is based solely on careful examination of the fundus and does not involve imaging modalities like OCT or FFA. This was more commonly used in the last decade where macular laser was the main indication of treatment.

The diagnosis of CSME depends on documenting any of the following:

- Retinal thickening at or within 500 μm of the center of the macula
- Presence of hard exudates at or within 500 μm of the center of the macula, along with thickening of the adjacent retina

A zone or zones of retinal thickening that are at least one disc area in size or larger, with any part of it located within one disc diameter of the center of the macula: It is preferable to start treatment for DME before performing scatter photocoagulation or cataract surgery to reduce the risk of DME worsening as a result of these interventions. Intravitreal injections of anti-VEGFs are the mainstay of treatment for macular edema. Intravitreal steroids can be considered for resistant cases. Focal/grid laser can be appropriate first-line treatment for eyes with DME if there is clearly focal leakage that can be specifically targeted by the laser. This approach may also be suitable for patients who are not ideal candidates for anti-VEGF therapy. Vitrectomy, on the other hand, is usually reserved for more challenging cases, such as those with epiretinal membrane (ERM) or vitreomacular traction. It is also important to advise optimization of blood sugar, blood pressure, and blood cholesterol as this was shown to improve long-term outcomes of retinopathy in type 1 and 2 DM.

22.3.4.1 High-Yield Notes

- The most common cause of a spontaneous vitreous hemorrhage is undiagnosed proliferative diabetic retinopathy.
- Differential diagnosis for asymmetrical diabetic retinopathy includes ipsilateral severe carotid atherosclerotic disease, increasing the diabetic retinopathy, history of cataract surgery, or history of BRVO in the affected side.
- Worsening of diabetic retinopathy and macular edema are expected following cataract surgery. For patients with severe NPDR or PDR, scatter photocoagulation should be considered either 1–2 months prior to cataract surgery or immediately after, depending on the clarity of the ocular media, to address these issues effectively. Patients with DME can undergo anti-VEGF injection during cataract surgery. Intravitreal steroid implants are contraindicated in aphakia, lens subluxation, rupture posterior capsule, and uncontrolled glaucoma.

22.4 Hypertensive Retinopathy

Risk factors for hypertensive retinopathy include African American ethnicity, advanced age, obesity, and noncompliance with antihypertensive therapy.

22.4.1 Pathogenesis

Normally, the autoregulation mechanisms respond to increased blood pressure by increasing the resistance of blood vessels in order to maintain a normal blood flow.

Initially, this is done by vasoconstriction, but if the increase in blood pressure is sustained, it will result in thickening of arterial walls due to hypertrophy of tunica media; this results in "arteriosclerosis," that is, hardening, sclerosis, and loss of elasticity of small vessel walls.

Also, damage to the endothelium from high blood pressure will initiate atherosclerosis and secondary luminal narrowing.

If blood pressure levels were severe enough that they become beyond the ability of autoregulatory mechanisms to correct, it will damage blood-retinal barriers causing exudates, edema, hemorrhage, and ischemic damage.

22.4.2 Stages of Hypertensive Retinopathy

Hypertensive retinopathy is graded as shown in Table 22.7.

22.4.3 Hypertensive Choroidopathy

It is typically seen with acute severe hypertensive crisis (malignant hypertension). Features include the following:

Elschnig spots: small hyperpigmented spots surrounded by hypopigmented halo. These spots result from choroid and RPE infarcts

Siegrist streaks: linear flecks along choroidal vessels caused by fibrinoid necrosis of the choroid

Exudative retinal detachment (see Retinal detachment below)

It is also important to note that hypertension can result in increased progression of diabetic retinopathy and also predisposes to other vascular disorders including retinal and vein occlusions, retinal artery macroaneurysm, NAAION, and other cranial nerve palsies.

Treatment of hypertensive retinopathy is mainly directed towards gradual controlled low-

Table 22.7 Stages of hypertensive retinopathy

Grade I	Generalized arteriolar narrowing and tortuosity	Seen with sustained chronic high blood pressure
Grade II	Grade I plus – AV nipping: focal narrowing of arteries at arteriovenous crossing points – Copper wiring: sclerosed and opacified arteriolar wall	
Grade III	Grade II plus – Retinal hemorrhages: Dot, blot, and flame shaped (Fig. 22.7) – Exudates: Cotton wool spots, macular star	Seen with emergency hypertension associated with end-organ damage
Grade IV	Grade III plus – Optic disc edema	

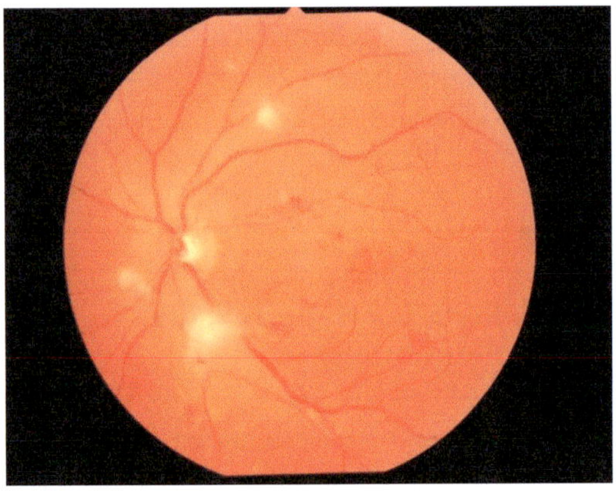

Fig. 22.7 Grade III hypertensive retinopathy (Courtesy of Retina Rocks®)

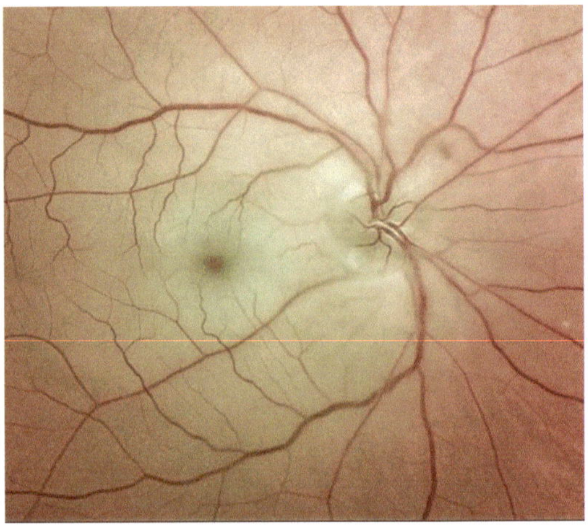

Fig. 22.8 Features of CRAO (Courtesy of Retina Rocks®)

ering of blood pressure. Most of the retinal findings resolve with treatment.

22.5 Retinal Vascular Occlusion

22.5.1 Central Retinal Artery Occlusion (CRAO)

- Though uncommon, this is an important cause of sudden vision loss.
- Usually an *embolic* occlusion of central retinal artery, rarely ophthalmic artery is involved.
- Retinal ischemia is irreversible after 90 min of occlusion.
- Typically associated with poor prognosis due to late presentation.

Source of Embolus

1. Carotid artery atherosclerosis (the most common) causing cholesterol (Hollenhorst) embolus
2. Valvular heart disease or arrhythmias (most commonly atrial fibrillation) causing the calcific embolus
3. Coagulopathies (the least common) causing the fibrin-platelet emboli

Signs of CRAO (Fig. 22.8)

- Attenuation, narrowing, and segmentation of arterioles
- Diffuse whitening of the retina
- Optic disc pallor
- Macular cherry red spots

Cilioretinal artery is a branch from short posterior ciliary artery present in 20–30% of population; if spared in CRAO (Fig. 22.9), the patient may have good central vision, but with significant field defect.

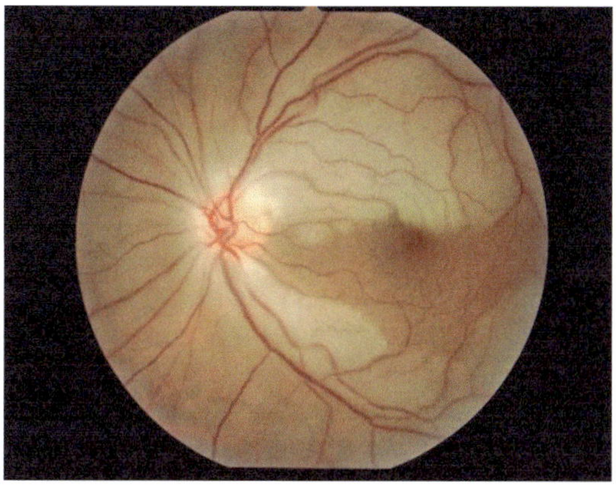

Fig. 22.9 Macular sparing CRAO with patent cilioretinal artery (Courtesy of Retina Rocks®)

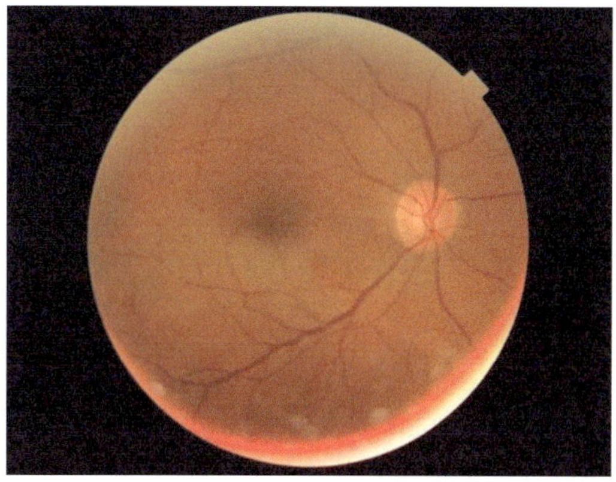

Fig. 22.10 Inferotemporal BRAO (Courtesy of Retina Rocks®)

22.5.1.1 Management of Central Retinal Artery Occlusion

Early intervention: Within the first 24 h, rescue treatment is usually recommended with the aim of providing more oxygen to the ischemic retina and moving the embolus towards a more peripheral branch. However, it is important to note that in most cases, this does not lead to improvement in vision. The initial steps involve:

- Keeping the patient in a supine position
- Performing digital ocular massage
- Using a rebreathing bag or a 95% oxygen, 5% CO_2 face mask
- Performing anterior chamber paracentesis
- Lowering intraocular pressure (IOP) using topical and systemic antiglaucoma medications

Other techniques such as intravenous prostaglandin therapy, intravenous and intra-arterial tissue plasminogen activator (tPA), and pars plana vitrectomy with surgical embolectomy have been attempted, but the results are generally uncertain.

Secondary prevention: Once the immediate situation is under control, long-term prevention becomes the focus. This typically involves collaborating with primary care providers to identify potential causes of central retinal artery occlusion (CRAO). The most common causes include giant cell arteritis (GCA) and emboli from the carotid artery or heart. It is crucial to optimize control of cardiovascular risk factors in these patients, including managing blood pressure, blood sugar, and cholesterol levels. Antiplatelet and/or anticoagulant therapy may be considered for cases attributed to atherosclerosis or atrial fibrillation. In some cases, centers may recommend an MRI scan of the brain to identify any concurrent stroke in patients with central or branch artery occlusion.

22.5.2 Branch Retinal Artery Occlusion (BRAO)

This is similar to CRAO in presentation, pathology, and management but involves one or two quadrants only (Fig. 22.10).

22.5.2.1 High-Yield Notes

- Complete vision loss to no light perception should raise suspicion of an ophthalmic artery occlusion especially if cherry red spots are absent.
- CRAO is associated with a decreased b-wave amplitude on ERG. Ophthalmic artery occlusion is associated with an extinguished ERG.
- Iris neovascularization develops approximately in 5–20% of eyes after acute CRAO. Hence, follow-up of patients is important for up to 6 months.
- CRAO is most commonly embolic in origin. However, giant cell arteritis accounts for approximately 1–2% of cases and can cause isolated cilioretinal artery occlusion as well.

- The leading cause of death in patients with retinal arterial occlusion is cardiovascular disease, and these patients also face an increased risk of strokes.

22.6 Central Retinal Vein Occlusion (CRVO)

It is the second most common retinal vascular disease after diabetic retinopathy.

22.6.1 Risk Factors

Hypertension (the most important risk factor), POAG, age, hypercoagulable state including polycythemia and leukemia, and prior RVO in one eye (increases the risk in the fellow eye to 7–10%). Anatomical factors also exist including optic disc drusen and peripapillary vascular loop.

22.6.2 Pathogenesis

Because central retinal arteries and veins share a common adventitial sheath, arteriolar atherosclerosis is associated with compression of venules at AV crossing points resulting in stasis, turbulent flow, and thrombotic occlusion of central or branch retinal veins. Venous occlusion results in engorgement and tortuosity of retinal veins with secondary leakage, hemorrhage, exudates, and macular and optic disc edema. Occlusion-induced ischemia results in infarction of neuronal bodies and hence development of cotton wool spots; it also stimulates VEGF release causing neovascularization and neovascular glaucoma (NVG). The peak for NVG is usually at 3 months, hence the name 100-day glaucoma.

CRVO can be perfused (75%) (Fig. 22.11) or ischemic (25%) (Fig. 22.12). Differences are demonstrated in Table 22.8. However, about 33% of perfused cases progress into ischemic within 3 years.

Macular edema is the most common cause for poor vision, with anti-VEGF therapy being the primary treatment. Steroid injections may be considered for cases resistant to anti-VEGF. In patients with CRVO, clinical and angiographic edema responded to grid laser treatment. There was no significant improvement in long-term visual acuity, so this treatment is no longer recommended.

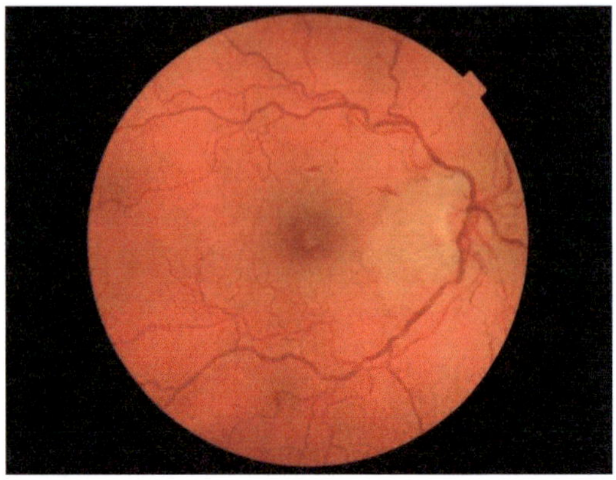

Fig. 22.11 Features of perfused CRVO (Courtesy of Retina Rocks®)

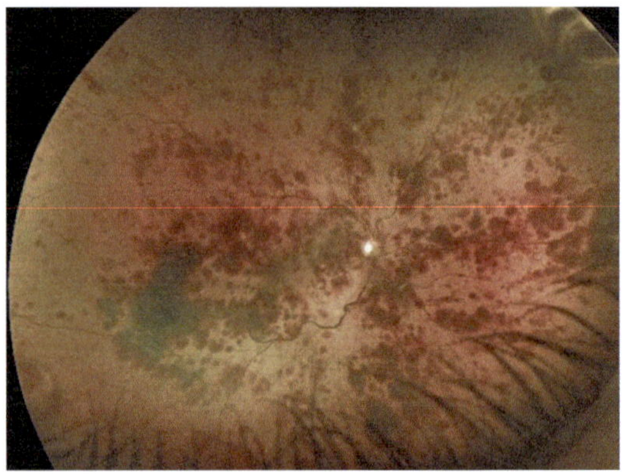

Fig. 22.12 Features of ischemic CRVO (Courtesy of Retina Rocks®)

22.6.3 Branch Retinal Vein Occlusion (BRVO)

It is similar to CRVO in presentation, pathology, and management but involves one or two quadrants only with the superotemporal quadrant being the most commonly involved (Fig. 22.13).

22.6.3.1 High-Yield Notes

- Neovascularization of the iris occurs in about 2% of eyes with BRVO. If these complications

Table 22.8 Comparison between ischemic and perfused CRVO

Comparison	Perfused (nonischemic) CRVO	Ischemic CRVO
Visual acuity	Better than counting fingers	Worse vision Counting fingers or worse
Relative afferent pupillary defect (RAPD)	Absent	Present
Severity of hemorrhages	Less severe	More severe, deeper, and extensive
Optic disc and macular edema	Mild	Severe
Rubeosis iridis/neovascular glaucoma	Rare	Common (50%)
Capillary perfusion (FFA)	Good	Extensive nonperfusion (>10 disc diameters)
Electroretinography	Normal	Low B–A wave ratio (<1)
Prognosis for vision	Good	Poor

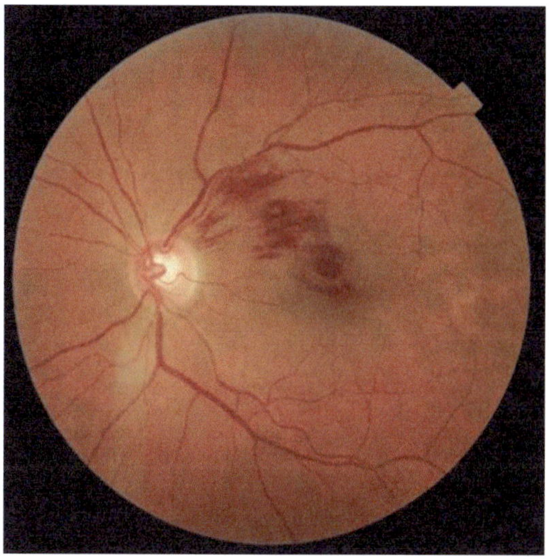

Fig. 22.13 Superotemporal BRVO (Courtesy of Retina Rocks®)

arise, scatter laser photocoagulation in the area of the occluded vein should be considered to prevent the progression to neovascular glaucoma. However, this treatment should only be performed if there is evidence of neovascularization.

- Systemic anticoagulation is not recommended for the treatment of RVO.
- Neovascularization of the disc (NVD) is characteristically common with hemiretinal vein occlusion but can also occur with CRVO and rarely BRVO.
- In retinal vein occlusion patients younger than 50 years and in the absence of common risk factors, an extensive workup for hypercoagulable conditions should be considered.

22.6.4 Ocular Ischemic Syndrome (OIS)

It is a progressive and chronic condition caused by atherosclerotic obstruction of carotid or ophthalmic artery, leading to progressive ischemic changes and visual acuity drop over weeks. Internal carotid stenosis (typically 90% or more) is the most common cause of ocular ischemic syndrome.

Presentation is with poor vision due to both retinal artery and cilioretinal artery obstruction, signs of anterior segment ischemia, iris neovascularization, and anterior chamber flare. IOP can be low, normal, or even high if patients develop neovascular glaucoma (NVG). The retinal findings often resemble those of a partial central retinal vein occlusion, with typical features including narrowed arteries, dilated but not tortuous veins, hemorrhages, microaneurysms, and neovascularization of the optic nerve head, retina, or both.

The most definitive treatment for OIS involves carotid artery stenting and endarterectomy, although the outcomes for visual acuity are variable.

22.7 Other Vascular Diseases

22.7.1 Sickle Cell Retinopathy

Retinopathy is most commonly seen with SC trait, to a lesser extent with S-thalassemia, and least likely with SS trait.

22.7.1.1 Ocular Manifestations of Sickle Cell Disease

As shown in Tables 22.9, 22.10, and 22.11, sickle cell disease can have manifestations affecting the anterior segment as well as retinopathy, which can be classified into non-proliferative and proliferative retinopathy.

22.7.1.2 High-Yield Notes

- Many neovascular complexes involute spontaneously as a result of auto-infarction, so the decision to treat proliferative sickle retinopathy (PSR) with scatter photocoagulation should be made cautiously especially because such treatment is associated with increased risk of tears and rhegmatogenous retinal detachment (RRD).
- It is recommended to avoid scleral buckles in sickle patients with retinal detachment (RD) as they are associated with high risk of anterior segment ischemia.
- All black patients presenting with a traumatic hyphema should be screened for sickling hemoglobinopathy due to increased risk of complications associated with the presence of rigid sickled erythrocytes.

22.7.2 Idiopathic Juxtafoveal Telangiectasia (Perifoveal Telangiectasia or mac-tel)

This condition is a degenerative, often asymmetrical disease that tends to affect both eyes. It is characterized by the development of telangiectatic vessels (abnormal, dilated blood vessels) at the temporal region of the macula.

Key risk factors for the condition include hypertension and diabetes. The earliest noticeable sign is typically a graying of the retina in the area temporal to the fovea. As the disease progresses, telangiectasia forms, which can eventually lead to macular edema (swelling) and fluid leakage. In the later stages, pigment migration can occur, leading to atrophy (wasting away) of the fovea. In rare cases, this can result in severe vision loss.

Table 22.9 Anterior segment manifestations of sickle cell disease

Conjunctiva	Corkscrew or comma-shaped vessels; most often in the inferior bulbar conjunctiva and fornix
Anterior chamber	Hyphema: tends to be aggressive and associated with high IOP and other complications
Iris	Patchy iris atrophy, rubeosis iridis

Table 22.10 Features of non-proliferative sickle retinopathy

Optic disc	Sickling sign (red blots resulting from small vessel occlusion)
Macula	Microaneurysms Epiretinal membrane (ERM) Depression sign (oval temporal thinning and irregular foveal reflex) Macular thinning best imaged by OCT
Peripheral retina	Salmon patches (intraretinal hemorrhages which may break into subretinal or preretinal space) Black sunburst (patches of degenerative retinal pigment epithelial changes resulting from resolved salmon patches) Angioid streaks reported clinically in up to 6% of cases
Retinal vasculature	Venous tortuosity and retinal venous occlusion Arterial silver wiring, corkscrewing, retinal arterial occlusions

Table 22.11 Stages of proliferative sickle retinopathy

Stage one	Arteriolar occlusion
Stage two	Arteriovenous anastomosis
Stage three	Sea fan neovascularization (Fig. 22.14)
Stage four	Vitreous hemorrhage
Stage five	Retinal detachment could be tractional or combined tractional rhegmatogenous detachment

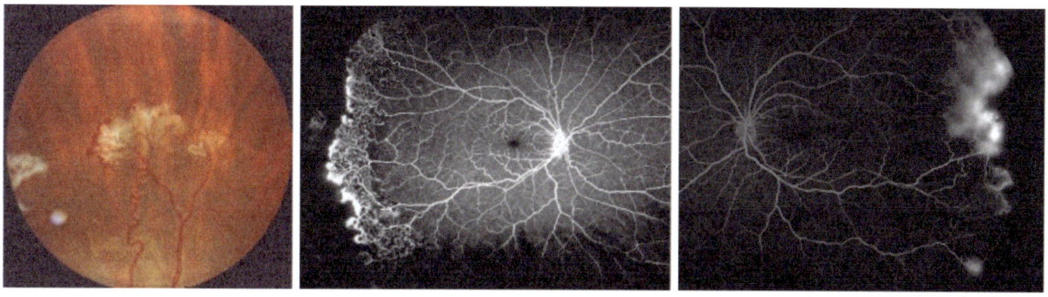

Fig. 22.14 Sea fan neovascularization in sickle retinopathy (Courtesy of Retina Rocks®)

Optical coherence tomography (OCT), especially en face OCT, can provide precise and reproducible measurements of photoreceptor loss, which often aligns significantly with functional loss as seen in microperimetry.

While macular edema may sometimes resolve on its own without the need for injections, regular monitoring is crucial to watch for the development of macular neovascularization (MNV). Treatments like photocoagulation and anti-VEGF are primarily aimed at managing MNV rather than edema.

Historically, three types of idiopathic juxtafoveal telangiectasia (IJFT) have been identified:

- Type I (also known as forme-fruste Coats' disease or Leber's miliary aneurysms) typically affects one eye and is more common in males. It causes vision loss primarily through macular edema and is usually diagnosed at around age 40.
- Type II is the most common form of IJFT. It affects both eyes and occurs in middle-aged people (between 50 and 70 years), with both sexes being equally affected. It is associated with metabolic dysfunction, leading to the loss of Muller cells and photoreceptors. It presents with less obvious telangiectasis, but characteristic vessel dilatation can be seen on fluorescein angiography (FFA) and OCT angiography (OCTA). A new imaging technique called macular pigment optical density can show a distinctive oval reduction in pigment optical density within 6 degrees of the fovea, suggesting that the disease is confined within the fovea.
- Type III (also known as occlusive telangiectasia) is very rare and is characterized by the progressive obliteration of the perifoveal capillary network. It usually occurs in association with a medical or neurological disease and typically carries a poor prognosis.

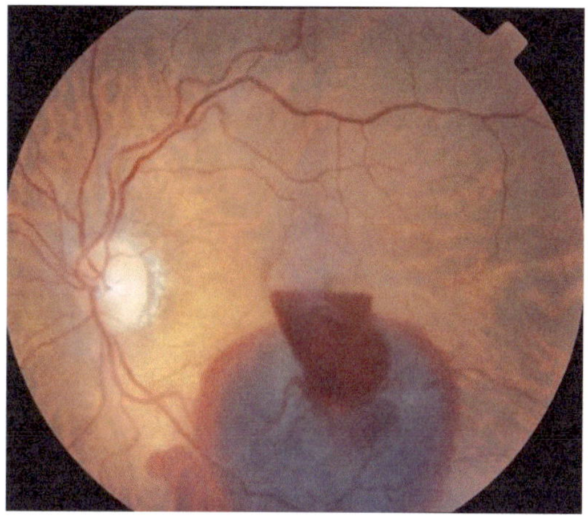

Fig. 22.15 Inferotemporal RAMA (Courtesy of Retina Rocks®)

22.7.3 Retinal Arterial Macroaneurysms (RAMAs)

Retinal arterial macroaneurysms (RAMAs) are localized, saclike dilatations of the retinal arterioles, most commonly found at points where these arterioles bifurcate or cross over veins, typically within the temporal arcades of the retina (Fig. 22.15).

RAMAs usually present in elderly females who have hypertension. Although typically unilateral and solitary, they can sometimes be found in both eyes or as multiple lesions in one eye.

These macroaneurysms can cause a variety of symptoms depending on how they affect the retina. In many cases, they result in chronic fluid leakage, leading to retinal exudates and macular edema. Alternatively, they may rupture, causing hemorrhage that can be intraretinal (within the retinal layers), subretinal (beneath the retina), or preretinal (in front of the retina). Such hemorrhages can lead to the development of complications such as epiretinal membrane (ERM) or macular neovascularization (MNV).

Interestingly, many RAMAs spontaneously regress over time due to fibrosis (scarring) or thrombosis (blood clot formation). Because of this, a common first-line approach to managing RAMAs is "watchful waiting" or observing the condition over time without intervening unless necessary.

When intervention is required, treatment options can include the following:

- Laser photocoagulation: This involves using a laser to cauterize the aneurysm, stopping fluid leakage and helping to reduce swelling and improve vision.
- YAG laser hyaloidotomy: This procedure uses a YAG laser to create a small opening in the hyaloid face (a membrane within the eye), allowing trapped blood from a preretinal hemorrhage to disperse.
- Anti-VEGF injections: These can be used to help reduce macular edema and inhibit the growth of abnormal blood vessels.
- Intravitreal gas or tissue plasminogen activator (t-PA) injections: These can be used to help displace a dense macular hemorrhage.
- Pars plana vitrectomy (PPV): This surgical procedure may be required for cases where there is significant vitreous hemorrhage or dense macular hemorrhage that does not respond to other treatments.

As with any eye condition, the choice of treatment should be individualized to each patient, taking into account their overall health, the specifics of their RAMA, and the potential benefits and risks of each treatment option.

22.7.4 Coats' Disease

This is an idiopathic unilateral acquired (not inherited) condition characterized by intraretinal and subretinal exudates (may progress to exudative RD) and primary retinal telangiectasia with tortuosity and aneurysmal dilatation.

It typically presents with unilateral decreased vision and leukocoria (or xanthocoria) in a male child <10 years.

Treatment options include laser or cryoablation of abnormal vessels, anti-VEGF or steroid injections, and external drainage of exudative detachment with or without PPV.

22.7.4.1 High-Yield Note

Histopathologic study of Coats' disease demonstrates that irregular dilatation of intraretinal blood vessels is associated with massive exudation of periodic acid-Schiff-positive (PAS-positive) material into the outer neural retinal layers.

22.7.5 Eales Disease

It is an idiopathic peripheral bilateral occlusive periphlebitis typically affecting young males, especially Indians, and thought to occur as a hypersensitivity reaction to tuberculosis protein.

Three overlapping stages of Eales are the following:

1. **Inflammatory stage**
   It is characterized by mild acute anterior uveitis (AAU) and retinal periphlebitis.
2. **Occlusive stage**
   This is characterized by branch retinal vein occlusion.
3. **Neovascular stage**
   It is characterized by neovascularization (NVEs, NVDs, and NVIs) causing recurrent self-limited vitreous hemorrhages.

Generally, macular involvement is rare, and prognosis is good; however, complications such as tractional retinal detachment (TRD), neovascular glaucoma, ERM, and cataract frequently need treatment.

22.7.6 Susac Syndrome (Retinocochleocerebral Vasculopathy)

It is an autoimmune endotheliopathy affecting the brain, retina, and inner ear. It is characterized by multiple branch retinal arterial occlusions and can be associated with hearing loss and, in rare cases, strokes. The condition is most commonly diagnosed in women in their third decade of life, and its cause is unknown. Treatment typically involves corticosteroids or immunosuppressive therapy. In the acute phase, treatment with intravenous immunoglobulin or plasma exchange seems effective.

22.7.7 Incontinentia Pigmenti (IP)

It is an X-linked dominant ectodermal disease, characterized by poorly developed peripheral retinal vasculature. It tends to be lethal for male fetuses in utero. It manifests at birth or early childhood. Ocular abnormalities occur in about 35% of cases and mostly include peripheral vascular occlusion and its sequel, including hemorrhages, neovascularization, and eventually retinal detachment. Systemic features include characteristic progressive skin lesions presenting soon after birth.

22.7.8 Trauma-Associated Retinopathy

22.7.8.1 Purtscher Retinopathy

It describes a chorioretinopathy associated with indirect non-ocular trauma such as compression to the thorax or head with a constellation of retinal findings including Purtscher flecken (areas of inner retinal whitening), cotton wool spots, and retinal hemorrhages (Fig. 22.16).

Optic disc usually appears normal, but optic disc edema might be occasionally seen.

Visual disturbance may appear synchronous with that event or be delayed up to 24–48 h and usually leads to irreversible vision loss.

When typical retinal findings occur in the complete absence of trauma, the term Purtscher-like retinopathy is used, with pancreatitis being the typical example.

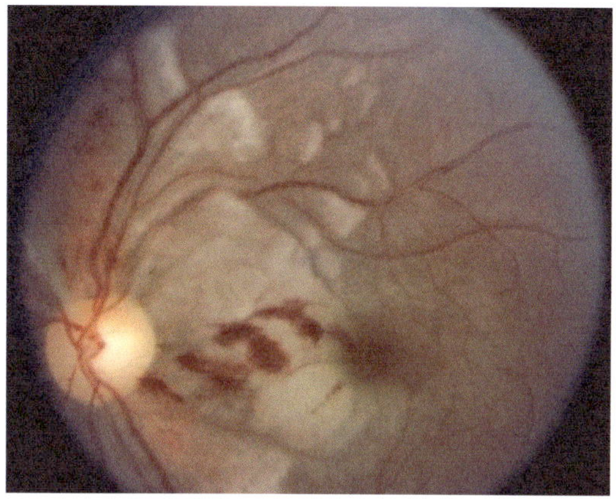

Fig. 22.16 Purtscher retinopathy (Courtesy of Retina Rocks®)

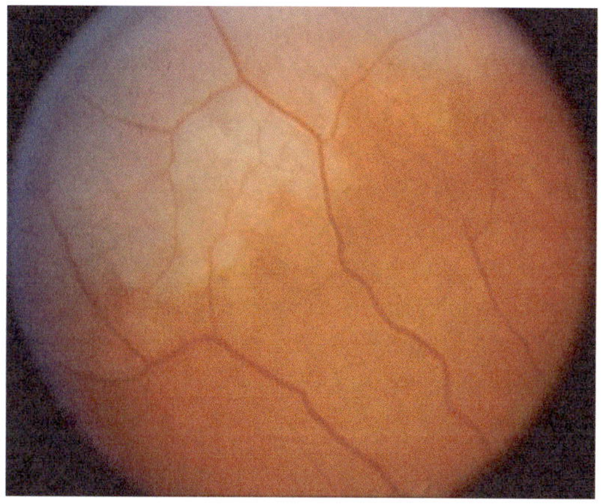

Fig. 22.17 Commotio retinae (Courtesy of Retina Rocks®)

Purtscher-like retinopathy can also be found in long-bone fractures, retrobulbar injection, systemic lupus erythematosus (SLE) (can be the presenting sign), thrombotic thrombocytopenic purpura (TTP), pancreatitis, and chronic renal failure.

22.7.8.2 Commotio Retinae

This represents an actual disruption or destruction of retinal photoreceptor in the outer layers of the retina, rather than retinal edema. It is usually caused by shock waves from blunt trauma or blast injury, primarily affecting the globe (Fig. 22.17). It usually progresses from outer to inner layers. The photoreceptor outer

Table 22.12 Comparison between Purtscher retinopathy and commotio retinae

	Purtscher	Commotio
Responsible injury	Chest or head compressive trauma	Direct or indirect globe trauma
Affected retina	Inner retina	Outer retina
Findings	Purtscher flecken, hemorrhages, and cotton wool spots	Grayish appearance
Visual acuity	Severely affected	Preserved, except with macular hole (few months after injury)

segment is always involved; damage to more inner layers requires more force. It appears as gray-white opacification of the neuroretina with occasional RPE mottling. Cherry red macular spot can be seen when commotio involves the fovea. It most frequently affects temporal fundus.

Table 22.12 demonstrates the major differences between Purtscher retinopathy and commotio retinae.

22.7.8.3 Terson's Syndrome

It is characterized by vitreous or retinal hemorrhage resulting from a sudden, spontaneous, or traumatic intracranial hemorrhage, such as subarachnoid or subdural hemorrhages. This condition is primarily caused by rapid increase in venous pressure and occurs in approximately 20% of patients with spontaneous or traumatic subarachnoid hemorrhages. In severe cases, PPV may be necessary to remove the hemorrhage.

22.7.8.4 Valsalva Retinopathy

A sudden increase in intrathoracic or intra-abdominal pressure such as from coughing, vomiting, heavy lifting, or straining during a bowel movement may raise intraocular venous pressure, leading to the rupture of small superficial capillaries in the macula, typically beneath the internal limiting membrane (ILM) (Fig. 22.18). Vision is usually only mildly affected, with an excellent prognosis and complete resolution typically occurring within months. The differential diagnosis for valsalva retinopathy includes conditions such as posterior vitreous separation, which can cause a similar hemorrhage, or a retinal macroaneurysm. Therefore, it is crucial to rule out a peripheral retinal tear or an aneurysm along an arteriole in all cases.

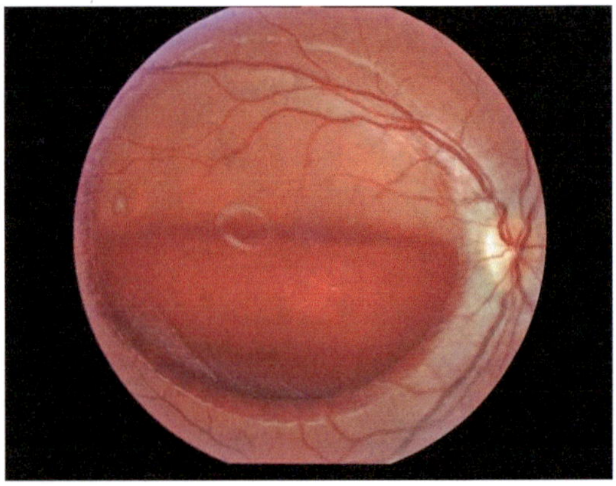

Fig. 22.18 Valsalva retinopathy (Courtesy of Retina Rocks®)

22.8 Pathological Myopia

Pathological myopia, also referred to as degenerative or malignant myopia, is a severe form of myopia where the eye grows excessively long from front to back (anterior-posterior elongation), causing mechanical stretching and structural changes in the scleral envelope of the eye.

Key Features

- Tessellated fundus: Due to diffuse thinning of the retinal pigment epithelium (RPE), larger choroidal vessels become more visible, giving the retina a tessellated or "tigroid" appearance.
- Chorioretinal atrophy: Areas of focal or patchy atrophy in the choroid and retina can develop.
- Anomalous optic discs: The optic disc may appear abnormal—being either larger or smaller than normal, tilted or twisted (torsional), or showing peripapillary atrophy (Fig. 22.19) or optic disc pits.
- Staphyloma: This is a localized, outward bulging (ectasia) of the sclera, which can occur around the optic nerve (peripapillary staphy-

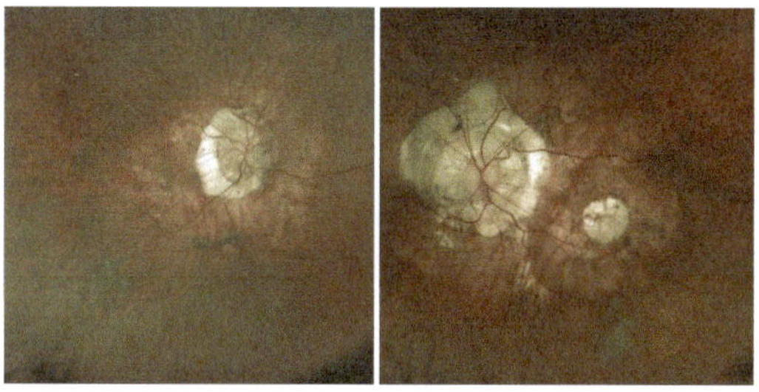

Fig. 22.19 Peripapillary atrophy and chorioretinal atrophy in pathological myopia (Courtesy of Retina Rocks®)

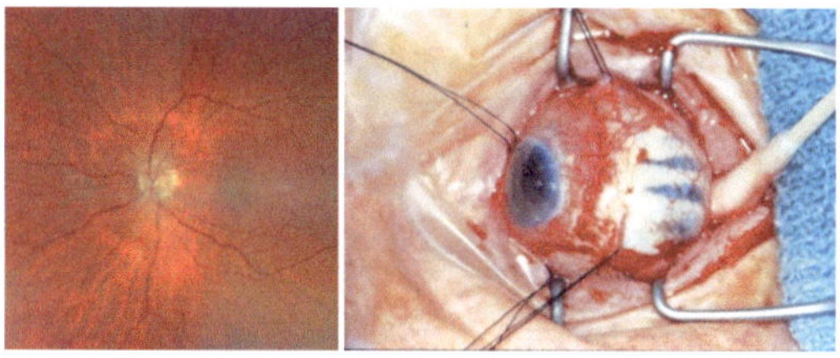

Fig. 22.20 Internal (Left) and external view (Right) of staphyloma in pathological myopia (Courtesy of Retina Rocks®)

loma) or the macula (macular staphyloma). Macular staphylomas are associated with macular holes and excavation of the macula (Fig. 22.20).

- Lacquer cracks: These are breaks in the RPE-Bruch's-choriocapillaris complex, appearing as irregular yellow lines crossing the posterior pole of the retina. They can lead to the development of myopic macular neovascularization (MNV) or can bleed, causing a subretinal hemorrhage. When this hemorrhage resorbs, it can leave a pigmented lesion known as a Fuchs spot or Foster-Fuchs spot.
- Intrachoroidal cavitation: Also known as peripapillary detachment in pathological myopia, this is a yellow-orange pocket that represents posterior bowing of the sclera around the optic nerve. It can be associated with visual field defects similar to those seen in glaucoma.

Associations with Pathological Myopia

- Retinal detachment: The incidence of retinal detachment is higher in patients with pathological myopia due to the presence of peripheral retinal degenerations (like lattice degeneration), stretched and thinned peripheral retina, increased frequency of posterior vitreous detachment and retinal tears, and an increased risk of vitreous loss during cataract surgery.
- Myopic maculopathy: This is the most common cause of vision loss in pathological myopia, with myopic macular neovascularization (MNV) being a key complication. The prognosis is relatively better than that of neovascular age-related macular degeneration (nAMD).
- Macular holes, shallow detachments, foveoschisis: These are all potential complications of pathological myopia.
- Cataract: Patients with pathological myopia have an increased risk of developing cataracts, especially posterior subcapsular cataracts, and lens subluxations.
- Glaucoma: Several forms of glaucoma, including primary open-angle glaucoma, pigment dispersion syndrome, and steroid-induced glaucoma, are more common in patients with pathological myopia. Measuring the retinal nerve fiber layer thickness with optical coherence tomography (OCT) can be challenging due to the varying shape of the eye.
- Amblyopia: This is a condition where vision in one or both eyes fails to develop properly during early childhood. It can be associated with severe forms of refractive error, including pathological myopia.

In pathological myopia, regular follow-up is crucial to monitor for the abovementioned complications and to initiate treatment as soon as possible to prevent further vision loss.

Acknowledgements None.

Conflict of Interest None.

References

Doft B et al (1995) Results of the Endophthalmitis Vitrectomy Study. A randomized trial of immediate vitrectomy and of intravenous antibiotics for the treatment of postoperative bacterial endophthalmitis. Endophthalmitis Vitrectomy Study Group. Arch Ophthalmol 113:1479–1496

Heeren TFC et al (2020) Macular telangiectasia type 2: visual acuity, disease end stage, and the MacTel area: MacTel project report number 8. Ophthalmology 127(11):1539–1548. https://doi.org/10.1016/j.ophtha.2020.03.040

Kanski JJ, Bowling B (2015) Kanski's clinical ophthalmology: a systematic approach. Saunders

Karampelas M, Malamos P, Petrou P, Georgalas I, Papaconstantinou D, Brouzas D (2020) Retinal pigment epithelial detachment in age-related macular degeneration—ophthalmology and therapy. Ophthalmol Ther 9(4):739–756. https://doi.org/10.1007/s40123-020-00291-5

Kertes PJ, Conway MD (1998) Clinical trials in ophthalmology: a summary and practice guide. https://doi.org/10.1604/9780683302059

Kim SJ (2021) 2021–2022 basic and clinical science course, section 12: retina and vitreous

Reed K (2001) Fluorescein Angiography Refresher Course. Fluorescein Angiography Refresher Course. https://www.reviewofoptometry.com/article/fluorescein-angiography-refresher-course

Scott IU, Campochiaro PA, Newman NJ, Biousse V (2020) Retinal vascular occlusions. Lancet 396(10266):1927–1940. https://doi.org/10.1016/S0140-6736(20)31559-2

Clinical Review of Retina and Vitreous Diseases: Part II

23

Mo'ath AlShawabkeh, Saif Aldeen Alryalat, Mohammed Abu-Ameerh, and Ahmed A. Sallam

Abstract

This chapter explores a range of retinal conditions, starting with hereditary retinal dystrophies. It categorizes these dystrophies into diffuse types, including rod-dominant and cone-dominant syndromes, and choroidal syndromes, detailing their genetic underpinnings and clinical manifestations. The chapter then examines retinopathy associated with systemic diseases, discussing conditions such as vitamin A deficiency, abetalipoproteinemia, Refsum disease, Jalili syndrome, albinism, disseminated intravascular coagulation, and others. Each condition is analyzed for its impact on retinal health. Next, the chapter addresses retinopathy related to drug toxicities, focusing on specific medications such as chloroquine, hydroxychloroquine, thioridazine, tamoxifen, sildenafil, and interferon, highlighting their potential retinal side effects. Finally, the chapter concludes with a discussion on retinal detachment, covering its types, causes, clinical features, and management strategies. This comprehensive overview support readers with critical insights into hereditary and acquired retinal conditions.

Keywords

Hereditary retinal dystrophies · Diffuse dystrophies · Choroidal syndromes · Systemic diseases · Retinal detachment

For readers interested in further more comprehensive and detailed information, the following references are useful (Kim 2021; Kanski and Bowling 2015; Kertes and Conway 1998; Karampelas et al. 2020; Scott et al. 2020; Heeren et al. 2020; Reed 2001; Doft et al. 1995).

23.1 Hereditary Retinal Dystrophies

Hereditary retinal dystrophies are a group of genetic disorders that result in the progressive loss of retinal cells and often lead to severe visual impairment. They can have autosomal dominant, autosomal recessive, and X-linked inheritance patterns. Below are key points to consider:

M. AlShawabkeh (✉)
Department of Ophthalmology, The Hashemite University, Zarqa, Jordan

S. A. Alryalat
Department of Ophthalmology, The University of Jordan, Amman, Jordan

The University of Colorado Anschutz Medical Campus, Aurora, CO, USA

M. Abu-Ameerh
The University of Jordan, Amman, Jordan

A. A. Sallam
Harvey and Bernice Jones Eye Institute, University of Arkansas for Medical Sciences (UAMS), Little Rock, AR, USA

S. A. Alryalat (ed.), *Ophthalmology Board and FRCS Part 2 Exams*,
https://doi.org/10.1007/978-981-96-1517-9_23

1. Bilateral symmetry: These diseases usually affect both eyes equally, though exceptions exist.
2. Progressive nature: Hereditary retinal dystrophies are characterized by progressive degeneration of the retina. However, total blindness is relatively uncommon, with many patients retaining some degree of vision.
3. Differential diagnosis: Before diagnosing a hereditary retinal dystrophy, it's important to rule out other treatable causes of retinal dysfunction. These include vitamin A deficiency, autoimmune retinopathies, paraneoplastic syndromes, and infectious retinopathies.
4. Pigmentary retinopathy: This term is often used when the etiology of a retinal disorder is unknown and no associated systemic disease is present. It refers to a group of conditions characterized by pigmented changes in the retina.
5. Unique phenotypes: Some hereditary retinal dystrophies have distinctive phenotypes that can help in their identification:
   - Retinitis punctata albescens: Characterized by deep retinal white dots or flecks.
   - Choroideremia: Marked by choriocapillaris atrophy. It's an X-linked recessive disorder characterized by progressive degeneration of the choroid, RPE, and photoreceptors.
   - Mutations in CRB1: These can lead to retinal thickening and loss of laminations, leading to conditions like retinitis pigmentosa and Leber congenital amaurosis.
   - Bietti crystalline dystrophy: Associated with crystalline deposits in the retina and is caused by mutations in the CYP4V2 gene.
   - CRB1-related retinopathy: Characterized by preservation of the para-arteriolar retinal pigment epithelium.

23.1.1 Diffuse Dystrophies

Disorders primarily affecting diffuse photoreceptor are classified separately from those predominantly involving the macula, as their symptoms and prognoses generally differ. The category of diffuse photoreceptor dystrophies c is further divided into subcategories based on rod-dominant, cone-dominant, and choroidal syndromes and diseases.

23.1.2 Diffuse Retinal Dystrophy

23.1.2.1 Rod-Cone Dystrophy (Retinitis Pigmentosa)

Nyctalopia is the main manifestation. Fundus examination will show arteriolar narrowing, disc pallor, and bony spicules, which are non-specific intraretinal pigment deposition by macrophages as part of the degenerative process (Fig. 23.1). Other manifestations include vitreous cells, CME, epiretinal membranes, optic nerve drusen, and posterior subcapsular cataract. Paracentral scotoma progresses peripherally and eventually leads to tunnel vision. AR is being the most common inheritance pattern. X-linked retinitis pigmentosa is the least common form of RP but the most severe. In female carriers of X-linked RP, manifestations may occur, and the ERG often shows a slight reduction or delay in b-wave responses (delayed implicit time).

In eyes with rod-cone dystrophies, the ERG response typically shows a loss or a significant reduction of rod-derived responses, more so than cone-derived responses. Both a-wave and b-wave amplitudes are usually reduced, and the ERG signal may become undetectable as the disease progresses. However, an undetectable ERG signal is not diagnostic; while it indicates severe retinal dysfunction, it doesn't necessarily correspond to the patient's level of visual function. High-dose daily vitamin A (15,000 IU/day) may decrease progression 20%/year, but with marked toxicity on liver and BIH.

Syndromic Retinitis pigmentosa (AR inheritance):

- Bardet-Biedl syndrome: pigmentary retinopathy with Bull's eye maculopathy. Systemic features including obesity, polydactyly, hypogonadism, and cognitive disability.
- Usher syndrome: RP with associated sensorineural hearing loss.

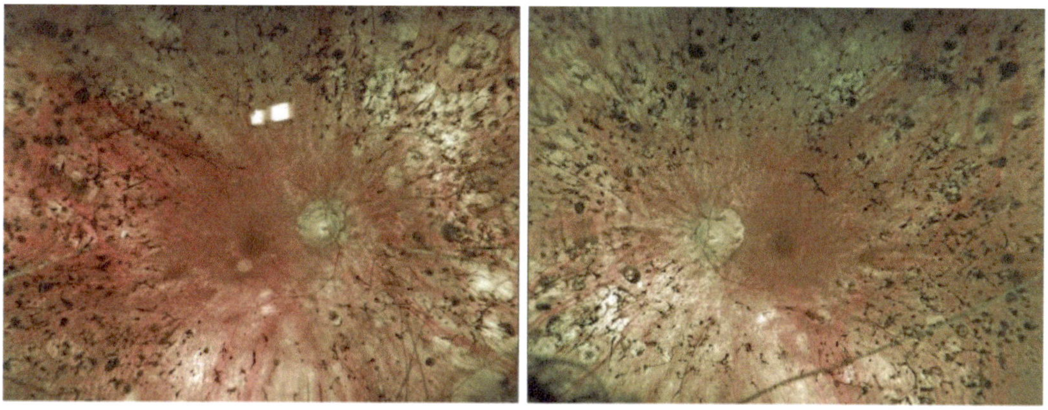

Fig. 23.1 Features of retinitis pigmentosa (Courtesy of Retina Rocks®)

Types I and III of Usher syndrome are characterized by vestibular dysfunction, and patients with profound deafness are more likely to exhibit cerebellar atrophy. Unilateral RP is generally sporadic. Usher syndrome, classified as a ciliopathy, is defined by the combination of retinitis pigmentosa and congenital sensorineural hearing loss. In retinitis pigmentosa, both the ERG and EOG show subnormal results. However, in conditions like sector retinitis pigmentosa, which affects only specific areas of the retina, the b-wave amplitude may be reduced, but the shape and timing of the waveforms produced by the unaffected, healthy regions of the retina typically remain normal.

Clinically, the ERG is the most critical diagnostic tool, as it provides evidence of the diffuse photoreceptor damage that characterizes the hereditary dystrophies grouped under RP.

23.1.2.2 Cone-Rod Dystrophy

The main manifestations are photophobia and day blindness (aka., hemeralopia), with symptoms onset typically occurring during the teenage years or later in adulthood. The fundus often appears normal although it may sometimes display a symmetric bull's-eye pattern of macular atrophy. Unlike macular dystrophies, cone dystrophies are more commonly associated with color vision issues and photophobia, necessitating differentiation from other. Diagnosis is confirmed when ERG reveals an abnormal or undetectable photopic ERG response, with a normal or near-normal rod-isolated ERG response, except in cases where rods are also severely affected. The defining feature of cone-rod dystrophy is that cone- derived full-field ERG responses are more impaired than rod ERG responses.

23.1.2.3 Leber Congenital Amaurosis (LCA)

LCA is a severe hereditary retinal dystrophy that manifests as profound vision loss or blindness at birth or within the first few months of life. It represents a heterogeneous group of conditions, with distinct subtypes defined by the specific causative gene involved.

Key Points

- Incidence: LCA is the most common cause of inherited blindness in childhood, contributing to more than 5% of all retinal dystrophies and leading to blindness in more than 20% of children attending schools for the blind.
- Clinical presentation: Infants with LCA usually have severely reduced vision, ranging from 20/200 to no light perception (NLP), along with nystagmus and photophobia. Some infants may also exhibit the oculodigital reflex, which includes eye-poking, pressing, and rubbing behaviors.
- Eye examination: Fundus examination is typically normal in the early stages of the disease although central macular atrophic lesions may be seen as the disease progresses. Despite poor vision, affected individuals often have high hyperopia (>+5).

- Diagnosis: Diagnosis is primarily established based on clinical features and confirmed by genetic testing. Electrophysiologic testing with ERG is characteristically "extinguished" or severely reduced in these patients.
- Associations: LCA is associated with early-onset cataracts, keratoconus, and, in certain cases, nephronophthisis, leading to end-stage renal disease (ESRD).
- Treatment: Gene therapy has shown promising results for certain types of LCA. In 2018, the FDA approved Luxturna, a gene therapy for the treatment of LCA caused by mutations in the RPE65 gene. This was a significant advancement, marking the first approval of a gene therapy for a genetic disease in the United States.

LCA should not be confused with Leber Hereditary Optic Neuropathy (LHON) (see Table 23.1) which is a mitochondrially inherited disease, so it mostly affects males (9:1 ratio). Initially unilateral, but then both eyes will be affected. Optic nerve edema occurs in acute attack and then progresses to pallor and atrophy later in the disease. Visual acuity might range from mild unilateral loss to severe vision loss, rarely NLP. In acute LHON, macular changes precede peripapillary retinal nerve fiber layer swelling.

23.1.2.4 Enhanced S-cone Disease (aka., Goldmann–Favre Syndrome)

Enhanced S-cone disease is an AR disease. The retina in this condition has no rods, but cones were increased two-fold, >90% are S cones. This condition is marked by early onset of night blindness, reduced bilateral visual acuity, and characteristic fundus changes, including progressive pigmentary peripheral degenerative changes, macular edema, and retinoschisis. The key feature is an enhanced S-cone function due to the loss of rod photoreceptors, which paradoxically leads to nyctalopia (night blindness) while increasing sensitivity to blue light. Additional associated findings include pigmentary changes and hyperopia. Macular (and sometimes peripheral) schisis may be present, overlapping the phenotype of X-linked retinoschisis.

The ERG response shows no detectable dim-flash, rod-specific signal, and delayed, simplified responses to brighter flashes that have similar waveforms under both dark-adapted and light-adapted conditions. Additionally, the flicker ERG response is of lower amplitude compared to the single-flash photopic a-wave.

X-Linked Retinoschisis

XLRS is a genetic eye disorder that affects males and typically presents in childhood or early adolescence. It is characterized by the splitting (schisis) of the layers of the retina, leading to visual impairment.

Key Points

- Etiology: XLRS is caused by mutations in the RS1 gene, located on the X chromosome. This gene is responsible for coding retinoschisin, a protein found in photoreceptor, Muller, and bipolar cells in the retina.
- Clinical presentation: Common symptoms include strabismus and nystagmus. Patients usually present around the age of 5–10 years.
- Eye examination: The characteristic finding in XLRS is bilateral progressive splitting of the nerve fiber layer in the central macula. Peripheral schisis may also develop but is usually non-progressive. In the early stages, a parafoveal spoke-wheel pattern may be observed.

Table 23.1 Comparison between Leber's congenital amaurosis (LCA) and Leber's hereditary optic neuropathy (LHON)

	Leber's congenital amaurosis	Leber's hereditary optic neuropathy
Affecting	Retina	Optic nerve
Inheritance	AR	Mitochondrial
Visual acuity	<6/60 to no light perception	Range from mild to severe
Age onset	Infants	10–30 years
Diagnostic investigation	Electroretinography	Visual evoked potentials

- Associations: Around 50% of individuals with XLRS also have peripheral retinoschisis. Retinal detachment occurs in 15–20% of cases, usually due to retinal breaks, which are more common in the inner than the outer retinal lamina. Retinal vessels may bleed, leading to vitreous hemorrhage, which can significantly impair vision. Sclerotic vessels may appear as "vitreous veils."
- Diagnosis: Diagnosis is established based on clinical features and confirmed by genetic testing. An "electronegative ERG," characterized by a reduced or inverted "b" wave compared to the "a" wave, is found in more than 80% of cases.
- Treatment: Early treatment with the topical medication dorzolamide may help reduce macular schisis and associated complications such as lamellar and full-thickness macular holes.

Females can be carriers of XLRS, but they typically do not exhibit clinical symptoms. ERG can be used to identify female carriers who cannot be clinically identified. Genetic counseling is recommended for families of affected individuals.

23.1.3 Choroidal Dystrophies

All manifest in RP-like pictures, including nyctalopia, paracentral scotoma, and decreased vision upon progressing to fovea. They differ by onset of symptoms.

23.1.3.1 Choroideremia

Choroideremia has similar manifestations, but better prognosis than RP. It manifests between third and fifth decade of life. It is X-linked, so, higher frequency in men, and carrier women are generally asymptomatic. It is caused by mutations in *CHM*. Initial changes occur in the retinal pigment epithelium in the mid-periphery of the fundus. The macula is generally preserved till later in the disease. Carriers of choroideremia are generally asymptomatic and typically have normal ERG results, unlike carriers of juvenile X-linked RP. In choroideremia, central acuity tends to be preserved until later in life, whereas in X-linked RP, central visual acuity may be affected earlier.

23.1.3.2 Gyrate Atrophy

An AR dystrophy is caused by deficiency in the enzyme ornithine aminotransferase (OAT) in chromosome 10. Nyctalopia within the first decade of life, with accelerated course of vision loss with macular edema is being a common finding (managed by acetazolamide). Paving stone appearance in the mid-periphery progresses to become a scalloped border between normal and abnormal RPE (Fig. 23.2). A key differential diagnosis to consider is paving stone degeneration, which usually does not extend posteriorly

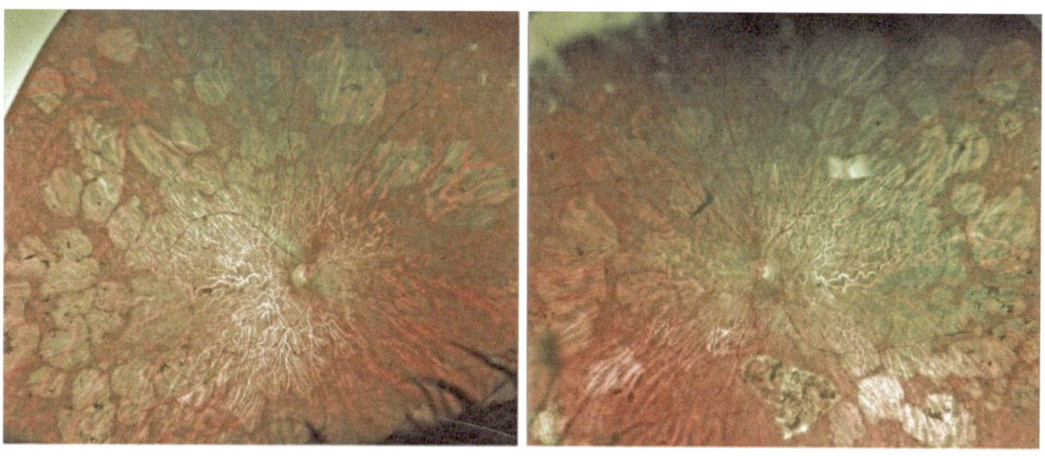

Fig. 23.2 Gyrate atrophy (Courtesy of Retina Rocks®)

beyond the equator. Unlike other dystrophies, moderate to marked myopia is common in most patients. The diagnosis is further supported by elevated plasma levels of ornithine and confirmed through genetic testing for mutations in the ornithine aminotransferase (OAT) gene. When initiated at a young age, aggressive dietary restriction of arginine intake and, in some cases, vitamin B6 supplementation can slow or even halt the progression of retinal degeneration. Progressive myopia and early cataract are also features. Gyrate atrophy does not affect intelligence or lifespan.

23.1.3.3 Bietti Crystalline Dystrophy

AR caused by mutations in the *CYP4V2* gene typically leads to nyctalopia in the second to fourth decades of life. Intraretinal yellow-white crystals can be observed in the posterior retina and in the peripheral cornea near the limbus, although these crystals tend to disappear as the disease advances. Over time, the condition progress to widespread retinochoroidal atrophy.

23.1.4 Macular Dystrophy

23.1.4.1 Stargardt Disease (aka. Fundus Flavimaculatus)

The most common inherited degenerative maculopathy is Stargardt disease. It causes progressive vision loss in late childhood due to accumulation of lipofuscin in the macula, with visual acuity ranges from 20/50 to 20/200, but usually most patients do not become legally blind (e.g., severe visual loss in both eyes).

Pathophysiologically, it is most caused by mutations in the *ABCA4* gene and inherited in an autosomal recessive manner. It is not diagnostic, as it is also present in 10% of the normal population. This mutation causes defects in the ATP-binding cassette transporter of the retina (or ABCR) protein, resulting in an accumulation of all-trans retinol in the outer segment discs of photoreceptor rods. The pisciform lesions observed in the posterior fundus are indicative of lipofuscin-like deposits at the level of the RPE cells. Juvenile foveal atrophy is surrounded by diffuse yellowish flecks at the level of the RPE, which might be mistaken as drusen. In other patients, these flecks can be scattered throughout the retina. Features include:

- **Retinal flecks:** The flecks spare the fovea in greater than 85% of patients (so still present in the macula in 15%), contrary to AMD that typically affects the fovea as part of its definition (Fig. 23.3).
- **Bull's eye maculopathy** with later atrophy, most evident on FAF.
- **Dark choroid:** on fluorescein angiography, 80% or more of patients with Stargardt disease have a "dark choroid," which refers to

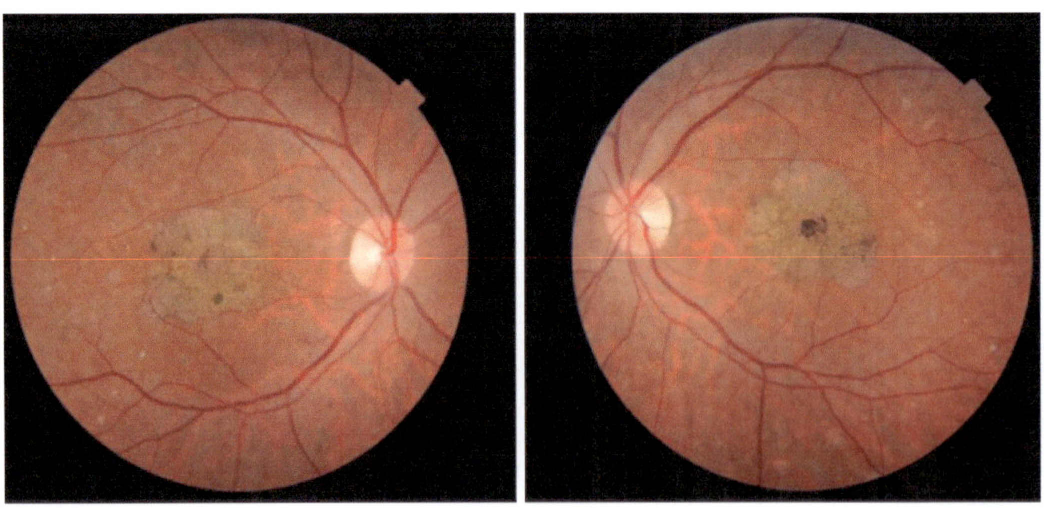

Fig. 23.3 Stargardt disease (Courtesy of Retina Rocks®)

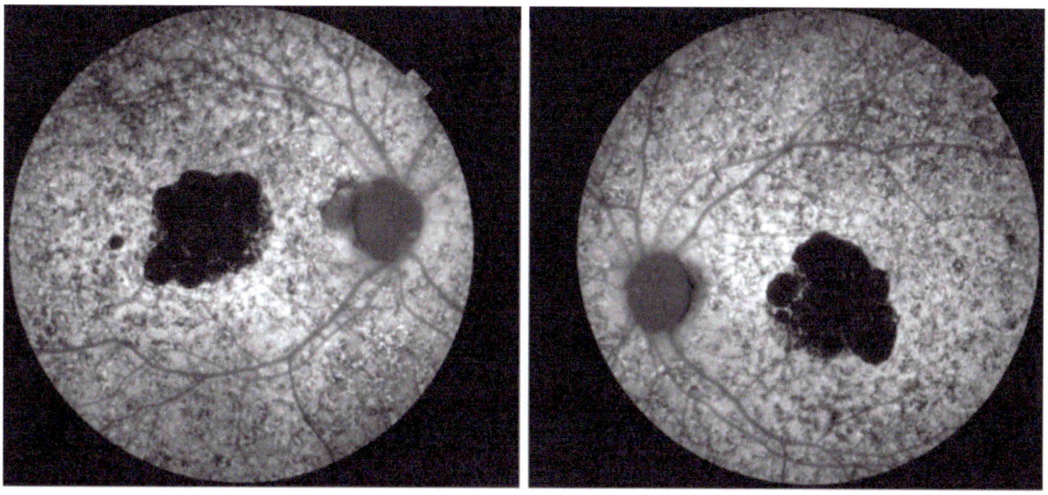

Fig. 23.4 FAF in Stargardt disease (Courtesy of Retina Rocks®)

the blockage of choroidal fluorescence that accentuates the retinal circulation due to the accumulation of lipofuscin in the mid-periphery. Full-field ERGs are typically not diagnostic for this condition, as they often appear normal. OCT shows outer retinal atrophy. On FAF, Stargardt disease appears as multiple hyper-autofluorescence lesions with hypo-autofluorescence around the fovea (Fig. 23.4).

Once thought a separate entity, fundus flavimaculatus (Fig. 23.5) is now considered a milder condition. Patients with fundus flavimaculatus often have a later disease onset and slower visual deterioration. Flecks are more in fundus flavimaculatus, but macular involvement is more severe in Stargardt.

An autosomal dominant Stargardt-like disease has been described. It is phenotypically similar to its autosomal recessive counterpart, with the exception of its inheritance pattern and associated mutated genes (*ELOVL4 and PROM1).*

The two conditions most commonly associated with bull's eye maculopathy are cone dystrophy and Stargardt disease (juvenile macular degeneration). Fluorescein angiography in Stargardt disease typically reveals the characteristic "dark choroid." Treatment for Stargardt is mainly supportive at this stage. It is important to note that unlike RP, vitamin A worsens the disease. Smoking should also be avoided and looking to direct sunlight.

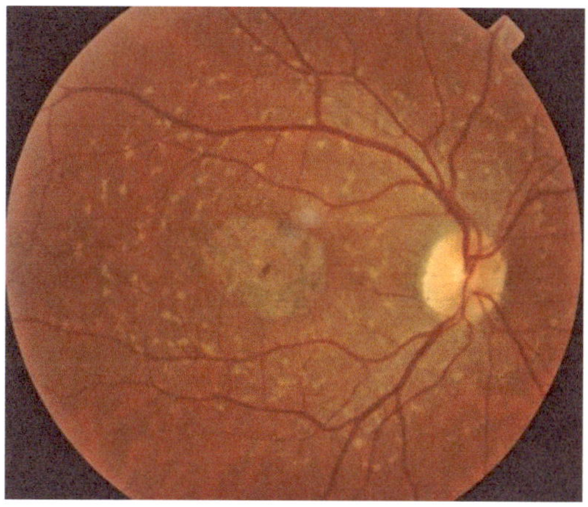

Fig. 23.5 Fundus flavimaculatus (Courtesy of Retina Rocks®)

23.1.4.2 Best Disease

Best disease is an autosomal dominant eye disorder that typically begins in childhood or adolescence and is characterized by lesions in the macula, the part of the eye responsible for central vision.

Key Points

1. Etiology: Best disease is caused by mutations in the BEST1 gene (also known as VMD2) on chromosome 11. This gene codes for the pro-

tein bestrophin, which plays a role in the normal functioning of the retina.

2. Clinical presentation: Characteristic feature includes a yellow, egg yolk-like (vitelliform) lesion in the macula. This lesion can break down over time, leaving a geographic atrophic appearance. About 30% of patients also have similar lesions outside the fovea.
3. Vision prognosis: Vision prognosis is generally good, with visual acuity ranging from 20/30 to 20/60 even in eyes with significant macular lesions. However, about 20% of patients may develop choroidal neovascularization (CNV) in one eye, which can lead to more severe vision loss. Most patients retain good vision in at least one eye throughout their lifetime.
4. Diagnosis: The diagnosis is established based on clinical features and confirmed by genetic testing. The full-field electroretinogram (ERG) is typically normal, but the electrooculogram (EOG) is almost always abnormal, showing a severely reduced or absent light rise (Arden ratio of 1.5 or less). This abnormal EOG can be present even in asymptomatic individuals with the causative genetic variant who have normal-appearing fundi. Table 23.2 demonstrates the major differences between Stargardt disease and Best disease.
5. Stages of Best disease:
   - Stage 0: Normal fundus appearance with an abnormal EOG.
   - Stage 1: Subtle retinal pigment epithelium (RPE) mottling.
   - Stage 2: Vitelliform stage characterized by "egg yolk" appearance or vitelliruptive "scrambled egg" appearance.
   - Stage 3: Pseudo-hypopyon stage, where the yellow material accumulates inferiorly.
   - Stage 4: End-stage, characterized by macular scarring or neovascularization.
6. Differential diagnosis: It's important to distinguish Best disease from Stargardt disease. While both are hereditary macular dystrophies, Best disease is autosomal dominant, often involves multiple family members, typically presents with an abnormal EOG (even in asymptomatic carriers), and the vision usually remains reasonable until middle age.

23.1.4.3 Pattern Dystrophy

Pattern macular dystrophies typically manifest between the fourth to sixth decade of life. Their autosomal dominant inheritance, relatively better visual outcomes, and later onset help distinguish these disorders from other macular dystrophies and degenerations. They generally have normal ERG and subnormal EOG (like but not as profound as in Best dystrophy).

Mutation in PRPH2 gene at chromosome 6 is characterized by reticular pigmentation at the level of RPE. The development of CNV is very rare, and the prognosis is generally good, with preserved visual acuity and normal electrophysiology. Subdivided into four major patterns according to the distribution of pigment deposits:

1. Adult-onset foveomacular vitelliform dystrophy
2. Butterfly-type pattern dystrophy
3. Reticular-type pattern dystrophy
4. Fundus pulverulentus (coarse pigment mottling)

Adult-onset foveomacular vitelliform dystrophy is a type of pattern dystrophy, despite its name suggesting a connection to best disease. Unlike Best disease, this condition is not associ-

Table 23.2 Comparison between Stargardt disease and Best disease

	Stargardt	Best
Inheritance	AR (ABCA4 gene)	AD (BEST1 gene)
Onset of symptoms	Earlier during late childhood	Later during early adulthood
Visual prognosis	Worse (as low as 20/200)	Better (as low as 20/60)
Diagnosis	Clinical, FAF & FA	Clinical, ERG followed by EOG

ated with an abnormal EOG. Patients with this disorder may initially present with a ring-like area of RPE clumping, which over time evolves into a yellowish lesion typically half a disk diameter or smaller, located in the central fovea. These lesions are notably smaller than those seen in Best disease. This disorder is more commonly associated with CNV than Best disease. Fluorescein angiography (FA) typically shows hypofluorescence in the area of the vitelliform lesion, surrounded by a ring of hyperfluorescence.

23.1.4.4 North Carolina Macular Dystrophy

Inherited as AD, abnormality at chromosome 6, characterized by macular abnormality that has been present since birth and ranges from as mild as subtle macular spots to coloboma-like lesions. These lesions represent well-demarcated atrophy of the RPE and choriocapillaris, and pigment deposition in the macular region. Both EOG and ERG (full field) are normal.

23.1.4.5 Early-Onset "Drusenoid" Macular Dystrophies

Drusen typically manifests at younger ages than do drusen in most cases of AMD (see AMD section).

23.1.4.6 Central Choroidal Areolar Dystrophy (CAD)

CAD is an AD hereditary retinal disorder caused by mutations in the *peripherin/RDS* gene. This conditions primarily affect the macula, leading to well-defined areas of atrophy in the RPE and choriocapillaris. CAD typically affects both eyes symmetrically and usually manifests between the second and fourth decades of life, which helps differentiate it from AMD.

23.1.4.7 Sorsby Pseudoinflammatory Fundus Dystrophy

When early-onset drusen is associated with CNV in young adulthood, the diagnosis of Sorsby macular dystrophy should be considered. The diagnosis can be confirmed by demonstrating a disease-causing mutation in the tissue inhibitor of metalloproteinase-3 (*TIMP3)* gene with autosomal dominant inheritance. The retinal changes appear in the third to fifth decades of life. It is characterized by the accumulation of a yellowish material, similar to drusen, in the posterior pole. This commonly progresses to choroidal neovascularization, hemorrhagic maculopathy, and even disciform fibrosis and atrophy which can extend beyond the macula.

23.1.5 Congenital Stationary Retinal Diseases (CSNB)

Congenital stationary night blindness is an early onset of non-progressive night vision difficulty; however, no histological evidence of rod abnormalities and normal fundus exam. Variable inheritance. It comprises the following: congenital stationary night blindness, color blindness, achromatopsia, Oguchi disease, and fundus albipunctatus.

23.1.5.1 Color Blindness

Dyschromatopsia is a color vision defect, while achromatopsia is absence of color discrimination. Whereas congenital color vision defects are stationary and usually affect both eyes equally, acquired color vision defects may be progressive and/or monocular.

Prefix: Prot- (red), deuter- (green), trit- (blue)

Suffix: -anomaly ranging from near normal to completely abnormal, -anopia (complete deficiency).

- Protanomaly 1% male and 0.1% female (X-linked).
- Deuteranomaly 6% male and 0.4% female (X-linked).
- Tritanomaly 0.01% in both (Ch.7).

Hereditary congenital color vision defects are most commonly X-linked-recessive, red-green abnormalities, affecting 5–8% of males and 0.5% of females. Acquired color vision defects are more frequently blue-yellow (tritan) and affect both males and females equally.

Individuals who require only two primary colors to make a color match have *dichromacy*, which suggests that they are missing one of the cone photopigments.

23.1.5.2 Achromatopsia

Achromatopsia means that any spectral color may be matched with any other solely by adjusting intensity. It represents disorders of photoreceptor function and includes two main forms: (Kim 2021) *rod monochromatism,* and (Kanski and Bowling 2015) *S-cone monochromatism (blue-cone monochromatism).* Both types typically present with congenital nystagmus, poor visual acuity, and photophobia. Electroretinography (ERG) is crucial in differentiating achromatopsia from other conditions such as congenital motor nystagmus or ocular albinism, which are associated with normal cone ERGs (see Table 23.3).

The early onset of photophobia and nystagmus points to a congenital cone dysfunction. Achromatopsia is indicated by an absence of photopic ERG response, including photopic flicker response, while rod function remains essentially normal. This condition results in complete color blindness due to a congenital absence of cone photoreceptors. It is inherited in an autosomal recessive manner and typically does not affect more than the current generation. Visual acuity usually ranges from 20/100 to 20/200 and is often better in dim lighting or with sunglasses.

Rod abnormality mainly manifests as nyctalopia or night vision difficulties and include:

23.1.5.3 Congenital Stationary Night Blindness (CSNB)

A non-progressive disorder of night vision, mostly X-linked, but also can be AR or AD. VA ranges from 20/200 to 20/20. Poor vision is usually attributed to myopia. Normal fundus compared to the below other rod disorders. Some individuals with CSNB have a paradoxical pupillary response in which the pupil constricts in response to decreased light.

A negative ERG is characterized by a bright-flash, dark-adapted ERG that shows a normal (or near-normal) a-wave but a markedly reduced b-wave. The normal a-wave indicates that there is no significant rod photoreceptor dysfunction. This pattern is key in differentiating CSNB from more severe, potentially blinding disorders like retinitis pigmentosa.

23.1.5.4 High-Yield Notes

- Melanoma-associated retinopathy (MAR) (see Miscellaneous) is the main differential diagnosis, which demonstrates an identical ERG pattern to CSNB.
- Duchenne muscular dystrophy produces negative ERG signal similar to CSNB (i.e., a normal a-wave but a reduced b-wave).
- ERG is normal in vitelliform dystrophy (and other pattern dystrophies), dominant drusen, X-linked ocular albinism (as only the macula involved, so not sufficient to affect ERG), and pattern dystrophy.

23.1.5.5 Fundus Albipunctatus

This is a form of CSNB results from a mutation in *RDH5* that encodes 11-*cis*- retinol dehydrogenase. Individuals with this condition experience night blindness from birth and typically present with yellow-white dots in the posterior pole that extends into the mid-periphery, while sparing the fovea. The ERG is abnormal.

Fundus albipunctatus can be distinguished from retinitis punctata albescens, an RP variant, by the normal vasculature seen in fundus albipunctatus, as opposed to the typically attenuated

Table 23.3 Comparison between rod monochromatism and S-cone monochromatism

	Rod monochromatism	S-cone monochromatism
Abnormality	Absence of all cones	Absence of L and M cones
Inheritance	AR	X-linked
VA	20/200–20/80	>20/80
Manifestations	Patients see only shades of gray	See in blue and black
ERG	Absence of cone response	Severely reduced cone flicker ERGs

vasculature found in retinitis punctata albescens. Fundus albipunctatus is a form of congenital stationary night blindness marked by distinctive yellow-white dots in the posterior pole. Patients typically have normal visual acuity and color vision. The rod ERG is minimal initially but normalizes after several hours of dark adaptation. This condition is non-progressive and should be differentiated from retinitis punctata albescens, a variant of retinitis pigmentosa.

23.1.5.6 Oguchi Disease

Oguchi disease is an AR form of CSNB with abnormal fundus color, most common in Japanese. After prolonged dark adaptation, the posterior pole reverts to a normal appearance, but shows a peculiar yellow iridescent sheen (i.e., golden color) alteration after exposure to even brief light (the *Mizuo–Nakamura phenomenon).* The characteristic electroretinogram (ERG) changes include un-recordable rod response and reductions of maximal response that improve with dark adaptation.

23.2 Retinopathy Associated with Systemic Diseases

23.2.1 Vitamin A Deficiency

Vitamin A deficiency retinopathy most commonly occurs in patients who have undergone gastric bypass surgery for obesity or small-bowel resection for Crohn's disease. These individuals often suffer from malabsorption of fat-soluble vitamins and may develop blind loop syndrome, where bacterial overgrowth depletes vitamin A. Patients experience night blindness (nyctalopia), and if left untreated, may suffer from vision loss and develop diffuse, drusen-like spots similar to those seen in retinitis punctata albescens.

23.2.2 Abetalipoproteinemia

Failure to synthesize apolipoprotein B results in abnormal absorption of fat and fat-soluble vitamins, leading to problems including retinal and spinocerebellar degeneration. Treatment with vitamins A and E is advised.

Familial adenomatous polyposis (FAP, also known as Gardner syndrome) is characterized by the presence of more than 4 widely spaced, small lesions (less than 0.5-disc-diameter) in each eye, with bilateral involvement. This condition is caused by mutations in the adenomatous polyposis gene (APC) and follows an autosomal dominant inheritance pattern.

23.2.3 Angioid Streaks

Angioid streaks represent discontinuities in Bruch's membrane, which has become abnormally thickened and calcified. These streaks most commonly radiate from the optic nerve head, but can also form a circumferential ring around the peripapillary area. Due to the associated atrophy of the overlying RPE, angioid streaks often appear as window defects on fluorescein angiography. Angioid streaks are idiopathic in 50% of cases, other associations include:

Pseudoxanthoma elasticum: An AR disorder caused by mutations in the ABCC6 gene. Characteristic findings include angioid streaks, optic nerve head drusen, and a "peau-d'orange" appearance of the retina. Patients often exhibit skin manifestations resembling a "plucked-chicken" appearance and are prone to widespread vascular malformations, with mucosal vasculature abnormalities in the stomach and bowel potentially leading to recurrent hemorrhages.

Paget disease: This condition encompasses a range of findings, most notably osteoclastic hyperactivity, especially at the base of the skull and in long bones, predisposing patients to pathologic fractures.

Ehlers–Danlos syndrome: A genetic disorder resulting from defective collagen synthesis characterized by hyperextensible joints and lax skin. Ocular manifestations may include dislocated lenses, retinal detachment, and blue sclera.

Sickle Cell Disease and Marfan Syndrome: Patients with angioid streaks are highly susceptible to choroidal rupture following even minor blunt injury. As a precaution, the use of safety glasses is recommended for these individuals.

23.2.4 Refsum Disease

Refsum disease is an AR deficiency in the enzyme phytanic acid 2-hydroxylase that leads to over-accumulation of phytanic acid. Patients have either have elevated plasma levels of phytanic acid or reduced phytanic acid oxidase activity in cultured fibroblasts. Ocular manifestations include pigmentary retinopathy (i.e., retinitis pigmentosa-like picture). Systemic features are polyneuropathy, cerebellar ataxia, deafness, anosmia, cardiomyopathy, and ichthyosis. Treatment is with plasmapheresis and maintaining a phytanic acid-free diet early on.

23.2.5 Jalili Syndrome

It is a type of cone-rod dystrophy with incomplete dentition and teeth enema development (aka, amelogenesis imperfecta) along with pigmentary retinopathy and macular coloboma.

23.2.6 Albinism

Albinism can manifest as ocular albinism (X-linked, so mainly affect males), or with skin and hair involvement, aka. Oculocutaneous albinism (AR).

Photophobia, iris transillumination, and hypopigmented fundus almost always present, but the most important feature is foveal hypoplasia, where if present, then reduced visual acuity and nystagmus develops (aka. True ocular albinism). They usually have high refractive errors.

The gold standard for diagnosis of true albinism is the finding of characteristic abnormalities of the flash and pattern visual evoked potentials (VEPs).

Oculocutaneous albinism has 2 forms with potentially lethal systemic implications:

- Chediak-Higashi syndrome is characterized by neutropenia causing recurrent infections and lymphoreticular malignancies.
- Hermansky-Pudlak syndrome is characterized by abnormal platelets and susceptibility to bleeding and bruising.

23.2.7 Disseminated Intravascular Coagulation (DIC)

DIC can lead to fibrinoid necrosis of the choriocapillaris, serous retinal detachments, and multiple areas of RPE changes. However, purtscher-like retinopathy, which includes numerous cotton-wool spots, sub-internal limiting membrane hemorrhages, and retinal hemorrhages, is uncommon in DIC.

White-centered hemorrhages, on the other hand, may be seen in conditions associated with septic emboli, such as endocarditis and Candida bacteremia, as well as in leukemia, and collagen vascular diseases.

23.2.8 Juvenile Neuronal Ceroid Lipofuscinoses (aka., Batten Disease)

This condition presents with vascular attenuation, optic atrophy, and peripheral pigmentary loss, alongside neurological symptoms such as seizures, and progressive dementia.

23.2.9 Aicardi Syndrome (AS)

AS is characterized by a triad of features: agenesis of corpus callosum, chorioretinal lacunae, and infantile spasms. Aicardi syndrome almost exclusively affects females and is believed to result from de novo mutation on the X chromosome, with homozygous being lethal in males. Chorioretinal lacunae, which are nearly universal in these patients, appears as well-defined, multifocal pale areas with minimally pigmented borders, typically clustered around the optic disc.

23.2.10 Mucopolysaccharidoses (MPSs)

AR conditions. Only those MPSs in which heparan sulfate is stored are associated with retinal dystrophy. These include:

- **MPS type I H** ***(Hurler syndrome)*** **and MPS type I S** ***(Scheie syndrome)***, these conditions present with clinical features such as coarse facies, cognitive disabilities, corneal clouding, and retinal degeneration. While the retinal pigmentary changes may be subtle, the ERG response is typically abnormal.
- **MPS type II** ***(Hunter syndrome)*** also presents with pigmentary retinopathy, but corneal clouding, if present, is usually mild. Patients often have coarse facies features, short stature, and may show cognitive disabilities.
- **MPS type III** ***(Sanfilippo syndrome)***, somatic stigmata are milder, but the pigmentary retinopathy is more severe.

23.2.10.1 Tay-Sachs Disease (Gangliosidosis Type 1) (Hexosaminidase A Deficiency)

This is the most common ganglioside storage disease, characterized by accumulation of glycolipids in the brain and retina. It leads to cognitive disabilities, blindness (often presenting with retinopathy and a cherry-red spot), and typically results in death between the ages of 2 and 5 years.

23.2.10.2 Gaucher Disease

Gaucher disease can also cause cherry-red spots, and it results in accumulations of glucosylceramide.

23.2.10.3 Niemann-Pick Disease

This condition results from the absence of various sphingomyelinase isozymes. In type A (acute neuronopathic) Niemann-Pick disease, a cherry-red spot is observed in about 50% of cases. **Cystinosis** causes crystalline depositions in cornea. Type 1 (aka., nephropathic) also causes retinal depigmentation.

23.2.10.4 Sjögren-Larsson Syndrome (SLS)

A neurocutaneous disorder with AR inheritance. Patients have ichthiosys, mental retardation, and spasticity. Crystalline maculopathy is typical, which leads to photophobia and variable decrease in visual acuity.

23.2.10.5 Chronic Progressive External Ophthalmoplegia (CPEO)

CPEO belongs to a group of diseases collectively termed mitochondrial myopathies and is associated with RP-like pigmentary retinopathy.

23.2.10.6 High-Yield Notes

- RPE degenerations have been identified in patients with Hunter, Hurler, Sanfilippo, and Scheie mucopolysaccharidoses.
- Maroteaux–Lamy syndrome is not usually associated with RPE degeneration.
- Nicotinic acid, a treatment for elevated cholesterol and triglycerides, can (rarely) cause a cystoid macular edema that demonstrates no leakage or staining on fundus fluorescein angiography.
- "Poppers" is a slang term for alkyl nitrites, which are a class of chemical used as recreational drugs. The chemicals are inhaled to induce euphoria and relax smooth muscles, usually in preparation for sexual activity. In rare cases, use can lead to acute central scotoma and vision reduction associated with a yellow, "vitelliform"-like macular lesion.

23.3 Retinopathies Associated with Drug Toxicities

23.3.1 Chloroquine and Hydroxychloroquine

These antimalarial drugs can lead to melanin deposition, within the RPE and iris. Usage of these drugs significantly increased during the

COVID-19 pandemic in 2019 and 2020. Chloroquine is generally more toxic than hydroxychloroquine at equivalent doses. Toxicity often manifests between ages 20 and 50 and is more common in females. The earliest sign of toxicity is bilateral paracentral scotoma, which on OCT appear as loss of the inner segment ellipsoid layer in a paracentral location. In the end-stage, the condition resembles retinitis pigmentosa (RP) with pan-retinal degeneration. Bull's eye maculopathy is a distinctive feature of this toxicity and is irreversible. Additionally, anterior subcapsular cataract and corneal epithelium deposits, though non-visually significant, may occur. Treatment should be discontinued at the first sign of toxicity. Vision loss due to hydroxychloroquine toxicity generally does not recover and can continue to progress even after the drug is stopped due to slow excretion. Obese patients may be at higher risk of toxicity due to potentially higher dosages, whereas lean patients are at greater risk per dose, because the drugs are not stored in fatty tissue. High-risk retinal toxicity occurs with:

- A cumulative dose of 460 g (note the "grams") chloroquine and 1000 g hydroxychloroquine
- Daily dose of >3 mg/kg chloroquine and >5 mg/kg hydroxychloroquine
- Duration of use (>5 years)
- Kidney disease
- Concomitant use of tamoxifen (fivefold increase)
- Concomitant retinal disease such as age-related macular degeneration (AMD)

OCT and VF are the usual screening modalities. Patients who are at risk of toxicity or have unclear symptoms can be further assessed with fundus autofluorescence and multifocal electroretinography (mfERG). Screening is done via VF 10–2, with a structural image (OCT mostly, but also fundus AF, or mfERG).

23.3.2 Thioridazine (An Antipsychotic)

Toxicity occurs with excessive (1–2 g per day) doses, it causes pigment granularity posterior to the equator, along with geographic areas of depigmentation and loss of choriocapillaris. Withdrawal of thioridazine soon after the onset of visual symptoms reverses the visual loss; however, the pigmentary changes in the fundus often progress. Symptoms include nyctalopia and a brownish discoloration of vision.

23.3.3 Corticosteroids

Considered the most common medications associated with the development of central serous chorioretinopathy (CSCR).

23.3.4 Aminoglycosides (*Amikacin* and *Gentamicin)*

When administered intraocularly, they can cause significant macular damage. They can lead to macular infarction and severe macular ischemia, resulting in irreversible central vision loss.

23.3.5 Tamoxifen

An anti-estrogen medication used as adjuvant therapy for breast cancer is the most common cause of crystalline retinopathy (Fig. 23.6). Although crystalline retinopathy is rare at standard doses (20 mg daily), it has been reported in patients receiving high-dose tamoxifen therapy, particularly those on daily doses exceeding 200 mg or cumulative doses greater than 100 g. Tamoxifen also may cause macular cavitary lesion most evident on OCT resembling macular telangiectasia type 2, laser pointer injury, solar retinopathy, popper's retinopathy, and cone dystrophy (Fig. 23.7).

23.3.6 Sildenafil

Sildenafil can cause transient blue tinting of vision and temporarily abnormal ERG responses, such as a delayed cone b-wave implicit time, in up to 50% of patients taking doses greater than 100 mg. However, these effects are temporary, and no permanent retinal toxicity has been reported. It has also been associated with CSCR.

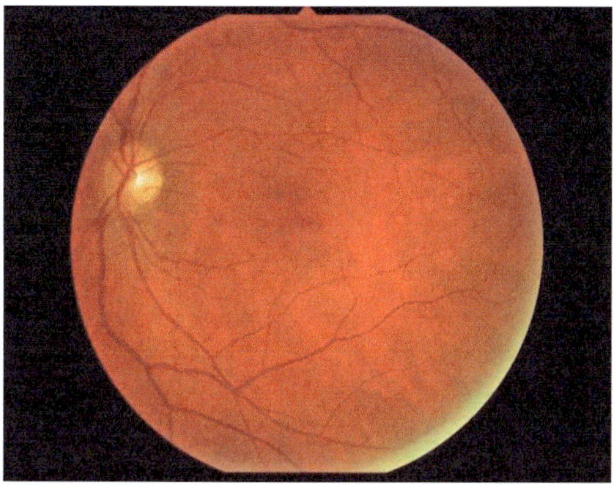

Fig. 23.6 Tamoxifen crystalline retinopathy (Courtesy of Retina Rocks®)

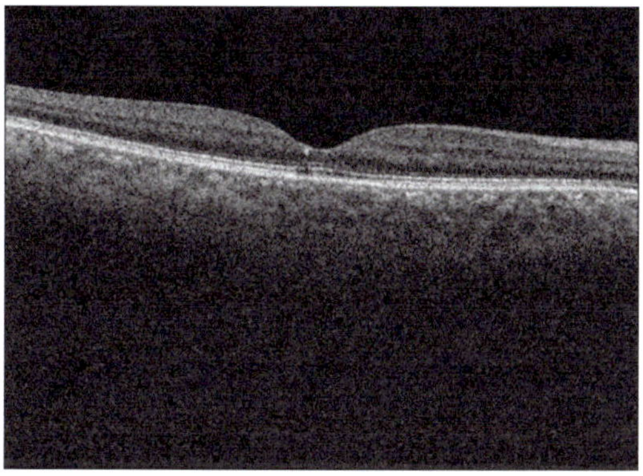

Fig. 23.7 Tamoxifen-related macular cavitary lesion (Courtesy of Retina Rocks®)

23.3.7 Digitalis

A cardiac glycoside causes reversible yellow tinting of vision, or *xanthopsia. Same side effect can be caused by voriconazole, an antifungal treatment.*

23.3.8 Isotretinoin

Used in the treatment of acne, studies have reported reversible poor night vision. Toxic optic neuropathy is a risk as well.

23.3.9 Silver

Ingestion might lead to blue discoloration of tears and hyperpigmentation of choroid.

23.3.10 Topiramate (and Occasionally Acetazolamide)

It has been associated with retinal and choroidal folds, which might lead to myopia, and if severe, to angle closure glaucoma.

23.3.11 Interferon

Commonly used in patients with a history of liver transplantation, can lead to characteristic retinal changes. In asymptomatic patients, interferon retinopathy is typically marked by multiple peripapillary cotton-wool spots.

23.3.12 Crystalline Retinopathy

Crystalline deposits in the retina consisting of irregular refractile yellow retinal deposits (similar to cotton-wool spots) are a toxic manifestation of:

- Tamoxifen
- Methoxy*flurane*
- Cantha*xanthin*
- Nitrofurantoin
- Talc
- Pentosan polysulfate sodium therapy for interstitial cystitis

The differential diagnosis of crystalline retinopathy also includes Bietti's crystalline dystrophy, Sjogren-Larsson syndrome, cystinosis, West-African retinopathy, and oxalosis.

23.3.13 High-Yield Notes

- Pigmentary retinopathy can be caused by quinine and phenothiazine, resulting in a pseudoretinitis pigmentosa picture.
- Phenothiazines, including chlorpromazine and thioridazine (severer) also bind RPE, patchy atrophy that may extend to mimic choroideremia in late stages.
- Desferrioxamine may also cause secondary macular edema caused by RPE toxicity.

Hemorrhagic occlusive retinal vasculitis (HORV) has been linked to the use of intracameral vancomycin for endophthalmitis prophylaxis, though such cases are rare. The pathogenesis of HORV is not fully understood but is thought to involve a type III hypersensitivity reaction, where antibody/antigen complexes deposit in small vessels, leading to vasculitis. Additionally, occlusive retinal vasculitis has been observed with intravitreal brolucizumab.

23.4 Retinal Detachment

Retinal detachment (RD) is defined as the separation of the neurosensory retina from the RPE. Normally, the retina remains attached due to factors like the continuous physiologic movement from the RPE into the choroid. This function, known as the retinal pigment epithelium pump, is disrupted when fluid passes through a retinal break, leading to retinal detachment. Retinal detachments are broadly classified into rhegmatogenous, tractional, or exudative types, with *rhegmatogenous retinal detachments* (RRDs) being the most common.

Primary retinal detachment occurs in a previously unaffected phakic eye, while recurrent retinal detachment reflects a failure to successfully repair the initial detachment. This may result from unsuccessful closure of the original breaks, development of new or missed retinal breaks, or more frequently, from scar tissue and retinal traction, a condition known as proliferative vitreoretinopathy (PVR), which occurs in about 75% of cases. Subclinical retinal detachment is defined as subretinal fluid extending at least 1 disc diameter from the break but not more than 2-disc diameters posterior to the equator. Since around 30% of these cases progress, treatment is often recommended.

23.4.1 Rhegmatogenous Retinal Detachment

Most cases are caused by anomalous PVD, resulting in undue peripheral retinal traction, retinal tear formation with fluid from the synchitic vitreous seeping under the retina causing it to deattach from the underlying RPE. In young patients <40 years, retinal detachment can occur without undue vitreous traction due to atrophic retinal holes or retinal dialysis that can be caused high myopia or pathological retina syndromes such as Marfan or due to trauma.

In general, a retina break can be found in 95% of RRD cases and in the remaining 5%, a presumed break may not found before the surgery. Lincoff's rules can be used to localize retinal break sites as the following.

Lincoff's Rules

- Inferior retinal detachment with an equal level of subretinal fluid progressing nasally and temporally suggests that a break is probably present at approximately 6 o'clock position.
- Inferior detachment with a higher fluid level on one side. Suggests the break is on the side with the higher fluid level.

Superior detachment, the break may be located anywhere between the 10 and 2 o'clock meridians, but it is most commonly between 10 and 12 o'clock positions. The vitreous base involves the full circumference of the peripheral fundus and measures about 3.2 mm in width. In terms of retinal breaks, they frequently occur along the posterior border of the vitreous base; however, in the case of traumatic detachment, breaks can be found along the anterior border as well.

23.4.1.1 Symptoms of Retinal Detachment

Symptoms of RRD include loss of peripheral visual field in relation to the detachment area as well as loss of vision if the macula is involved. In many cases, patients complain of floaters and flashes of light occurring due to anomalous PVD. In most cases, the onset is acute but sometimes it happens gradually over weeks. Cases due to atrophic retinal holes or retinal dialysis have slower progression as the vitreous is usually healthier and tamponade those breaks.

23.4.1.2 Signs of Rhegmatogenous Retinal Detachment

Shafer's sign (aka., tobacco dust) Small clumps of pigmented cells frequently present in the anterior vitreous.

Convex and corrugated appearance of the retina that undulates with eye movements. This differentiates RRD from other types of retinal detachment including tractional and exudative types (Fig. 23.8).

RAPD occurs only in extensive RD.

Typically, retinal detachment is associated with **low IOP.** However, Schwartz-Matsuo syndrome is a specific case where a rhegmatogenous retinal detachment results in photoreceptor outer segments being liberated into the anterior chamber, mimicking inflammatory cells. In these cases, IOP may be elevated because the photoreceptor outer segments are phagocytosed by endothelial cells in the trabecular meshwork, leading to secondary open-angle glaucoma. **Proliferative vitreoretinopathy** (PVR) folds—discussed later.

Retinal thinning, demarcation line, subretinal precipitates, and retinal atrophy are signs of chronic RD.

23.4.1.3 Considerations in RRD

- Duration of the retinal detachment.
- Current level of vision and previous vision level before the retinal detachment which gives an indication on the visual potential of the eye.

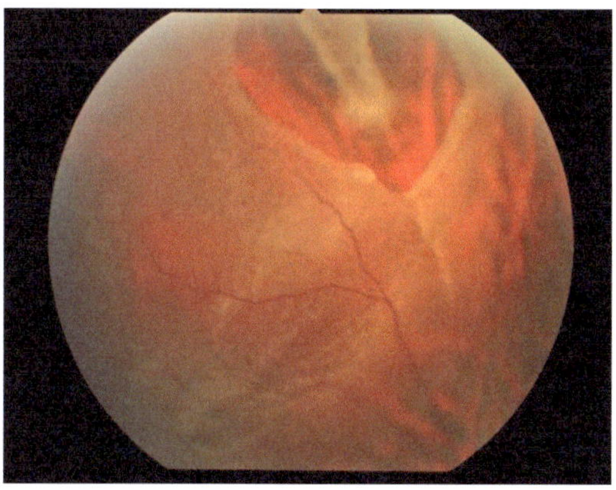

Fig. 23.8 Rhegmatogenous retinal detachment (Courtesy of Retina Rocks®)

- Confirm the diagnosis by checking the characteristics of detached retina (see signs of RRD), finding retina break(s), and checking for the presence of PVR.
- Status of the posterior hyaloid whether it is detached or not.
- Status of the macula.
- Status of the crystalline lens.

23.4.1.4 Risk Factors

The incidence of retinal detachment is 1:10000. Retinal detachment in the fellow eye (associated with the highest risk), male gender, myopia, aphakia or pseudophakia, and incomplete PVD (the most common risk factor) are the risk factors. Peripheral retinal lesions are classified into those associated with high risk of RRD (predisposing retinal lesions) and innocuous (non-predisposing) lesions.

23.4.2 Predisposing Retinal Detachment Lesions

1. **Posterior vitreous detachment (PVD)** (see vitreomacular traction below) occurs in fewer than 10% of patients under age 50 years but in >60% of those over age 70 years. The most important point is to exclude the presence of retinal break most commonly in the superotemporal quadrant. The risk of retinal break with:

   Acute PVD alone: 15%

   Acute PVD with vitreous hemorrhage: 50–70%

   With Shafer's/tobacco dust sign: 90%

   PVD is more prevalent in older age, female gender, myopes, vitreoretinal diseases (Stickler's syndrome, retinitis pigmentosa, posterior uveitis), post-menopause (due to low estrogen), high vitamin B6 intake (due to its anti-estrogen effect), surgeries, lasers, or trauma around vitreous.

   High-risk PVD patients for tears: aphakia or pseudophakic, myopia, fellow eye history, family history of retinal detachment, and Stickler syndrome.

   The risk of breaks decreases upon the occurrence of complete PVD, which is usually made on the basis of the presence of the Weiss ring, a 1.5 mm ring of glial tissue seen attached to the posterior hyaloid anterior to the optic disc (Fig. 23.9).

High-Yield Note

Differentiating RD from PVD is not difficult if there is a good view to the fundus. In the presence of poor view such as in cases of dense cataract or vitreous hemorrhage, B scan ultrasonography can help differentiating. Table 23.4 helps to differentiate posterior vitreous detachment from retinal detachment.

2. **Lattice degeneration** is characterized by localized retinal thinning, which occurs alongside vitreous liquefaction, and marginal vitreoretinal adhesion. In this condition, the vitreous directly above the lattice degeneration is liquefied, while the formed vitreous remains attached at the margins of the degenerated area. Additionally, the internal limiting membrane is discontinuous, and the inner retinal layers become atrophic. The condition is found in 5–10% of the general population. Bilateral in up to 50% of cases; 30% of RDs have underlying lattice, while only 1% of patients with lattice develop RD.

Clinically, any retinal lesion with borders that show an "abrupt, discrete irregularity of the otherwise smooth surface of the retina" should be considered lattice degeneration. The presence of white lines is not required for diagnosing lattice degeneration (Fig. 23.10).

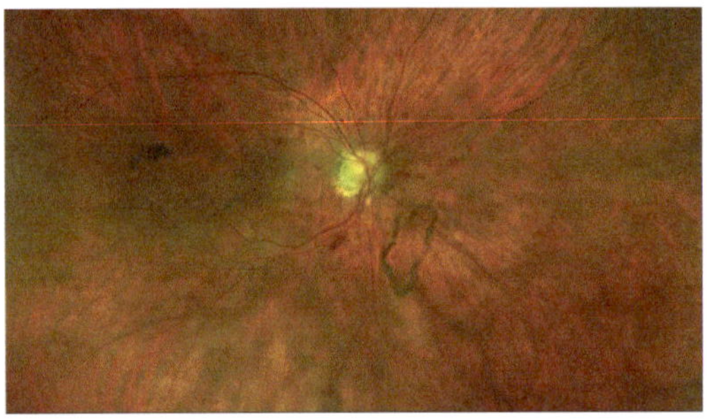

Fig. 23.9 Weiss ring in complete PVD (Courtesy of Retina Rocks®)

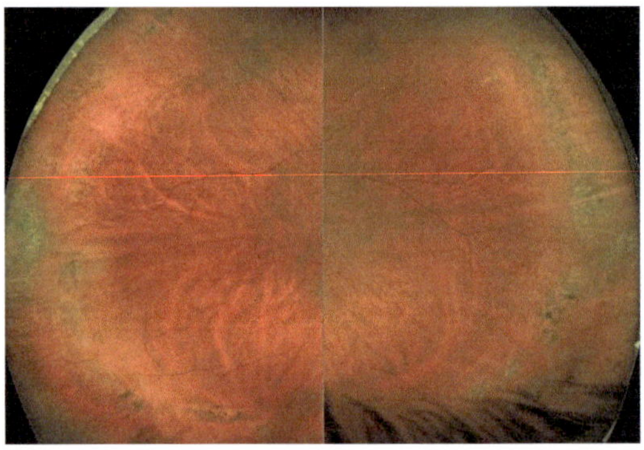

Fig. 23.10 Lattice degeneration (Courtesy of Retina Rocks®)

Table 23.4 Comparison between retinal detachment (RD) and posterior vitreous detachment (PVD)

	Retinal detachment (RD)	Posterior vitreous detachment (PVD)
Location	Attached to the optic disc at both sides	May or may not be attached depending on the degree of PVD (see later)
Shape	Thick folded membrane. May be smooth	Usually fine, smooth/folded membrane. May be thick especially in cases with neovascularization of disc/fibrovascular proliferation
Amplitude of Echo	100% compared to choroid-sclera	Usually less than 100%
Persistence in low gain (around 40–50 decibel)	Persists	Disappears
After-movements	Limited	High
Associated features	May have macrocysts (hemorrhagic or non-hemorrhagic), peripheral membrane also has 100% amplitude	Peripheral/anterior part of membrane usually has <100% spike, may be attached to the ocular coats (retina) at areas other than disc (at neovascularization of retina)
Doppler	Vascular	Usually avascular. The fibrovascular proliferations with attached vitreous membranes may have active vascularity

Lattice is associated with atrophic holes and retinal tears. The latter are associated with some risk of RD but is still the risk is low. Atrophic holes can occur in about 80% of patients.

Generally, in the absence of progressive subretinal fluid or risk factors such as a prior RD in the fellow eye especially in the context of retinal syndromes such as Marfan or Stickler, laser prophylactic treatment is not required for atrophic holes or lattice degeneration.

3. **Cystic retinal tufts** present in 5% of the population and have an increased risk of RD. But as with lattice, there is no need for prophylactic lasers in isolated tufts. Retinal tufts are small, peripheral, focal areas of elevated glial hyperplasia with vitreous attachment, and they may be surrounded by hyperplasia of the RPE.
4. **Retinal breaks**
   - Retinal break that are at high risk for progression to RD included those with an acute onset, superior location, large size, and the presence of surrounding subretinal fluid. They may be classified as *retinal holes* that generally do not require treatment unless symptomatic, caused by trauma, or for patients with history RD in the fellow eye. Retinal holes are generally atrophic, and do not result from traction by overlaying vitreous. Atrophic retinal holes are associated with a family history of such holes, lattice degeneration, increasing age, and axial myopia.
   - *Operculated holes* usually originate in focal areas of vitreoretinal abnormalities. Although the risk of retinal detachment is lower than horse tears (16%), laser treatment is required for symptomatic operculated tears to decrease the risk of retinal detachment.
   - *Horseshoe retinal tears (HSRT)* are full-thickness breaks in the neurosensory retina caused by vitreous traction, often due to PVD. These tears are the primary cause of most RRDs. If symptomatic horseshoe tears are left untreated, they can result in RD in about 50% of cases. All HSRT should be surrounded by a laser especially at their posterior edge soon after diagnosis. *Giant retinal breaks* are large, full-thickness tears that extend at least three clock hours (90′). Patients with a giant retinal tear in one eye have a very high risk, about 50%, of retinal detachment in the fellow eye. PVD is usually present.

Retinal dialysis is a circumferential, linear break that occurs at the ora serrata, with the vitreous base remaining attached to the retina posterior to the tear's edge. PVD is typically absent in these cases. Non-traumatic retinal dialysis is most commonly occurs in the superonasal quadrant, while dialysis resulting from blunt trauma is usually found in the inferotemporal quadrant. Traumatic retinal breaks are often multiple and are commonly located in the inferotemporal and superonasal quadrants. The most frequent type of injury associated with trauma is retinal dialysis, though breaks can happen in other location as well. Avulsion of the vitreous base, which may accompany retinal dialysis, is considered pathognomonic of ocular contusion.

Treatment of Retinal Breaks

Treatment of retinal breaks is typically prompted by factors such as the acute onset of symptoms, e.g., flashes or new floaters, and the presence of vitreous traction, e.g., in cases of flap tear. Conversely, the incidence of clinical retinal detachment is generally low in association with round holes in lattice degeneration and asymptomatic retinal tears, with or without an operculum. Therefore, treatment is usually not indicated for these types of breaks. Closing retinal breaks is the most important step, which should be done by creating adhesions between surrounding retinal layers. Two approaches currently present:

- Argon blue-green laser photocoagulation (532 nm laser) leads to adhesion within few days to 1 weeks but is ineffective if extensive subretinal fluid is present. This is usually delivered via the slit lamp or the indirect ophthalmoscope.

- Transscleral cryopexy performed by a probe with very low temperature leads to adhesions within 2 weeks. Cryopexy is useful in cases where laser is not possible due to cataract interfering with a crips view and in pale fundi where the uptake of laser is not ideal. However, cryotherapy can be a stimulating factor for postoperative proliferative vitreoretinopathy (PVR) if treatment is extensive.

  High Yield Note

  Laser retinopexy for symptomatic HSRT cuts down the risk of retinal detachment from 50% to 5%. Subsequent retinal breaks may occur after treatment in about 5–10%, usually within 6 weeks.

5. **Meridional Folds, Enclosed Ora Bays, and Peripheral Retinal Excavations:** Meridional folds are folds of redundant retina, usually located superonasally, and they may sometimes have a small retinal hole at its apex. These folds are often associated with dentate processes but can also extend posteriorly from ora bays. Tears associated with PVD may occur at the most posterior limit of the folds. Peripheral retinal excavations are areas of firm vitreoretinal adhesions, found adjacent to, or up to 4-disc diameters posterior to, the ora serrata, often aligned with meridional folds.
6. **Retinal white with/without pressure (WWOP)** is a common bilateral retinal condition occurring in up to 30% of the general population. It is less likely to affects inferonasal quadrant and has a higher incidence in individuals who are black, myopic, or older (reaching 70% in above 70 years). WWOP appears as a translucent white to gray area, often bounded posteriorly by a reddish-brown line (Fig. 23.11). This condition can mimic the appearance of a shallow retinal detachment, and its size, shape, and location may change over time.

   In white with pressure, the retina may appear normal without indentation. In white without pressure, retina appears white without indentation, and accentuated if scleral indentation is done.

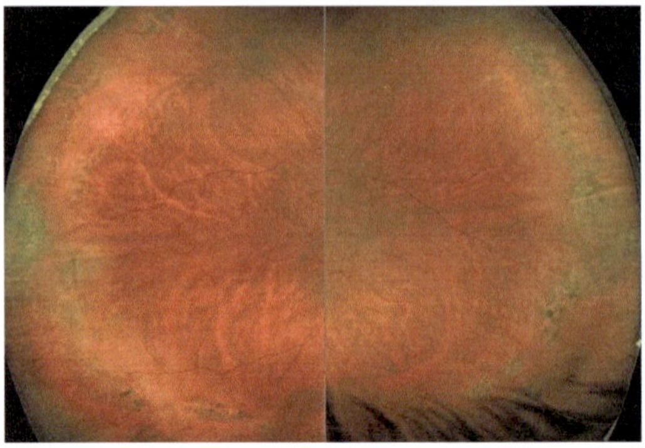

Fig. 23.11 White without pressure lesions (Courtesy of Retina Rocks®)

Table 23.5 Summary of lesions predisposing to RD and their respective RD risk

Lesion	Risk of RD (%)
RRD in the general population	0.0001
PVD	15
PVD with associated VH	50–70
PVD with Shafer's sign	90
Giant tear in the fellow eye	50
RRD in the fellow eye	10
Symptomatic horseshoe tear	50
Symptomatic operculated tear	16
Aphakia and Pseudophakia	1–3

A rare form known as *Dark-Without-Pressure* describes a brown fundus lesion with well-defined margins. OCT findings show hyperreflectivity of the ellipsoid zone.

Summary of predisposing retinal lesions and risk of RD is shown in Table 23.5.

23.4.3 Non-retinal Detachment Predisposing Retinal Lesions

Paving stone degeneration. Most commonly found at the inferior quadrants, characterized by peripheral, small, discrete areas of atrophy of the RPE and outer retina; it appears in 22% of individuals older than 20 years.

RPE hyperplasia occurs at the site of previous inflammation or traction.

RPE hypertrophy occurs with aging and congenital hypertrophy of RPE (CHRPE) (Fig. 23.12).

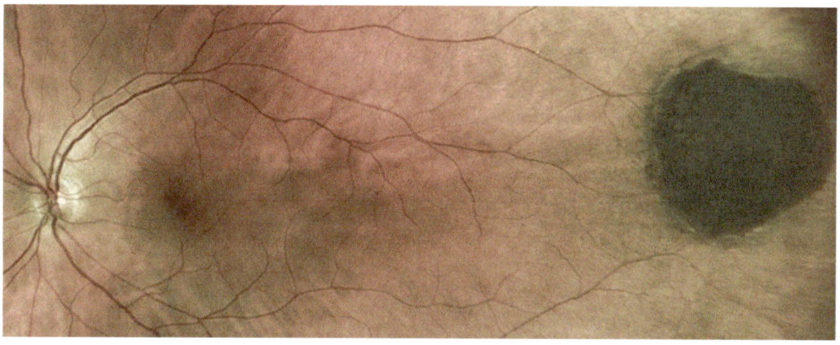

Fig. 23.12 RPE hypertrophy (Courtesy of Retina Rocks®)

Peripheral cystoid degeneration is characterized by zones of microcysts in the far-peripheral retina and is present in almost all adults over the age of 20 years. When these microcysts coalesce, they can lead to the formation of typical retinoschisis. Although retinal holes may develop within these areas of degeneration, they rarely lead to retinal detachment. **Pars plana cysts** rare lesions, usually temporally located and associated with no risk of RD.

Retinoschisis is splitting within the layers of neurosensory retina. It can be degenerative (typical and reticular senile retinoschisis) or congenital-Juvenile X-linked retinoschisis(JXLR). Sclerotic vessels present predisposing patients to VH.

Degenerative retinoschisis is often bilateral (50%–80%), symmetric, and bullous, frequently occurring in the inferotemporal quadrant. It is commonly associated with hyperopia, in contrast to RD. The splitting of retinal layers typically occurs at the outer plexiform layer. Adult retinoschisis usually appears inferiorly, between the equator and the ora serrata, but may extend into the pars plana (Fig. 23.13). In the region of the lesion, the choriocapillaris is usually absent, and chorioretinal scar formation is common. Retinal breaks may develop in the inner or outer retinal layers, or even in the adjacent full-thickness retina. Retinal detachments can occur if there is an outer layer retinal break, either alone or in conjunction with an inner layer break. Therefore, the presence of an outer layer break is a key factor in the development of retinal detachment in cases of retinoschisis.

The reticular form of senile retinoschisis involves splitting at the level of the nerve fiber layer and is typically associated with a more aggressive course.

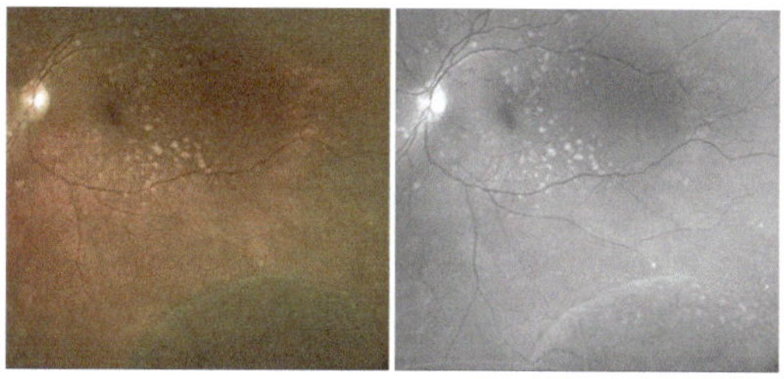

Fig. 23.13 Degenerative retinoschisis (Courtesy of Retina Rocks®)

In retinoschisis, the underlying retinal pigment epithelium remains normal, with no atrophy, demarcation line, or subretinal strand formation, unless a combined rhegmatogenous retinal detachment is present. Both rhegmatogenous retinal detachment and retinoschisis produce scotomas, but in retinoschisis, the scotoma is absolute, whereas in RRD, it is relative. Laser photocoagulation applied to the retina under a retinoschisis cavity whitens the retina, but it causes no reaction in cases of RRD.

Most cases of posterior retinoschisis will not progress beyond 3-disc diameters from the macula. Sclerotic vessels present predisposing patients to vitreous hemorrhage. Retinal detachments associated with senile retinoschisis are rare, typically progress slowly but are difficult to repair. RD may occur in two forms:

- When holes develop only in the inner surface (i.e., inner retina). This type of retinoschisis detachment usually does not progress, or it progresses slowly and seldom requires treatment. A demarcation line in an eye with retinoschisis or outer retinal atrophy suggests that

a full-thickness detachment is present or was formerly present and has spontaneously regressed.
- When holes develop in both layers. The schisis cavity may collapse, and a progressive RRD may result. Such detachments often progress rapidly and require treatment.

Observation only is recommended for most cases of retinoschisis without progressive retinal detachment. Prophylactic laser for schisis itself was not shown to decrease the risk of retinal detachment and is not recommended.

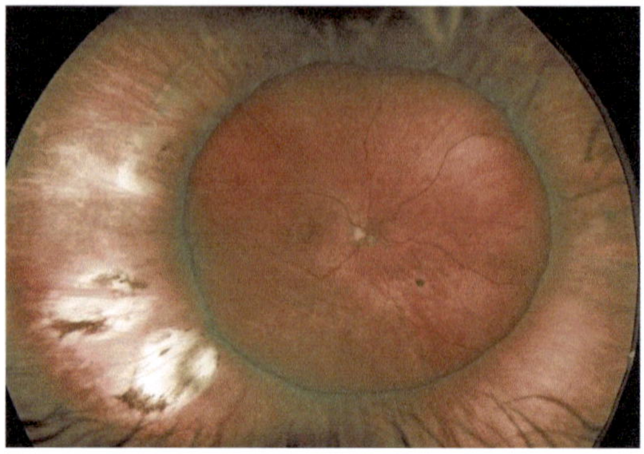

Fig. 23.14 Scleral buckle in RRD (Courtesy of Retina Rocks®)

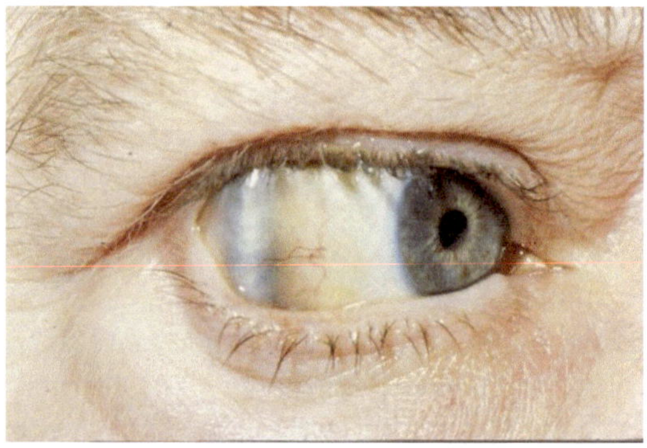

Fig. 23.15 Extrusion of scleral buckle (Courtesy of Retina Rocks®)

23.4.3.1 RRD Management

The most important prognostic factor in RRD repair is the presence and duration of macular detachment. Urgency of surgery mainly depends on the status of the macula. If the macula is not detached yet (macula on RRD), urgent surgical repair is indicated ideally within 24 h. When the macula detached, retrospective studies have shown a worsened prognosis in cases for which surgery was delayed for about 7 days or more from the time of diagnosis.

The goal of treating retinal breaks is to close them by bringing the RPE and choroid into contact with the retina long enough to create a permanent chorioretinal adhesion, which seals off the subretinal space. The three principal methods used to achieve retinal reattachment are scleral buckling, vitrectomy, and pneumatic retinopexy. *Scleral Buckling Surgery,* an extraocular approach indents the eye wall to help restore contact between the detached retina and the underlying tissues. In this procedure, a piece of silicone with an appropriate configuration is positioned on the external sclera under the retinal breaks and secured with sutures (Fig. 23.14).

Scleral buckles have an overall reattachment rate of at least 90%. Postoperative myopic shift is expected. Choroidal effusion, high IOP, diplopia, and CME are common early complications that in most cases resolve without treatment. Late complications include buckle extrusion (Fig. 23.15), intrusion, and infection. Scleral buckling can be tailored according to the number and position of the breaks, circular, radial or segmental indentation may be used. It is usually combined with cryopexy and, in some cases, external fluid drainage is needed. It can be combined with other surgical techniques. The main indication of scleral buckling nowadays is retinal detachment in young patients due to atrophic retinal holes or retinal dialysis. These patients have clear lens, and PPV will cause cataract. However, the main reason for selection of buckle surgery in these cases is that the vitreous is very adherent to the retina which makes vitrectomy surgery difficult and associated with higher complications risk.

Pars plana vitrectomy (PPV) is an intraocular surgical approach used to treat retinal detachments by relieving traction on the retina. This is achieved by removing the vitreous gel that is attached to the retinal breaks. While PPV avoids some of the complications associated with scleral buckling, it can accelerate cataract formation, leading to cataract surgery in about 50% of patients within 2 years of the procedure, and in 90% of patients over the age of 50 years. Other potential complications include glaucoma, retinal tears, and disturbances in the retinal pigmented epithelium, though these occur in less than 5% of cases. It is the preferred approach for pseudophakic patients, especially if it is not possible to locate the breaks, if the breaks are posterior, in giant tears, re-detachments, in cases of advanced proliferative vitreoretinopathy or when there is media opacity. The most common complication for PPV overall is cataract, while the most common short-term complication is rise in IOP. Nowadays, PPV is the commonest approach for treating primary RRD in old patients. *Pneumatic retinopexy* can be considered in cases of small breaks in the upper 2/3rds of the retina, and breaks are within 1 clock hour. Breaks must be identified with certainty, not pursued if no apparent breaks are observed. It is a procedure performed in the ophthalmologist's office that utilizes the ability of a small bubble of pure sulfur hexafluoride (SF6) or perfluoropropane (C2F6), injected intravitreally, to expand over the course of 1 or 2 days. This expansion occurs as the bubble absorbs tissue nitrogen and other gasses. Subretinal fluids will be drained by pumping mechanisms of RPE over months, so visual acuity gain is slow. After retinal apposition (the fluid is usually reabsorbed in 6–8 h), laser retinopexy or cryopexy can be performed. Contraindications for pneumatic retinopexy are as follows:

- Presence of retinal breaks within the lowest 4 clock hours of the inferior quadrants with detached retina, as even after full expansion of a 0.3-mL bubble of pure perfluoropropane (C3F8) to 1.2 mL, the inferior retina will not be covered by the gas bubble unless the patient assumes an extreme head position.
- Presence of proliferative vitreoretinopathy grade C or D.
- Noncompliance with required head positioning.
- Severe glaucoma.
- Hazy media or prior vitrectomy.

23.4.3.2 High-Yield Notes

- Total or bullous RD is not a contraindication for pneumatic retinopexy, as we are concerned by the break position and extension, rather than the detached part.
- The single operation success rate of scleral buckle is slightly higher (90%) than para plana vitrectomy (805); however, selection bias does exist as most cases operated with scleral buckle now are more straightforward than those operated by PPV. Pneumatic has a slightly lower single procedure success rate (75%).

23.4.3.3 Vitreous Tamponading Agents

Vitreous tamponades including intraocular gas and silicon oil are generally used during vitreoretinal surgeries in order to primarily tamponade retinal breaks long enough until laser or cryoretinopexy adhesions develop.

The most used intraocular gasses are sulfur hexafluoride (SF6), perfluoroethane (C2F6), and perfluoropropane (C3F8). Physical properties of these agents are summarized in Table 23.6.

Postoperatively, patients with intraocular gasses in situ should be advised against air travel or traveling to high altitudes in order to avoid gas expansion and IOP rise.

As C3F8 has the highest expansile rate for any intraocular gas. It can cause dramatic increases in IOP in the early postoperative period.

Silicone oil, when placed in a fluid-filled eye, has a lower specific gravity compared to the sur-

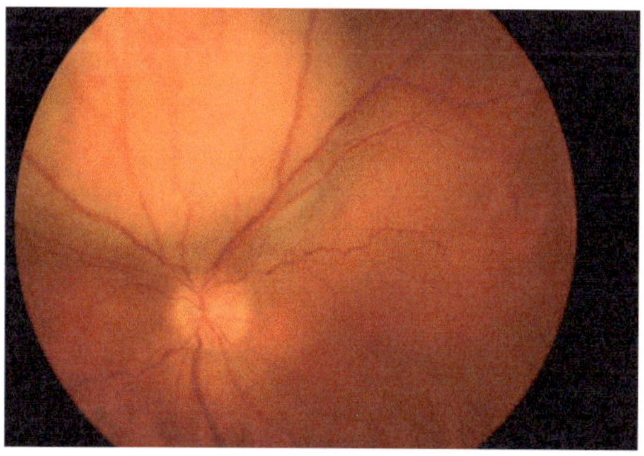

Fig. 23.16 Exudative RD in choroidal melanoma (Courtesy of Retina Rocks®)

rounding fluids. Its surface tension is significantly less than of all gasses, including air.

According to the Silicone Oil Study Group, reattachment rates and visual outcomes were worse when SF6 used as a tamponade agent, compared to either C3F8 or silicone oil. Furthermore, in cases of PVR, no significant difference in outcomes was observed between eyes undergoing primary vitrectomy and those that had been previously vitrectomized when either silicone oil or C3F8 gas was used as the tamponade. Current practice is to use gas for primary RRD due to better tamponade properties and to use SO in surgery for recurrent retinal detachment with scarring due to its long-term effect.

Proliferative vitreoretinopathy (PVR) is a proliferative, contractile cellular membranes that form in the vitreous and on both sides of the retina, resulting in tractional retinal detachment with fixed retinal folds. PVR is characterized by proliferation of retinal pigment epithelium (RPE) cells that is independent of the vitreous in a preexisting RRD. This is compared to fibrovascular tissue in PDR.

Ocular manifestations of PVR include macular pucker, marked vitreous flare, increased stiffness, and decreased undulation of the detached neural retina and star folds.

The mainstay of the management of PVR is surgical, with PPV with epiretinal membrane peeling and long-acting tamponade with SO or C3F8 gas being the primary procedure. In some cases, removing contracted retinal tissue (retinectomy) is necessary to allow retinal reattachment. Several medical agents were investigated to prevent PVR including corticosteroids and anti-proliferative agents (e.g., 5-fluorouraci and mitomycin) but definite benefit was not demonstrated.

23.4.4 Tractional Retinal Detachment

Contraction of fibrovascular membrane pulling the neurosensory retina from the RPE typically occurs with advanced PDR, sickle cell retinopathy, ROP, and trauma. Compared with RRD, TRD has a regular, immobile surface, concave configuration, and less subretinal fluid that rarely extend from disc to ora serrata. Many, if not most, tractional retinal detachments begin distant from the fovea and are typically asymptomatic unless they have recently converted to a combined rhegmatogenous-tractional retinal detachment.

23.4.4.1 Crunch Syndrome

In eyes with PDR and TRD, anti-VEGF may be used as tool before vitrectomy surgery to decrease the risk of intraoperative and early postoperative bleeding. Anti-VEGF crunch syndrome describes the worsening of tractional retinal detachment that may occur following intravitreal anti-VEGF therapy in this context. The onset is usually after 10 days from the injection. It is therefore important when using anti-VEGF preoperatively to operate within a week of the injection and not later.

23.4.5 Exudative Retinal Detachment

Accumulation of subretinal fluid in the absence of retinal breaks and traction. The most serious underlying cause is choroidal tumor (Fig. 23.16). For this reason, exudative RD should be considered to be caused by intraocular tumor until proven otherwise. Exudative retinal detachment is characterized by fluid shifting, a feature not present in RRD, so the patient should be exam-

Table 23.6 Physical properties/dynamics of commonly used vitreoretinal surgery gasses

Gas	Molecular weight	Maximal expansion (h)	Duration	Nonexpansile concentration (%)	Expansivity (times)
Air	29	–	5–7 days	–	0
Sulfur hexafluoride (SF6)	146	24–48	1–2 weeks	20	2
Perfluoroethane (C2F6)	138	36–60	4–5 weeks	16	3.3
Perfluoropropane (C3F8)	188	72–96	6–8 weeks	12	4

ined using a slit lamp, then in supine position with an indirect ophthalmoscope to confirm diagnosis. Management of exudative RD is directed to the underlying cause.

Acknowledgment None.

Conflict of Interest None.

References

Doft B et al (1995) Results of the Endophthalmitis Vitrectomy Study. A randomized trial of immediate vitrectomy and of intravenous antibiotics for the treatment of postoperative bacterial endophthalmitis. Endophthalmitis Vitrectomy Study Group. Arch Ophthalmol 113:1479–1496

Heeren TFC et al (2020) Macular telangiectasia type 2: visual acuity, disease end stage, and the MacTel area: MacTel project report number 8. Ophthalmology 127(11):1539–1548. https://doi.org/10.1016/j.ophtha.2020.03.040

Kanski JJ, Bowling B (2015) Kanski's clinical ophthalmology: a systematic approach. Saunders

Karampelas M, Malamos P, Petrou P, Georgalas I, Papaconstantinou D, Brouzas D (2020) Retinal pigment epithelial detachment in age-related macular degeneration. Ophthalmol Ther 9(4):739–756. https://doi.org/10.1007/s40123-020-00291-5

Kertes PJ, Conway MD (1998) Clinical trials in ophthalmology: a summary and practice guide. https://doi.org/10.1604/9780683302059

Kim SJ (2021) 2021–2022 basic and clinical science course, section 12: retina and vitreous

Reed K (2001) Fluorescein angiography refresher course. Fluorescein angiography refresher course. https://www.reviewofoptometry.com/article/fluorescein-angiography-refresher-course

Scott IU, Campochiaro PA, Newman NJ, Biousse V (2020) Retinal vascular occlusions. Lancet 396(10266):1927–1940. https://doi.org/10.1016/S0140-6736(20)31559-2

Clinical Review of Retina and Vitreous Diseases: Part III

24

Mo'ath AlShawabkeh, Saif Aldeen Alryalat, Mohammed Abu-Ameerh, and Ahmed A. Sallam

Abstract

This chapter discusses vitreous and vitreomacular surface disorders, outlining their stages and implications for visual health. It also addresses congenital vitreoretinal diseases, exploring their characteristics and management. The chapter further delves into imaging techniques used in retinal diseases, including optical coherence tomography, fundus autofluorescence, fundus fluorescein angiography, and indocyanine green angiography, highlighting their roles in diagnosis and monitoring. Additionally, a summary of landmark trials in retinal diseases is presented, offering insights into the evidence that shapes current clinical practice. High-yield notes on photocoagulation lasers are included to emphasize their significance in treatment strategies. The chapter includes a miscellaneous section covering choroidal diseases, pseudophakic cystoid macular edema, various retinopathies, and endophthalmitis, providing a well-rounded understanding of the complexities in retinal health.

Keywords

Vitreous disorders · Imaging techniques
Choroidal diseases · Landmark trials
Miscellaneous

M. AlShawabkeh (✉)
Department of Ophthalmology, The Hashemite University, Zarqa, Jordan

S. A. Alryalat
Department of Ophthalmology, The University of Jordan, Amman, Jordan

The University of Colorado Anschutz Medical Campus, CO, USA

M. Abu-Ameerh
The University of Jordan, Amman, Jordan

A. A. Sallam
Harvey and Bernice Jones Eye Institute at the University of Arkansas for Medical Sciences (UAMS), Little Rock, AR, USA

For readers interested in further more comprehensive and detailed information, the following references are useful (Kim 2021; Kanski and Bowling 2015; Kertes and Conway 1998; Karampelas et al. 2020; Scott et al. 2020; Heeren et al. 2020; Reed 2001; Doft et al. 1995).

24.1 Vitreous and Vitreomacular Surface Disorders

24.1.1 Vitreomacular Surface Disorders

Normally, the vitreous gel is loosely adherent to the retina except at the following sites (strong vitreoretinal attachments): vitreous base, optic disc, macula, and blood vessels.

S. A. Alryalat (ed.), *Ophthalmology Board and FRCS Part 2 Exams*,
https://doi.org/10.1007/978-981-96-1517-9_24

The normal aging process of the vitreous causes development of the posterior vitreous detachment (PVD); liquefaction of the vitreous gel (synchysis) results in formation of fluid-filled cavities (lacunae) which enlarge and coalesce with time and eventually condense (syneresis) and access preretinal space causing separation of the posterior vitreous from the retina. PVD occurs in the following stages:

Stage 1: Vitreous detaches from the perifoveal area but still attached at fovea, peripheral retina and optic disc.
Stage 2: Vitreous detaches from fovea but still attached at peripheral retina and optic disc.
Stage 3: Vitreous detaches from peripheral retina and still attached at optic disc.
Stage 4: Vitreous detaches from optic disc, this stage is called complete PVD and is characterized clinically by the Weiss ring.

Normal PVD should result in a "clear" and "complete" separation of cortical vitreous and posterior hyaloid membrane from the ILM. Any deviation from the normal stages of normal PVD is called anomalous PVD.

Clear separation means there should be no residual vitreous layer attached to the ILM, otherwise, this vitreoschisis could result in epiretinal membrane or macular hole development.

Complete separation means that vitreous should detach from all vitreoretinal attachment sites up to the vitreous base, otherwise, retinal tears or vitreomacular traction can develop.

24.1.1.1 Vitreomacular Adhesion (VMA)

VMA is a condition characterized by detachment of the posterior vitreous from the perifoveal area while still attached to fovea within 3 mm from the center of the macula and with no changes of retinal architecture or distortion of foveal contour.

Can be classified as focal (≤1500 μm) or broad (>1500 μm).

Can be classified as isolated (with no other abnormalities) or concurrent (when associated with other pathologies such as diabetic retinopathy, retinal vein occlusion, or AMD).

VMAs are considered one of the stages of normal PVD, usually asymptomatic and only needs observation.

24.1.1.2 Vitreomacular Traction Syndrome (VMT)

VMT is a condition characterized by detachment of the posterior vitreous from the perifoveal area while still attached to fovea within 3 mm from the center of the macula and with distortion of the foveal contour and secondary retinal structural changes such as macular thickening, pseudocyst, leak, detachment, or CME. VMT can also result in the development of macular hole.

VMT can be classified in a similar way as in VMA but VMT is usually symptomatic and needs treatment.

Treatment Options

1. Observation

   This is the main line of treatment for cases with no to mild symptoms. Spontaneous separation may also occur in approximately 30% especially focal and mild VMT.
2. Pharmacological vitreolysis

   Ocriplasmin (Jetrea®), a recombinant human plasmin targets fibronectin and laminin in the vitreoretinal interface. When given intravitreally, success rate is low at 30–40% for mild and focal VMT. Concerning side effects include lens subluxation and diffuse retinal dysfunction
3. Pneumatic vitreolysis

   A small gas bubble (e.g., SF6 or C3F8 gas) is injected into the eye in the office with sitting up positioning for few days.
4. Pars plana vitrectomy (PPV)

   This is currently the main line of treatment for VMT with significant symptoms.

24.1.1.3 Idiopathic Macular Hole (MH)

Foveal interruption of all retinal layers from ILM to RPE (Fig. 24.1).

MH is usually unilateral in presentation. The risk of fellow eye involvement is around 10% unless complete PVD had occurred, and patients with fellow eye vitreomacular traction have a higher rate of up to 40%.

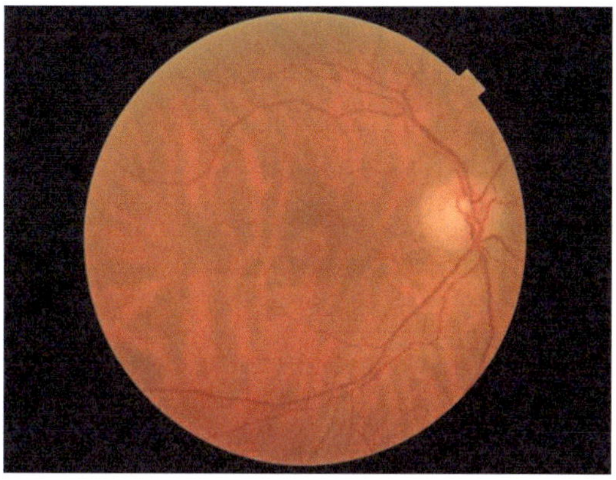

Fig. 24.1 Macular hole due to vitreomacular traction (Courtesy of Retina Rocks®)

MH is twice more common in female than male and typically presents between the sixth and seventh decade of age.

Classifications of Idiopathic MH

AS demonstrated in Table 24.1, MH can be staged according to Gass classification (biomicroscopy-based) and Hee and Puliafito classification (OCT-based).

24.1.1.4 Management of MH

1. Observation

   This is indicated only in stage 0–1 where 50% of stage one MHs close spontaneously, observation is indicated at this stage.
2. Pharmacological vitreolysis

   Patient with Stages up to 1B can be offered intravitreal ocriplasmin which is most effective in eyes with focal adhesions. As mentioned before, there has been a significant decline for ituse in VMT and MH.
3. PPV

   Detaching the posterior hyaloid (the most important step), ILM peeling, gas injection and face down position. Indicated for stage 2 and more, with a success rate up to 90% or greater for a recent- onset MH.

24.1.1.5 Lamellar/Partial Thickness Macular Hole

Partial defect of inner retina with intact photoreceptors.

Proposed mechanisms include:

- Aborted stage of FTMH development
- Secondary to chronic CMO
- Anomalous PVD and pseudocyst

Most cases of lamellar macular hole are not symptomatic or have only mild symptoms and are therefore only observed.

24.1.1.6 Epiretinal Membrane

Sheet-like fibrocellular structure on/above the surface of the retina that develops as a result of complete but not clear PVD. It is thought to that the separating vitreous leaves a residual vitreous tissue (vitreoschesis) for subsequent proliferation of glial cells derived from posterior hyaloid (in primary ERM) or pigment cells derived from RPE (in secondary ERM). Contraction of ERM causes wrinkling, puckering, elevation, and pseudocyst of the macula.

Primary ERM is idiopathic, usually milder and can be bilateral in 10% of cases.

Secondary ERM can develop after retinal tears, RD repair surgery, laser photocoagulation, retinal vascular occlusion, posterior uveitis, and other ocular pathologies.

24.1.1.7 ERM Presentations

Cellophane Maculopathy

Irregular translucent sheen on ILM, best seen on green (red-free) filter.

Macular Pucker

Variable striae and distortion due to contraction of cellular elements of ERM.

Table 24.1 Stages of idiopathic macular hole

Stage 0	Vitreomacular adhesion	Represents vitreomacular adhesion VMA (see above)
Stage 1a	Impending macular hole/VMT	Characterized clinically by yellow spot and loss of foveal depression Detached inner retinal layers with foveal cyst but intact photoreceptors
Stage 1b	Occult macular hole/VMT	Characterized clinically by yellow ring Detached inner and outer retinal layers with separation of photoreceptors Vitreous is still attached to the foveal center
Stage 2	Small full thickness macular hole with VMT	Eccentric full thickness defect, smaller than 400 μm at the narrowest point Incomplete detachment and attached operculum at one side
Stage 3	Full thickness macular hole with VMT	Central round full thickness defect >400 μm Vitreous detached completely from the fovea but still attached at optic disc
Stage 4	Full size macular hole with complete PVD	FTMH regardless of size Complete detachment of posterior vitreous from optic disc (Weiss ring)

Macular Pseudohole

Distortion of perifovea into heaped edges without actual loss of retinal tissues.

ERMs are generally observed unless they are progressive or if the patient is affected by reduced visual acuity or metamorphopsia. Vitrectomy with ERM peeling is the method of treatment.

24.1.2 Congenital Vitreoretinal Diseases

24.1.2.1 Hyaloid Artery Remnants/Tunica Vasculosa Lentis Remnants

Mittendorf dot, Cloquet's canal, and Bergmeister papilla are remnants of hyaloid artery at posterior capsule, vitreous, and optic disc, respectively.

24.1.2.2 Prepapillary Vascular Loops

Normal retinal vessels extend into the Bergmeister papilla before returning to the retina. These loops are not derived from hyaloid artery and typically extend less than 5 mm into the vitreous. The majority of these loops 95% are arterial while a small percentage (5%) is venous. Complications associated with these prepapillary vascular loops include branch retinal artery obstruction, amaurosis fugax, and vitreous hemorrhage.

24.1.2.3 Persistent Fetal Vasculature (PFV)

Sporadic and unilateral condition (90%). Microphthalmos is a common association.

Two types:

1. *Anterior PFV*: White vascularized fibrous retrolental mass is present and elongated ciliary processes are attached to it. Leukocoria is often present at birth. May be complicated by lens swelling, angle closure glaucoma, and cataract, leading to deprivation amblyopia. The most important differential diagnosis is retinoblastoma.
2. *Posterior PFV* may be associated with anterior PFV. Remnants of the hyaloid artery attached to the optic disc inferiorly. The condition may lead to retinal detachment in children.

24.1.2.4 Hereditary Hyaloid-Retinopathies

A collection of AD-inherited diseases is characterized by early liquefaction of the vitreous (synchysis). This condition leads to formation of a thin cortical vitreous layer behind the lens, along with thread-like membranes that attach to the retina. Fundoscopic examination often reveals equatorial and perivascular (radial) lattice degeneration. Additionally, the ERG response may be reduced. These include:

- *Stickler's syndrome* (the most common): (aka. Hereditary arthro-ophthalmopathy)
  Caused by COL2A1 gene mutation resulting in abnormal synthesis of mainly type II collagen, but also type XI or IX. Manifesting as bilateral giant retinal tears, cleft palate, severe myopia, and severe arthritis. Ocular associations include glaucoma, cataract, myopia, radially oriented lattice lesions, and optically empty vitreous (Fig. 24.2). Systemic association includes joint anomalies and orofacial anomalies (cleft palate and a small lower jaw). These features are part of the Pierre Robin sequence. Marfanoid habitus can be observed. Stickler's syndrome is the most common inherited cause of RD in children.

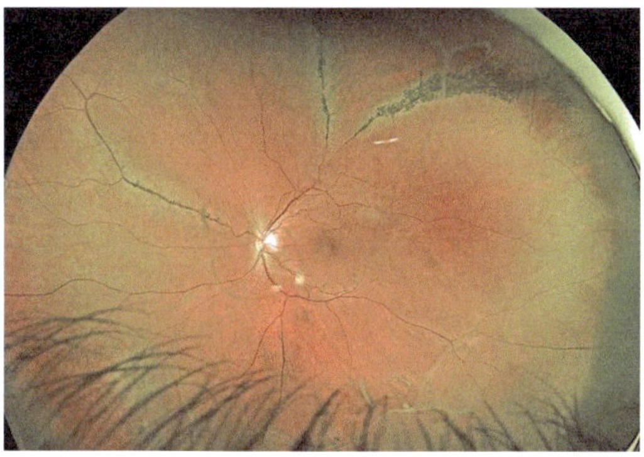

Fig. 24.2 Stickler's syndrome (Courtesy of Retina Rocks®)

- *Jensen's syndrome*: Similar to stickler's but with no systemic associations, the risk of retinal detachment is high.
- *Wagner's syndrome*: No systemic associations or retinal detachment risk. Associated with cataract, strabismus, and myopia.

24.1.2.5 Asteroid Hyalosis

Calcium pyrophosphate freely mobile precipitates within the vitreous gel (Fig. 24.3). Mostly unilateral (75%) and increase in incidence with age. Although it may impede the fundus exam, they are usually visually non-significant. There may be an association with asteroid hyalosis and both diabetes mellitus and hypertension, but not hypercalcemia.

24.1.2.6 Cholesterolosis (Synchysis scintillans)

Cholesterolosis is seen almost exclusively in eyes with repeated or severe accidental or surgical trauma as a result of chronic vitreous hemorrhage. Unlike asteroid hyalosis, cholesterol tends to sediment inferiorly as the vitreous is syneretic.

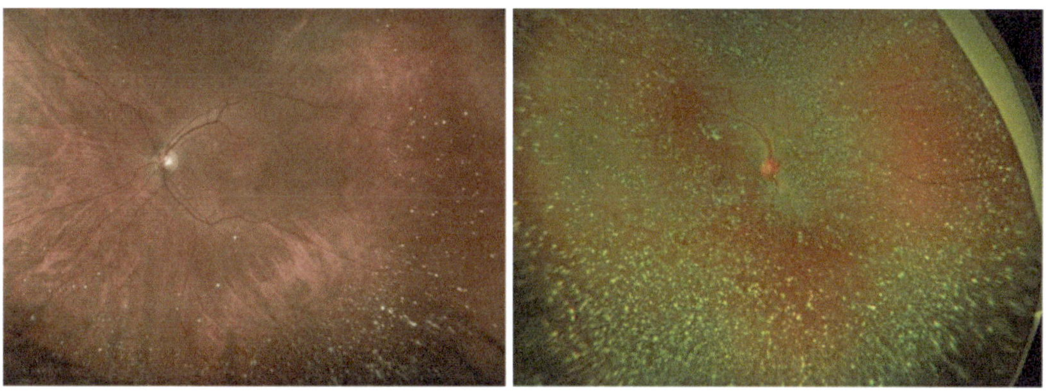

Fig. 24.3 Asteroid hyalosis (Courtesy of Retina Rocks®)

24.2 Fundus Imaging

Adaptive optics (AO) is an additive feature that can be added to either OCT or SLO and allows visualization of the human photoreceptor mosaic and for a lateral resolution of up to 2 μm.

24.2.1 Optical Coherence Tomography (OCT)

24.2.1.1 Overview

Both SD-OCT and SS-OCT generate A-scan through tissue. B-scans are made up of multiple A-scans collected across a plane of tissue, while a volume scan comprises numerous B-scans.

Optical coherence tomography operates on the principle of low-coherence interferometry, where infrared light backscattered from the ocular tissue is a reference beam.

Three main advances, first is time domain (TD), then spectral domain (SD), and finally swept source (SS) (see Table 24.2). SD and SS both depend on Fourier transformations.

The clinical benefits of SS-OCT over SD-OCT are not yet well defined. While SS-OCT provides better visualization of the choroid and structures beneath the RPE, the practical implications of these improvements still need further investigation.

Remember that higher wavelengths mean more penetration, but lower resolution.

OCT interpretation steps

- Check patient identifying data, laterality of the eye (OD vs. OS).
- Check scan quality, either numeric via SSI (Signal Strength Index) or via observing the clarity of layers. A signal strength of 6 and above is desired in Ziess, and 20 or above in Spectralis-Heidelberg.
- Upper quantitative thickness maps.
- Lower macular qualitative maps.

Here are the normal retinal anatomical layers as appearing on OCT (Fig. 24.4), with ellipsoid zone and RPE/Bruch complex being most important for distinction:

24.2.1.2 Important Tips

There are four hyper-reflective lines in the outer retina; they are (from outer to inner):

- Bruch's/RPE complex
- The interdigitation zone (formed by apical processes of the RPE and the cone outer segments)
- Ellipsoid zone (formed by mitochondria containing part of photoreceptors)
- External limiting membrane

Disruption of any of the above-mentioned lines is a poor prognostic sign for treatment response.

Hyper-reflective structure: cell bodies (inner and outer plexiform layers) including, retinal pigment epithelium and epiretinal membrane.

Intermediate reflectivity: axons.

Nuclear layers are generally hypo-reflective, while plexiform layers are generally hyper-reflective.

24.2.1.3 OCT-Angiography

In a series of images taken at regular intervals, a moving object will appear at different positions in the successive images. Comparing these images pixel by pixel reveals that stationary regions remain unchanged, while moving objects create areas with high variance.

Table 24.2 Types of optical coherence tomography (OCT) imaging

	Time domain	Spectral domain	Swept source
Principle	Moving reference mirror	Spectrometer using Fourier transform principle	Laser scanning using Fourier transform principle
Number of A-scans	<100 A-scans/s	40,000 A-sans/s	>100,000 A-scans/s
Infrared wavelength		800 nm	1200 nm

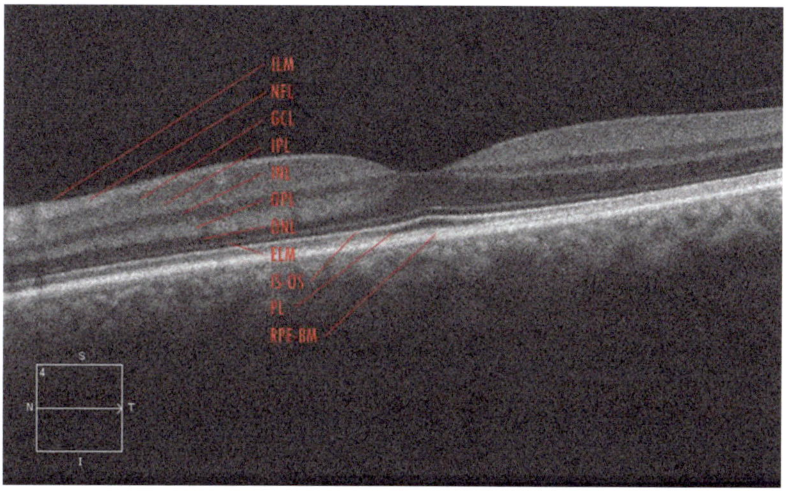

Fig. 24.4 Normal retinal anatomy on OCT (Courtesy of Retina Rocks®)

Table 24.3 Comparison between fundus fluorescein angiography (FFA) and OCT-angiography

	FFA	OCTA
Emergence	Old	New
Principle	Reflection from fluorescence pigment	Capturing moving pixels in white, and stationary in black
Depth	Only superficial plexus	Superficial and deep plexuses, and even choroidal vessels
Motion artifact (i.e., patient movement during imaging)	Little interference	Huge interference

Assigning black to areas of low variance (non-moving) and white to areas of high variance (moving) results in an image that highlights motion known as motion contrast. The retina itself is stationary, except for the flow of blood. High resolution retinal images can thus capture the movement of blood through the retina.

Unlike fluorescein angiography, which only visualizes the superficial capillary plexus, OCTA can image all capillary layers, including the superficial plexus, the radial peripapillary capillary network, and the deep vascular plexus (see Table 24.3).

Other artifacts that may affect OCTA include projection artifact, which occur when light passing through a blood vessel off a deeper reflective structure. This reflected light can mimic the appearance overlying blood vessel, resulting in an image with two levels of the same vessel: one at its actual location and another at the depth of the reflective structure.

24.2.2 Fundus Autofluorescence (FAF)

Uses blue light excitation, to capture emissions within a preset spectral range, creating a brightness map that reflects the distribution of lipofuscin, a major fluorophore found in the RPE. This imaging can be performed with a fundus camera equipped with special filters, or with scanning laser ophthalmoscopy (SLO).

Lipofuscin, located in the RPE, is a key macular fluorophore that absorbs blue light with a peak excitation wavelength of 470 nm and emits yellow–green light with a peak wavelength of 600–610 nm. Its autofluorescent properties are due to bisretinoid compounds, metabolic by-products of vitamin A, and the visual cycle.

Autofluorescent patterns are influenced by the interaction between fluorophores such as lipofuscin, which emit the autofluorescent signal, and other elements such as melanin and rhodopsin, which absorb the excitation light and reduce autofluorescence.

Lipofuscin increases in degenerative disorders, such as age-related macular degeneration (AMD), and macular dystrophies such as Best and Stargardt disease.

FAF has recently been added to the imaging studies recommended by the National Eye Institute (National Institutes of Health, USA) to investigate and follow patients suspected of chloroquine retinopathy.

FFA, ICG, and FAF (respectively below) can be differentiated by the color of the vessel and the disc on the image.

24.2.3 Fundus Fluorescence Angiography (FFA)

24.2.3.1 Overview

Fluorescein angiography has traditionally been imaged with a fundus camera or an SLO after administration of the dye.

The dye can be either 2–3 mL of a 25% solution, or 5 mL of a 10% solution is injected in the antecubital vein.

The dye is typically visible in the retinal circulation within 12–14 s of injection, rapidly filling the arterial system. If it takes >15 sec, this might indicate heart disease.

After 30 s, the dye will be out of the eye (aka. transient phase). Can capture one eye, then after the re-circulation, the other eye can be captured.

About 80% bound and 20% free, the free form is the one useful for imaging.

Choriocapillaris (i.e., small choroidal vessels) permeable to free, so FFA is not useful to study choroid.

Renal clearance is within 36–48 h.

The only absolute contraindication is allergy to fluorescein. Relative contraindications: Pregnancy, lactation, and for kidney failure, the concentration should be lower.

All patients injected with fluorescein experience a temporary yellowing of the skin and conjunctiva that lasts 6–12 h.

The most common adverse effects include nausea and vomiting (occurring in about 5% of injections) and the development of hives (also around 5%).

Although there are no identified teratogenic effects, many ophthalmologists avoid using FA in pregnant women during the first trimester unless necessary. In lactating women, fluorescein is present in breast milk.

For children and patients with difficult IV access, FA can be performed using oral fluorescein, which produces assessable image but with reduced quality.

24.2.3.2 Autofluorescence

Autofluorescence is the fluorescence observed with the excitation and barrier filters in place before the injection of fluorescein dye. It results from the natural fluorescence of tissue components, such as the accumulation of outer segments, lipofuscin, or optic nerve head drusen.

24.2.3.3 Hypofluorescence

Occurs when normal fluorescence is reduced or absent and present in 2 major patterns:

- *Vascular filling defects* happen when retinal or choroidal vessels fail to fill due to an intravascular obstruction, resulting in nonperfusion of an artery, vein, or capillary, and this is seen as delay in or complete absence of filling of the involved vessels.
- *Blocked fluorescence* occurs when the visualization of the fluorescein is obstructed by fibrous tissue, pigment, or blood, which prevents normal retinal or choroidal fluorescence in the affected area. The depth of a lesion can be determined by correlating the level of the blocked fluorescence with details of the retinal circulation; for example, if lesions block the choroidal circulation, but retinal vessels are visible above the defect, then the lesions are located above the choroid and below the retinal vessels.

24.2.3.4 Hyperfluorescence

Occurs when the fluorescence is abnormally excessive, typically extending beyond the borders of recognized structures:

- *Leakage*, such as from NVEs, is characterized by a gradual and significant increase in fluorescence over the course of the study due to fluorescein molecules seeping across the blood–retina barrier. When the outer blood–retina barrier is compromised, the dye can cross the pigment epithelium into the subretinal space or neurosensory retina. If the inner blood–retina barrier is affected, the dye leaks through the vascular walls into the retinal parenchyma, fibrotic tissue, and cystoid spaces. Additionally, dye can leak through the posterior blood–retina barrier (the RPE) and accumulate in the subretinal space, fibrotic tissue, or directly into the retina, if the external limiting membrane of the retina is compromised.
- *Staining,* such as with drusen, refers to a pattern of hyperfluorescence where the fluorescence increases in intensity through transit views, and persists in late views, but the borders remain intact throughout the study. This occurs when fluorescein enters solid tissue or materials, such as a scar, drusen, optic nerve tissue, or sclera, which retain the fluorescein.
- *Pooling,* seen in conditions like CSCR or RD, describes the accumulation of fluorescein in a fluid-filled space within the retina or choroid. As fluorescein leaks into this space, the margins trap the dye, making the edges of the space appear distinct, for example, as seen in an RPE detachment in central serous chorioretinopathy.
- *Transmission defect,* or *window defect,* is observed when normal choroidal fluorescence is visible through a defect in the RPE. Hyperfluorescence appears early as the choroidal circulation fills, reaching peak intensity during choroidal filling. The fluorescence does not change in intensity or shape and usually fades in the later phases as the choroidal fluorescence is diluted by non-fluorescein-containing blood. The fluorescein remains confined to the choroid and does not enter the retina.

Notes

In the choroidal phase, there will be a patchy filling of choroidal circulation (ground glass).

Cilioretinal will be filled in venous phases.

In the arteriovenous phase, the lamina of the artery is filled first then the central artery after 1–2 s.

For astrocytic hamartoma and disc drusen, there will be auto-florescence at the optic disc.

NVEs and NVDs are retinal neovessels that lack the normal tight junctions of retinal vessels, so leaky early.

Note that choroidal shunts do not leak, IRMAs mildly leak and NVEs leak profusely. In CSCR, expanding point of fluorescein leakage with late pooling into a serous detachment.

To differentiate ischemic and non-ischemic CRVO on FFA, more than 5 disc diameter ischemia represents ischemic CRVO.

Leakage occurs with bleeding in non-confined space, so appear diffuse and irregular (e.g., NVEs and NVDs) increasing throughout images.

Pooling occurs with bleeding in a confined space, so regular border (e.g., pigment epithelial detachment), and increase in intensity with time.

Choroidal leakage will be irregularly diffused, while retinal (subretinal) leakage is regularly confined.

24.2.4 Indocyanine Green (ICG)

Because of its physical properties, ICG is retained in the choroidal circulation more than FA and thus help to better image and characterize choroidal diseases. ICG is important in the diagnosis of certain diseases such RAP and PPCV, inflammatory uveitis with choroiditis (e.g., white dot syndromes) as well as choroidal hemangioma. Differences between it and the FFA are demonstrated in Table 24.4.

Note that both excitation and emission are within visible light for FFA, but within IR for the ICG, so ICG needs digital sensors, not just cameras.

There is no reason to suspect that a shellfish allergy should preclude the use of ICG, as the allergy in seafood is due to proteins within them, rather than to iodine.

In case of anaphylaxis, a 0.3–0.5 mL IM injection of 1:1000 adrenaline should be administered.

Table 24.4 Comparison between fundus fluorescein angiography (FFA) and indocyanine green (ICG)

	FFA	ICG
Protein bound	80%	98%
Peak excitation	465–490 nm	790–805 nm
Peak emission	520–530 nm	825–835 nm
Optic disc appearance	White	Black
Leakage through small choriocapillaris vessels	Yes (limiting its use in choroidal diseases)	No (as it is more protein bound and has a large molecular weight)
Leakage through retinal and large choroidal vessels	No	No
Iodine content	No	Yes
Incidence of adverse reaction	Relatively higher (5%)	Lower (<1%)
Excretion	Renal	Liver

Table 24.5 Clinical trials in retinal vein occlusion

Clinical trials in RVO	Main conclusions
BVOS	Macular laser photocoagulation is superior to observation in macular edema secondary to BRVO Sectoral laser is indicated only if neovascularization develops
CVOS	Macular laser photocoagulation is not beneficial in macular edema secondary to CRVO Prophylactic PRP does not prevent NVI and is not recommended PRP is indicated only if neovascularization develops
SCORE	Intravitreal triamcinolone is superior to observation in CRVO Intravitreal triamcinolone is not superior to macular laser in BRVO, and laser has better safety profile
GENEVA	Intravitreal dexamethasone implant (0.7 mg and 0.35 mg) is better than sham in macular edema secondary to CRVO and BRVO at 3 months but equally effective at 6 months
CRUISE	Intravitreal ranibizumab (0.3 and 0.5 mg) is superior to sham in macular edema secondary to CRVO at 6 months
BRAVO	Intravitreal ranibizumab (0.3 and 0.5 mg) is superior to sham in macular edema secondary to BRVO at 6 months
HORIZON and RETAIN	Extension for CRUISE and BRAVO studies to 1 and 4 years, respectively
COPERNICUS and GALILEO	Intravitreal aflibercept is superior to sham in macular edema secondary to CRVO
VIBRANT	Intravitreal aflibercept is superior to laser in macular edema secondary to BRVO

24.3 Summary of Retinal Diseases Landmark Trials

Summary of the major conclusions of landmark trials in retinal vein occlusion, AMD, diabetic retinopathy, and DME and in endophthalmitis are demonstrated in Tables 24.5, 24.6, 24.7, and 24.8, respectively.

24.3.1 High-Yield Notes About Photocoagulation Laser

- Classified as type 4 lasers.
- Absorption spectra of the key pigments found in ocular tissues:
  - *Melanin* effectively absorbs green, yellow, red, and infrared wavelengths.

Table 24.6 Clinical trials in age-related degeneration (AMD)

Clinical trials in AMD	Main conclusions
Macular photocoagulation study (MPS)	Focal laser is superior to observation in preventing severe vision loss in classic extrafoveal or juxtafoveal MNV Subfoveal MNV with good vision is not a good candidate for laser
TAP	PDT is more effective than observation in preventing vision loss in predominantly classic subfoveal MNV caused by nAMD
VIP	PDT is more effective than observation in preventing vision loss in subfoveal myopic MNV and in occult MNV caused by nAMD
ANCHOR	Intravitreal ranibizumab (0.3 and 0.5 mg) is superior to PDT in predominantly classic MNV caused by nAMD
MARINA	Intravitreal ranibizumab (0.3 and 0.5 mg) is superior to PDT in minimally classic and occult MNV caused by nAMD
CATT and IVAN	Intravitreal bevacizumab is non-inferior to ranibizumab in nAMD if given at the same regimen (PRN or monthly)
VIEW 1 and VIEW2	Intravitreal aflibercept is non-inferior to ranibizumab in nAMDmonthly or every 2 months aflibercept is equally effective to monthly ranibizumab
HAWK and HARRIER	Intravitreal brolucizumab is non-inferior to aflibercept in nAMD

Table 24.7 Clinical trials in diabetic retinopathy (DR) and diabetic macular edema (DME)

Clinical trials in DR and macular edema	Main conclusions
DCCT	**Tight control of blood sugar level in type 1 DM,** HbA1c value of around 7% reduced the risk of retinopathy progression as well as renal and neurological complications of DM
UKPDS	Similar to DCCT, UKPDS shown reduction in retinopathy progression in patients with type 2 DM with intensive blood sugar control
DRS	PRP reduces the risk of vision loss by 50% in high-risk PDR
ETDRS	Scatter laser photocoagulation may be considered for severe NPDR and early PDR Focal laser should be considered for CSME with any DR Aspirin does not reduce progression of DR bit also does not have harmful effects on vision
DRVS	Early vitrectomy provides prompt visual recovery in type one diabetes with moderately severe neovascularization
Protocol T	Aflibercept, ranibizumab, and bevacizumab are effective in treating DME If VA > 20/50, all are equally effective If VA ≤ 20/50, aflibercept is superior at year one but equally effective to ranibizumab at year two Bevacizumab arm was less likely to get anatomically dry macula
Protocol S	Intravitreal ranibizumab is non-inferior to PRP in high-risk PDR and is associated with less visual field loss
Protocol I	Intravitreal ranibizumab with focal laser is superior to focal laser alone in DME Intravitreal triamcinolone with focal laser is superior to focal laser alone in DME in pseudophakic patients but with risk of increased IOP
Protocol V	In central-involving DME with good vision, strategies other than anti-VEGF (such as observation) should be initiated first
RISE & RIDE and RESOLVE	Intravitreal ranibizumab is safe and more effective than sham for DME
RESTORE	Intravitreal ranibizumab alone or with focal laser is superior to focal laser alone in DME
DAVINCI	Intravitreal aflibercept is superior to macular laser in DME
VIVD & VISTA	Intravitreal aflibercept is safe and superior to macular laser in DME
BOLT	Intravitreal bevacizumab is superior to laser in DME
KESTREL & KITE	Intravitreal brolucizumab is non-inferior to aflibercept in DME with fewer number of injections

Table 24.8 Clinical trials in endophthalmitis

Clinical trials in endophthalmitis	Main conclusions
EVS	No proven benefit from intravenous/systemic antibiotics in the treatment of endophthalmitis Vitrectomy is better than conservative treatment for VA < hand motion Vitrectomy is equally effective to conservative treatment for VA ≥ hand motion
ESCRS	Intracameral cefuroxime is associated with reduced risk of endophthalmitis Scleral tunnel incision reduces the risk of endophthalmitis Temporal incision, intraoperative complications and silicon-type IOLs are associated with increased risk of endophthalmitis

  - Macular *xanthophyll* primarily absorbs blue light but absorbs yellow and red wavelengths minimally.
  - *Hemoglobin* easily absorbs blue, green, and yellow, with minimal absorption of red wavelengths.
- The *green laser* (e.g., Argon) is commonly used due to its effective absorption by melanin and hemoglobin, with less absorption by xanthophyll, thus reducing macular damage.
- The *red laser* (e.g., Krypton) is beneficial for penetrating nuclear sclerotic cataracts and moderate vitreous hemorrhages more effectively than lasers with other wavelengths. In addition, it is minimally absorbed by xanthophyll, making it suitable for treatments near the fovea, though it can cause more discomfort, due to its deeper penetration.
- The *krypton red laser* is least absorbed by hemoglobin or red blood cells. Krypton red (647 nm) laser photocoagulation is particularly advantageous for treating branch retinal vein occlusion (BRVO), particularly in cases with extensive intraretinal hemorrhage or media opacities like vitreous hemorrhage or cataract.
- Blue light is absorbed by macular xanthophylls, while green light is absorbed well by melanin and hemoglobin. Red light is absorbed well by melanin but poorly by hemoglobin, and Krypton red light penetrates more deeply than argon green light.
- Optical scattering is less from longer wavelengths than from shorter wavelengths, making diode red relatively advantageous in terms of light scattering.
- Xenon-arc photocoagulation, although similar in effect to argon laser photocoagulation for reducing severe visual loss, is no longer used due to slightly increased side effects.
- Risk of a Bruch membrane rupture and laser-induced MNV is higher with small spot size, high intensity, short duration, and red-type lasers.

24.4 Miscellaneous

24.4.1 Choroidal Diseases

24.4.1.1 Central Serous Chorioretinopathy (CSCR)

Idiopathic localized serous detachment of the sensory retina at the macula caused by leakage from choriocapillaris through hyperpermeable RPE sites.

Typically affects young Caucasian male.

Risk Factors

Stress, type A personality, steroids use, pregnancy, sleep apnea, and *H. pylori* infection.

Presentation

- Unilateral central vision loss, metamorphopsia, micropsia, and dyschromatopsia associated with a hyperopic refractive shift.
- Appears clinically a round elevation of detached retina at the macula with clear or turbid SRF with or without PED (Fig. 24.5).
- Typical appearances on fluorescein angiography include: early hyperfluorescence that enlarges gradually (called inkblot appearance (31%)) or hyperfluorescence that forms a vertical column called smokestack pattern (12%).

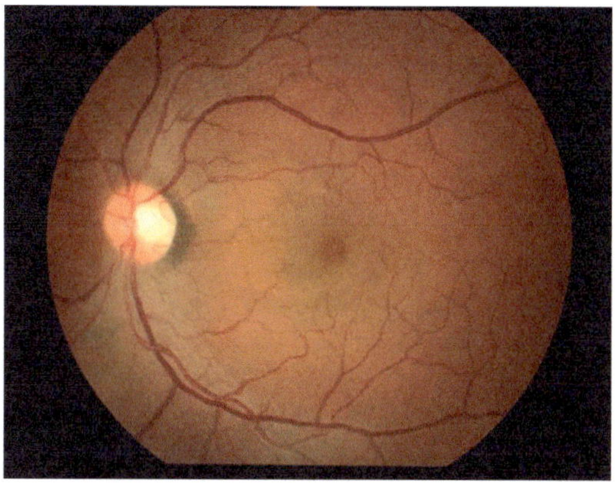

Fig. 24.5 Central serous chorioretinopathy (CSCR) (Courtesy of Retina Rocks®)

Important differential diagnosis: include optic nerve pit, PPCV, choroidal tumors including hemangioma and metastases, as well as inflammation including scleritis and Vogt–Koyanagi–Harada (VKH) disease.

Prognosis

- Majority (80%) show spontaneous resolution within 3–6 months.
- Few develop chronic course with RPE and photodetectors atrophic degeneration.
- Recurrence rate ranges 30–50%, MNV develops in 20% of patients.

24.4.1.2 Treatment

1. Observation

   With minimizing risk factors should always be considered especially that most cases resolve and laser treatment is associated with risks such as RPE rips or MNV.
2. Medical treatment

   Spironolactone, eplerenone (a mineralocorticoid receptor antagonist) topical CAI (e.g., Trusopt) may reduce subretinal fluid and choroidal thickness. However, their efficacy is not consistent.
3. Laser treatment

   Conventional macular laser can be used for lesions where leaking points are outside the foveal avascular zone. Micropulse laser applied to leakage sites may be an effective treatment for foveal involving lesion.
4. Photodynamic therapy

   Currently, the main line treatment for chronic cases helps to reduce subretinal fluid, choroidal thickness, and possibly recurrences.

Indications for treating CSCR with laser or PDT:

- Persistent serous detachment (>3–4 months) is the main indication.
- Occupational or other demands for rapid recovery of binocular function.
- Prior episodes of CSCR that have been associated with permanently decreased visual acuity.
- Permanent visual loss due to CSCR in the contralateral eye.

24.4.1.3 Choroidal Folds

Parallel horizontal striae that cross the posterior pole and are typically secondary to ocular or orbital diseases. Thyroid eye disease is a common cause, as are external forces such as an indenting tumor, which can lead to choroidal folds. Posterior scleritis can thicken the sclera, causing crowding and folding of the choroid. Hypotony, such as following glaucoma surgery, is also a significant cause. Additionally, choroidal folds can occur in middle-aged adults with hyperopia although this cause is relatively common and poorly characterized.

24.4.1.4 Uveal Effusion Syndrome

Abnormal scleral composition or thickness impairs transscleral aqueous outflow, disrupting fluid movement through the posterior eye wall. This can lead to choroidal and ciliary body thickening, RPE alterations, and exudative retinal detachment. The causes include malignant hypertension and inflammation such as scleritis. For young hyperopic patients diagnosed with CSC or retinal detachment without a retinal hole or tear, idiopathic uveal effusion syndrome should be considered. In some patients, intravitreal triamcinolone may help resolve fluid. Short axial length (<23 mm) strongly correlated with the development of choroidal effusion due to increased resistance to fluid outflow from the suprachoroidal space. Medical management typically includes cycloplegia and steroids, either systemic or intravitreal steroids, if inflammation is suspected. In idiopathic cases, partial sclerectomy to improve choroidal drainage is often necessary.

24.4.1.5 Bilateral Diffuse Uveal Melanocytic Proliferation (BDUMP)

A relatively rare paraneoplastic disorder affecting the choroid is characterized by bilateral proliferation of benign melanocytes and mostly associated with cancers of the ovary, uterus, and lung.

24.4.1.6 Choroidal Infarcts

The choroidal infarcts appear as wedge-shaped hyperpigmented areas in the fundus, reflecting the lobar anatomy of choroidal blood flow. Differential diagnosis for choroidal infarction includes accelerated (malignant) hypertension, such as that seen in pregnancy-related toxemia. Other potential causes are disseminated intravascular coagulation, and inflammatory conditions such as SLE and polyarteritis nodosa.

24.4.1.7 Choroidal Ruptures

Crescent-shaped white break of choroid, Bruch's membrane, and RPE that is concentric with the optic disc are usually a consequence of blunt ocular trauma (but not penetrating), which stretches the sclera and choroid to the point where Bruch's membrane (and the choroid) breaks. The presence of adjacent subretinal hemorrhage is common. Choroidal ruptures are more common in young, male patients and those with angioid streaks. They affect the post-equatorial retina and, in a small percentage of patients, they can cause choroidal neovascularization later on. Provided there is no central macular involvement, the visual prognosis is favorable.

24.4.1.8 Choroidal Detachment and Suprachoroidal Hemorrhage

Accumulation of fluid or blood in the potential suprachoroidal space. It can be divided into serous choroidal detachment (aka. choroidal effusion) and hemorrhagic choroidal detachment (see Table 24.9). The former is most commonly resulting from hypotony particularly after large incision cataract surgery and glaucoma surgeries. Risk factors include hypertension, advanced age, glaucoma, myopia, aphakia, and cardiovascular disease.

Retina may appear elevated, mimicking RD when B-scan can help to distinguish between these entities. Initial management with observation, cycloplegia, and steroids is usually sufficient for simple serous detachment; however, surgical drainage is indicated in the following cases that are more likely to be encountered with suprachoroidal hemorrhage:

- Corneo-lenticular touch with decompensation
- Kissing choroids: appositional choroidals (due to the potential for retinal adhesion formation and subsequent visual impairment)
- Long-lasting choroidal effusions (no signs of improvement within 4 weeks)
- Decreased vision due to macular involvement with the choroidal detachment
- Suspected suprachoroidal hemorrhage.

Table 24.9 Comparison between serous and hemorrhagic choroidal detachment

Serous choroidal detachment	Hemorrhagic choroidal detachment
Shallow anterior chamber	Shallow anterior chamber
Low IOP	High IOP
Painless	Painful
Normal transillumination and low echogenicity of fluid on B-scan	No transillumination and high echogenicity of fluid on B-scan
Good prognosis	Worse prognosis

24.4.1.9 Sclerochoroidal Calcifications

Represent deposits of calcium pyrophosphate in the sclera and/or choroid, typically found in elderly white individuals. These deposits appear as irregular, yellow chorioretinal lesions, often located superotemporally near the superior vascular arcade. They generally have no significant clinical consequences. Because of systemic association in some case, it is important to assess calcium and phosphorus level.

24.4.2 Pseudophakic Cystoid Macular Edema (CME)

CME is originally known as Irvine–Gass syndrome. The incidence of clinically detected cystoid macular edema is in the range of 1% in uneventful phacoemulsification while the incidence of CME after extracapsular cataract surgery was previously reported as high as 15–30%.

The risk is higher after posterior capsular rupture and in eyes with pre-existing uveitis and epiretinal membrane. Diabetics are at higher risk that is proportional to the degree of retinopathy ranging from 2% in mild NPDR to up to 10% in PDR cases. A causative role of prostaglandin analogues was questionable in recent studies which found no significant to minimal impact. Generally, CME rate peaks at 6–10 weeks surgery, and it resolves spontaneously in 95% of cases within 6 months. Clinically, the patient usually reports a decrease of vision 1-month post-surgery with present of macular edema on slit lamp biomicroscopy and OCT. Intraocular lens implantation at the time of cataract extraction does not change the incidence of CME. Pseudophakic CME typically demonstrates a fluorescein angiographic hyperfluorescent cystic ("petaloid") pattern but this is usually not required for diagnosis. Treatment is usually in the form of topical steroids plus NSAIDs eye drops. Resistant cases are usually treated with periocular steroids. Intravitreal steroids are reserved for CME that is persistent despite periocular steroids. Short-term acetazolamide tablets could also be used in some cases. The prophylactic use of NSAIDs showed a better preventive impact than steroids and should be considered in high-risk cases.

24.4.3 Retinopathies

24.4.3.1 Radiation Retinopathy

Microangiopathic changes that clinically resemble diabetic retinopathy are typically observed around 18 months after treatment with external-beam radiation and earlier with brachytherapy. An exposure to doses of 30–35 grays (Gy) or more is usually required to develop clinical symptoms. Increasing steadily at doses greater than 45 Gy; occasionally, however, retinopathy may develop after as low as 15 Gy of external-beam radiation. Comorbidities such as diabetes, hypertension, simultaneous chemotherapy, and pregnancy are associated with an increased risk of radiation retinopathy. Risk factors for developing proliferative radiation retinopathy include younger age, pre-existing diabetes mellitus, and shorter tumor distance to the optic disc. Hyperfractionation (dividing dose) of external-beam radiation has been associated with a decreased incidence of radiation retinopathy. Exposure of radiation is thought to cause preferential loss of vascular endothelial cells with relative sparing of the pericytes (opposite to DR pathophysiologically, but similar clinically). The earliest fundus manifestations of radiation retinopathy are discrete foci in the posterior pole of occluded capillaries with surrounding irregular dilatation of neighboring microvasculature.

The lens is the most radiosensitive structure in the eye, followed by the cornea, the retina, and the optic nerve. Cataract formation is the most likely initial complication of radiation exposure with an average latent period for the development of radiation-induced cataracts of 2–3 years.

24.4.3.2 Autoimmune Retinopathy

Broadly separated into neoplastic and non-neoplastic:

Cancer-associated retinopathy (CAR) is an autoimmune paraneoplastic syndrome due to the development of anti-retinal protein antibodies. Patients present with progressive deterioration of vision, with eventual bilateral involvement and severe visual loss. On examination, patients with CAR usually have prominent cone dysfunction with a markedly decreased visual acuity, loss of color vision, and central scotomas. In MAR, color vision and central visual acuity have more peripheral visual field loss. Fundus examination is usually normal untill advanced stage of the disease characterized by atrophy of the retinal pigment epithelium as well as optic atrophy. Some cases also develop vascular sheathing and vitreous cells.

ERG is almost always abnormal, due to the preferential rod involvement. Melanoma-associated retinopathy (MAR) is another autoimmune retinopathy characterized by auto-antibodies that have activity against bipolar cells. Table 24.10 demonstrates the major differences between CAR and MAR.

24.4.4 Solar Retinopathy

It is aaused by photochemical retinal injury. Initially, visual acuity is mildly reduced, and small scotoma can occur. Vision usually improves spontaneously to 20/20–20/40 within 6 months, although scotoma and even metamorphopsia can persist. No treatment currently available for eclipse retinopathy.

24.4.5 Endophthalmitis

Endophthalmitis is an inflammatory condition of the anterior and posterior segment with involvement of the aqueous and vitreous humor. While non-infectious causes exist, the term "endophthalmitis" is mainly coined to inflammation caused by infection, mainly bacterial and fungal.

Types of endophthalmitis are discussed in Table 24.11.

24.4.5.1 Presentation of Endophthalmitis

- Painful significant drop of vision. The onset is usually acute in exogenous endophthalmitis and more gradual in endogenous cases particularly those caused by fungi

Table 24.10 Comparison between cancer-associated retinopathy (CAR) and melanoma-associated retinopathy (MAR)

Cancer-associated retinopathy (CAR)	Melanoma-associated retinopathy (MAR)
Cone dysfunction and rod dysfunction	Bipolar cells dysfunction with rod more than cone dysfunction
Auto-antibodies against recover in retinal antigen	Auto-antibodies against 22-kd neuronal antigen and transducin
Symptoms usually precede diagnosis of malignancy	Symptoms usually start after diagnosis of malignancy
ERG is abnormal early	a-wave preserved (negative ERG)
Most commonly small cell lung cancer	Cutaneous melanoma
Poor visual prognosis	Good prognosis

Table 24.11 Types of endophthalmitis

Exogenous endophthalmitis	Caused by direct inoculation of the eye by the pathogen, can occur after surgery or penetrating trauma or by spread of an external infectious focus		
	Post-operative endophthalmitis	The most common type	Early (<6 weeks): the most common cause is *S. epidermidis* Late (>6 weeks): the most common cause is Strep. species
	Posttraumatic endophthalmitis	The most severe form with the worst visual prognosis	The most common cause is Bacillus. species
Endogenous endophthalmitis	The eye is involved as part of a systemic infection that reaches intraocular tissue via blood stream. Systemic immunosuppression increases the risk of infection The most common cause is Candida species		

- Lid edema
- Anterior segment: chemosis, corneal edema, AC cells, hypopyon, corneal infiltrates
- Posterior segment: vitritis, decreased red reflex, retinitis, and vasculitis

24.4.5.2 High-Yield Note

Care should be taken to differentiate endophthalmitis from toxic anterior segment syndrome (TASS). Table 24.12 shows the major differences between these entities.

24.4.6 Management of Endophthalmitis

1. Confirming the diagnosis:

   Endophthalmitis is a clinical decision. In the context of post-surgical endophthalmitis, the diagnosis should be considered when the severity of inflammation is more than expected for a given surgery, and the vitreous is involved. Vitreous biopsy with microbiological evaluation is advised but the yield is in the range of 50% only. Samples of aqueous have much poorer yield.

   B-scan ultrasonography can be used to confirm vitreous involvement if view is poor and assess the retinal status. In endogenous endophthalmitis, physician input to look for a source of infection is important, and assessment usually includes direct questioning about intravenous drug use, recent surgery or hospital admission, blood culture, and echocardiography.

2. Medical/Conservative treatment

   Exogenous endophthalmitis

   The main line of treatment for exogenous endophthalmitis is intravitreal antibiotics. Adjuvant treatment includes topical and subconjunctival injection.

   No benefit was demonstrated with the use of systemic amikacin or ceftazidime but quinolones such as moxifloxacin were shown to have good ocular penetration.

   Steroids can be given as eye drops or subconjunctival injections.

   Systemic and intravitreal steroids can only be used but are better held off in cases where when fungal infection is suspected.

   Endogenous endophthalmitis.

   Systemic antibiotic is the main stay of treatment. Intravitreal antibiotics are also important.

3. Surgical treatment with vitrectomy. Indicated when:
   - There is no or poor response to conservative treatment.
   - Condition is worsening despite conservative treatment.
   - Presenting visual acuity is worse than hand motion in post cataract surgery cases.
   - Significant and severe vitreous involvement.

24.4.6.1 High-Yield Notes

- The reported incidence of endophthalmitis following:
  - Cataract surgery: 0.04%
  - PPV: 0.05%

Table 24.12 Comparison between toxic anterior segment syndrome (TASS) and endophthalmitis

	TASS	Endophthalmitis
Onset	Within hours of surgery	3–7 days after surgery
Pain	None to mild	Severe*
Lid swelling	Absent	Present
Pupils	Fixed dilated	Reactive ± RAPD
Corneal edema	Diffuse limbus-to-limbus	Focal/segmental
AC reaction	++ Fibrinous exudates ± Cells and hypopyon	± Fibrinous exudates ++ Cells and hypopyon
Vitritis	Absent	Present
IOP	Elevated	Normal/slightly elevated
Management	Topical ± systemic steroids	Intravitreal antibiotics ± PPV

- Intravitreal injection of anti-VEGF: 0.017–0.025%
- Posttraumatic endophthalmitis 3%. The risk is higher with intraocular foreign body, wounds contaminated with organic lens matter and lens capsule disruption 7

- Immediate vitrectomy only beneficial for light perception (LP) vision or worse on presentation.
- Current standard protocols for intravitreal antibiotics injections are empirically based and typically involve the peptide antibiotic vancomycin (1.0 mg/0.1 mL) for Gram-positive coverage, combined with the β-lactam antibiotic ceftazidime (2.25 mg/0.1 mL) for Gram-negative coverage. For patients who are sensitive to β-lactam drugs, amikacin (400 μg/0.1 mL), an aminoglycoside antibiotic, may be used instead of ceftazidime, though amikacin has been associated with some degree of retinal toxicity.
- After an intravitreal injection of triamcinolone, pseudo-endophthalmitis may develop, characterized by drop in vision immediately or soon after injection, heavy staining of the anterior vitreous with particles and strands that may impede fundus view, no pain and swelling, and no to mild anterior chamber reaction. Spontaneous resolution is within 1–2 months.
- Important conclusions from endophthalmitis vitrectomy study results:
  - Approximately 25% of eyes with endophthalmitis had no pain at presentation.
  - There was no difference in final visual acuity/media clarity whether or not patients received systemic antibiotics.
  - Hand motions or better visual acuity on presentation did equally well whether immediate vitrectomy was performed in addition to the intravitreal antibiotic injections or not.
  - Eyes with light perception–only vision had much better visual outcome with immediate vitrectomy.
  - Most eyes (>90%) became sterile, not requiring a second injection regardless of whether immediate vitrectomy was performed or not.
  - The EVS clearly demonstrated that neither amikacin nor ceftazidime offers any therapeutic advantage when given systemically.

Acknowledgment None.

Conflict of Interest None.

References

Doft B et al (1995) Results of the Endophthalmitis Vitrectomy Study. A randomized trial of immediate vitrectomy and of intravenous antibiotics for the treatment of postoperative bacterial endophthalmitis. Endophthalmitis Vitrectomy Study Group. Arch Ophthalmol 113:1479–1496

Heeren TFC et al (2020) Macular telangiectasia type 2: visual acuity, disease end stage, and the MacTel area: MacTel project report number 8. Ophthalmology 127(11):1539–1548. https://doi.org/10.1016/j.ophtha.2020.03.040

Kanski JJ, Bowling B (2015) Kanski's clinical ophthalmology: a systematic approach. Saunders

Karampelas M, Malamos P, Petrou P, Georgalas I, Papaconstantinou D, Brouzas D (2020) Retinal pigment epithelial detachment in age-related macular degeneration. Ophthalmol Ther 9(4):739–756. https://doi.org/10.1007/s40123-020-00291-5

Kertes PJ, Conway MD (1998) Clinical trials in ophthalmology: a summary and practice guide. https://doi.org/10.1604/9780683302059

Kim SJ (2021) 2021–2022 basic and clinical science course, section 12: retina and vitreous

Reed K (2001). Fluorescein angiography refresher course. Fluorescein angiography refresher course. https://www.reviewofoptometry.com/article/fluorescein-angiography-refresher-course

Scott IU, Campochiaro PA, Newman NJ, Biousse V (2020) Retinal vascular occlusions. Lancet 396(10266):1927–1940. https://doi.org/10.1016/S0140-6736(20)31559-2

25 Clinical Review of Laser and Refractive Surgery

Saif Aldeen Alryalat, Mo'ath AlShawabkeh, Ayat Alni'mat, and Muawyah Al Bdour

Abstract

This chapter provides a comprehensive overview of refractive surgery options, beginning with non-surgical alternatives for vision correction. It then explores corneal collagen cross-linking as a vital treatment for conditions like keratoconus, enhancing corneal stability. The discussion extends to incisional surgeries, detailing the effects of radial keratotomy and incisional correction of astigmatism on visual outcomes and corneal integrity. Corneal refractive surgeries are categorized into surface ablation techniques and flap-based procedures, with a thorough examination of their methodologies and indications. Additionally, miscellaneous options such as corneal rings and collagen shrinkage procedures are discussed, highlighting their role in refractive correction. The chapter also covers lens-based refractive surgeries, outlining the various techniques and their applications. Finally, a stepwise approach to refractive surgeries is presented, providing a structured framework for clinicians to optimize patient outcomes.

Keywords

Refractive surgery · Non-surgical options · Vision correction · Astigmatism correction · Corneal refractive surgeries

S. A. Alryalat (✉)
Department of Ophthalmology, The University of Jordan, Amman, Jordan

The University of Colorado Anschutz Medical Campus, Aurora, CO, USA

M. AlShawabkeh
Department of Ophthalmology, The Hashemite University, Zarqa, Jordan

A. Alni'mat · M. Al Bdour
The University of Jordan, Amman, Jordan

25.1 Overview

Ideally when the light enters the eye, it will be collected on the retina forming the images that we see, however when this does not occur correctly, we call the eye to have an optical aberration.

Optical aberrations are imperfections of the eye that result in light being unable to focus on the retina effectively. It is divided into low-order aberrations and high-order aberrations.

Low-order aberrations include refractive errors (myopia, hyperopia, and regular astigmatism) and other non-visually significant aberrations.

High-order aberrations are measured with wave front aberrometer and expressed in terms that describe the shape and severity of the deviated light rays, and they include most importantly coma, spherical aberration, and trefoil.

S. A. Alryalat (ed.), *Ophthalmology Board and FRCS Part 2 Exams*,
https://doi.org/10.1007/978-981-96-1517-9_25

Glasses and contact lenses are non-surgical options for refractive error correction but when the patient has high-order aberrations (i.e., uncorrectable via non-surgical options), or wants to get rid of glasses, surgical options are available.

After a brief overview of the high-yield information about the non-surgical options for vision correction, laser and refractive surgery chapter discusses various procedures used in the treatment of different refractive disorders including collagen cross-linking, incisional surgeries such as radial keratotomy and astigmatic keratotomy. This is followed by a thorough overview of the corneal refractive surgery where it is divided into surface ablation procedures, flap-based procedures, and miscellaneous procedures which include Intrastromal corneal rings and conductive keratoplasty.

Lens-based refractive treatments are also discussed here with special attention given to the most important notes about phakic intraocular lens and refractive lens exchange procedures.

While maintaining a high-yield design in highlighting important notes that have appeared or may appear in ophthalmology exams, comparison tables were used to differentiate conflicting points between important entities, together with point-by-point design useful for exam revisions.

Finally, as ophthalmologists should know and master how to approach patients with refractive disorder, a detailed stepwise approach to refractive surgery is given at the end of this chapter. This includes history taking, examination, investigations, and planning surgical options.

For readers interested in more detailed information, the following references are useful (Kim 2021; Elkington 2023; Sinjab 2014; Sinjab 2021; Hafezi and Randleman 2013; Vinciguerra et al. 2022; Hafezi et al. 2021; Ambrósio and Wilson 2003; Feder and Rapuano 2007; Gomes et al. 2015).

25.2 Non-surgical Refractive Options

Before considering any refractive surgery, one should discuss non-surgical alternatives for patients with refractive error. These include spectacles and contact lenses. As they have the advantages of being available, affordable, and usually effective and safe vision correction options.

25.2.1 Considerations in Glasses Prescription

- Back vertex distance (BVD) is the distance between the back of the lens and the cornea. It should be specified with prescriptions over 5 diopters.
- Interpupillary distance should be measured accurately in order to align the center of the spectacles with the center of visual axis.
- Anisokonia (difference in the size of images between the two eyes) is associated with glasses correction in anisometropia (difference in the refractive error between the two eyes) can be problematic and may affect binocular vision and stereopsis.
- The spherical equivalent (SE) is the sum of the sphere power to half of the cylinder power; it reflects closest overall spherical effect of an astigmatic lens.

Contact lenses used in ophthalmology can be refractive and nonrefractive.

Refractive contact lenses are most commonly worn as an alternative to glasses in those who perceive glasses as non-attractive or inconvenient. In some cases, they can provide better vision than glasses like in high degree of astigmatism, irregular astigmatism, and anisometropia.

The refracting power of the optical (central) zone of a contact lens is influenced by its anterior with the posterior curvatures, thickness, and refractive index. Contact lenses can be either spherical, with the same radius of surface curvature in all meridians, or spherocylindrical (toric). The posterior surface of the optical zone is characterized by its posterior central curvature (PCC), commonly referred to as the base curve.

The base curve represents the steepest part of the contact lens, similar to the normal central cornea. Moving toward the periphery, the lens gradually flattens, with the secondary curve being less steep than the base curve, and the peripheral curve being the flattest.

Table 25.1 Comparison between soft and rigid contact lenses

Soft contact lenses	Hard contact lenses
Low oxygen permeability—diffusion coefficient (Dk value) <30	High oxygen permeability—diffusion coefficient (Dk value) >60
HEMA material	Fluoropolymer and silicon acrylate material
Very comfortable	Less comfortable
Easy to adapt	Longer adaptation time
Suitable for occasional wear	Not suitable for occasional wear
Cannot correct irregular astigmatism	Can correct irregular astigmatism

The fit of the contact lens on the cornea, as well as its movement with each blink, is determined by the base curve and the lens diameter. Maintaining the base curve but increasing the lens diameter will result in tighter fit of the contact lens on the eye. Similarly, decreasing the base curve while keeping the diameter constant will also lead to a tighter fit. A lens with a tighter fit tends to be less mobile, which can compromise the limbal area and cause increased injection, conjunctival indentation, and redness. On the other hand, signs of a loose-fitting lens include edge lift, excessive lens movement, and decentration of the lens. Contact lenses can be classified according to the materials used in manufacturing into soft, rigid, or hybrid. Table 25.1 demonstrates the major differences between soft and rigid contact lenses.

Ideal contact lens material characteristics include meeting corneal oxygenation requirements, physiologically inert, biocompatible, excellent wetting in vivo, and resisting spoliation.

To meet corneal oxygenation requirements, the material should be oxygen transmissible.

Oxygen transmissibility depends on permeability of the lens material and thickness of the lens.

Soft contact lenses can be of daily use or extended. Because of the significantly increased risk of infection with extended-wear use, the FDA has mandated that soft lenses can only be used for up to 7 days.

Hybrid contacts are made of rigid central optical zone and soft peripheral part (skirt), and they are more comfortable than totally rigid contacts.

Nonrefractive contact lenses can be for therapeutic reasons as the bandage contact lenses used after refractive surgeries or to accelerate healing of corneal epithelial defect or seal small perforation. They can be used also for cosmetic reasons as the painted contact lenses in aniridia.

25.2.1.1 High-Yield Notes

- Cautions should be taken with the use of contact lenses in order to avoid serious complications particularly bacterial keratitis especially acanthamoeba and pseudomonas infections.
- Swimming with contact lenses increases the risk of acanthamoeba keratitis.
- Contact lens wearers are advised to use them no longer than 8 h a day, clean them with appropriate solution. Never bath or sleep with contacts, replace them regularly and to see their doctor if they experience any unusual feeling.
- Contacts should be stopped 2–4 weeks prior to corneal topography or corneal refractive surgery.

25.3 Corneal Collagen Cross-Linking

Cross-linking is commonly used in the polymer industry to enhance the rigidity and stability of materials. Corneal collagen cross-linking (CXL) is the first surgical technique that has been shown to effectively stop the progression of corneal ectatic disorders, such as keratoconus and postrefractive corneal ectasia.

The most widely used CXL techniques were developed in Europe by researchers at the University of Dresden/Germany in the late 1990. First patients were treated in 1998.

It was approved by the US FDA in 2016 for two indications: the treatment of progressive keratoconus and post-refractive ectasia. Other non-approved indications can include pellucid marginal degeneration, fungal and bacterial keratitis, corneal melting, and bullous keratopathy.

The procedure involves applying riboflavin (vitamin B2) solution to the cornea, followed by exposure to ultraviolet A (UV-A) light of 370 nm. With riboflavin present, about 95% of the UV-A light is absorbed within the anterior 300 μm of the corneal stroma. To prevent corneal endothelial damage, a minimum corneal thickness of 400 μm after epithelial removal is recommended.

CXL is generally advised for eyes with mild to moderate keratoconus (maximum *K* value <65 D) that exhibits progression in adults or at the time of diagnosis in children. If the corneal thickness is less than 400 μm after epithelial removal, the standard Dresden protocol should be avoided.

Complications can include temporary stromal edema, transient or permanent haze, corneal scarring, sterile infiltrates, infectious keratitis, diffuse lamellar keratitis in a post-LASIK patient, and endothelial cell damage, likely due to oxidative damage from the reactive oxygen free radicals generated during the interaction.

Contraindications for CXL: Include corneal thickness less than 400 μm at the thinnest location (after epithelial removal), a history of herpetic infection (to prevent viral reactivation), active infection, severe corneal scarring or opacification, poor wound healing history, severe ocular surface disease, and a history of autoimmune disorders.

If a patient is not suitable for standard protocol CXL due to advanced disease or other conditions, deep anterior lamellar keratoplasty or full thickness corneal transplantation may be considered as alternative treatments.

25.3.1 Procedure

- Riboflavin is used as the photosensitizer. It is safe for systemic use. It is effectively absorbed by the corneal stroma when applied topically and can be adequately absorbed by the corneal stroma topically.
- UV-A light absorption: Riboflavin has an absorption peak at 370 nm, making UV-A light ideal for CXL (Fig. 25.1). This wavelength ensures effective cross-linking while protecting other ocular structures. The total fluence delivered during the procedure is 5.4 J/cm^2.
- Oxygen role: Oxygen is crucial for effective CXL as it facilitates the generation of reactive oxygen species necessary for the cross-linking process.
- Formation of covalent bonds: Upon exposure to UV-A light, riboflavin generates reactive oxygen species, leading to the formation of covalent bonds between collagen molecules and between collagen molecules and proteoglycans as the corneal structure.

25.3.2 Alternative Protocols

The Bunsen–Roscoe law (photochemical effect would be the same provided that the total fluence remains constant) has formed the principle of additional protocols for CXL which uses different combinations of the intensity and duration of UV-A exposure to generate the same overall effect.

Accelerated protocol: The goal is to deliver a target UV energy of 5.4 J/cm^2. The standard Dresden protocol achieves this with a 30-min exposure at an irradiance of 3 mW\cm^2. Newer accelerated protocols aim to reduce the duration of UV-A exposure while maintaining the same

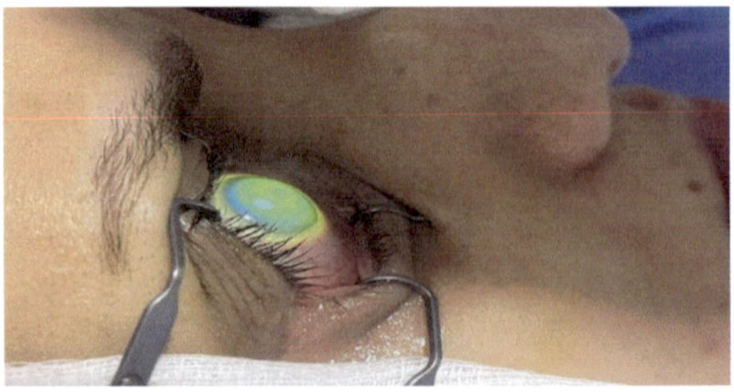

Fig. 25.1 Ultraviolet light exposure during collagen cross-linking

total energy dose. For example, 30 min at 3 mW\cm^2 is equivalent to 3 min at 30 mW\cm^2 or 10 min at 9 mW\cm^2.

Studies have shown that the 10-min exposure protocol is not inferior to the traditional 30-min exposure in terms of effectiveness.

Epithelial on protocol: For effective transepithelial CXL, several parameters must be adjusted. One of the key differences between epi-off and and epi-on CXL is that the corneal thickness requirement of 400 μm includes the epithelium in epi-on procedures. This means that patients with a corneal thickness that falls below 400 μm only after epithelium removal, who might be excluded from epi-off CXL, can still be eligible for epi-on CXL.

25.3.2.1 Riboflavin Solutions

Investigators have experimented with different riboflavin solution concentrations to enhance riboflavin absorption through an intact epithelium during epi-on CXL. Examples of these solutions include hypotonic riboflavin solution 0.1% without dextran, hypotonic riboflavin solution 0.5% without dextran[, riboflavin 0.1%, dextran 15.0%, trometamol, and EDTA. However, the literature still lacks comprehensive in vivo trials comparing the efficacy of these various riboflavin solutions and additives in epi-on CXL.

25.3.2.2 Iontophoresis-Assisted Epi-on CXL

Iontophoresis involves the use of an electrical gradient to move charged particles across epithelium. The negativly charged hydrophilic riboflavin is an ideal candidate to be drived across the lipophilic corneal epithelium via iontophoresis.

It entails the use of riboflavin solution with 0.1% riboflavin. The corneal iontophoresis electrode generates a constant current of 1 mA (the total dose of 5 mA/5 min is monitored by the generator) for 5 min. UV-A irradiation parameters of 10 mW for 9 min for a total energy dose of 5.4 J/cm^2 (Fig. 25.2).

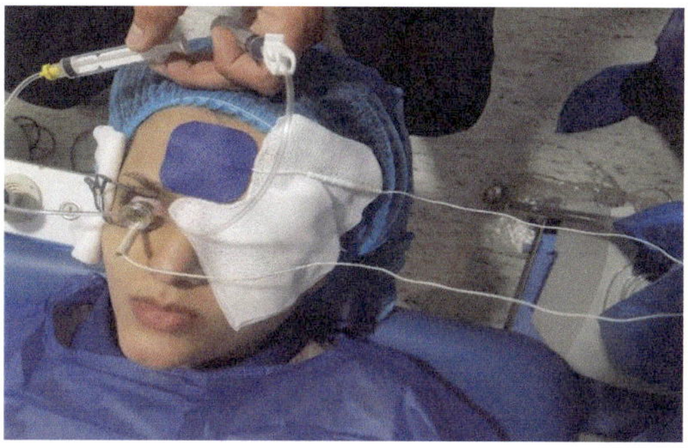

Fig. 25.2 Iontophoresis-assisted CXL

25.3.3 Sub400 Protocol

The sub400 protocol involves various techniques designed to modify stromal thickness to safely and effectively perform CXL on thin corneas. For example, hypotonic riboflavin solutions can be used to swell the cornea to a thickness greater than 400 μm, or contact lens-assisted CXL can artificially thicken the stroma by placing a contact lens over the cornea. However, these techniques have significant limitations and lack standardization.

To address these issues, Hafezi et al. developed an algorithm that adapts the overall UV-A fluence during the CXL procedure based on the patient's stromal thickness. This algorithm tailors the irradiation settings according to the minimal corneal thickness measured at the end of riboflavin soaking but just before UV-A exposure, ensuring that the corneal endothelium is protected from harmful UV-A radiation .

This approach introduces the concept of individualizing the total energy delivered during CXL according to intraoperative pachymetry, marking a significant advancement in CXL protocols.

25.3.3.1 High-Yield Notes

- The estimated success rate of CXL in halting progression of keratoconus and postrefractive ectasia is around 80%.

- CXL mainly stiffens anterior 200–250 μm of the stroma which is characterized by the demarcation line on OCT.

25.3.4 Incisional Surgeries and Sutures Effects

In principle, focal corneal steepening caused by sutures yields a positive astigmatism at the same axis and focal flattening as with incisions or releasing sutures yields negative astigmatism at the same axis.

Clear corneal cataract incisions can act similarly to arcuate incisions used to correct astigmatism. These incisions flatten the cornea in the direction of the incision, while simultaneously steepening the cornea 90° away due to the "coupling" effect. The impact of this correction depends on two factors: the size of the optical zone and the length of the incision. Surgeons who perform clear corneal cataract procedures often choose to make the incision on the steep meridian. Temporal incisions smaller than 3.5 mm, located within 0.5–1.0 mm of the limbus, typically correct up to 1.25 D of astigmatism. By adding a peripheral arcuate incision 180° opposite, it is possible to correct 2 or more diopters of astigmatism.

25.4 Radial Keratotomy (RK)

It is a method of irreversibly flattening the central corneal curvature to reduce its refractive power and correct myopia.

The process of making 8 radial incisions with a depth of 85–90% of the corneal thickness, leaving a circular clear optical zone with diameter of 3.00, 3.50, or 4.00 mm, based on the level of preoperative myopia, where it can correct myopia from −2.00 D to −8.75 D. These incisions will lead to flattening in the optical zone, leading to hyperopic shift up to one diopter continues over the next few years.

25.4.1 Complications

- The refraction might be stable for 3 months, but may result in progression afterward.
- The incisions might leave scars that cause glare symptoms.
- Diurnal fluctuation of refraction, where the cornea swells from hypoxic effect of eye closure, leading to hyperopic shift.

25.4.1.1 High-Yield Notes

- PRK is more suitable than LASIK for post-RK refractive correction, due to flap-related complications.
- After cataract surgery on eyes that had prior RK, short-term flattening of the cornea and hyperopic shift are frequently noted as a result of the corneal edema after surgery. Therefore, in the event of a **refractive surprise**, neither an intraocular lens (IOL) exchange nor PRK should be considered in post-RK eyes until the cornea and refraction stabilize, which can take several weeks to months.

25.5 Incisional Correction of Astigmatism

Incisions in cataract surgery should be made at the axis of the steep keratometry (K2). Note that subjective refraction astigmatism comprises both lenticular and corneal astigmatism, so should not be depended on when deciding on correcting astigmatism in cataract surgery, as the lenticular part will be removed after surgery.

Done using adjustable diamond blade at the astigmatism meridian:

- Either tangential (transverse/straight) keratotomy or arcuate (curved) keratotomy (AK), in which incisions are typically placed in the cornea at the 7-mm optical zone
- Or limbal relaxing incisions (LRIs), which are placed at the limbus

Arcuate, or astigmatic, keratotomy incisions typically done 6–9 mm from the center, leaving an optical zone of 7–9 mm, while a 4-mm optical zone is too narrow and would have a high incidence of irregular astigmatism. The incisions will flatten the cornea in the meridian of the incision and steepen the cornea 90° away when performed in an arcuate fashion, which is the most common pattern used for astigmatism.

Arcuate keratotomy (AK) incisions have been made at various optical zones. Limbal relaxing incisions (LRIs) are placed closer to the limbus than AK incisions. In general, to achieve a similar effect, LRIs should be longer than AK incisions, although this is not specific to the definition. In addition, the cornea is thicker in the periphery; therefore, LRIs should generally be deeper than AK incisions for the equivalent refractive result.

25.5.1 Astigmatic Keratotomy for Astigmatism Correction

Incisions are made perpendicular to the steep meridian of the astigmatism within 5–7 mm optic zone, with incisions can be lengthened up to 90′ of arc.

The incision must stop just peripheral to the central clear zone. Causes a flattening in the meridian of the incision. The goal is to correct about two-thirds of the astigmatic error, rather than all astigmatism.

Coupling defined as the compensatory steepening occurring simultaneously in the meridian 90° away from the meridian that is flattened as a result of an astigmatic incision.

The number, type, and length of the incisions are considered the most important factors influencing the coupling ratio.

25.5.1.1 High-Yield Notes

- AK can be done with the cataract surgery to correct around 2D astigmatism. Before proceeding with the keratotomy with cataract surgery, make sure that the astigmatism to be corrected is not lenticular, as correcting such lenticular astigmatism after cataract extraction would yield to manifest astigmatism.
- AK incisions require more time to stabilize than do radial incisions (degree of correction depending on age), so enhancement should be deferred for a minimum of 6 weeks after the primary procedure. Overcorrection can be managed by interrupted 10–0 nylon suture at incision site left for 4 months.

25.6 Refractive Surgeries

Refractive surgeries can treat myopia, hyperopia, compound and mixed astigmatism, but not irregular astigmatism.

Classified as:

Cornea-based
- Photoablation lasers
- Incisional procedures
- Intrastromal corneal rings

Lens-based
- Phakic IOL
- Refractive lens exchange

Combination
- The combination of corneal and intraocular refractive surgery, termed *bioptics.*

25.6.1 Photorefractive Laser

Excimer stands for "excited dimer," a photoablative laser that generates light using the interaction of argon (Ar) and fluoride (F-). This excimer laser generates a UV in corneal photoablation. Photoablation results in the cleavage of covalent chemical bonds in tissue proteins.

The femtosecond laser (FS) is an infrared laser. FS laser-like Nd: YAG laser works by producing photo disruption or photoionization of the optically transparent tissue such as the cornea. Table 25.2 shows the major differences between these types of lasers.

In addition to the use of FS laser in LASIK flap creation, other ocular surgeries involving FS laser include astigmatic keratotomy (AK), intrastromal corneal ring segments (ICRS), small-incision lenticule extraction (SMILE), corneal grafting, cataract surgery particularly wound construction, capsulorrhexis, and nuclear fragmentation.

Cornea-based refractive surgeries can be divided into either:

- Surface ablation based, where epithelium is removed, and laser applied to Bowman and underlying stroma. Includes PRK, LASEK, and epi-LASIK.

Table 25.2 .The major differences between femtosecond and excimer laser

Comparison	Femtosecond laser	Excimer laser
Effect	Photodisruption	Photoablation
Penetration	High through transparent tissues	Limited
Wavelength	1053 (near infrared)	193 (far ultraviolet)
Need for suction	Required	Not required

Table 25.3 Comparison between surface ablation and flap-based surgeries

	Surface ablation	Flap-based
Corneal biomechanics	Better	Worse
Post-op pain and recovery	Slower	Faster
Preferred in	Myopia	Hyperopia
Advantages	Better in irregular or thin corneas. Epithelial basement membrane disease. Previous corneal surgery (e.g., RK). After LASIK surgery. Deep set eyes where flap is difficult to create	Faster recovery, faster stable vision (within 3 months). Sooner re-enhancement can be done
Disadvantages	Potential of corneal haze (reduced by mitomycin). Slow recovery (up to a week)	More dryness symptoms
Dry eye post-op	Less	More
Ectasia risk	Lower	Higher
Endophthalmitis and corneal perforation rates	Lower	Higher
Technique	Exposure of the Bowman layer	Exposure of midstroma

- Lamellar ablation based, where a flap is created that includes the epithelium and the Bowman layer, then excimer laser is applied to the superficial stroma. Includes LASIK, Femtosecond/SMILE (see Table 25.3).

25.6.2 High-Yield Notes

- Surface ablation has therapeutic and refractive benefits for patients with epithelial basement membrane dystrophy (EBMD).
- PRK tends to lead to initial temporary myopic overshoot, which can be followed by a hyperopic regression over months to years.
- Ectasia is far more common after LASIK than after PRK. This is related to the residual stromal bed (RSB) thickness, which is far less after LASIK flap creation than after surface ablation.
- The primary force preventing flap dislocation in the immediate postoperative period following LASIK is endothelial-pump function. Central and peripheral fibrosis are responsible for late flap adherence.
- SMILE is a refractive procedure involving the use of FS laser to make and extract a lens-shaped corneal tissue from the optical zone, it has the advantages of faster recovery, more biomechanical stability, and less damaging effect to the corneal nerves compared with LASIK.

25.6.3 General Contraindications for Cornea-based Refractive Surgery

- Age below 21 years (relative CI)
- Unstable topography for 6–12 months
- Pregnant or lactating women within 3 months
- Uncontrolled DM
- Dryness or recent isotretinoin use (within 6 months)
- Vigorous jobs that may lead to flap dislodgement
- Myopia and astigmatism more than 10 D
- Glaucoma (in flap based for its suction, and for both due to corneal thinning)

25.6.4 Procedures

25.6.4.1 Surface Ablation Procedures

Exposure of the Bowman layer for surface ablation chemically (e.g., alcohol), mechanically (microkeratome), or via laser.

Variants for the PRK

- **LASEK** the epithelium is preserved, by the use of with 20% alcohol for 20 seconds loosens the epithelium and folds back an intact sheet of epithelium and replace it after excimer ablation.
- **Epi-LASIK** the same principle as in LASEK; however, the epithelial flap is fashioned mechanically with a blunt epikeratome.
- **Trans-PRK** where epithelial and stroma are both removed by laser.

25.6.4.2 High-Yield Note

Epi-LASIK and LASEK were not proved to be significantly superior to PRK in reducing corneal haze. However, intraoperative mitomycin C (0.02% or 0.2 mg/mL) application is broadly adopted to lessen this complication.

25.6.4.3 Epithelial Removal in Ablation Procedures

Mechanical: This method involves using a blunt spatula to scrape off the epithelium from the periphery toward the center. After scraping, a wet sponge is used to hydrate and wipe across the cornea.

Alcohol: A 20% alcohol solution is applied to a 6- or 7-mm area of the cornea. After 20–30 s, the surface is irrigated with BSS to reduce toxicity to the limbal germinal epithelium. The epithelium is then easily removed, with generally rapid healing within 2–3 days.

Laser: The "laser-scrape" technique uses a laser to remove 38–45 μm of epithelial cells. Any residual debris is then mechanically removed with a spatula. Prior to ablation, the tear film is irrigated with BSS to ensure a smooth and homogeneous surface.

25.6.4.4 Flap Creation Procedure

A microkeratome is used where it has a suction ring that hinge on sclera, a disposable blade that cut the surface of the cornea up to the midstroma.

Adequate suction must be adequately checked before flap creation through the following signs:

- IOP measured to be >65 mmHg (most accurate).
- The patient reports dimming of vision.
- Pupil dilates and remains so.

Note that conjunctival vessels blanching is not a reliable sign for adequate suction.

After the laser is applied, the field is irrigated with BSS, then the flap is restored.

The LASIK flap will be thinner if:

- The faster the microkeratome head passes (aka., translation speed) to create a flap.
- Microkeratome reuse in the second eye, where the average corneal flap is thinner in the second eye than the first eye, presumably due to the microkeratome blade getting duller after the first pass.
- Thick cornea.

However, if plate thickness increases, the flap will be thicker. The meniscus flap is thicker in the periphery and thinner in the center.

25.6.4.5 Correction Limits

Correction of myopia and astigmatism is generally effective within a central diameter of 6 mm, whereas hyperopia correction works best within a diameter range of 6–9 mm.

Most studies use hyperopic treatment zones with transition zones extending to 9.0–9.5 mm Research shows that larger ablation zones can achieve good results for refractive errors up to +4.00 D with conventional treatments. However, the predictability and stability of LASIK treatments for hyperopia decrease significantly beyond this level. Consequently, most refractive surgeons avoid treating hyperopia at the highest levels approved by the FDA for conventional treatments.

25.6.4.6 Correction Re-enhancement

Only surface ablation can be used for re-enhancement. Retreatment rate is higher for patients with hyperopia and high astigmatism. Before considering re-enhancement makes sure that the refractive error is stable which requires 3 months after Lasik surgery, 6 months after surface ablation. Surface ablation procedure for retreatment closely mirrors the technique used for the primary surface ablation. In LASIK retreatment, the approach depends on whether you lift the existing lamellar flap to apply additional ablation to the stromal bed or perform surface ablation directly on the LASIK flap. When opting for surface ablation on the flap, it is important to avoid using a rotating brush to remove the epithelium from the LASIK flap.

25.6.5 Complications

Ectasia occurs 4.5 times more frequently after LASIK compared to surface ablation procedures. This condition is observed in patients who either have an underlying predisposition to corneal ectatic disorders or who have a significantly reduced residual stromal bed (RSB) following ablation. Although the exact incidence of ectasia is not precisely known, reported cases of postrefractive ectasia in eyes without preoperative risk factors are as follows: 20 per 100,000 eyes in PRK (0.02%), 90 per 100,000 eyes in LASIK (0.9%), and 10 per 100,000 eyes in SMILE (0.01%).

For managing postoperative ectasia, corneal cross-linking (CXL) is increasingly recognized as the first-line treatment globally.

Overcorrection: if significant stromal dehydration develops before starting, the excimer treatment can lead to refractive regression. Myopic or hyperopic surface ablation typically experiences some degree of refractive regression over a period of 3–6 months. Might be prevented with Mitomycin C use. Regression might occur after PRK due to re-epithelialization for PRK (12–18 months), this regression will lead to myopia.

Regression or under correction after myopic laser refractive surgery is the development of myopia or an increase in myopic after surgery. Mostly with high ametropia levels.

Occur after 7% of excimer laser surgeries. Factors that lead to regression include small optical zone (<6.00 mm), high error corrected (> −5D), the use of Mitomycin and unstable fixation during laser ablation, abrupt discontinuation of corticosteroids will result in myopic regression after PRK. After LASIK, surgery risk factors include flap thickness, keratometry readings, significant astigmatism, and age over 40 years.

High-order aberrations: Including glare, ghost images, and halos. Risk factors include treatment with smaller ablation zones (<6.0 mm in diameter), higher spherical and cylindrical correction, and patients with symptoms prior to refractive surgery. These problems likely compromise night vision.

Decentered ablation: The primary concern of a decentered LASIK flap is proximity of the flap edge to the visual axis.

Corticosteroid-associated IOP elevation is more likely to occur after surface ablation when corticosteroid therapy may be used for 2–4 months to prevent postoperative corneal haze, or in cases of complicated LASIK cases.

Central toxic keratopathy is a rare condition characterized by acute, noninflammatory central corneal opacification, which can develop within days after an otherwise uneventful LASIK or PRK procedure. This opacification results in flattening of the anterior corneal curvature without changes to the posterior curvature, as seen in in anterior segment tomography. Patients may experience a hyperopic shift, which typically resolves over time.

Infectious keratitis*: It is more common following surface ablation procedures. The most frequently encountered pathogens are gram-positive organisms, including *Staph. aureus*, MRSA, Strep. pneumoniae, and Strep viridans. If an infection is suspected after LASIK, the surgeon should lift the flap, scrape the stromal bed for culture and sensitivity testing, and irrigate with antibiotics before repositioning the flap. Intensive treatment with topical antibiotic drops should be initiated pending culture results. Keep in mind the possibility of fungal infection.

25.6.5.1 Unique for Surface Ablation

Corneal haze: The most common complication of PRK, typically peaking in intensity at 1–2 months, and gradually diminishing or disappearing over the following 6–12 months. Surgeons generally recommend waiting at least 6–12 months for the haze to improve spontaneously before considering a repeat surface ablation.

Persistent epithelial defect: Treated with aggressive preservative free lubrication, topical cyclosporine, temporary punctal occlusion, amniotic membrane grafting, and autologous serum drops in severe cases.

Sterile infiltrate: May sometimes be mistaken for infection. Any infiltrate should be carefully monitored and managed. If an infectious keratitis is suspected, the cornea is usually scraped and cultured to identify any organisms.

25.6.5.2 Unique for Flap-Based Surgeries

Microkeratome related: Include defects in the blade, poor suction, or uneven progression of the microkeratome across the cornea, which can result in an irregular, thin, or buttonhole flap. Although a new flap can usually be created safely with a deeper cut after at least 3 months of healing, many surgeons prefer a surface ablation technique instead.

Flap folds (stria): Microstria is common and occurs spontaneously. Macrostria occurs with flap movement and eye rubbing. The first step in evaluating a patient with corneal folds is determining the BCVA. Folds are not treated if the BCVA and the subjective visual acuity are good. If large, and visually disturbing, flap reposition can be tried. About 95% of flap striae are noted by 1 week postoperatively. Risk factors include excessive irrigation under the flap at the time of surgery, thin flaps, or large ablations with subsequent mismatch of the flap to the underlying stroma. The best way to prevent flap folds, or *macrostriae,* is meticulous flap realignment with minimal irrigation.

Flap dislocation: It might occur due to adhesion with the upper lid due to dryness, rubbing, or due to eye trauma.

Hypoesthesia: After LASIK, corneal sensitivity is decreased in the central cornea for as long as 6 months or more.

Diffuse lamellar keratitis: It describes inflammatory infiltrates beneath the corneal flap interface that develops 1–2 days following refractive surgery and typically resolves 5–8 days after the initiation of appropriate therapy. They are usually peripheral in early stages. Includes all the following:

- Mild and moderate DLK (mild to moderate peripheral cellular infiltration) is treated with an increase in topical steroids and close follow-up.
- Severe DLK (dense, undulating central and peripheral cellular infiltration, associated with decreased vision and photophobia) with a possible infiltrate should be treated with flap lift, scrapings to remove inflammatory material, and for smears and cultures, interface antibiotics and steroids, postoperative steroids and antibiotics, and close follow-up, oral steroids may be helpful in severe DLK.

So, flap lifting is indicated in clumped, white, granular haze—densest in the central lamellar interface (stage 4).

LASIK infectious keratitis: Characterized by haze around flap with corneal edema. Infections occurring within 10 days of surgery are typically bacterial, with the preponderance being from gram-positive organisms.

Epithelial ingrowth: Epithelial ingrowth occurs in less than 3% of LASIK cases. Epithelial defects along the flap edge are a major risk factor, as stromal edema can impair flap adherence early post-surgery. Isolated nests of epithelial cells in the peripheral lamellar interface that are not advancing and not affecting vision typically do not require treatment. However, if the ingrowth affects vision, it should be managed by lifting the flap, scraping the epithelium from both the underside of the flap and the stromal bed, and then repositioning the flap. Some surgeons also remove epithelium from the periphery of both the flap and the stromal bed to improve flap adherence before the epithelial edge reaches the flap edge.

Steroids do not prevent epithelial ingrowth. Care should be taken during flap lift retreatment to be certain the stromal bed is free of epithelium. Ingrowth can lead to blurred vision and to flap melting and should be treated if progressive or if >2 mm from the flap edge.

Filamentary keratitis is rare, but occurs when operated eye has been patched rather than contact lens use after PRK.

25.6.5.3 High-Yield Notes

- Granular infiltrates and conjunctival injection can be seen with DLK and infectious keratitis; however, keratic precipitates are usually seen only with infectious keratitis and are not part of the clinical findings of DLK.
- Excessive energy settings are the most common cause of post-LASIK diffuse lamellar keratitis (DLK), other risk factor is epithelial basement membrane dystrophy (EBMD) increases the risk for DLK.
- Some patients may have prolonged pupillary dilatation after refractive surgery, resulting in HOA. Topical brimonidine for night vision is well tolerated and will result in a mild pupillary constriction.

25.6.6 Miscellaneous Corneal Refractive Surgeries

25.6.6.1 Intrastromal Corneal Ring Segments (ICRSs)

A potentially reversible procedure in which a PMMA split ring is placed into a tunnel within the mid-peripheral corneal stroma concentric with the limbus. It causes flattening of the central corneal curvature to treat low myopia and astigmatism. The main indication for ICRS placement is keratoconus and other forms of ectatic corneal diseases since it is FDA approved to treat myopia at levels ranging from −1.00 to −3.00 D spherical equivalent among KC patients.

The segments are available in various thicknesses and arcs. The degree of correction achieved is related to the thickness of the ring segments.

25.6.6.2 High-Yield Note

The appropriate depth for placement of ISCRs in a myopic cornea is around 80% of stromal thickness. Too deep or too shallow can result in erosion and sub-optimal effect, respectively.

25.6.7 Collagen Shrinkage Procedures

Conductive keratoplasty is a procedure that is performed by applying heat to cause collagen shrinkage. It works by radiofrequency shrinkage of collagen lamellae in the cornea. It is approved by the FDA for the treatment of hyperopia and presbyopia, not myopia.

In laser thermal keratoplasty, a Holmium: YAG laser instead of just thermal probe is applied to the cornea. The optimal temperature for avoiding stromal necrosis while still obtaining corneal collagen shrinkage is approximately 58°–76 °C, applied 6–8 mm from the center. However, long-term results showed almost complete regression to the pre-treatment status.

25.6.7.1 Lens-Based Refractive Surgeries

Including

- Phakic intraocular lens implantation (PIOL), including iris-fixated and posterior chamber (sulcus) lenses for myopia.
- Refractive lens exchange (RLE) is the removal of the crystalline lens with IOL implantation for the primary purpose of correcting refractive error.

25.6.7.2 Phakic Intraocular Lens Implantation (PIOL)

PIOLs are available for powers between −3.00 D and −20.00 D and for correcting hyperopia up to +10.00 D.

PIOL Advantages
- Correct a broad range of refractive errors
- Reversible
- Preserve natural accommodation
- Crystalline lens barrier is preserved, and vitreous destabilization is minimal
- Lower risk of endophthalmitis and postoperative retinal detachment

Disadvantages
- An intraocular procedure with all associated potential risks
- Postoperative astigmatism
- Cataract formation
- Risk of glaucoma, persistent uveitis, and endothelial cell loss

Prerequisites

An inner anterior chamber depth of >3.2 mm.

An endothelial cell count ≥2000 cells/mm^2.

An anterior chamber angle ≥30°.

No cataract, glaucoma, or uveitis.

25.6.8 Refractive Lens Exchange (RLE)

Surgeons need to differentiate between corneal and lenticular astigmatism, as only corneal astigmatism will persist postoperatively.

Small amounts of corneal astigmatism (less than1.00 D) may be reduced by placing the incision in the steep meridian.

For residual corneal astigmatism of less than 2.00 D, limbal relaxing incisions or arcuate keratotomies—whether performed with a blade or a femtosecond laser—can be used to correct it.

The "piggyback" IOL system involves inserting two posterior chamber IOLs: One in the capsular bag and the other mostly in the ciliary sulcus. To account for the posterior shift of the posterior IOL, the combined power of the IOLs may need to be increased by +1.50 to +2.00 D of astigmatic changes.

The light-adjustable IOL is a 3-piece silicone-optic posterior chamber monofocal IOL that can be modified post-implantation using ultraviolet light through a slit-lamp delivery system. This adjustment can occur 1–2 weeks after implantation and allows for changes in the IOL's shape and power. Initial studies show that this system can induce up to 5.00 D of spherical and up to 2.00 D of astigmatic changes.

25.6.8.1 High-Yield Notes

- PIOL is FDA approved for myopia and not hyperopia.
- Most surgeons recommend implanting an IOL after RLE in patients with high myopia rather than leaving them aphakic, even if minimal or no optical correction is needed. Plano power IOLs are available if necessary. The IOL serves as a barrier to prevent anterior vitreous prolapse and helps maintain the integrity of the aqueous–vitreous barrier, which is beneficial if Nd: YAG laser posterior capsulotomy becomes necessary.

25.6.9 Stepwise Approach to Refractive Surgeries

25.6.9.1 Preoperative Assessment

Generally speaking, young, healthy patients with healthy eyes are the ideal candidates for refractive surgery. However, in real practice we will encounter patients with criteria that is totally different!

Therefore, proper patient selection is the most important initially.

Select patients who are motivated psychologically to the procedure, with realistic hope and views regarding the operation, with good reasoning for risks and able to show on follow-up visits.

25.6.9.2 Patient History

Past Medical History

In general, some systemic diseases like diabetes and hypertension have the potential to affect the decision toward refractive surgery since they can affect refractive stability and corneal healing. Table 25.4 summarizes important medical diseases affecting refractive surgery decision.

25.6.9.3 Medications

Medications with important considerations are demonstrated in Table 25.5.

25.6.9.4 Occupational History

Determine the visual demands of the patient as certain jobs require optimum distant vision (like soldiers, fire fighters, and drivers); while other professions require optimum near vision. This might be disrupted in myopic patient with postoperative emmetropia since they are used to see perfectly at near without the use of near glasses like jeweler and sculptor. Sports and recreational activities affect the decision regarding the type of refractive surgery. For example, a SA may be preferable to a LA for a patient who wrestles, boxes, or rides horses and is at high risk of ocular trauma.

Ocular History

This includes refractive history, dry eye, tearing, chronic infections, chronic allergies, use of CLs, ocular trauma, previous surgeries, ectatic corneal disorders, and other pathologies.

1. **Refractive history:** It is important to address the age of onset of the refractive error, refractive error stability, anisometropia, and presbyopia.
2. **Use of contact lens:** Important information includes the type of lens; the wearing schedule; the type of cleaning, and how old the lenses are.

   Using CLs should be stopped 2–4 weeks prior to examination since it can alter corneal

Table 25.4 Medical conditions with important refractive surgery considerations

Medical conditions	Consideration
Diabetes	Unstable refraction with blood sugar fluctuation, poor healing process, other diabetic eye disease features
Hypertension	A relative contraindication for refractive surgery when malignant or uncontrolled
Allergy and atopic disease	Risk of haze, eye rubbing, KC, flap complications
Collagen vascular diseases and autoimmune diseases	Less predictable wound healing and greater potential for corneal melting
Pregnancy and nursing	Unstable refraction due to hormonal changes
Cardiac pacemakers and implanted defibrillators	Unknown effects of the laser's electromagnetic emissions
Epilepsy	Must be good controlled with 1-year seizure free prior to surgery
Hepatitis B and C	Contraindications due to the potential risk to surgical staff

Table 25.5 Medications with important considerations in refractive surgeries

Medications	Consideration
Anticoagulants	Increased risk of expulsive suprachoroidal hemorrhage during intraocular refractive surgery
Isotretinoin and vitamin A	Significantly decreased tear production—should be stopped for at least 6 months before surgery
Amiodarone, hormone replacement therapy, and antihistamines	Significant impact on corneal epithelial healing especially with surface ablation
Triptans	Risk of vascular occlusion when IOP is raised during application of suction ring—should be stopped for at least 1 month before treatment
Immunosuppressants and steroids	Risk of infection and delayed healing

topography, induce hot spots and irregular astigmatism, change the amount, type and axis of astigmatism, and change corneal thickness.

3. **Ocular trauma:** Asking the patient about previous ocular trauma (even minor) is necessary because it may explain faint corneal opacities and scars, iridodonesis, cataract, lens subluxation, and retinal tears.
4. **Previous surgeries:** Identifying and evaluating a patient's previous ocular surgery status are crucial for the success of any subsequent refractive surgery (Table 25.6).
5. **KC and ectatic corneal disorders:**

   The patient should also be asked about a family history of ectatic corneal disorders.
6. **Glaucoma and previous glaucoma surgery: multiple issues should be addressed:**
   - Bleb may cause of irregular astigmatism and may interfere with suction ring application.
   - The application of the suction ring is associated with very high IOP for relatively significant period of time.
   - Steroids after refractive surgery may impact the IOP, especially when used for a long period
7. **HSV or HZV keratitis** not good candidates for SA procedures. This is due to significant risk of recurrence of keratouveitis and the common presence of underlying neurotrophic corneas in these individuals.

25.6.9.5 Ocular Examination

You have to examine the patient eyes fully; this examination should include visual acuity measurement, refractive error, anterior segment exam, dilated fundus exam, pupil exam, ocular motility and alignment, and IOP measurements.

25.6.9.6 Clinical Refraction

In general, achieving refractive stability after discontinuing CL use takes longer for hard contact lens (HCL) users compared to soft CL (SCL) users. The time to stability is influenced by both the duration and frequency of lens wear. For patients who have used soft contact lenses (SCL) for 10 years, a typical recommendation is to stop wearing the lenses for 2 weeks. For those who have worn hard contact lenses (HCL) for the same duration, a longer abstinence period of 4 weeks is often advised. Extended periods of lens wear generally necessitate even longer breaks to achieve refractive stability. General rules in the refraction for refractive surgery candidates are as follows:

- The least myopic correction that gives the best corrected visual acuity is given (Do not over minus).
- The most hyperopic correction that gives the best corrected visual acuity is given.
- The manifest refraction for myopes should not differ from the cycloplegic refraction by more than 0.50 D.
- The manifest refraction for hyperopes should not differ from the cycloplegic refraction by

Table 25.6 Considerations in different previous ocular surgeries and their relation to refractive procedures

Ocular surgery	Consideration
Pterygium surgery	Risk of recurrence, scar can cause of irregular astigmatism
PRK surgery	Residual refractive error and postoperative aberrations can cause impaired vision
Cataract surgery	Ensure refractive stability—No surgery before 6 months post phaco or 1 year post ECCE
Scleral buckle surgery	Buckles alter the refractive status of the eye and may interfere with suction ring application
Vitrectomy surgery	Refractive index is altered by the silicone oil together with refractive shift
Squint surgery	Risk for phoria to become tropia

more than 0.75 D, otherwise post mydriatic test is indicated.

- The axis of cylinder should not differ by more than 15° between manifest and cycloplegic refraction.
- Anisometropia is one of the preoperative risk factors for ectasia, especially, if it is on the account of astigmatism.

25.6.9.7 Pupillometry

Accurate pupil measurement is crucial before laser surgery, as even 1 mm difference can significantly impact the amount of corneal tissue that needs to be ablated.

Pupil size should be evaluated under both mesopic and scotopic light conditions. Typically, the OZ diameter is set to be 0.5 mm larger than the scotopic pupil diameter to reduce the risk of glare, ghost images, and halos after the procedure. Larger pupil size necessitates a larger OZ and more corneal tissue removal, which may make some eyes unsuitable for treatment if the stromal bed thickness drops below 270 μm, as this can increase the risk of ectasia. Pupil measurement can be done by tomography.

Patients with large pupils (scotopic more than 6.5 mm) are at increased risk for glare, haloes, and night vision symptoms. Low-dose pilocarpine (0.5–0.3%) can be helpful in reducing them.

25.6.9.8 Presbyopia and Monovision

The age of a refractive surgery candidate is a key factor in predicting postoperative satisfaction. It is important to discuss the potential loss of near vision with aging. Typically, patients younger than 40 years do not need reading glasses for near vision. However, those older than 40 years should be aware achieving emmetropia through refractive surgery will likely necessitate the use of reading glasses for near tasks. Monovision involves targeting the dominant eye for distance vision, and the non-dominant eye for near vision by leaving a residual myopic error (−0.75 D to −2.5 D) in the near eye, based on the surgeon's preferences and patient's needs. It should be discussed with presbyopic patients as it can improve near vision but may also lead to loss of depth perception and increased anisometropia in some cases. To assess suitability, trial of monovision with contacts in various settings should be performed preoperatively. This trial helps determine the preferred eye for near vision, which is usually but not always the non-dominant eye.

25.7 Imaging

This is the technical distinction between topography and tomography as in Table 25.7.

25.7.1 General Principles in Interpretation of Corneal Tomography

- At first, correctly identify your patient's demographic data, and confirm the validity of the image. Then study the numerical values on the left of the display and then the four refractive

Table 25.7 Comparison between corneal topography and corneal tomography

Comparison	Topography	Tomography
Dimensions	Two dimensions	Three dimensions
Measurement	Anterior corneal surface only	Anterior and posterior corneal surface
Examples	Orbscan, atlas	Pentacam, Galilei
Principle	Placido disc evaluates the cornea based on the reflection of concentric rings (mires)	Scheimpflug imaging evaluates the cornea using a camera that captures cross-sections of the cornea as it rotates
Popularity	Less common nowadays	More widely used

maps (axial curvature map, anterior and posterior elevation maps, and pachymetry map).
- When considering the tomography of a normal cornea, it is necessary to remember that there is a wide spectrum of normality.
- Always when evaluating one eye, look at the other eye since normally it would be the mirror image, this phenomenon is called enantiomorphism. The knowledge of this fact is useful to decide whether a cornea is normal or not, by comparing it with the map of the contralateral eye.

25.7.2 Abnormalities in Numerical Values

- Bearing in mind that roughly correcting each diopter of myopia reduces the flat K (K1) by 0.75 D, an expected postoperative k1 less than 34 D is considered risky.
- Bearing in mind that correcting each diopter of hyperopia increases the steep K (K2) by 1.20 D, an expected postoperative K2 more than 48 D is considered risky.
- Mean k readings (Km) less than 40 D (flat cornea) is associated with increased risk of free flap during LASIK.
- Km more than 46 D (steep cornea)is associated with buttonhole during LASIK.

25.7.2.1 Abnormalities in Axial Curvature Map

- There are several patterns of corneal curvature, some can be normal and accepted, while others are considered risky patterns for photorefractive surgery or indicators for ectasias. Corneal axial map may appear as round, oval, superior steep, inferior steep, or irregular pattern. Other less common patterns include symmetric bow-tie with or without skewing, asymmetric bow-tie with superior or inferior steep or skewing, and butterfly or claw pattern.

25.7.3 High-Yield Notes

- Angulation (skewing) is considered clinically significant when it exceeds 22°.
- In asymmetric bow-tie with the inferior steep, if the difference between symmetric values on the 5 mm center is more than 1.5 D, it is considered significant.
- In asymmetric bow-tie with the inferior steep, If the difference between symmetric values on the 5 mm center is more than 2.5 D, it is considered significant.
- Claw pattern is associated with low K readings, hyperopia, pellucid marginal degeneration (PMD), or in pellucid-like keratoconus (PLK).

25.7.3.1 Abnormalities in Elevation Maps

- These maps are generally considered better in assessing both corneal surfaces than curvature maps as they are less affected by tear film disturbance and corneal warpage.
- Anterior elevation value in best fit toric ellipsoid (BFTE) more than 12 μm is considered risky.
- Posterior elevation value (BFTE) more than 15 μm is considered risky.

25.7.3.2 Abnormalities in Pachymetry Map

- Cone pattern is characteristic for keratoconus; bell pattern is characteristic for PMD.
- When comparing the symmetric superior and inferior values within the central 5 mm circle, value greater than 30 μm is considered suspicious.
- Difference in thickness at thinnest location between both eyes more than 30 μm is suspicious.

An example of normal corneal tomography is shown in Fig. 25.3, and an example of KC tomography is shown in Fig. 25.4.

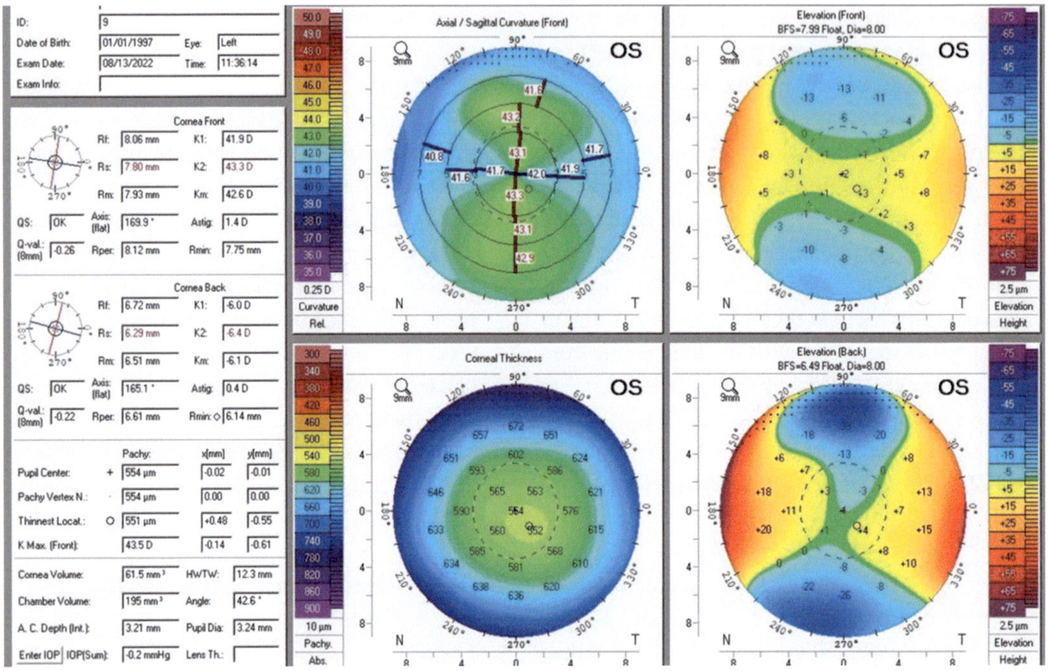

Fig. 25.3 Normal corneal tomography with with-the-rule astigmatism

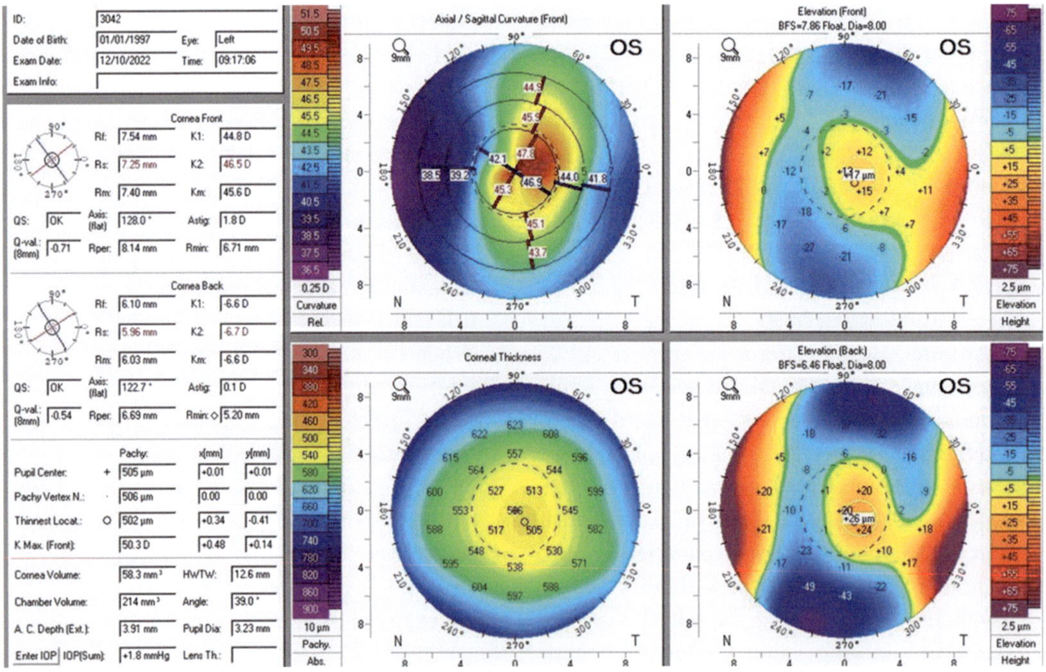

Fig. 25.4 Keratoconus corneal tomography

25.7.4 Summary of the Most Important Conclusions from Global Consensus on Keratoconus and Ectatic Diseases

- The diagnosis of keratoconus necessitates abnormal posterior elevation, abnormal corneal thickness distribution, and clinical noninflammatory corneal thinning.
- Posterior corneal elevation abnormalities should be present to diagnose early or subclinical keratoconus.
- Keratoconus and PMD are different clinical presentations of the same disease while keratoglobus is a different entity.
- The location and pattern of thinning differentiate keratoconus, PMD, and keratoglobus.
- True unilateral keratoconus does not exist.
- Tomography is the most accurate and widely adopted diagnostic modality to detect early keratoconus.
- Currently, there is no clinically adequate classification system for keratoconus.
- Central pachymetry is the least reliable indicator for diagnosing keratoconus.
- Keratoconus can be present in a cornea of normal central thickness.

Ectasia progression is defined by a consistent change in at least two of the following parameters, with changes exceeding the normal variability of the testing system. These parameters include progressive steepening of both the anterior and posterior corneal surface and progressive thinning of the cornea, or an increase in the rate of corneal thickness change from the periphery to the thinnest point.

25.7.4.1 Important Considerations in Flap-Based Surgeries

- Roughly consider 15 μm decrease in corneal thickness for each diopter correction.
- The RSB should be more than 55% of the preoperative thinnest location thickness.
- The ablation depth should be less than 20% of the preoperative thinnest location thickness.
- The Munnerlyn formula is used to estimate ablation depth as the square of optical zone diameter multiplied by third of the dioptric correction. So, roughly ablation depth is 12 μm/D for myopia correction with a 6.0-mm treatment zone and 15-μm/D for a 6.5-mm treatment zone.
- Decreasing the optical zone diameter decreases the ablation depth but compromise the quality of vision due to glare.
- The full laser correction is applied only to the optical zone; however, the pupil dilates at night beyond the optical zone inducing optical aberrations such as halos and glare compromising the contrast sensitivity. These issues are addressed by a ***blend zone*** that is intended to taper the laser treatment to reduce the sharp transition from the optical zone to the untreated area of the cornea.

25.7.4.2 High-Yield Notes

- Flap thickness ranges between 120 μm in conventional LASIK and 100 μm in femtosecond LASIK.
- Data on preoperative astigmatism may differ between topography, cycloplegia, and manifest refraction. The most accurate one to use is the mansifest refraction power and axis.
- For patients with high astigmatism, night symptoms related to high-order aberrations (HOA), BCVA less than 6/6 or reduced quality of vision, consider doing wavefront-guided ablation.
- Roughly an ablation zone of 6–6.5 mm is used for myopia. Hyperopic treatment needs a treatment zone of 9.0 mm. Mixed astigmatism treatment also needs an ablation zone of 9.0 mm.
- The maximum ablation diameter approved by the FDA is 9.0 mm.

Acknowledgment None.

Conflict of Interest None.

References

Ambrósio R, Wilson SE (2003, January) LASIK vs LASEK vs PRK: advantages and indications. Semin Ophthalmol 18(1):2–10

Elkington A (2023) E-book clinical optics 3rd edition 1999. Ebook Malahayati

Feder RS, Rapuano CJ (2007) The LASIK handbook: a case-based approach. Lippincott Williams & Wilkins

Gomes JA, Tan D, Rapuano CJ, Belin MW, Ambrósio R Jr, Guell JL et al (2015) Global consensus on keratoconus and ectatic diseases. Cornea 34(4):359–369

Hafezi F, Randleman JB (2013) Corneal collagen cross linking. Slack

Hafezi F, Kling S, Gilardoni F, Hafezi N, Hillen M, Abrishamchi R et al (2021) Individualized corneal cross-linking with riboflavin and UV-A in ultrathin corneas: the Sub400 protocol. Am J Ophthalmol 224:133–142

Kim SJ (2021) 2021–2022 basic and clinical science course, section 13: refractive surgery

Sinjab MM (2014) Five steps to start your refractive surgery: a case-based systematic approach. JP Medical Ltd.

Sinjab MM (2021) Corneal tomography in clinical practice (Pentacam system): basics and clinical interpretation. JP Medical Ltd.

Vinciguerra R, Legrottaglie EF, Tredici C, Mazzotta C, Rosetta P, Vinciguerra P (2022) Transepithelial iontophoresis-assisted cross linking for progressive keratoconus: up to 7 years of follow up. J Clin Med 11(3):678